Tuning the Brain
Principles and Practice
of Neurosomatic Medicine

OTHER BOOKS BY JAY GOLDSTEIN

Betrayal by the Brain: The Neurologic Basis of Chronic Fatigue Syndrome, Fibromyalgia Syndrome, and Related Neural Network Disorders

Chronic Fatigue Syndromes: The Limbic Hypothesis

Chronic Fatigue Syndrome: The Struggle for Health

Symptoms and Solutions

ADDITIONAL TITLES OF RELATED INTEREST
FROM THE HAWORTH PRESS

A Companion Volume to Dr. Jay A. Goldstein's Betrayal by the Brain: A Guide for Patients and Their Physicians by Katie Courmel

A Parents' Guide to CFIDS: How to Be an Advocate for Your Child with Chronic Fatigue Immune Dysfunction by David S. Bell, Mary Z. Robinson, Jean Pollard, Tom Robinson, and Bonnie Floyd

The Pharmacotherapy of Common Functional Syndromes: Evidence-Based Guidelines for Primary Care Practice by Peter Manu

CFIDS, Fibromyalgia, and the Virus-Allergy Link: New Therapy for Chronic Functional Illnesses by R. Bruce Duncan

Chronic Fatigue Syndrome and the Body's Immune Defense System by Roberto Patarca-Montero

Chronic Fatigue Syndrome, Genes, and Infection: The ETA-1/OP Paradigm by Roberto Patarca-Montero

Concise Encyclopedia of Chronic Fatigue Syndrome by Roberto Patarca-Montero

Phytotherapy of Chronic Fatigue Syndrome: Evidence-Based and Potentially Useful Botanicals in the Treatment of CFS by Roberto Patarca-Montero

Chronic Fatigue Syndrome, Christianity, and Culture: Between God and an Illness by James M. Rotholz

Stricken: Voices from the Hidden Epidemic of Chronic Fatigue Syndrome edited by Peggy Munson

Tuning the Brain
Principles and Practice of Neurosomatic Medicine

Jay A. Goldstein

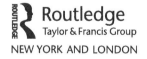

Routledge
Taylor & Francis Group

NEW YORK AND LONDON

First published by
The Haworth Press, Inc.
10 Alice Street
Binghamton, N Y 13904-1580

This edition published 2011 by Routledge

Routledge
Taylor & Francis Group
711 Third Avenue
New York, NY 10017

Routledge
Taylor & Francis Group
2 Park Square, Milton Park
Abingdon, Oxon OX14 4RN

PUBLISHER'S NOTE

This book has been published solely for educational purposes and is not intended to substitute for the medical advice of a treating physician. Medicine is an ever-changing science. As new research and clinical experience broaden our knowledge, changes in treatment may be required. While many potential treatment options are made herein, some or all of the options may not be applicable to a particular individual. Therefore, the author, editor, and publisher do not accept responsibility in the event of negative consequences incurred as a result of the information presented in this book. We do not claim that this information is necessarily accurate by the rigid scientific and regulatory standards applied for medical treatment. **No warranty, expressed or implied, is furnished with respect to the material contained in this book. The reader is urged to consult with his/her personal physician with respect to the treatment of any medical condition.**

Cover design by Brooke R. Stiles.

Library of Congress Cataloging-in-Publication Data

Goldstein, Jay A.
    Tuning the brain : principles and practice of neurosomatic medicine / Jay A. Goldstein.
      p. ; cm.
    Includes bibliographical references and index.
    ISBN 0-7890-2245-1 (hard : alk. paper) — ISBN 0-7890-2246-X (soft : alk. paper)
    1. Chronic fatigue syndrome. 2. Fibromyalgia. 3. Psychoneuroimmunology. 4. Neural networks (Neurobiology) 5. Limbic system. [DNLM: 1. Psychophysiologic Disorders—therapy. 2. Neuropsychology—Personal Narratives. 3. Psychosomatic Medicine—Personal Narratives. WM 90 G624t 2003] I. Title.

RB150.F37G653 2003
616.8—dc21

2003007556

To Jordan,
the son who lights my way
and gives meaning to what I do

ABOUT THE AUTHOR

Jay A. Goldstein, MD, has seen over 20,000 patients at the Chronic Fatigue Syndrome Institutes in Anaheim Hills and Santa Monica, California.

Dr. Goldstein has specialized in chronic fatigue syndrome and related disorders for the past sixteen years and has been interested in the illness since 1985. He has written three books on the topic, *Betrayal by the Brain: The Neurologic Basis of Chronic Fatigue Syndrome, Fibromyalgia Syndrome, and Related Neural Network Disorders* (1996), *Chronic Fatigue Syndromes: The Limbic Hypothesis* (1993), and *Chronic Fatigue Syndrome: The Struggle for Health* (1990). He is also the author of *Symptoms and Solutions,* published by Berkeley Press. He was a contributing editor to the *CFS Encyclopedia, The Clinical and Scientific Basis of Myalgic Encephalomyelitis/Chronic Fatigue Syndrome,* published in 1992. Since 1988, Dr. Goldstein has been a regular contributor of articles to the *CFIDS Chronicle* and more recently, to the *National Forum,* and has had over forty publications in peer-reviewed journals.

Dr. Goldstein has organized annual international conferences about the neurobiology of chronic fatigue syndrome and broadened the scope of these meetings to include other disorders of regulatory physiology caused by dysfunction of the limbic system. Referring to these illnesses as "neurosomatic," he includes fibromyalgia, irritable bowel syndrome, migraine headaches, interstitial cystitis, sleep disorders, and premenstrual syndrome in this category.

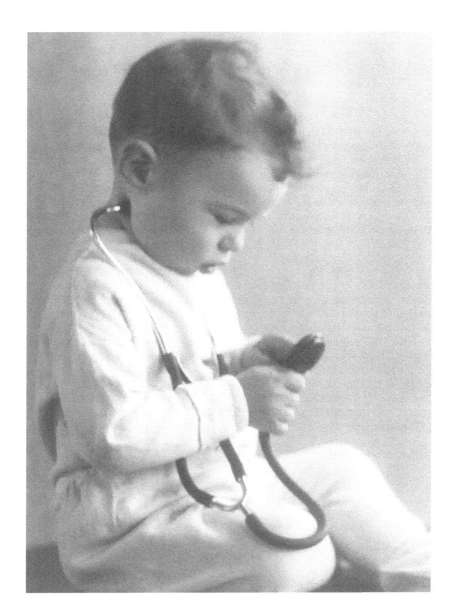

CONTENTS

Foreword

Tuning the Brain may be considered the third volume of a trilogy that began with *Chronic Fatigue Syndromes: The Limbic Hypothesis,* which was followed by *Betrayal by the Brain,* all published by The Haworth Press. I did not intend to write a trilogy—it just turned out that way.

For anyone trying to understand neurosomatic medicine, it would be helpful to read the three books in chronological order, since I assume a knowledge of previous works when writing subsequent ones. *Limbic Hypothesis* describes basic neuroanatomy and discusses the multiple presentations of the neurosomatic disorder chronic fatigue syndrome (CFS). It has a psychoneuroimmunological focus, reflecting my approach in the early 1990s. *Betrayal* sets the stage for *Tuning the Brain.* It focuses heavily on pathophysiology and treatment but could obviously not reflect the advances in neuroscience that have occurred since 1996. *Betrayal* elaborated the notion of neurosomatic medicine, viewing disorders lumped into "psychosomatic medicine" in a neurobiological perspective, without recourse to outmoded psychodynamic concepts. It introduced my finding that neurosomatic disorders may be ameliorated quite rapidly, still a novel concept in an era when patients wait weeks for antidepressants to take effect. Despite evidence to the contrary, antidepressants are the treatment of choice, along with cognitive-behavioral therapy, for neurosomatic disorders in mainstream medical practice at the present time.

Tuning the Brain incorporates (I hope) many of the advances in neuroscience that have occurred between 1996 and 2003. I have tried to present a fairly unified hypothesis of dysregulated attentional and regulatory processes to explain my approach to treatment. I use the same paradigm I have always employed when teaching: What is the normal physiology? How is it deranged by illness (pathophysiology)? How may the derangement be most appropriately corrected?

I have learned a great deal about how to treat neurosomatic disorders, and I wish to pass along this knowledge. The best way to accomplish this goal would be an apprenticeship with me, because I have not written down many of my "tricks of the trade." However, such a process is not feasible since I have no means to fund it. Thus, I write books.

It has become fashionable of late to bemoan the dearth of new treatment entities in neuropsychopharmacology. The bases for most medications used today were serendipitously discovered in the 1950s and 1960s. Many more therapeutic agents are available if one looks at the pharmacological mode of action rather than the indication for use in the *Physician's Desk Reference.* Almost all patients I see have consulted many other health care practitioners and have tried "standard therapy," yet most of them are significantly improved after coming to my office. A physician does not need to venture too far "out of the box" in order to practice neurosomatic medicine, yet numerous financial, cultural, and medicological disincentives to do so exist. It must be more cost effective to treat a patient intensively for four days than to have that person be ill for several years. It is certainly more humane.

Tuning the Brain will be a difficult read for most people once they reach the scientific sections. I recognize this problem, but I cannot help the fact that neuroscience is complicated and becomes more so every day. It has been fairly observed that the brain is the most complicated object to study in the universe. I have tried to proceed from the simple to the complex in my explanations, but I have not intended to write a textbook of clinical neuroscience, although this book may have turned out that way. *Tuning the Brain* is too dense for most readers to absorb in one sitting, but I hope that dipping into it from time to time will prove to be a rewarding experience.

Jay A. Goldstein, MD
Orange, California

Preface

During the past five years I have greatly expanded my therapeutic armamentarium to the point where I can significantly help almost every patient. I shall discuss these new treatments along with refinements and further understanding of previous treatments in this book. I have tried to make this book more reader friendly, but doubt that I have succeeded. What I thought to be a rigorous scientific justification of a new but almost self-evident paradigm in my book *Betrayal by the Brain* seemed to be either too difficult or too demanding even for many a scientifically educated reader (Goldstein JA, 1996); *Tuning the Brain* was to be an easier read. Even though *Betrayal* has gone through several printings, its technical complexity "suppressed sales" as my publisher politely phrased it. Many lay readers were able to understand only the introduction and the case histories, and some had trouble with the introduction. A companion guide to *Betrayal* was written by Katie Courmel (1996). It was something like Cliffs Notes, and it helped some people.

Nevertheless, there has been an explosion of knowledge in neuroscience recently, primarily because of advances in functional brain imaging, but also in computational and cognitive neuroscience, as well as molecular genetics and neuropharmacology. I shall allude to these developments in future chapters on attentional mechanisms and instantaneous neural network reconfiguration. *Tuning the Brain* will explain the practice of neurosomatic medicine and desribe its treatment in some detail. I shall incorporate the constantly accelerating developments in neuroscience into the text, which I hope will be user friendly.

These intervening years have been replete with triumphs and tribulations, some of which I discussed in a column (Goldstein JA, 1998) I wrote for a new publication, *The National Forum,* edited by Gail Kansky and reprinted as follows.

THE PILGRIM'S PROGRESS
(WITH APOLOGIES TO JOHN BUNYAN, 1678)

As I write this article, I have recently returned from a CFS conference in Sydney, Australia titled "The Clinical and Scientific Basis of Chronic Fatigue Syndrome: From Myth Towards Management," February 11-13, 1998. Prior to my leaving, I had resolved to attend no more CFS conferences (I may go to another fibromyalgia syndrome (FMS) conference—many attendees there know that they don't know, but at least would like to know). Gail and I have organized five CFS conferences, all of which patients and professionals found quite informative, I was told. To paraphrase Lawrence "Yogi" Berra, "It's déjà vu over, and over, and over again." I feel as if I have been to the same conference 15 or 20 times. The Sydney conference was no different (except for a few quality speakers who are also my friends), but at least most of the Australians know they are as clueless as everyone else.

At the end of the proceedings, the earnest but pedantic chairman of the Australian committee to define CFS management guidelines said words to the effect of, "We think there might be something wrong with the brain, but we don't know what it is or how to treat it." I was not permitted to speak at this conference, although I was "snuck in" to a question-and-answer session about treatment. I had the opportunity to say that CFS was quite understandable and treatable, and that neurally mediated hypotension was a disorder of central cardiovascular homeostasis, in other words, more of a symptom than a cause. I also chimed in that many current National Institutes of Health (NIH)-funded experiments had been done unofficially by clinicians years ago (prednisone and Florinef being prime examples), with resultant lack of support for the various hypotheses. Had clinicians been consulted, other experiments might have been performed that had some, albeit minuscule, chances at a positive outcome. It is quite common to encounter funded researchers who are incredibly arrogant about their knowledge for no reason that I can discern. One prominent neuropsychologist at the conference (whose name shall be shrouded in mystery) summed up his finding as if those of other researchers were pitiable and antediluvian, like a room full of monkeys with typewriters composing the *Encyclopædia Britannica*. He stated that his montane group had not learned much yet about his chosen topic, implying that the other groups of benighted dullards such as myself were predictably far behind, mired in eternal oblivion. The research he discussed was largely that which our group had done about ten years before. Then he said (more or less), "Five major questions remain," displaying them on a slide. How soon they would be answered (if ever) was left unsaid. During the "question" period (as if I had any), I remarked that we had already solved these conundrums, and described the results, hoping that he would use this information to take the next steps. His only reply was, "Do you have a question, Dr. Goldstein? If not, sit down and give someone else a chance to ask one."

Why, you may wonder, did my resolve waver enough to attend the conference "down under"? There were five reasons:

1. My patients from Australia described the medical environment for CFS as a "vast wasteland," although some progress was being made in educating individual physicians. Most sufferers were poorly diagnosed (a good deal of the meeting was about diagnostic techniques) and untreated. Experienced American clinicians can diagnose CFS in about two minutes by asking key questions and then listening to the answers: "I was fine until October 17, 1989, when I got the worst flu of my life . . .," etc. My patients from Australia had been asking me to visit their country for several years and wander like Johnny Appleseed, planting bits of relevant information and intervention in the hope that some would sprout and take root.
2. There was an airfare war, enabling me to go at half price.
3. I had heard Sydney was a beautiful city and that the people were very friendly (both true).
4. Patients organizing this conference informed me that one of the principal speakers made it a precondition of his acceptance that I not be invited. I was told (by more than one person) that this researcher, whom I had never met, was urged to take this stance by an acolyte of the "dark side of the Force," who in the past derided the very existence of CFS until the sheer weight of information made him shift to a more politically profitable position.
5. My wife, a psychologist and registered nurse, insisted that I go. I believe the pettiness and groupthink of supposed professionals rankles her far more than it does me.

It no longer particularly bothers me to be passively, or even actively, ignored by academic panjandrums, but when I was informed of this spineless maneuver, I thought, like Popeye before he swallows that can of spinach, "Dat's all I can stans; I can't stans n' more." A friend urged me to pull an end run and display some research posters, and so away I went.

The situation in Australia is tragic. Many patients with CFS are derided by their physicians, unlike in the United States, where they are treated by at least a few establishment physicians with benign condescension. Because in Australia few treatments are known, few are offered. Offices that provide vitamins, colonics, and other holistic therapies are swamped as a result. Patients and physicians eagerly took two hundred of my treatment protocols, and The Haworth Press, Inc. generously donated 40 copies of *Betrayal by the Brain,* which is difficult to obtain in Australia.

The researchers, with whom I hoisted a few at intimate soirees of a hundred or so, are mostly a gregarious lot, who freely admit that they don't really have much of an idea what they are doing. I did learn to speak some

Australian phrases, however, possibly even fooling some natives. A psychiatrist whom I had met elsewhere confided that she must treat CFS patients sub rosa, lest her stature in the medical community be markedly diminished.

I had been told previously that various reasons for my ostracism by the worldwide academic CFS community were that

1. I was unscientific.
2. No one understood my work.
3. Others were jealous.
4. My conclusions were too "premature."
5. I was a loose cannon, even an outright lunatic.

In Australia, I learned that many researchers in the erstwhile commonwealth considered me rude as well. This alleged incivility stemmed from three visits to conferences in the British Isles, most recently in Dublin. After being stupefied by the usually yawn-provoking procession of meaningless facts casting pseudolight on poorly defined problems, I stood up to state that time and money being spent on viral immunology (useful to a degree in CFS) and muscle pathophysiology (valueless in FMS) were missing the point and that these disorders were caused by improper gating of the information in the brain. For this shocking breach of propriety, I was henceforth regarded as a boorish lout in certain circles, yet another blot on my escutcheon.

I must say that the British CFS researchers (with very few exceptions), even more than their counterparts in the United States, don't know they don't know and wouldn't care if they did. They seem to slavishly regard cognitive-behavioral therapy as the Holy Grail of CFS. Publications around the fringes of neurobiology are infrequent in number and trivial in their implications.

Meanwhile, back in the States, I met a currently prominent CFS grandee at a conference a few years ago. "I didn't realize you knew anything about CFS," I said. "I don't know a thing about CFS," he replied, "but I sure know a lot about how to write grants."

These attitudes were unknown to me when I ingenuously entered the "EBV" (Epstein-Barr virus) arena in 1984-1995, having previously published a report that Tagamet could cure acute infectious mononucleosis in a day or two (Goldstein JA, 1983). I felt rather like the kid who blurted out "The emperor has no clothes!" to the horror of all. Seeing an increasing number of individuals with "chronic EBV," I thought that I might help to figure out what was wrong and find out how to fix it. I naively believed that there must be numerous scientists here and abroad who knew much more about what was going on than I did, and that we could work together to reach the common goal. It took at least seven years for this idealistic enthusiasm to be squelched. Although many clinicians shared my agenda, it appeared that few researchers did. So, except for the help of certain academic colleagues (who were often told by peers that working in CFS would end their careers), the intellectual excitement of my quest has been fairly solitary, making me an unwilling "master of my domain." The tenets of this domain are so simple that they almost seem self-evident truths: In CFS and related disorders the brain does not handle information properly. As a result, a patient experiences sensations and cognitions that are not appropriate to his or her stimulus environment. If the input is incorrect, so is the output ("garbage in, garbage out"), and physiology regulated above the level of the brainstem may be dysfunctional. The corollary to this theorem, which is not as self-evident, is that the brain can be tuned to enhance the signal (salient information) and eliminate the noise (irrelevant stimuli), much like tuning a radio to hear the music and not the static. This process can often occur immediately—some researchers use the word instantaneously, but I have been advised not to (yet)—with the proper intervention. A few papers in scientific journals are beginning to address this common phenomenon, such as

> Marder E (1997), Computational dynamics in rhythmic neural circuits. *The Neuroscientist* 3(5):295-302.
> Nicolelis MAL (1997), Dynamic and distributed somatosensory representations as the substrate for cortical and subcortical plasticity. *Seminars in Neuroscience* 9:24-33.
> Glanz J (1997), Mastering the nonlinear brain. *Science* 277:1758-1760.

G'digh 'til the next issue, maights!

Because more and more doctors will probably be practicing neurosomatic medicine in the future, I thought it would be interesting for them to read about the path I took to become a neurosomaticist, as well as what I have experienced since I became one. Because neurosomatic medicine is such a novel approach that many physicians, even those who are employed by regulatory agencies, might not understand it, I discuss my difficulties in this regard. Hopefully others will profit from my autobiographical narrative.

ABBREVIATIONS

2-AG	2-arachindonylglycerol
3-HK	3-hyrdokyneureine
5-HT	serotonin, or 5-hydroxytryptamine
12-HPETE	12-hyrdoperoxyeicosatetraenoic
AA	arachidonic acid
AACFS	America Association for Chronic Fatigue Syndrome
AC	adenyl cyclase
ACC	anterior cingulate cortex
ACE	angiotensin-converting enzyme
Ach	acetylcholine
ACTH	adrenocorticotropin
ADC	arginine decarboxylase
ADD	attention-deficit disorder
ADHD	attention-deficit hyperactivity disorder
ADP	adenosine diphosphate
ADR	adverse drug reaction
AED	antiepileptic drug
AgRP	agouti-related peptide
AII	angiotensin II
ALS	amyotrophic lateral sclerosis
AMA	American Medical Association
AMP	adenosine monophosphate
AMPA	alpha-amino-3-hydroxy-5-methyl-4-isoxazole proponic acid
ANB	atrial natriuretic factor beta
ANS	autonomic nervous system
APO	apomorphine
APTT	activated partial thromboplastin time
ARAS	ascending reticular activating system
ART	adaptive resonance therapy
AST	aspartate aminotrasferase
ATP	adenosine triphosphate
BBB	blood-brain barrier
BDNF	brain-derived neurotrophic factor
BEAM	brain electrical activity mapping

BH_4	tetrahydrobiopterin
BK	bradykinin
BMS	burning mouth syndrome
BST	bed nucleus of the stria terminalis
BZD	benzodiazepine
cADPR	cyclic adenosine diphosphate ribose
cADPR	cyclic ADPribose
CaMKII	calcium/calmodulin kinase II
cAMP	cyclic adenosine monophosphate
CART	cocaine- and amphetamine-regulated transcript
CB	cannabinoid
CBT	cognitive-behavioral therapy
CCK	cholecystokinin
CCU	coronary care unit
CDS	clonidine-displacing substance
CFS	chronic fatigue syndrome
CFTR	cystic fibrosis transmembrane conductance regulator
cGMP	guanosine3,5-cyclic monophosphate
CGRP	calcitonin gene-related peptide
CICR	calcium-induced calcium response
CKII	casein kinase II
CMV	cytomegalovirus
CNS	central nervous system
CNTF	ciliary neurotrophic factor
CO	carbon monoxide
COMT	catechol-orthomethyltransferase
COX	cyclooxygenase
CPAP	continuous positive airway pressure
CPK	creatine phosphokinase
CR	conditional response
CREB	cAMP-response element-binding protein
CRF	corticotropin-releasing factor
CRH	corticotropin-releasing hormone
CS	conditioned stimulus
CSTC	corticostriatal-thalamocortical
DA	dopamine
DAG	diacylglycerol
DAT	dopamine transporter
DDAVP	desmopressin acetate
DEA	Drug Enforcement Agency
DH	dorsal hypothalamus
DHEA	dehyroepiandrosterone

DLPFC	dorsolateral prefrontal cortex
DMH	dorsomedial hypothalamus
DMHN	dorsomedial hypothalamic nucleus
DNIC	descending nociceptive inhibitory control
DRN	dorsal raphe nucleus
DSI	depolarization-induced suppression of inhibition
EAA	excitatory amino acid
EBV	Epstein-Barr virus
ECT	electroconvulsive therapy
EDGF	edothilial-derived growth factor
EDS	excessive daytime sleepiness
EEG	electroencephalogram
ELISA	enzyme-linked immunosorbent assay
EMDR	eye movement desensitization and reprocessing
EMG	electromyogram
EMS	emotional motor system
ENK	enkephalin
EPSC	excitatory postsynaptic current
EPSP	excitatory postsynaptic potential
ER	endoplasmic reticulum
ERK	extracellular signal-related kinase
ERN	error-related negativity
ET	endothelin
EtOH	ethanol
FASPS	familial advanced sleep phase syndrome
FDA	Food and Drug Administration
FDOPA	fluorodopa
FEF	frontal eye field
FGF	fibroblast growth factor
FMRF	Phe-Met-Arg-Phe
FMS	fibromyalgia syndrome
FRA	fos-related antigen
FS	fast spiking
FSH	follicle-stimulating hormone
GABA	gamma-aminobutyric acid
GABAR	GABA receptor
GAD	generalized anxiety disorder
GAT	GABA transporter
GBL	gamma butyrolactone
GBP	gabapentin
GC	guanylyl cyclase
GDNF	glial-derived neurotrophic factor

GDP	guanosine triphosphate
GH	growth hormone
GHB	gamma hydroxybutyrate
GHRH	growth hormone-releasing hormone
GHT	geniculohypothalamic tract
GI	gastrointestinal
GIRK	G-protein-activated inwardly rectifying K^+ channels
GnRH	gonadotropin-releasing hormone
GP	globus pallidus
GPCR	G-protein-coupled receptor
GPe	globus pallidus externa
GPi	globus pallidus interna
GR	glucose responsive
GRP	gastrin-releasing peptide
GSNO	S-nitrosoglutathione
GSR	galvanized skin response
GSSG	oxidized glutathione
GTP	guanosine triphosphate
GWS	Gulf War syndrome
H_2S	hydrogen sulfide
HA	histamine
HCG	human chorionic gonadotropin
hCK1ε	human casein kinase 1 epsilon
HMGCoA	3-hydroxy-3-methylglutaryl coenzyme A
HMO	health maintenance organization
HPA	hypothalamic-pituitary-adrenal
HPT	hypothalamic-pituitary-thyroid
HSP	heat-shock protein
IBS	irritable bowel syndrome
ICV	intacerebroventricular
IEG	immediate early gene
IGF-1	insulin-like growth factor 1
IGL	intergeniculate leaflet
IL	interleukin
INH	isoniazid
IP	intraperitoneal
ITR	inhibitory temporalis reflex
IV	intravenous
IVIG	intravenous gamma globulin
KOR	kappa-opioid receptor
LA	lateral amygdala
LC	locus coeruleus

LDHA	lactate dehydrogenase
LDT	laterodorsal tegmental nucleus
LH	luteinizing hormone
LHA	lateral hypothalamic area
LHBT	lactulose hydrogen breath test
LHRH	lutenizing hormone-releasing hormone
LLPDD	late luteal-phase dysphoric disorder
LPFC	lateral prefrontal cortex
LPS	lipopolysaccharide
LRF	lateral reticular formation
LSD	lysergic acid diethylamide
LTD	long-term depression
LTG	lamotrigine
LTP	long-term potentiation
mAchR	muscarinic acetylcholine receptor
MAO(I)	monoamine oxidase (inhibitor)
MAPK	mitogen-activated protein kinase
MCH	melanin-concentrating hormone
MCL	mesocorticolimbic system
MCS	multiple chemical sensitivity
MD	mediodorsal
MDD	major depressive disorder
MDMA	3,4-methylenedioxy-N-methylamphetamine
MFB	medial forebrain bundle
mGluR	metabotropic glutamate receptor
MMAI	5-methoxy-6-methyl-2 aminoindan
mPFC	medial prefrontal cortex
MPH	methylphenidate
MPOA	medial preoptic area
(f)MRI	(functional) magnetic resonance imaging
MRN	median raphe nucleus
MRS	magnetic resonance spectroscopy
MS	multiple sclerosis
MSH	melanocyte-stimulating hormone
NAAG	*N*-acetyl-aspartate glutamate
NAALADase	N-acetylated alpha-linked acidic dipeptidase
NAc	nucleus accumbens
nAchR	nicotinic acetylcholine receptor
NAD	nicotinic adenine dinucleotide
NADPH	nicotinamide adenine dineuclotide phosphate
NCAM	neural cell adhesion molecule
NE	norepinephrine

NGF	nerve growth factor
NIH	National Institutes of Health
NMDA	N-methyl-D-aspartate
NMDAR	NMDA receptor
(n)NOS	(neuronal) nitric oxide synthase
NO	nitric oxide
NP-B	natriuretic peptide type B
NPY	neuropeptide Y
NRI	norepinephrine-reuptake inhibitor
NRM	nucleus raphe magnus
NSAID	nonsteroidal anti-inflammatory drug
NT	neurotrophin
NTS	nucleus tractus solitarii (nucleus of the solitary tract)
NTX	naltrexone
OCD	obsessive-compulsive disorder
ODC	ornithine decarboxylase
OFC	orbitofrontal cortex
OMPFC	orbitofrontal/medial prefrontal cortex
OR	orienting response
OSA	obstructive sleep apnea
OTC	over the counter
OTR	oxytocin receptor
OXT	oxytocin
PAF	platelet-activating factor
PAG	periaqueductal gray
PAR	protease-activated receptor
PCP	phencyclidine
PDD	pervasive developmental disorder
PDE	phosphodiesterase
PDEI	phosphodiesterase inhibitor
PDGF	platelet-derived growth factor
PDR	Physician's Desk Reference
PDV	primary disorder of vigilance
PET	positron-emission tomography
PFC	prefrontal cortex
PHI	peptide histidine isoleucine
PI	personal injury
PI-3K	phosphatidyl insitol-3 kinase
PIN	posterior intralaminar nucleus
PI-PLC	phosphoinositide-specific phospholipase C
PKA	protein kinase A
PKB	protein kinase B

PKC	protein kinase C
PLA$_2$	phospholipase A$_2$
PLC	phospholipase C
PLO	pluronic organogel
PMd	dorsal premammillary nucleus
PMDD	premenstrual dysphoric disorder
PMLS	periodic leg movements in sleep
PMS	premenstrual syndrome
PNS	peripheral nervous system
POA	preoptic area
POAH	preoptic anterior hypothalamic
POMC	propopiomelanocortin
PP	phophatase
PPI	prepulse inhibition
PPM	parts per million
PPN	pontine parabrachial nucleus
PRL	prolactin
PSD	postsynaptic density
PTSD	post-traumatic stress disorder
PVN	paraventricular nucleus
RAIC	rostral agranular insular cortex
rCBF	regional cerebral blood flow
REM	rapid eye movement
RHT	retinohypothalamic tract
RLS	restless leg syndrome
RSD	reflex sympathetic dystrophy
rTMS	repetitive transcranial magnetic stimulation
RTN	reticular nucleus of the thalamus
RVLM	rostral ventrolateral medulla
RyR	ryanodine-sensitive receptor
S1	primary somatosensory cortex
SAMe	*S*-adenosylmethionine
SCG	superior cervical ganglion
SCN	suprachiasmatic nucleus
SIBO	small intestinal bacterial overgrowth
SN	substantia nigra
SNAP-25	synaptosomal-associated protein 25
SNARE	soluble *N*-sensitive factor attachment protein receptor
SNpc	substantia nigra pars compacta
SNr	substantia nigra pars reticulata
SNR	signal-to-noise ratio
SOD	supraoptic decussation

SON	supraoptic nucleus
SP	substance P
SPECT	single photon emission computed tomography
SS	somatostatin
(S)SRI	(selective) serotonin reuptake inhibitor
STN	subthalamic nucleus
SUR	sulfonylurea
SWS	slow-wave sleep
SynGAP	synaptic Ras-GTPase activating protein
TCA	tricyclic antidepressant
TD	tardive dyskinesia
TENS	transcutaneous electrical nerve stimulation
TGF-beta	transforming growth factor beta
TH	tyrosine hydroxylase
THC	tetrahydrocannabinol
THT	trigeminohypothalamic tract
TMD	temporomandibular dysfunction
TMJ	**temporomandibular joint**
TMN	tuberomammillary nucleus
TMS	transcranial magnetic stimulation
TNF-á	**tumor necrosis factor-alpha**
tPA	tissue plasminogen activator
TRH	thyrotropin-releasing hormone
Trk	tyrosine kinase
TrkA	tyrosine kinase A
TrkB	tyrosine kinase B
TRN	thalamic reticular nucleus
TrypH	tryptophan hydroxylase
TST	thyroid-stimulating hormone
TTX	tetrodotoxin
UARS	upper airway resistance syndrome
US	unconditioned stimulus
VA	ventral anterior
VBST	ventral bed nucleus of the stria terminalis
Vc	ventralis caudalis
VIP	vasoactive intestinal peptide
VL	ventral lateral
VLPO	ventrolateral preoptic area
VMAT	vesicular monoamine transporter
VMH	ventromedial hypothalamus
VMpo	posterior ventral medial nucleus
VP	ventral pallidum

VPA	valproic acid
VPR	vasopressin
VR	vanilloid receptor
VSCC	voltage-sensitive calcium channel
VSUB	ventral subiculum
VTA	ventral tegmental area
WDR	wide-dynamic range

Part I:
Inventing Neurosomatic Medicine: Rewards and Satisfactions versus Problems and Pitfalls

It's not easy bein' me.

Rodney Dangerfield (1921-)

There are three major rewards for the physician practicing neurosomatic medicine: (1) Patients who have been miserable and nonfunctional for years can get significantly better in days. (2) Because this branch of medicine is largely terra incognita, someone who has learned its database (which takes several years) can greatly advance knowledge of pathophysiology and treatment with appropriately targeted interventions, which need not be very complicated. I am reminded of the possibly apocryphal story of Nikola Tesla, the inventor of the dynamo, and widely regarded as a genius in his era (1880s). A large power-generating corporation could not make its giant transformers operate, despite legions of expert consultants. Finally, they called in Dr. Tesla. He looked at the banks of machines, went over to one, and kicked it. Immediately, the entire system became operational again. "Thank you, Dr. Tesla," said the chairman of the board. "What is your fee?" "$100,000," replied Tesla. "$100,000!" exclaimed the chairman (a lot of money in those days, about $10 million today). "It only took you a minute to kick the machine!" "Ah," said Tesla, "kicking the machine only cost you a dollar. Knowing *where* to kick it cost you the rest." The same can be said for the practice of neurosomatic medicine—it is usually fairly easy if you know "where to kick" (Seifer MJ, 1998). Unlike the case of Tesla, however, moguls are not lining up with millions so that I can fix their neuroelectric systems. (3) You don't have to be part of managed health care. Indeed, it is virtually impossible for a primary care physician in a health maintenance organization (HMO) to adequately care for a neurosomatic patient. The physician (or the company) receives $10 to $20 per month to take care of each patient. This allocation means rationing not only expensive tests and consultations, none of which are really necessary if one understands neurosomatic medicine, but also rationing *time,* the most precious commodity. Physicians must listen to their patients, educate them, and treat the underlying dysfunction. A Beverly Hills woman was referred to me by her psychiatrist after seeing ten other doctors. She arrived at the office with her mother and her medical records. I reviewed the records, and said, as I usually do, "Would you like to start treatment while we are talking, or would you like to talk first?" A look of consternation passed across her face. "You mean you're not going to check my T cells?" "No, I'm not, there's no reason to do so. You've had that test before, and the T-cell count was normal. I'd just like to help you to feel better." "Come on mother, we're getting out of here," she exclaimed, looking at me as if I were deranged. She later reported me to the California Medical Board, an occupational hazard of the practice of neurosomatic medicine.

For a brief period around 1983 I was medical director of the local HMO started by a group of neighboring physicians. I eventually had to resign because I couldn't tolerate financial considerations dictating the nature of the doctor-patient relationship. I found myself being angry at patients who talked too long or had too many questions, and I abhorred the adversarial relationship I necessarily found myself in with patients who had expensive illnesses and/or wanted expensive health care, because I had to pay for it. If I did not see patients quickly enough, or spent too much money on their care, either I would go bankrupt, or later, when managed health care became more pervasive, I could be dismissed from a health plan, losing possibly a thousand patients because of "overutilization." I lay awake too many nights wondering whether I had missed a life-threatening problem by not ordering a certain expensive test, such as a CT scan. Today flow charts called "algorithms" instruct doctors how to manage almost every common medical problem, so compliant physicians do not feel that they are placing their careers in jeopardy in a difficult case as long as they go by the cookbook. Neurosomatic patients are not in the cookbook, take up a lot of time, and can tremendously overutilize medical resources if the physician does not understand how to manage them, which he or she almost always does not. They are thus frustrating to deal with, and many physicians shun them. About three years ago I gave a lecture on CFS to doctors at a large local hospital. The following is how I was introduced by the moderator: "Ladies and gentlemen, we all have two or three "patients from hell" in our practices. Dr. Jay Goldstein, here to talk to us about chronic fatigue syndrome, has two or three *thousand.*"

Medical practice algorithms are very useful to maintain a basic level of competence among primary care physicians. When I opened my office in 1975 for family medicine, I was the first physician in the county (as far as I knew) to have had residency training in this "specialty." I had also had training in psychiatry.

There were tremendous abuses of patient care and insurance billing in this bygone era, now regarded as the "Golden Age of Medicine" by physicians who were in practice then, because the insurance companies paid for everything that was billed. This policy was like Nirvana for most physicians. Those who were primarily interested in providing the best care for their patients could do so, because medical ethics provided that the physician had a fiduciary responsibility, i.e., they would charge a fair price for services and not overutilize them for personal gain.

Many, perhaps most, primary care physicians from Pasadena to San Diego that I encountered during these years abused the system unconscionably for maximum monetary gain. I knew lots of them who became quite wealthy. For example, during my family practice residency, a friend and I moonlighted at a local community hospital owned by obscenely wealthy doctors where we were paid $100 to cover the emergency room and $10 each to perform a history and physical exam on each newly admitted patient. Although the compensation was low, the work was easy. Hospitals that were so busy that moonlighters had to stay awake all night paid more, but one was exhausted the next day. My friend and I used to tell each other horror stories that eventually became amusing because they were so commonplace.

Doing surgery paid a lot more than caring for patients medically. Some doctors would admit entire families to have their tonsils removed. One doctor in particular, who did a lot of surgery, apparently had such a poor technique that he got a wound infection on every single patient we saw while we were there. We even made a wager of $100 for the first one of us who examined a female patient over thirty years of age at this hospital who had not had a hysterectomy. After a year, the money was unclaimed.

It seemed that every patient, no matter what the diagnosis, had several thousand dollars worth of tests. The patients thought they were getting the best care ("I wanted to go into the hospital and have a *complete* physical to find out what's wrong with me"), and the doctors who owned the hospital (almost all of those who admitted patients there) made a fortune, since the tests were done there. Since then, state regulations have been tightened, limiting self-referrals. That is, a doctor cannot refer his or her patient to his or her own lab, etc.

Because I made two or three urgent calls a night to physicians who had totally botched a patient's care, I eventually came to formulate the rule that a primary care physician's income (above a certain reasonable level) was inversely related to his or her competence in medicine. This rule remained unchanged while I was in private practice, and was true to a certain extent for specialists as well, since incompetent specialists tended to receive referrals from incompetent generalists.

The public seemed generally unable to discriminate between good and bad physicians and went to see a doctor because he or she was convenient or likeable. Although at one time I had the largest solo family practice in my part of the county, cared about my patients, and was on call every single day because even then no other physician could deal with my unusual mix of "treatment-resistant patients." Some other physicians whom I knew seemed to have primarily a pecuniary orientation. They made ten or twenty times as much money as I did, largely by performing unnecessary tests and procedures. I shall not belabor this point, except to say that most family doctors in 1975 had no additional training past internship and that the amount of medical knowledge doubles every five years. I'll talk about psychiatrists, the other group of physicians with whom I am most familiar, a little later. In the meantime, I describe my "education" as a neurosomaticist in Chapter 1.

Chapter 1

The Education of a Neurosomaticist

To understand other aspects of my early life please refer to *Portnoy's Complaint,* by Philip Roth (1969). I am ten years younger, my father was a doctor, and my sex life was far more mundane. Otherwise, the depictions are fairly accurate.

I went to medical school solely to get my ticket punched for a psychiatric residency because I became fascinated as a teenager by how the brain worked. I realized that psychologists knew a lot about how the brain worked as well, but they could not prescribe medication, which I saw as a necessary partner to psychotherapy in helping people to feel better. Chlorpromazine (Thorazine) was invented in 1951, when I was nine years old, and by the time I was in my teens had made a tremendous impact on psychiatric practice, even though no one knew how it worked in the treatment of schizophrenia.

I started to read psychiatry, which in those days consisted of psychoanalysis and psychoanalytically oriented psychotherapy, which was just psychoanalysis done once or twice a week, not four or five times a week, for five years or so. Although there were different brands of psychoanalysis ("schools," they were called), psychiatry consisted of learning psychoanalysis, using medications which worked by unknown mechanisms, and doing electroconvulsive therapy (ECT). Insulin shock therapy was on its way out, as was hydrotherapy, or wrapping a difficult patient in wet towels for a long time. Prefrontal lobotomy, popular for a time and performed more or less by putting an ice pick into the brain through the nostrils and wiggling it around, was also losing favor.

In high school I read the collected works of Sigmund Freud. Because I was a tabula rasa at that time when it came to psychiatry, almost all of it just soaked in, although it didn't seem like any other kind of science I had learned before.

Although I went to high school, I spent most of my time playing basketball, posing purposely ridiculous arcane intellectual arguments to my teachers, and trying to score with girls who preferred to be "friends" with me. I also dated cheerleaders but didn't know what to say to them. They usually got headaches and had to go home early. Because I was a curious child who regularly read two or three books a day, I regarded high school itself as an outlet for adolescent urges, as did almost everyone else I knew.

The Ivy League university I attended made the mistake of putting me into a special program in which I could pretty much do anything I wanted for four years. My being in this program was like giving a loaded gun to a child (a simile only in those days!), since I was far too undisciplined to make good use of the opportunity. I chose this college because the girl who allowed me to be the most "friendly" with her was going there. As soon as we matriculated, she informed me that she had fallen in love with a wealthy medical student, although she still wanted to be my friend, just less "friendly" than before.

While in college I did little but play basketball and show up for exams. I would usually spend one day cramming for each exam and otherwise ignore the class. Besides wasting four years of possible learning, I dropped in on some of my classes on the day that a midterm was being given, without warning from my usually reliable sources. Usually I could fake it well enough to at least get a C, but not in my calculus course, since I had somehow neglected to learn calculus in my preteen years when I was reading most of the books in the neighborhood library. I had a chance to snatch a passing grade from the jaws of ignominy by getting a good mark in my final exam, but calculus was my last final of six in the semester. I crammed well enough to get As and Bs in the first five, but found to my horror that after being awake for 48 hours, I could not cram four months of calculus into the next 24 hours. I got a D minus on the exam and failed the course. I repeated it the next term and actually went to class fairly regularly, getting a B. I took the precaution of intellectually seducing the female instructor by discussing on several occasions how the calculus invented by Newton was different from that devised by Leibniz. I believe this practice is still called "sucking up." I thought the damage had been done though—I would never get into medical school, and there were no other plausible scenarios.

The rest of college dissolved into a blur of basketball, parties, and card games, since I thought I had already learned most of the remaining courses. But I was torpedoed by one crucial previously unsuspected disorder which could have completely ruined my changes of becoming a "real" doctor, although I had been offered admission to the graduate school of history, a subject which I study to this day. My latent and potentially lethal defect was that I could not bore holes in corks.

The "make-or-break" course in most colleges for getting into medical school is organic chemistry, a subject that was easy for me to learn. Unfortunately, a laboratory section of the course involved being given an unknown substance and through a process of chemical tests, some of which involved distillation, figuring out what it was and handing in the result at the end of the lab. Distilling something often entailed heating the unknown so that it became a gas which traveled through glass tubes from one corked flask to another. Often several flasks and sets of tubes were involved. I don't know whether mechanical cork borers existed in those days, but my college didn't have any. I found that I was apparently congenitally unable to bore a hole in a straight line through a cork with a manual cork borer, which was a hollow metal tube with a handle. It worked on the principle used by the device that opens wine bottles (if the cork was held in the hand), but for me it was unworkable. The corks would break, the holes would come out on the side of the cork, I would cut my fingers on the cork borer—it seemed that I was cursed to never bore a cork so that I could insert the glass tubes for distillation and start performing the necessary tests. Everyone else in the lab was finishing up the experiment while I was still engaged in this frenetic exercise in futility. Eventually, the lab instructor, whom I had befriended and drove home every night, bored the corks for me for each experiment (in about a minute). If not for him, I would be teaching history, which really is not such a bad second choice. Thank you, Mr. Seasonwine, wherever you are.

It was still by no means a sure thing that I was going to get into medical school, because there was that F in calculus standing out like a disgusting fungus among all my flowery rows of As and Bs. I had stopped growing at an inconvenient time, ending at 5'11" rather than 6'7", so my chances of going to the NBA were nil. Moreover, in those days before Lyndon Johnson doubled the number of medical students and admitted large numbers of foreign medical graduates to correct a real or imagined physician shortage, it wasn't all that easy to get into a medical school. Today, as it becomes less and less attractive to be a physician, some schools almost have to beg for applicants.

My incipient descent into oblivion was fortuitously halted by the Medical College Admission Test (MCAT), which is like an SAT for would-be doctors. I have a knack for doing well on these tests, and fortunately one medical school in the United States decided that year to weigh MCAT scores higher than grades. I was thus summarily snatched from the abyss, and away I went for four more years of self-destruction.

Medical school was much more difficult than college, particularly since I had no prior self-education in most of the course material, except psychiatry. People also used to flunk out, a practice which is almost unheard of today. "Look at the person on your right, and then look at the person on your left," many deans would instruct the alphabetically assembled first-year students on orientation day. "One of you won't be here in four years," he continued, eliciting the predictable shudder from the group.

There was a lot to learn. I had to start studying for exams several days in advance. The volume of material was too much to cram. Fortunately, my roommates took very good notes, because I found that lectures caused me to go to sleep almost instantly. If I had studied this hard in college, I would have gotten an A on every test. My roommates felt the same way. Furthermore, I still had my "basketball jones." A basketball player is at the peak of his ability (says Shawn Kemp, an NBA player who ought to know) when he is 27 years old. I was still getting better every day. Although I was now watching Bill Bradley playing for the Knicks, rather than at the Palestra at Penn, I was doing just as well in the low minors of intramurals. Somewhat like a very pale version of Elgin Baylor, the Michael Jordan of my era, I could go right and left, inside and outside, hit the fadeaway jumper, shoot hook shots with both hands (a lost art since Kareem retired), and occasionally dunk.

I was blessed with gross anatomy partners who actually enjoyed dissection (it had to be done), while I learned Gray's *Anatomy*. Our anatomy professor was Dr. Nicholas Cauna, a magisterial Lithuanian who had helped to discover the Pacinian corpuscle, a sensory structure in the skin. He spoke like a kindlier version of Count Dracula. "Remember forever and never forget," he would enjoin us when making a point that would certainly be on the next exam. We thought he knew everything there was to know about anatomy. Following the example of Case Western Reserve, our medical school was attempting to introduce clinical relevance to the first and second years, which were traditionally devoted to basic science. One day an orthopedic surgeon was talking about some operation on the leg and showing slides. After the lights went out, but before my eyes closed, the orthopedist, discussing the muscles of the thigh, could not remember the name of one of them. "ADDUCTOR MAGNUS *(mahgnoose)*" boomed a voice from the back of the room like an Old Testament prophet.

Because all I wanted to do in life (I thought) was be a psychiatrist, I "passed through" medical school just as I had college, making sure, however, not to flunk anything. By the time I reached my psychiatry rotation I was ready to jump in and do what I had been preparing for since I was 15. I had even worked summers as a ward attendant in a psychiatric teaching hospital so that I could go to all the resident seminars. I plunged right into the arcane world of psychoanalysis with vigor and enthusiasm, which became less, and less, and less, since the patients stubbornly resisted resolving their transferences. I was advised to not expect so much, because the process usually took at least five years. I knew that, but I couldn't see why it had to take so long, and in the end I didn't really understand how resolving a transference could make someone better anyway.

In the meantime, the rest of medical school was going by. I don't remember much of it now, but one occasion when rounds were going to be made by the chief of medicine has stuck in my mind. Days were spent preparing for this event. The chief resident, the senior residents, the junior residents, the interns, and the lowly medical students were all prepared to answer any possible question about the patients we were presenting. Charts were impeccably organized. We all came to the hospital an hour early, wearing clean shirts and ties and freshly laundered white coats. The medical student presenting a case, which was done in a very formal, stylized manner then, spent days rehearsing it. For most of the rounds, the chief, who even then was developing a diagnostic computer program that thought like he did, would nod his head and ask a few pointed questions of the patients and the house staff. At least once during each session of rounds he would find a patient who, despite everyone's best efforts, had been inadequately diagnosed and/or treated. Then he began to teach in his own inimitable way. Starting with the medical student assigned to the patient, he would ask a question. If the medical student did not know the answer, he went up the line to the intern and eventually the chief resident. If no one could respond to this by now obvious question, he would exclaim "This man (or woman) needs a doctor!" and we would repair to a conference room to discuss our deficiencies in a Socratic dialogue. I found myself using the exact same expression twenty years later when I was making inpatient rounds with house staff who apparently couldn't care less if they knew the answers to any of my questions or not. But *I* really meant it.

One day in 1966, the chief, waxing somewhat philosophical in response to our overly zealous diagnostic efforts for a certain patient, eerily prophesied, "If you doctors don't stop ordering so many expensive tests, some day you'll find that the government will be telling you what you can and can't do." Such a notion was inconceivable to us young princes, and we exchanged knowing glances that the chief was perhaps entering geezerdom a little early.

I began to explore other avenues of helping people psychiatrically. I spent one summer doing hypnosis research with Martin Orne, testing subjects for hypnotic susceptibility and reading their electroencephalograms (EEGs) while they were hypnotized. Orne devised the concept of "demand characteristics," which encouraged the experimental subject to try to produce the results which he or she perceived the experimenter wanted. Because Orne was trying to define the neurophysiological basis of hypnosis, which has not been done to this day (Gruzelier J, 1996), he also hired actors who were not at all susceptible to hypnosis to pretend that they were hypnotized. Even though it now appears that hypnosis involved shifting of attentional neural networks, we did not possess the neuroscientific background or the electronic technology to make such a discovery.

During the summer of 1967 I did research at Langley Porter Neuropsychiatric Institute, a part of the University of California San Francisco School of Medicine. The summer of 1967 was also "The Summer of Love" in Haight-Ashbury and Golden Gate Park, which was just down the street. Not only was that summer my first experience of girls with long ironed hair and tie-dyed T-shirts, Janis Joplin, Jimi Hendrix, The Jefferson Airplane, the Fillmore, and altered states of consciousness, it was also my initial sampling of the numerous alternatives to psychoanalytic psychotherapy. Behavior therapy (fairly Skinnerian at that time) was opposed by Gestalt therapy à la Fritz Perls and his "hot seat" at the Esalen Institute. I returned for my fourth year of medical school prepared to use some of the new therapeutic tools I had acquired.

Lest the reader think from what follows that I was studying at some backwater institution, the then-current presidents of the American Psychiatric and Psychoanalytic Associations, respectively, were professors there. One could thus assume that the nature of psychiatry practiced by these men and their associates epitomized that of 1967 to 1968.

In the fourth year at my medical school we were permitted to choose our course of study. I elected to sample everything the department of psychiatry had to offer and became an acting psychiatry resident for most of the year, as well as spending two months each being an acting intern on the medicine and pediatric services.

The main event of each month in the psychiatric/psychoanalytic institute was the presentation of the case of a patient who had completed his or her analysis by one of the psychoanalysts completing his or her training. My fourth year virtually began with one of these conferences, which were attended by at least 100 psychiatrists from hither and yon. The analysand that day was a middle-aged construction worker, who, about five years previously, was involved in a serious accident when the ball of a wrecking crane struck him and a co-worker, killing the latter and causing the patient to be hospitalized with multiple fractures. When he was discharged and completed physical therapy, he found he was unable to return to work because he was afraid of cranes. Being disabled, his income fell, his children had to drop out of college, and he lost his house. Accordingly, he presented himself to the outpatient psychiatry department and began daily 50-minute hours of analysis.

The presenting psychiatrist recounted the subtle details of the five-year analytic process, relating the patient's unconscious conflict to being locked in a closet when he was four years old, a trauma that was abreacted while the transference was brilliantly resolved. The audience was asked whether there were any questions, and everyone prepared to leave since there was obviously no doubt that the process was beyond reproach. From the back row, I raised my hand. Everyone stopped, perhaps incredulous that a medical student would be neurotic enough to intrude on such an august assemblage. I should parenthetically mention that in those days disagreement with analytic dogma was interpreted as evidence of an unresolved unconscious conflict, rather than an effort to refine the science, since psychoanalysis was so patently unscientific that it was actually a cult, as I was soon to realize. The lack of an experimental foundation for the tenets of this discipline has begun to be rectified in recent years (Schore AN, 1994).

I asked whether the patient had been able to return to work as a result of the analysis, a reasonable therapeutic goal which I naively thought the presenter had neglected to mention. Quiet consternation ensued, which perplexed me. Those who have not had training in an analytic institute will think the following responses are so bizarre that the inmates were running the asylum unless they have read *Mount Misery,* the recent sequel to *House of God* by the pseudonymous Samuel Shem, MD, which took place (I would guess) about twenty years later.

The question was considered by all to be completely irrelevant. The only salient information was how the analysis was conducted. Outcomes were never even considered. Because daily psychoanalytic sessions were the summum bonum of psychiatry, whatever transpired in the patient's actual life could not be altered, and discussion of it might even contaminate the analytic process.

The psychiatrist was not sure whether the patient had returned to work or not. Thinking that I had somehow not asked my question clearly, I restated it: "This man had a posttraumatic crane phobia. Shouldn't a successful analysis have resolved the phobia so that he could work again?" "I did all that could be done," replied the psychiatrist. "What else is there?"

"Behavior therapy could have eliminated his phobia in a few hours," I replied, suspecting that this experience couldn't really be occurring and I was having some sort of "flashback" hallucination that I had heard of in San Francisco, but no such luck. *"What's behavior therapy?"* asked the psychiatrist of me and everyone else in the assembly hall. Not one other person there had ever heard of it. I was asked by one of the professors to explain behavior therapy in the remaining five minutes, and I outlined the basic principles as I understood them. "People aren't rats," he stated and dissolved the conference, leaving me at the blackboard with my tongue hanging out. No one asked me a single question about behavior therapy for the rest of the year, even though I was routinely using it with my patients.

By this time I had been studying psychoanalytic theory for ten years, but I began to look at it in a more critical light. Numerous case conferences I attended were like miniature versions of the monthly extravaganza. I began to observe the process by which decisions were reached about the psychodynamics of the patient being presented (although I never had ample evidence that such discussion had relationship to any reality). As a bright, narcissistic, and mildly sociopathic psychiatric colleague of mine (who later went on to franchise a wildly successful chain of inpatient eating disorder clinics) observed: "Learning psychoanalysis is like learning to fly a dirigible. Both are very difficult and take a long time, but dirigible flying may have *some* practical value."

In these case conferences, the correct decision was made by either the most senior psychiatrist attending or by the person who offered the most esoteric explanation of the unconscious forces at work (which, of course, needed to be discovered by the patient). Because I was always the most junior person at these conferences, I concluded that I should offer the most esoteric interpretation. I searched my memory for the most ludicrous analytic concept and came up with the "oral impregnation fantasy," which is just what it sounds like. Like every other analytic principle, there were reams of commentary about this (alleged) process. I quickly read what was available about oral impregnation in the medical library and was able to locate other libraries in the country that contained further discourses. I was allowed to take a two-week vacation that year and spent it going to every major library that had articles about the topic. My three years of learning German in college was put to its only use during this time.

When I returned to the institute, I was probably one of the world's leading experts on the oral impregnation fantasy, certainly one of the signal distinctions of my life. I then proceeded to interpret every case in every conference as an oral impregnation fantasy. This feat is not as difficult as one might think. After learning the analytic lingo and the basically hydraulic relationships between the id, ego, superego, and the aggregation of lesser reifications, it is possible to metaphorically turn a sow's ear into a silk purse and back again in a few minutes. In the novels of Chaim Potok about discussions of the Talmud in the yeshiva, such meaningless intellectual grandstanding is called *pilpul* in Yiddish. I have never been in another situation where the use of this word was appropriate.

For the first week of oral impregnation interpretation (at different conferences, with different participants) I always carried the day, and I was beginning to be regarded as a wunderkind. When I succeeded in turning all case conferences of the next week into oral impregnation fantasies also (there was no way to refute this explanation), people began to get uncomfortable. I fortunately had the good sense to stop while I was ahead, or else I would have been invited to the dean's office much sooner.

After spending various amounts of time on every psychiatric service available at the time (inpatient, child, prison, developmental disorders, etc.), I rotated through the medical inpatient service (since I thought I should know a little bit about being a "real" doctor) at the local Veteran's Adminis-tration hospital (VAH). Physicians reading this book will know that experi-ence at a VAH is different than any other kind of hospital, but that they are all generically similar.

I also served as an acting intern in the local children's hospital for two months. Besides learning more about pediatrics, I had two notable experi-ences there. A 13-year-old boy was admitted with an unusual movement disorder which had been diagnosed as hysterical but had not responded at all to four years of child psychoanalysis (yes, five days per week). I noted that he had myoclonic jerks and coprolalia (uttering obscene words) and imme-diately diagnosed him as having Gilles de la Tourette disorder. I had never seen a case but had certainly read about it. I promptly administered a low dose of haloperidol (the only pharmacologic treatment available at the time), and the boy was virtually symptom free in less than an hour. His par-ents were amazed and grateful, and their child was discharged the next day after a period of observation. What I did not consider was that they might be really angry at the analyst.

The chief of child psychiatry called me in the next day and vigorously reprimanded me. I can recall only befuddlement about why he would be so upset about my helping a long-suffering patient. "What do you know about Tourette's syndrome?" he challenged me, as if it were inconceivable that a medical student would have the effrontery to make such a (then) rare diag-nosis. I briefly told him the history of the disorder since it was eponymously named for a French neurologist of many years ago, and that it could not have responded to psychoanalysis because it was a neurologic disease. Remem-ber that this era was one when psychiatry *was* psychoanalysis, which was the appropriate, best, and *only* treatment for virtually every disorder that even had a trace of psychiatric flavor added to it (even asthma, ulcers, and headaches, as well as schizophrenia and mania). I had not yet (and would not for decades) realized that it was not whether you won or lost, but how you played the game.

Two days later a teenaged patient of this chief was randomly admitted to me on the regular intern rotation. She had anorexia nervosa, had been treated for two or three years by the chief, and was at an alarmingly low weight. Even in those days we knew that anorexic patients could die from malnutrition and dehydration, although some controversy existed about how this outcome should be averted. Aggressive (and ultimately humane) psychiatry departments of this era would feed the patients through a nasogastric tube, doing a feeding gastrostomy if necessary to save the pa-tient's life. Psychotropic medications were not routinely used in these pa-tients, nor were they used in *any* patient by many psychoanalysts for fear of contaminating the transference by pharmacologic interaction. Later I found that most psychoanalysts knew next to nothing about psychopharmacology, but I still regarded these practitioners with a large degree of respect, if only because they were the leaders of American psychiatry. No one could expect to advance very far unless he or she had finished analytic training.

I noted that this girl behaved rather differently from the other anorexics I had known in medical settings. She acted quite inappropriately, appeared to be hallucinating at times, had conversations with angels who came into her room, and was suicidal. Not wanting to make the mistake again of making the patient better too rapidly, I tried to page the chief, but he was unavailable and it was nighttime. Thus, I diagnosed her as having a schizoaffective disorder (in an era when adolescents never had schizophrenia, they had "adjustment reactions"). I placed her on haloperidol and an antidepressant, lithium and other mood stabilizers being either unavailable in the United States or not known to have such an effect (e.g., carbamazepine). Rapid neuroleptization would not be done in this country for another ten years or more.

The next morning the chief went ballistic when he read my history and physical. The patient did not need medication, never did, and definitely was not psychotic. He countermanded all my orders and took me off the case. During our "discussion," the chief resident, somewhat bespattered, entered the room to inform the chief that his patient had declared that she was one of God's angels and then proceeded to hurl feces in his face, onto another resident, and all over the walls of her room. While transferring her to the institute, the chief remonstrated that she had engaged in this behavior because my ill-informed jejune diagnosis had made the staff relate to her as if she were psychotic and that she had responded to their reinforcements. In other words, this syndrome was produced by my diagnosis, the most behavioral formulation I had ever heard while I was in medical school. I was upset by the interaction but viewed it primarily as another instance when I was wrong for being right. Anyway, I was graduating in three weeks and would be putting this Kafkaesque series of events behind me.

Or was I graduating in three weeks? The next day I was summoned to the dean's office. I had never said one word to the dean and had scarcely even glimpsed his august personage since his welcoming speech four years earlier. He was perturbed that I had acted impetuously, and he questioned my readiness for internship. A pediatric researcher, he knew next to nothing about psychiatry. Although I was usually unsure of myself, and even anxious in many other situations, I always felt quite confident with intellectual challenges, especially when they were on familiar turf. Just a few years later, when I began to teach and do research, I genuinely longed for them, because no one seemed willing to engage me, either adversarially or collegially. I explained to the dean what had transpired, and he could see (I thought) that even if I were some young whippersnapper, I would soon be someone else's problem. Avuncularly dismissing me with advice about obeying the "captain of the ship" no matter what, he abjured me to keep my nose clean. I didn't just keep it clean, I kept it invisible. For three weeks I was the phantom of the senior class, reappearing only for graduation ceremonies, which were mandatory to receive the diploma. Otherwise, I would have been long gone.

My family arrived for the ceremony. One line from this visit deserves to be immortalized. I have neither the time nor the inclination to explain the subtleties of Jewish-American discourse, except to note that nothing is ever as it seems, and not in the way of the Sufi, the Hindu mystics, or even the *brujos* of Carlos Castaneda. No unequivocal statement can ever be made, no doctrine can remain unquestioned, and everyone has an opinion, knowledge about the subject under discussion being no criterion whatsoever. As my family and my girlfriend walked out of the auditorium, my mother turned to the assemblage and uttered the defining sentence of our relationship: "Well, nowadays everyone's a doctor."

It was no easy task for me to graduate from medical school when my basketball skills were peaking. Most courses except psychiatry had little interest for me, some appeared to be specially prepared for dull normals (Ob/Gyn and anesthesiology, although lucrative, traditionally attracted the bottom fifth of each class), and some, such as various forms of surgery, I had no aptitude for whatsoever. The diagnosis part was easy, but the technical aspects of the craft eluded me to the point that I disdained them. Tying surgical knots, viewing structures in three dimensions, making anastomoses or flaps with such a tedious emphasis on perfection drove me to distraction. The technical aspect of performing the surgical task is the most important in the outcome, followed by preoperative diagnosis and choice of procedure, and then postoperative management, usually relegated to flunkies. Although intraoperative judgment was sometimes important, I saw no reason why most operations could not be done well by mechanics, or *feldschers,* as they were called in Russia, technicians trained to do only one or two operations and then do them over and over again. I have assisted in hundreds of operations, and I must modify my callous viewpoint to an extent. An excellent surgeon, of whom I saw almost nothing in all my medical training, dissects tissue planes like they were butter, controls bleeding to the extent that there almost is none, finishes the operation in about one-fifth the time as it took at a university medical center, and almost never has a postoperative complication. I even eventually became as good at surgical assisting as a competent third-year medical student, although for routine cases the surgeon really did not need me. A surgical nurse could have done better. There was a rule for a while that the assistant had to be an MD, in the event the primary surgeon became incapacitated. Although this event never transpired in my career, my presence at the operating table would never have saved anyone's bacon.

I applied for internships only in San Francisco. "What, they don't have internships in Hawaii?" asked my father, wondering how far away from Philadelphia I could go. This question was only the second I can recall him asking me. An osteopathic general practitioner who grew up during the Depression, he solved problems in higher mathematics at the dining room table when he wasn't working, sleeping, or eating. The first question was asked repeatedly, since he viewed me as something of an overindulged slacker. It was asked especially when I came home from playing basketball, a sport which he regarded as totally frivolous. "Well, Jay, did you have *fun* today?" My wife, Gail, still asks that of me on occasion (lest I forget). She can never get the exact intonation of fun (long, drawn out, and conveying "funnnn" as reflecting a certain lack of character) quite right.

I graduated in the bottom fifth of my medical school class, and getting any internship in San Francisco at that time was very competitive, except for the one hospital (which no longer exists) that accepted me. This hospital happened to be my first choice, since it was known to be the easiest internship in San Francisco. I had no desire to be awake, on call, every other (or every third) night, which was the custom in those days.

This hospital offered a "rotating" internship, which required me to spend various amounts of time on all the medical and surgical specialties. It was entirely inpatient. I traded most of my surgical months for medical ones but was still required to spend one month on general surgery. I recall hesitantly doing my first appendectomy. "Be bold, Goldstein, be bold!" urged the resident as I was barely nicking the skin with my scalpel. Because my ineptness and disinterest in surgery was by then almost legendary, the surgery department took a picture of me holding up the extirpated appendix in a hemostat as if I had just caught a large fish.

For the rest of the year I did medicine and psychiatry. After a month or two of becoming acclimated to ward and intensive care medicine, I began to become bored with it. Most disorders seemed fairly straightforward in their diagnosis and treatment, so I began to learn eponyms. Eponyms are diseases and disorders that are known by the name or names of the person who first described them. They have been largely expunged from contemporary terminology in favor of more descriptive terms, e.g., hereditary hemorrhagic telangiectasia for Osler-Weber-Rendu disease. A few, such as Parkinson's and Alzheimer's diseases, linger on.

Thus, on rounds, I could ask the teaching physicians whether they had considered Grawitz tumor, Hallervorden-Spatz disease, the otolithic crisis of Tumarken, and hundreds of other colorful diagnoses. Because my patients usually did well, this eccentricity was tolerated. On the other hand, when I had my hair permed into an Afro and wore wire-rimmed glasses, bell-bottoms, and psychedelic shirts and ties, older members of the staff would cross to the other side of the hall when they saw me coming.

This hospital had no psychiatric service, although obviously, many of the patients had psychiatric problems. One psychiatrist came in to do consultations, but the house staff didn't like him. I soon found myself the recipient of almost every psychiatric consultation, an unusual position for an intern, but a great opportunity for on-the-job training.

Until then, I had learned very little about psychotropic medication. There was an obvious void in such expertise at my medical school, and psychiatric journals of the era primarily discussed psychoanalytic theory. Because the patients were usually in the hospital for a fairly short time, psychotherapy was out of the question, and so I became a de facto psychopharmacologist. I did hundreds of psychiatric consultations and treated many of these patients fairly successfully, primarily with tricyclic antidepressants. I often used behavior therapy as well, and even found the time to teach half of a graduate course in behavior therapy at a local university (as I said, this was an easy internship).

I could fill up the rest of this book with experiences in San Francisco, but I want to go on to the next year of training, my first as a psychiatric resident. I applied for psychiatry residencies in my senior year of medical school and wanted to go to Massachusetts General Hospital, which was beginning to investigate what would later be known as biological psychiatry.

If acquisition of the corpus of knowledge were any criterion for being accepted, I should have been notified on the spot, which, indeed, I was. "We're looking forward to seeing you in 1969," I was told by the director of residency training, and I received a confirmatory letter soon after. I can only assume that he encountered some of my medical school professors at a meeting, because two months later I received a strange letter from him informing me that I had been accepted in error. They had twelve residency positions, and I was the thirteenth accepted. I hastened to apply to Stanford and Langley Porter, but was rejected there also. I ended up at Los Angeles County-USC Medical Center, the largest hospital in the country for more (as it turned out) on-the-job training.

Ludicrous as it sounds today, schizophrenics were still being treated psychoanalytically in 1969. The fact, again, that this therapy had absolutely no benefit and often made patients worse was not even considered. I rapidly started inventing new psychotherapies. One of these, altering a patient's delusional system by entering it and using cognitive dissonance therapy, I discussed in my previous book, *Betrayal by the Brain*. For using this treatment I was put on probation for an indefinite period. Prior to that point I had a standing offer to remove any schizophrenic delusion in twenty-four hours or less (I had gotten fairly good at it).

Several schizophrenics were admitted every few months for bizarre behavior and were resistant to the standard neuroleptics of the day. I asked that they all be assigned to me, which was fine with the other residents. When one of these patients was admitted, I would typically walk up to him or her and introduce myself in a scenario that went something like this: "Hello, I'm your new psychiatrist, Dr. Goldstein. I see that this is your fifth admission here this year. As you know, this is a public, tax-supported institution, and it is expensive to keep you here. We have lots of visitors, many of whom have never seen a crazy person before. (This was before ill-advised humanitarian zeal forced closure of many state mental hospitals.) Since you are obviously one of the craziest people in Los Angeles, I'd like you to be the Ward Crazy Person. To fill this position, all you have to do is act just as you are now. Talk so no one understands you, gesture strangely with your hands and face, and act inappropriately. You may have five minutes each day to talk to me and act normally, so that you can make requests for various things like different food or calling your brother, but all the rest of the time you must behave as the Ward Crazy Person. As long as you do, you may stay here as long as you like. If you decide you don't want to be the Ward Crazy Person any more, you can talk to me about it and we'll see about your being discharged."

The ward staff was instructed to positively reinforce "crazy" behavior and negatively reinforce "normal" behavior, a direct application of Skinnerian operant conditioning which was much easier to provide than the "token economy" that had just begun at Patton State Hospital, where patients were given various colors of poker chips (I think) for "emitting" appropriate responses, in the jargon of the day.

The course of every schizophrenic patient treated in this way was the same (it made manic patients worse, a disaster in this era before lithium [1970] and subsequent mood stabilizers). Day #1—patient acted crazier. Day #2—more or less returned to baseline. Day #3—had to be prodded by the staff to act crazy. Day #4 or #5—patient behaved much more appropriately, asked to be discharged, was observed for several hours, and left the hospital. Although none returned while I was still a resident, many of them did not know enough about appropriate social behavior. I next planned to do what is now called "social skills training" on these people, but instead, I was inducted into the Navy at the beginning of my second year of residency.

Although I was designated a general medical officer (GP), there was more of a need for psychiatrists, so I practiced military psychiatry for two years. I tried to keep as low a profile as possible, which was not difficult, since my commanding officers had no idea what psychiatrists did and were satisfied if we processed the patients and paperwork correctly. Doctors who did not "get along" were often shipped to Vietnam, a much worse fate than being on probation in a psychiatry residency.

The military psychiatrists with whom I worked confirmed my suspicions that my completing any psychiatry residency would be a waste of time. Their consensus was that I knew as much psychiatry as anyone else. I tested myself on a practice version of the psychiatry board exams and scored in the top 1 percent. Thinking I should specialize in a type of medicine which was so broad I could never learn it all, I chose family practice, which had just begun to offer residency training. Prior to that time, family physicians went into practice right out of internship. To this day, most people don't realize that there is a difference between a family physician and a general practitioner.

I prepared for my residency by working for several months in an emergency hospital in the Compton area of Los Angeles, in a workers' compensation clinic in downtown Los Angeles, and in a family practice clinic in the San Fernando Valley. After these experiences I was aware of what lacunae in my database of medical knowledge needed to be filled, since I felt uncomfortable when I could not provide the best possible service to each patient.

The director of the family practice residency at Harbor-UCLA Medical Center was quite accommodating. Accustomed to selecting residents just out of medical school, he told me that I could essentially stay there as long as I wanted (at least a year) and choose whatever specialty rotations I desired, since I had a good deal of prior training. This opportunity was exactly what I wanted, and I took advantage of it for eighteen months, leaving with no gaping holes in my medical database.

At that time (1975) there was no physician surplus, and physicians could still start a practice where they wanted to live. I wanted to live in Los Angeles for the excitement and cultural opportunities, and in Laguna Beach because it was beautiful, laid back, and, most important, had a basketball court right on the beach next to the ocean. Choosing to teeter on the brink of chronic bankruptcy, I lived in both places and practiced in between, in a new planned community called Anaheim Hills, in Orange County, where I was the first family doctor.

Practicing there afforded me the opportunity of meeting for the first time, on a sustained basis, the type of people I had hitherto encountered only on the pages of Sinclair Lewis novels. Individuals with such prosaic occupations as fireman, middle-management, and engineer were almost legends to me. In a year or two I got to know thousands of people in the area who came to me as patients. My fantasy as a family doctor was to walk down the street and be hailed, "Hi, Doc!" (which actually happened quite frequently) and to reply "Hi, Clem—heard the mare foaled last night!" (this particular encounter never happened, though).

As a result of my family practice residency, I figured out what I didn't know, and I spent the next five years assiduously teaching it to myself. In 1977, I began to teach medical students and residents in family practice programs, starting at the University of California at Irvine. I made inpatient rounds one morning a week and taught in the clinic one afternoon a week. The best way to learn a subject is to teach it, so this experience was helpful for my patient care. I also hoped to help the young physicians I was teaching to be better doctors.

Figuring they could always look up facts in a book, I tried to teach them how to think about a patient the way I did: (1) What is the normal physiology? (2) How is the normal physiology deranged by the illness? (3) How does treatment correct the derangement and restore normal physiology? To my surprise, this approach was not what most residents wanted (although they would save up their most difficult cases to present to me).

Two residents were so incompetent and seemingly of such very limited intelligence that I recommended that they at least repeat a year, if not be dropped from the program entirely. This suggestion was almost unprecedented, although I did not know so at the time. I had the (apparently erroneous) belief that practicing medicine had such a potential for help or harm that physicians should be well qualified to render care.

I think the coup de grâce came when I was making rounds with the residents in the coronary care unit (CCU). A teenage girl with obvious, yet undiagnosed, viral myocarditis was presented to me. She was hospitalized with an irregular heartbeat (cardiac arrhythmia) for which she was being given digitalis gradually ("digitalized"). This treatment would have been appropriate if she did not have myocarditis, but her arrhythmias were becoming more potentially lethal every day. She was the patient of a prominent cardiologist, who did not seem to recognize what was happening. I told the resident to stop the digitalis immediately and explained to everyone why it was dangerous to give digitalis to a patient with myocarditis. I'm sure this occasion was not one of those when I echoed "This patient needs a doctor!" Nevertheless, two weeks later I received a letter from the chairman of the department that my clinical faculty appointment was terminated. He said that the level at which I taught was more appropriate for graduate medical education. This scenario was repeated almost identically at UCLA and at a private teaching hospital.

After being dismissed from the faculties of three family practice residencies, I thought I would try my hand at teaching psychopharmacology at UC Irvine. By 1979 I had taught myself quite a bit about it and was beginning to understand it on a molecular basis. Most psychiatry departments were still analytically oriented. I gave a lecture covering the field (not too hard to do in one hour in those days). Only one professor stood up to ask a question: "Why do we have to know about this stuff anyway?" I do not recall my reply.

Fortunately, about two years later, a real psychopharmacologist came in to head the department after losing a turf war at the National Institute of Mental Health. He brought several of his minions with him, highly regarded in their own right. We began to have scientific lecture series. I can't say that I learned many facts, since I already kept up with the literature, but I did learn more about how researchers in biological psychiatry *thought,* which was helpful to me. In addition to teaching normal psychological development and introduction to psychopathology to medical students, I cochaired a psychopharmacology problem-case conference and taught an elective in my office on molecular neurobiology. There were no textbooks on this topic at the time, so I had to make up the course as I went along. I also gave lectures from time to time on matters of general interest and frequently participated in a journal club, in which we would choose journal articles to discuss with one another. I was put up for clinical professorships twice but was rejected by the clinical faculty appointment committee both times. Nevertheless, I continued to teach for ten years, using the same principles as I had in teaching family medicine (i.e., what is the normal physiology, how is it deranged to produce the pathophysiology, and how does treatment attempt to restore pathophysiology to normal). The function of the brain is very complicated, and as I learned more and more about it, the answers to these questions became more complicated also. Eventually, I was told in 1989 by several faculty members that no one (including them) could understand what I was talking about.

As it happened, by 1989 I did not have the time to go to the university to teach any longer. I had married the love of my life, Gail, in 1979. By the early 1980s I had the largest family practice in my area of Orange County and was on the staff of six hospitals. It was not unusual on an average day for me to see 20 to 25 patients in the office and make rounds on all those in the hospital, as well as assist in surgeries. I also had a considerable practice in biological psychiatry and was developing one in what I called "treatment-resistant patients," people who did not know what was wrong with them and/or how their illnesses should be treated. By 1981 I thought that my self-education in medicine was complete. This evaluation was validated when I scored in the top 0.1 percent in that year's family practice boards. Thus, I began developing new treatments by using existing medications for new purposes. One of the first was giving H_2-receptor antagonists (such as Tagamet—see *Betrayal by the Brain*) for mononucleosis, which resolved all symptoms in one or two days in about 90 percent of the patients. Since 1997,

H_2-receptor antagonists have also been found to be N-methyl-D-aspartate (NMDA)-receptor antagonists, an increasingly common mode of action for many agents that are effective in neurosomatic disorders. The H_2 receptor modulates NMDA-receptor function in the neostriatum through a H_2-receptor-mediated regulation of potassium channels (Colwell CS, Levine MS, 1997). About 90 percent of patients I treated with acute infectious mononucleosis responded rapidly, and eventually those from elsewhere who had not been treated, but had not recovered, began to seek me out.

Chapter 2

The Office Practice
of Neurosomatic Medicine

BANKRUPTCY DESPITE
A THREE-MONTH WAITING LIST

"Tut, tut, child," said the Duchess. "Everything's got a moral if only you can find it."

Lewis Carroll (1865)
Alice's Adventures in Wonderland

I began seeing CFS patients when I thought they had chronic mononucleosis, a rather uncommon disorder. They had negative Monospot tests, however. I began to treat them with H_2-receptor antagonists, as I had previously done in those with acute infectious mononucleosis, a treatment still not part of mainstream medical care, although I have published its pharmacology in numerous journals and books. This discovery has lain fallow for so many years (since 1980) that I am even tired of complaining about it. H_2-receptor antagonists can even treat pseudoseizures, a common neurosomatic problem (Sanne P et al., 1997).

By 1985 I was deluged with CFS patients, and even more so after 1986 when I published that some of them, as well, responded to H_2-receptor antagonists. I still tried to schedule them as I would family practice patients, but I was running further and further behind in my schedule.

I started to bring in ancillary personnel and by 1987 had to move to larger quarters. Unfortunately, for me and my patients, the late 1980s marked the end of the "Golden Age of Medicine," when insurance companies paid without question for everything a physician billed. I was still operating under this assumption when I tripled my office space, bought a $250,000 BEAM (brain electrical activity mapping) scanner to objectively measure cerebral dysfunction, and added every conceivable health care professional and piece of equipment that I thought might benefit my patients. We were doing ambulatory polysomnography, computerized neurobiofeedback, cog-

23

nitive-behavioral therapy with two psychologists, chiropractic, massage, acupressure, herbal medicine, nutritional counseling, and pain management. I had discovered few effective pharmacologic treatments at that time, but two of them were intravenous (IV) ascorbate (vitamin C) and intravenous gamma globulin (IVIG), which worked better than intramuscular gamma globulin. In what now seems like the blink of an eye, I had 25 people working in my office. We had also switched to the fairly new technique of computerized billing and added a computer-billing specialist to the now bloated payroll.

The result was chaos. I was still scheduling CFS patients for the same 15- to 20-minute office visits as I had family practice and biological psychiatry patients, but found that I was always two or three hours behind and had to run from room to room. Desperate patients would lie slumped in the hallway outside the office door hoping for a cancellation. Competent office staff was impossible to obtain. Most high school graduates trained as medical assistants whom we interviewed were nearly illiterate. Those whom we did hire made so many errors that I became inured to inefficiency and would confess to numerous irate or puzzled patients that my efforts to correct the situation could only be partially successful because of the inferior quality of the clay I was trying to mold. Some patients who had experience in medical administration offered to work gratis for me, but the code of medical ethics forbids having any business or social relationship with a patient. Physical contact beyond a handshake is discouraged ("Hug a patient, call a lawyer"). When grateful women patients would be terribly offended if I refused their embrace, I had to make sure that witnesses were present. In extreme situations, I allow a patient to hug me but keep my arms noticeably outstretched.

Sometimes I told patients, usually complaining about what seemed to be incredibly stupid errors of omission or commission, that my office was a sheltered workshop for developmentally disabled medical assistants. Such efforts at drollery sometimes helped to defuse a potentially unpleasant situation. We hired three office managers, but libel laws prohibit me from discussing their often quite strange individual foibles. My current staff of several years is quite competent.

My wife Gail attempted to oversee the management of the office, but found this task so demanding that she at first had to stop seeing new patients, and then had to gradually terminate those who remained. This course of action was presciently well timed, however, because as I discovered new rapidly acting treatments at an accelerating rate, the need for psychotherapy diminished. Both Gail and her colleague practiced cognitive-behavioral therapy, which was quite inferior in its results to the treatment options I was evolving for CFS.

Eventually it became apparent to me that I could not serve two masters. My long-time patients could be cared for in fairly well-delimited segments of time, while CFS patients required open-ended appointments to discuss their numerous problems. Managed health care was attempting to make large incursions in dictating how I must treat my patients and demanding mountains of documentation on everyone I saw. This trend was antithetical to why I was practicing medicine and totally discouraged any innovative thought. Finally, I had to withdraw from all managed health care participation. This decision resulted regretfully in the loss of most of my family practice patients, many of whom were becoming frustrated anyway with waiting two hours to see me and weeks to get a nonemergency appointment. I also restructured my practice so that each patient could consult with me for practically as long as was necessary. This type of scheduling worked well except with the occasional patient with severe borderline personality disorder who seemed to have a complex life crisis on a daily basis. Some would even saturate my voice mail with 20- to 35-minute messages in a day so that no one else could get through.

The primary problem in the office was insurance billing. During the rapid change from indemnity insurance (seeing any physician the patient wants for anything that he or she needs) to managed health care, the payment criteria of the indemnity insurers changed so unpredictably that I felt like Alice in Wonderland. There seemed to be no fixed rules. We hired billing consultants by the score who proclaimed that we were doing everything properly, but in a practice that treated 20 to 25 patients a day, we were receiving two or three checks per diem.

From what I had heard from other physicians during the "Golden Age," insurance companies paid according to billing codes, or numbers used to describe the length of any office visit or any procedures performed. The most financially successful of these physicians apparently manipulated the billing codes so that they would receive the most money for whatever was done. For example, a common problem was an ingrown great toenail. The standard treatment at the time for this diagnosis was a "quadrant resection," a very brief procedure that involved doing nerve blocks on the great toe and then removing vertically the one-quarter of the nail that was growing into the skin next to it with a scissors and a hemostat (a type of locking tweezers). I charged $50 to $75 for a quadrant resection. Some physicians and podiatrists would divide this procedure into five or ten separate miniprocedures and bill for each one, so that they could charge $500 to $1,000 for the same thing. This practice is known by the quaint term "unbundling" and is illegal. Office managers who were experienced at manipulating billing codes were a highly prized commodity, and some of them were the aforementioned consultants to my practice. One of them I dubbed "Queen of the

Codes" and even made up a song about her to the tune of "Queen of the Hop," to Gail's obvious irritation. During the Golden Age we refused to engage in such practices because we thought they were fraudulent, unethical, and disgusting. Despite all our efforts, we were still hemorrhaging money that we did not have.

Our accountants were singularly unhelpful. Eventually we discovered one of the problems. The computer biller we hired was doing almost no billing even though she always said she was completely up to date. Bills from a year or two ago had not been submitted and were too old by then to be paid. Gail and I were not computer literate and were naive enough to believe the so-called billing "experts."

An even greater problem was intravenous gamma globulin. This treatment seemed quite effective in the early days when my pharmacologic treatment options were limited. Despite conflicting studies in the medical literature on the use of IVIG in CFS, in fairly low doses it often worked when nothing else did. On some occasions, patients became hypomanic after receiving IVIG, an indication that it had a potential mood-altering effect and that it affected brain chemistry. I have discussed this phenomenon in earlier works. This result still has not been reported in the literature. The patients could not have become hypomanic by fulfilling my nonverbally communicated expectations ("demand characteristics," as they were termed in the 1960s by Martin Orne), because I was totally surprised when this change occurred. Nonpsychiatrists who use IVIG might be unaware of this mood alteration, and psychiatrists never use IVIG (although they should). Neurologists sometimes administer it for intractable epilepsy of childhood or neuroimmune disorders, although they do not understand the mechanism of action, still viewing it in immunologic terms. When successful, IVIG increases norepinephrine (and probably dopamine) levels, along with their longer-acting cotransmitters, just like every other effective treatment. It may have antiepileptic activity by blocking a glutamate receptor, perhaps even that for NMDA.

IVIG is very expensive. A physician may attempt to document the need for IVIG by doing lab tests such as IgG subclasses or checking immune response to certain vaccines. I did these tests at first but found their results had no relation to therapeutic response, which, despite the validity of the science of psychoneuroimmunoendocrinology, was to be expected. IVIG can act as a neuropsychopharmacologic agent. I decided that it was fraudulent to treat patients according to the results of these tests, and I stopped doing them.

Whether the patients had positive tests or not, or whether they had a good response to IVIG or not, most insurance companies soon put all my claims under medical review and stopped paying for them. Some companies, such as Blue Cross, stopped paying all my claims entirely. In a miraculous gesture of honesty, a physician who had read my first book and was a senior vice president of Blue Cross called me up and confessed that his company would go bankrupt if they paid all CFS claims. I had been red flagged by the insurance companies, a kiss of death.

I was faced with an insoluble crisis. I had never stopped a treatment that was helping someone, particularly if there were no alternatives available. Every patient who received IVIG had failed on numerous other treatment trials, including all of the psychopharmacologic agents and combinations that were available at the time, as well as many nutritional supplements, which I tried extensively in the 1980s before abandoning them for relative lack of efficacy. Medical review usually took two to three weeks. Months were going by with no answer. I had about 30 patients a week receiving IVIG and others receiving IV vitamin C. Some got both. The pharmacology of IV vitamin C, or IV ascorbate, is discussed in *Betrayal by the Brain* and later in this book. I was losing $30,000 to $40,000 a month. I agonized over what to do, but after we refinanced our house and there was no end in sight to this catch-22, I decided that I had to stop giving IVIG unless patients could pay for it at the time of service, which almost none could. I discussed this problem with other physicians, one of whom suggested that I should call my malpractice insurer before I took such an unprecedented (for that era) step.

The claims representative I spoke to said she had never heard of such a dilemma and that she would consult legal counsel (we were all blissfully ignorant of future managed care practices). She called back two days later to inform me that discontinuing an effective treatment while reimbursement was not denied but was still being reviewed would constitute *patient abandonment,* and that each and every patient who stopped IVIG therapy could sue me.

If I knew then what I know now about medicolegal affairs I would have sought a second opinion, but I naively took the company's word as law. We had to ask the patients to try to pay some of their bills, since almost all of the medical reviews, which lasted up to a year, decided against reimbursement. Two patients became so irate that they reported me to the California Medical Board in 1989, the interminable saga which is discussed in a subsequent chapter. (See Mene, Mene, Tekel, Upharsin, in Chapter 3.) All the others left the practice. Only one paid anything, and she sends me $75 per month to this day.

I lost several hundred thousand dollars in one year, much more than my net worth. We took out all the loans that we could, and when we could get no more, obtained about 50 credit cards and maxed them out. We let almost all our employees go, which really was okay from my standpoint since I had become so adept in treating CFS pharmacologically that I did not need them anymore, and moved to a much smaller office. Gail was borrowing from Peter to pay Paul, and usually our bills for rent, supplies, telephone, accounting, taxes, etc., were much in arrears. We could not afford medical or dental insurance for our employees or ourselves. Sometimes employee paychecks bounced, which is the next-to-last thing that should ever happen in any business. Several of my friends advised me to declare bankruptcy, but this idea was anachronistically abhorrent to me. Fourteen years later, we have just recovered from this disaster. For many years, most of my income went to pay interest charges, which at least was a good tax write-off until the government disallowed credit card interest deductions. During several years, although working six days a week, ten to twelve hours a day, my net income was negative. Gail still refers to my CFS practice as my "expensive hobby" or, more recently, as a "folly." The twenty-fifth anniversary of my last vacation was in 1999. Gail forsook psychology and obtained a BS in nursing, after which she became probably the most qualified school nurse in the world, being credentialed as a teacher, educational administrator, educational psychologist (in which she has a doctorate), and marriage, family, and child counselor. She had a steady income and excellent health benefits. Her income kept us afloat while my practice tanked.

SOLVING THE PROBLEMS AND AVOIDING THE PITFALLS

Don't nobody here know how to play this game?

Casey Stengel (1962)
Manager of the expansion team,
cellar-dwelling, New York Mets

As I write this book, the office runs about as smoothly as it can with what I can afford to pay the employees. They are earnest and hard working, dealing with often desperate patients to whom they must explain the nature of my medical practice. A well-organized Web site to which patients are referred helps this process considerably.

Patients are told they should be prepared to stay in the office for at least four hours per visit, unless they are feeling completely normal (my endpoint), in which case I see them once or twice a year. Because I receive referrals from all over the world, telephone consultations or faxing may substitute for face-to-face encounters in selected individuals. New patients are advised to come in as frequently as possible for sequential medication trials until the right pharmacologic buttons are pushed and they feel perfect or as nearly perfect as they would like. About one-fourth of the patients approach this endpoint after the first visit. Three office visits is the average time to achieve this result. It requires about ten office visits to administer all treatments that have an immediate effect. By this time, perhaps 75 percent of the patients have achieved the desired result. The remaining 25 percent must then try medications that have a longer onset of action. It takes about four years presently to try every available option. There are still about 2 to 3 percent of patients I have not been able to help as much as they and I would like, but few have exhausted the therapeutic choices yet. Several patients have tried up to 100 treatments with little benefit and have suddenly reached the endpoint with treatment 101. Many, of course, become discouraged with the process. Some new patients now feel frustrated if they are not better after the second day, since they see so many others having seemingly miraculous remissions. Sometimes, when I'm on a roll and have made five new patients better the first day, I try pushing on the foreheads of relative nonresponders to cast out demons, but I am about zero for thirty with this approach.

I know that there are many other methods of practicing neurosomatic medicine, and I know what almost all of them are. I have tried many other techniques to help patients besides those I use now. After practicing this specialty for 15 years, I genuinely believe that not only is my way the best way, but also that it is the only way that makes sense. Physicians can do quite well by just cookbooking the treatment protocol, but of course better results can be obtained by understanding why the patients are sick and how the treatments make them better.

To my dismay, no one I have ever met in the entire world (and I have spent many years looking) has the requisite background in family practice, biological psychiatry, cognitive neuroscience, sleep disorders, pain management, and psychoneuroimmunology to have an in-depth understanding of neurosomatic medicine. This vain search has made my work a very lonely endeavor. My friends in academia tell me that I can't guest lecture at their various departments anymore, because the last time I was there, no one understood what I was talking about. I try to keep my lectures as simple as possible. Several years ago, a well-published professor at a leading medical school went to a talk that I gave to physicians and one that I gave to patients. He advised that I abandon the presentation I gave to physicians and use the one I did for patients for the physicians as well. I followed his advice at a continuing medical education seminar in the South about four years ago. I was invited to talk about CFS. The evaluation forms indicated that only 16 percent of the physicians in the audience understood the lecture. Those who understood it rated it as excellent. I rarely show my slides anymore. I just talk to audiences of patients for two or three hours (with intermissions) and then answer questions. I have given up lecturing to physicians. If they are really interested, they can read my books and then come to the office for a few days to get hands-on experience. About 20 have done so, and I have about an equal number of physicians as patients, so they can learn neuro-somatic medicine on the receiving end as well. These physicians know the most and make the best neurosomaticists.

I have made numerous mistakes in my transition from a family practitio-ner-psychopharmacologist to a practitioner of neurosomatic medicine. Some of them have almost destroyed my marriage and family as well as my career. These errors were a result of

1. my not understanding the medicolegal-financial system well enough;
2. an extremely rapid and unpredictable change in the health care deliv-ery and reimbursement process;
3. not having a sufficient understanding of the different needs of a neurosomatic patient versus those of a general medical or psychiatric patient;
4. my being oblivious to the real dangers of exploring the terra incognita of neurosomatic medicine, i.e., "boldly going where no man has ever gone before"; and
5. the process of readjusting my priorities in
    a. meeting the needs of neurosomatic patients (which can sometimes be virtually infinite) by rendering the best care possible,
    b. educating myself by reading books and journals (forget CFS con-ferences),
    c. teaching (almost a nonissue currently),
    d. doing complex targeted research with intelligent, compatible asso-ciates and no money, and
    e. having a loving, sharing, caring relationship with my wife and son as well as
    f. maintaining doctor-patient relationships where it often seems that *I am the only physician in the world* who can help some individuals.

Perhaps one more medication trial at 7:30 p.m. might improve their lives forever, since they are returning to Kokomo or Walla Walla the next morn-ing, and they can't afford plane fare to return any time soon, or ever, and I am reluctant or unable to prescribe this medication over the phone or by fax. Let's look at these issues one by one.

Goldstein in Wonderland: Standard of Care, Regulatory Agencies, and Malpractice Claims Made

"I don't think they play at all fairly," Alice began, in a rather complain-ing tone, "and they all quarrel so dreadfully one can't hear oneself speak—and they don't seem to have any rules in particular; at least, if there are, no one attends to them."

Lewis Carroll (1865)
Alice's Adventures in Wonderland

The basic standard of care for most neurosomatic illnesses is to do nothing, prescribe an antidepressant, refer the patient to multiple other specialists (if the patient has indemnity insurance), see him or her for a few minutes every few months for reassurance, refer him or her to a mental health practitioner, or discharge him or her from the practice. I do not see how most neurosomatic disorders can be diagnosed and treated in a managed-care environment, especially by physicians who are not employing the proper paradigm to understand what they are diagnosing or trying (sometimes) to treat. The situation can become somewhat dicey for the physician if the patient's chart is being reviewed by a third party for possible improprieties. These potential improprieties may include insurance billing, the patient seeing another physician, the insurance company decides that the physician is using medications improperly, disability claims, maloccurrences (as opposed to malpractice), real or imagined post-traumatic disorders (especially motor vehicle accidents, slips and falls, or possible toxic exposures), or if a patient doesn't understand the neurosomatic diagnostic and treatment process and files a complaint instead of asking me to explain it again. Also, someone or something may have made a patient angry about which the physician is completely unaware, a situation unfortunately too common in a patient population with an overrepresentation of those with borderline personality disorder. On the other hand, very few (maybe one out of a thousand) patients that I see are sociopaths, less than in the general population. These patients may either try to set the physician up for a malpractice suit and, on occasion, extortion. They may also attempt to get controlled drugs and then abuse them or sell them, bringing unwelcome attention from the Drug Enforcement Agency (DEA). Many are extremely creative in their attempts to cadge controlled substances from doctors. Some bipolar patients may have sociopathic relatives who may threaten the physician in various ways, particularly if the patient is wealthy. Doctors should particularly beware of the patient who is not very intelligent or well educated but thinks he or she knows more than the physician does. If the doctor does not exactly comply with his or her wishes (e.g., "I want you to treat my systemic candida—it's acting up") and he or she doesn't understand why the doctor won't, despite his or her best efforts at dispensing verbal and written information, it is prudent to terminate the relationship with such a patient at the first visit before attempting treatment. Such a course of action has been difficult for me to take in the past because these patients usually feel very sick, and I have known that I could help them as easily as everyone else. One such patient was an attorney who came to the office with her boyfriend to be treated for "my candida." After taking Nimotop she was able to run around the block and said that she felt virtually normal. I never saw or heard from her again. She reported me to the California Medical Board, which, in due course, reflexively accused me of negligence and gross incompetence in treating chronic fatigue syndrome.

Chronic noncancer pain, fatigue, disorders of excessive sleepiness, and cognitive dysfunction are major symptoms a neurosomaticist must treat. Most neurosomatic patients do not respond well to opioids or stimulants, but some of them (maybe 30 percent) do. After I have tried 50 or so other medications without much success, I will administer opioids and/or stimulants. After I have tried 70 or 80, I may use delta-9-tetrahydrocannabinol (THC), or Marinol, one of the ingredients of marijuana. I discuss updates on the pharmacology of these controlled substances in the treatment section of the book, but often one of these drugs is far and away the most effective treatment. Any medication, whether dependence on it may develop or not, is worth giving to a severely afflicted neurosomatic patient whose precarious condition seems to me and the patient like "living death."

When they are effective (they make many patients more fatigued), stimulants improve energy and alertness to varying degrees but rarely decrease pain. Opioids and Marinol improve all symptoms in many patients. It is well known (or it should be) that opioids can have a stimulatory effect. Methadone is far and away the best opioid because it also blocks the serotonin transporter (like Prozac) and the NMDA receptor (like ketamine). Remember that methadone has a very long half-life and can cause respiratory depression if you do not start low and go slow. Some patients, of course, will prefer other opioids, but not very many do. A physician cannot be prosecuted in California for prescribing opioids for chronic pain if the indication for them is well documented. Because every patient's chart is a "legal document," I must unfortunately transcribe almost every word a patient says and do not look at him or her nearly as much as I would like. Like Nixon, I have thought of recording and transcribing every word spoken in the office so that I could have a normal face-to-face conversation and not get blisters on my fingers when I grasp my pen, but the costs would be prohibitive. Sometimes I wonder whether patients mind seeing the top of my head so much.

I have had no adverse contact with the Food and Drug Administration (FDA) either. Although almost all the medications I prescribe are legally sold in the United States, they are mostly for "off-label" indications. Forty percent of all medications are prescribed this way. Patients may have a problem because their insurance company may say that any off-label use is experimental, so they don't have to pay for such drugs. Such a policy keeps health care costs down, particularly when some pills cost $20 each. A physician is allowed to prescribe medications available in other countries (as I understand it) as long as he or she does so rarely and does not sell them. Theoretically, a physician can prescribe anything he or she deems to be in the patient's best interest unless it is expressly forbidden (such as heroin or, until recently, thalidomide) by the FDA. In actuality, it appears to be dangerous for doctors to design their own drugs (and I have never done so), not just from the standpoint of safety and efficacy, but also because if the FDA perceives that a doctor has violated a statute their agents may enter his or her office with drawn guns without warning. I try to be as careful as I can not to pull on any tigers' tails. Unfortunately, physicians are not taught the do's and don'ts of the various regulatory agencies in their training, and may sometimes violate rules of which they are completely unaware. It is sometimes difficult, or even impossible, to find rules and regulations governing physician behavior in any publication. Even I, who had been actively involved in medical education at various levels for many years, exclaimed on several occasions while storm tossed on the sea of troubles "How was I supposed to know that? Where is this rule written? I want to abide by the rules, but where and what are they?" The American Medical Association (AMA) has recently published a monograph about medical ethics, but most of the material, although useful to know, does not help me much with how to practice neurosomatic medicine. Is it possible that no one knows?

For a claims adjuster or physician reviewer for a particular malpractice insurance company, not only do I appear to continuously violate the "standard of care" in the most flagrant manner, but also my "practice profile" attracts the most litigious patients imaginable. In 30 years as a physician I have never lost or settled a malpractice suit. Only one has gone to arbitration and trial, a case in which a patient alleged posttraumatic constipation after developing a bleeding ulcer when taking a drug similar to Motrin. He stated that he was so afraid that blood would be in the toilet bowl after having a bowel movement that he was afraid to defecate and that this problem (several years after the acute incident, which I diagnosed and treated promptly) rendered him unemployable.

I have about one malpractice claim filed every three or four years. As the attorneys involved learn more about their clients and review the patient charts, the claims are always dropped, except for the one in the previous paragraph. Usually the litigious patients do not understand what I am doing, despite the torrent of information they receive. One or two patients seem to have sued every physician they have ever seen. Sometimes a local doctor tells a patient from another state that I am a quack, that I am crazy, or that I am a danger to the public, and the patient wonders why I am prescribing these unusual medications. Borderline personality disorder patients may occasionally demonize me. One of them filed a claim because I refused to have an affair with her, although she complained about some other apparent misdeed. Despite this virtual minefield, my malpractice premiums were lowered four years ago because my rate of claims made and settled (zero) was lower than the average physician.

About a year before I wrote this page, a patient for whom I bent over backward filed a claim. I gave him greatly reduced fees, prescriptions after telephone consultations, long office visits to discuss his problems, samples of medications that completely relieved his symptoms which he could not afford and/or obtain in his state, and generally tried to help him in any way I could. One day he called with some very unusual symptoms that could not have been related to the medications he was taking. Because I knew he was unemployed and indigent, I prescribed a medication over the phone and told him to call back in an hour. Otherwise, he would have gone to the emergency department, where he went anyway without filling the prescription. After being hospitalized for several days, I received a call from his new doctor who spoke to me as if I were from another planet for prescribing the medications the patient was taking. He had been feeling fairly well prior to this incident. I never heard from this patient again except through his attorney who filed a claim. The suit was withdrawn after discovery (analysis of medical records).

As I had always done in the past, I reported these events to my malpractice carrier, who, as per usual, requested a copy of the records. This time, however, they actually had someone read them (a pharmacist and a family doctor), both of whom predictably "freaked." I received an urgent call from the claims adjuster almost ordering me to settle the case since I had not followed the standard of care. I actually had to tell him to shut up or I would hang up the phone. When he did, I informed him that I had not committed malpractice, and whatever problems the patient had were not of my doing. I saw an attorney selected by the company who agreed with me. As usual, the case was dropped. What was unusual, however, was that my malpractice insurance was terminated. I have never heard of termination when the physician had no malpractice judgments against him, had only one suit in his life that wasn't dropped, and had just had his premiums *reduced*. My appeal, with mounds of supporting data, was summarily rejected. I easily got malpractice insurance with another company. Be advised, though, that most physicians view a neurosomatic patient as a malpractice suit waiting to happen, especially if they diagnose a serious comorbid personality disorder.

TAKING CARE OF BUSINESS

Physicians who do not pay their office overhead each month will not be able to stay in business. Most physicians must also make a profit to some degree. A neurosomatic practice presents several problems in practice management that are unique.

I see an average of eight patients per day, most of whom I am treating simultaneously with a new medication every 30 to 45 minutes until they feel normal. Reviewing records, taking a history, and doing receptor profiling on a new patient takes 90 to 120 minutes. Seeing more than eight patients per day, unless some are receiving IV infusions, means making highly complex decisions too rapidly, particularly when dealing with patients who recognize that time is limited but nevertheless wish to monopolize it.

As I have alluded to before, the better a physician is, the less money he or she may make. Also, an ethical physician will usually almost go bankrupt. When I first began to practice neurosomatic medicine, I did not understand the illnesses very well and had few treatment options. I therefore ordered many tests, most of which were expensive, and gave intravenous infusions fairly frequently. I had many therapeutic modalities to offer my patients. If insurance reimbursements hadn't changed, I would have become fairly wealthy while practicing what I considered to be good, ethical medicine.

Now, all non-Medicare patients must pay cash for what they receive, since insurance reimbursement is poor to nonexistent. I rarely do any tests—none are usually necessary because patients bring records from previous physicians. I knew many physicians who charged each new patient several thousand dollars for in-house testing. As I developed more treatments, it became less necessary to treat people with intravenous infusions, which I now do infrequently. I devised numerous therapeutic eyedrops, nasal sprays, and transdermal gels, but medical insurance would not reimburse my office for dispensing them. They would pay for medicines, even those compounded, only if they came from a pharmacy.

I use few nutritional supplements, finding pharmacologic agents far superior in most circumstances. Many physicians, particularly holistic ones, insist that their patients buy hundreds of dollars of supplements from their office only. Many patients like the idea of "natural" remedies anyway.

A few physicians have a wealthy clientele and charge accordingly. A very few are extremely well known. Patients make appointments with them because they don't know any alternative, even if the cost is $8,000, or over $25,000 if surgery is involved.

I could do many unnecessary tests, procedures, and treatments that would quintuple my income at least. However, I cannot view practicing medicine as a business, and this proclivity has contributed to my downfall.

The patient would never know. I could make at least 70 percent of my patients feel much better with intravenous therapy. Should I treat all of them this way when pills would work just as well?

Should I insist that patients buy compounded products from my office, for which their insurance would not pay anything? Should I have a functional brain imaging machine that would take pretty pictures to impress the patients but have a dubious effect on my treatment decisions? Should I sell nutritional supplements in the office when I know most of them don't work very well compared to what I do now?

Can my patient population afford to pay more than $800 for an initial office visit and $225 to $300 for a revisit, when the average office stay is six hours? Will the insurance companies understand the charges? They rarely pay me anything as it is. Should I stop seeing Medicare patients? I can't just keep the ones I have and not allow new ones. Either the doctor participates or not. Medicare pays about 30 percent of what I charge. I lose money, more or less, on each one. I have heard a physician can "opt out" of Medicare. I am investigating this option, because I believe my services are worth more than what Medicare will pay.

The bulk of my practice is from out of town. I allot four days to treat a new patient, although only about 75 percent will feel normal by the end of the fourth day. I follow them by telephone with sample medications. Few can afford to stay into the next week. An occasional patient demands (about once a year) a refund if he or she is not well or does not remain well. I can scarcely refuse, because reporting me to the medical board will always be worse than giving a refund.

It has become more than an occasional occurrence that a new patient feels normal after one and a half days. I am glad for the patient, but I lose $600 to $900 as a result of this happy occurrence (I couldn't think of an antonym for malpractice). As I write this section, it is late Wednesday afternoon. Everyone in the office felt entirely normal before 2:00 p.m. (an admittedly unusual outcome). I am a victim of my own success.

At present, I must make $2,500 per day to break even and pay my personal bills. I almost never make that much. I find it impossible to renege on my fiduciary responsibility to my patients and overcharge them. I really need to be subsidized, but no latter-day Lorenzo de Medici has come forth to do so. Solving this problem will be up to each neurosomatic physician in his or her own practice. Right now, I owe the pharmacy that supplies me with compounded medicines I use for receptor profiling, the IRS, payroll taxes, malpractice insurance, and pharmaceutical suppliers. We are continually behind on telephone bills, but fortunately rarely bounce payroll checks. I deeply appreciate my staff for their patience and forbearance.

This miasma is my situation. I hope yours will be different.

Chapter 3

Lawyers and Litigation

"Beware the Jabberwock, my son! The jaws that bite, the claws that catch!"

Lewis Carroll (1872)
Jabberwocky, from *Through the Looking-Glass*

When I began to practice neurosomatic medicine, I knew more about wielding a vorpal blade to slay a manxome foe in the tulgey wood than about using it to fence with lawyers in the medicolegal arena. I personally know attorneys who are honest, good, kind, and intelligent and who are well prepared when they depose a witness or try a case in court. Unfortunately, encounters with such individuals professionally in the context of neurosomatic medicine are exceptions. The lawyers with whom I am friendly do not usually specialize in personal injury or disability litigation. Posttraumatic fibromyalgia and denial of disability payments for neurosomatic illnesses are the two main issues that bring me into contact with the legal profession, putting aside for the moment spurious allegations of my own negligence or (gross) incompetence in the case of my patients.

I have been called as an expert witness on numerous occasions, a task that is unappealing to me. I restrict testimony to my own patients and refuse to be a "hired gun" who renders opinions at the behest of attorneys who pay for the proper analysis on any case. I have even been retained as the same expert witness by attorneys for the opposing sides, each of whom tried to put just the right spin on what I was saying. In this particular case, in cross-examination reminiscent of medieval scholastic arguments about how many angels could dance on the head of a pin, my deposition was scheduled for two hours. By hour number eight, I cracked. "If you guys ask me one more question I'm going to immolate myself," I exclaimed after having the issue restated in a slightly different way for the eighteenth time. They then had mercy on me, or I would be a "crispy critter" now after spontaneous combustion.

The facts of the cases are fairly typical.

1. Ms. Jones was in a minor motor vehicle accident with mild damage to her car and subsequently developed fibromyalgia syndrome. How could such minor trauma cause such a disabling set of symptoms? or
2. Mr. Smith develops CFS. He asks his private disability insurer to compensate him because he is unable to work. The insurance company, which does not want to pay claims, argues that (a) Mr. Smith is malingering, (b) there are no objective data to use in rating his degree of disability, or (c) CFS is depression or another sort of psychiatric illness and is either not covered by the policy or the policy covers psychiatric disability for only 24 months. Meanwhile, Mr. Smith is living in a cardboard box under a bridge.

The following is a suggested pathophysiology for posttraumatic fibromyalgia and can be adapted to fit the circumstances of an individual patient. Opinions are best supported by objective data, such as neuropsychological testing looking for encoding (making new memories) problems, a functional capacity evaluation as described by Diane Barrows (Barrows D, 1995) and single-trial auditory evoked-response testing coupled to functional magnetic resonance imaging (MRI) with special attention to the N-100 wave. Performing an encoding task with helpful cues during the latter procedure should further highlight the nature and extent of the deficit.

SAMPLE PATHOPHYSIOLOGY
OF POSTTRAUMATIC FIBROMYALGIA

This patient was predisposed to develop this disorder, i.e., posttraumatic fibromyalgia. She had a history of other disorders that are caused by inappropriate handling of sensory and cognitive information by the brain, i.e., premenstrual syndrome (PMS), irritable bowel syndrome (IBS), and migraine headaches. The accident she suffered could have induced posttraumatic fibromyalgia by several mechanisms.

1. The patient may have had minimal traumatic brain injury. Such an injury disturbs the microvasculature of the cerebral cortex and alters brain function in a way that would not be apparent on a macroscopic magnetic resonance scan.
2. The patient may have congenital cervical spinal stenosis. This possibility can be assessed by doing a cervical MRI scan that measures the diameter of the cervical spinal canal and determines whether there is

any compression of the spinal cord. This finding would be relevant because

 a. The cell bodies of the neurons of the spinothalamic tract, which conducts pain, originate in the upper cervical spinal cord, and if there were little room for the spinal cord to move after impact, these could have been traumatized.

 b. The upper cervical nerve roots form about half of the volume of the mesencephalic tract of the trigeminal nerve, one of the main integrators of sensory input in the brainstem. If the nerve roots or the cell bodies of the nerves were damaged by the impact, this trauma could lead to altered function of the mesencephalic tract.

3. This patient has a developmental and perhaps a genetic reason to misinterpret sensory and cognitive information. The mere fact that she had an accident in her car could have caused a degree of stress sufficient to reconfigure her neural networks so that sensory information, particularly pain, would be misinterpreted, i.e., normal sensory input would be interpreted as being painful. Her history after the accident is quite typical of a patient who develops posttraumatic fibromyalgia involving what is called widening of receptive fields. The patient typically develops a localized or regional pain which is termed a regional myofascial pain syndrome, but the representation of this pain in the corticostriatal-thalamocortical network, which also includes the cingulate gyrus, hippocampus, and the amygdala, is expanded, somewhat analogous to a person hitting his or her thumb with a hammer. The thumb is painful for a period of time, perhaps a week or two, and during this time the brain remodels itself so that the representation of the sensory neurons from the thumb becomes larger. In the due course of events, in a person who is nonpredisposed to develop fibromyalgia, this neural representation returns to normal, although the brain retains a memory of the pain, which can often be evoked by electrode stimulation in the appropriate region of the brain many years later. Women have felt pains of childbirth 20 years later while having electrode stimulation of a region of the posterior thalamus during brain surgery.

In fibromyalgia patients, the neural representation of the pain does not slightly grow but keeps expanding to encompass the entire body. This phenomenon is another way to understand how a local injury can produce a diffuse pain syndrome by widening of receptive fields. Areas of the brain that are receptive to noxious stimulation reinterpret normal sensory input as being painful and recruit neurons called "wide-dynamic range (WDR) neurons" that are more likely to code for pain messages. Also, it appears that the thalamus, the main switchboard for sensory input in the brain, is dysregulated by other regions of the corticostriatal-thalamocortical (CSTC) network, particularly the anterior cingulate gyrus, the posterior caudate nucleus, and the dorsolateral prefrontal cortex. Appropriate functional brain imaging in this individual would probably reveal hypoperfusion in these regions, since we and others have seen these defects in hundreds of such patients previously. However, these tests are too expensive to perform on many individuals.

Patients with fibromyalgia always have cognitive impairment, even if they are not aware of it. This disorder mainly presents with problems with short-term memory or encoding, the making of new memories. Encoding data is very fragile in neurosomatic disorders and is extremely easily disrupted by additional cues, even those that would be helpful to a normal person. Too much information may enter the processing network because it is inappropriately gated, harkening back to the abused child's need to be aware of every stimulus in his or her environment. Genetic predisposition, which can be strong, weak, or anywhere in between, also contributes. If the genetic predisposition is strong, the patient will develop such disorders as fibromyalgia, irritable bowel syndrome, migraine headaches, and premenstrual syndrome, as well as a host of other related disorders, no matter what happens. If the genetic predisposition is less than robust, then environmental influences pre- and postnatally determine the susceptibility to develop such illnesses. Although the patient may have had illnesses related to fibromyalgia prior to her motor vehicle accident, they did not seem to be disabling because she was successfully employed. Diffuse pain was usually not one of her primary complaints. Thus, the motor vehicle accident for a summation of reasons can be held responsible for triggering an apparently new illness, i.e., fibromyalgia syndrome, which did not exist prior to the accident unless there were medical records suggesting its existence, of which I am unaware.

Disability issues in CFS have been well covered in a recent monograph by Klimas and Patarca-Montero and will not be further discussed here (Make B, Jones JM, 1998).

I have written this section to give pointers to the novice or unwary neurosomatic physician. Although it pains me to advise this attitude, because it does not reflect the way I would like the world to be, *don't trust a lawyer.* Demand that depositions or testimony be paid for at least two weeks in advance with a half-day minimum plus travel time. Doctors should arrange that the lawyers come to their office, not the doctor to the lawyer's office. If the time of the deposition exceeds that which has been agreed upon, stop testifying until the lawyer issues another check. No lawyer has ever sent me additional payment for time exceeding that which was agreed upon. Several lawyers have taken my testimony and then stiffed me. Some lawyer's checks have bounced. If not paid by two weeks prior to testimony but you wish the deposition to proceed anyway, demand that the attorney bring a cashier's check for the agreed amount. Lawyers will often cancel a deposition or a trial at the last minute, leaving the doctor with most of a working day open.

Do not be intimidated or obfuscated by a lawyer or a paralegal lackey. Lawyers have subpoena power—they can compel people to appear in court or to give a deposition. Anyone who does so unwillingly should firmly establish that he or she will be a *percipient,* as opposed to *expert,* witness. A percipient witness need only read what is written in the chart and is not required to offer opinions, factual knowledge, or logical reasoning. Attorneys will try to delay establishing the terms of one's testimony, will haggle with experts about the price, and will threaten with contempt of court if they do not give expert testimony when not being paid to do so. Doctors should stick to their guns and tell the lawyer to "shove it" if arrangements are not being made the way that is expected. Be courteous but firm. Nice guys (like me) are exploited.

I have always been a witness for my patients. To the extent possible, I try to protect them from the possible incompetence of their attorneys. It is essential that the attorney have the physician's curriculum vitae and be able to present relevant sections to the judge or arbitrator. There are very few experts in neurosomatic disorders, but if the judge does not know that the doctor is one, he is apt to regard any testimony as less credible than the local internist. He might be completely ignorant of disorders such as CFS and have an a priori attitude that they are bogus, and that the doctor is, too.

The attorneys for both sides will usually know little about neurosomatic disorders, unless they have done their homework, which is not the common practice in my experience. The patient's attorney should always interview the doctor before testimony so that he or she is well prepared and knows about what the doctor knows. He or she should submit into evidence relevant articles or books the physician has written, and he or she should have tried to read them. In the past year I saw a slam dunk disability case go down in flames because the lawyer was totally unprepared and seemed to have walked into court like a person off the street. I felt sorry for my patient.

CFS cases are not usually personal injury (PI) matters. Premorbid function, which is rarely objectively quantified anyway, is not at issue. Causation, a critical element in FMS PI, is not particularly relevant. CFS litigation is almost entirely devoted to whether the patient should receive disability compensation for his or her illness. How disabled is the patient? How should functional capacity be measured? Is the patient malingering? Has the patient conveniently become disabled just prior to a layoff or just after a business reversal? Is CFS depression? Is it a real illness? Is it a physical disease or a "nervous and mental disorder"?

As a physician, I do not take a history to determine whether my patient is malingering, but rather to establish the diagnoses with a reasonable certainty. Most CFS patients will have had some milder intermittent symptoms of one or more neurosomatic disorders for many years prior to the severe disabling onset of CFS, and many of them have a premorbid psychiatric history that can blur considerations of causality in PI cases. Such conundrums may be difficult for a judge and/or jury to resolve. Some judges appear to be far from impartial and show bias I would like to attribute only to intellectual rigidity. It is, in any event, a lengthy, expensive, and difficult task for a single patient to sue an insurance company. Sometimes it seems to me that more funds are allocated to legal fees than would have been awarded to the patient if no action had been brought.

MENE, MENE, TEKEL, UPHARSIN

MENE; God hath numbered thy kingdom, and finished it.
TEKEL; Thou art weighed in the balances, and art found wanting . . .

Daniel 5:25-28

"Someone must have traduced Joseph K., for without having done anything wrong, he was arrested one fine morning."

Franz Kafka (1883-1924)
The Trial

My pain management techniques in 1989 were quite primitive compared to today. I had learned how to do acupuncture and trigger-point injections in the 1970s, when the practice was quite uncommon. I recall seeing patients with fibromyalgia in those days, although I didn't understand what was wrong with them. Sometimes I would give these individuals 40 to 80 trigger-point injections in a session. They usually did not work very well or last very long. By 1989 I had learned what fibromyalgia was and hired a chiropractor and an acupressurist to treat patients with this disorder, in conjunction with other available therapeutic modalities. Intravenous vitamin C and IVIG were effective treatments for some patients. For a short period of time I treated supposed late Lyme disease with intravenous antibiotics. Until 1987 I treated some patients with intravenous acyclovir for putative Epstein-Barr virus infection. In 1989 I had only one patient receiving this treatment. She was quite unaffected by other measures and stated that IV acyclovir relieved her symptoms considerably. To administer these intravenous treatments I had to hire nurses, at first one, then more. "Every time I turn around you've hired a new nurse!" Gail exclaimed in frustration and bewilderment.

We received hundreds of telephone calls every day, many from current or prospective patients, but also from persons seeking a regional clearinghouse for information about CFS. There was also a blizzard of paperwork, including medical reports and requests for copies of patients' charts. I had become a consultant-specialist, and these requirements were several orders of magnitude greater than being a family doctor. Handling this volume of information required much more office personnel to answer phones, file charts, put information in charts, fill prescriptions, order supplies, do computerized and manual billing, pay bills, write down messages for me, and write down patients' presenting complaints: allergies, medications, and vital signs (height, weight, temperature, blood pressure, respiration) on every visit. It was necessary to hire an office manager to supervise and coordinate these operations.

All these changes occurred in an era of severe patient desperation. Patients with neurosomatic illnesses were told nothing was wrong with them and/or that their problems were psychiatric. Because most people still had insurance that paid for them to see the physician of their choice, I had a three-month waiting list for new patients.

I was totally overwhelmed by all this. Working 16-hour days was not unusual. I could not find a physician to join me unless I were to pay him $100,000 a year to start, quite a bit more than I had made at any time in my career. Hiring a nurse practitioner was a less expensive option, but everyone we interviewed rejected the position, stating that the job was too demanding and stressful, or that I didn't give them enough leeway in examining the patient or prescribing.

When I could, I recruited academic colleagues to help me figure things out. We began collaborating on research in about 1987 and continue to do so until this day. I started to write a column for a newsletter from Charlotte, North Carolina, called *The CFIDS Chronicle*. The newsletter initially consisted of several loose-leaf pages stapled together, but there was nothing else like it at the time. As miserable as things were, these were also exciting times, rather like the 1960s redux, but with the medical community as the establishment to protest against. I spoke at conferences, began work on my first book, and was organizing the first of several international meetings to bring together researchers in chronic fatigue syndrome, fibromyalgia, and other neurosomatic disorders with those doing relevant basic science. The best of times . . . the worst of times.

Into this ferment of patient care, intellectual exploration, research, literary efforts, and chaotic near-bankruptcy in the office was added, late in

1989, a request for copies of charts of two patients from the Medical Board of the State of California. Horror and stupefication were two emotions that I recall experiencing at that time.

Gail and I, already reeling from the pressures of the practice, consulted one attorney who, seeing that I looked shell-shocked, empathetically told me that I would probably get a TRO (temporary restraining order) forbidding me to practice medicine. He said that things looked bad, indeed, and that he needed a $25,000 retainer to go any further. He commented that once the medical board targets a doctor, they never let go. The next attorney we saw, Robert Gans, was also a physician and had worked for the medical board before going into private practice. He appeared to know the territory.

What we learned was that the board was under great political pressure to discipline incompetent physicians, and that by merely requesting my records they had already decided to prosecute me. As he reviewed the records of these two patients, the main deficiency he noted was that I didn't use the SOAP notation system: S = subjective, O = objective, A = assessment, P = plan. The physician should write down what the patient's complaints were, what the physical findings were, what his or her diagnosis was, and what the next steps were to be. I had known about SOAP notes for many years, but since they hadn't been invented yet when I was a medical student, I became comfortable writing chart notes in a different format. I mistakenly thought that the chart notes were primarily for my benefit in caring for a patient and that SOAP notes were an optional alternative, not the standard of practice. If I had known that there were rules about how to practice my specialty, I would have followed them, a refrain I was to echo several times over the next nine years. Although I intellectually knew that lack of knowledge of a law is no defense, somehow these various edicts had escaped my notice in the 20 years since receiving my license to practice medicine in the state of California. During this time I had been enrolled in two residency programs and had educated medical students, residents, and practicing physicians. If a medical Justinian code had been promulgated in the state or country, I should have known about it.

I was also using nonstandard diagnostic and treatment approaches. If the standard ones would have worked, I would have used them. Before rushing pell-mell into innovative medicine, I asked a good friend of mine, who was also a consultant to the medical board, about what criteria the board used to judge whatever innovative techniques were appropriate. "If there is a scientific rationale for what you are doing, then it's okay," she advised me. I used this maxim, as well as a risk to benefit assessment ratio, in developing new approaches. At that time, about 1979, cost to benefit ratios were scarcely heard of, because it was, or at least I thought it was, the standard of care to help every patient as much as possible. Outcome measures at that time were almost unheard of. I know, because I researched an article about them in the early 1980s for a newspaper column I wrote to convey my disgust with the shoddy way medicine was practiced by many physicians. Although treatment algorithms are all the rage to judge the standard of care today, few existed for any disorder in 1989, much less neurosomatic ones.

One of the problems was that by 1989 I had become quite accustomed to seeing patients with neurosomatic disorders, and I could diagnose them in a minute or two. A ten-year history of fatigue, malaise, diffuse pain, cognitive dysfunction, exertional relapse, and 30 other symptoms starting "October 27 in 1982 when I got the worst flu of my life which never went away" is not very likely to be anything else, particularly after the patient had seen 20 other physicians and had been to the Mayo Clinic and/or Scripps. I have reviewed records of other physicians who somewhat specialize in CFS, but because one only prescribes doxepin (and that's all), and others treat with similar fairly innocuous substances, they have not been haled before the bar of justice. Their records consist of a few scrawled lines on one page of progress notes. Patients inform me that such consultations take about five minutes, which is all the time that is really necessary if the doctor places a premium on efficiency in diagnosis, has little intellectual curiosity, has no knowledge of neuroscience, and has almost no treatment to offer. It would appear that this method fits within the standard of care of American medicine.

Dr. Gans advised me to not speak to anyone from the medical board unless he was present. He said they already had their minds made up, and anything I said at this point, without a judge being present, would only be used to ensnare me in a web of duplicity and nonstandard responses that would put one more nail into my coffin.

In reviewing the charts myself with a hypercritical eye, aside from not having SOAP notes, I could find no major error. The SOAP information was in the progress notes but not in SOAP format. I would always think, "well this could have been a little better, I could have said more here," but remember that I was dealing with a population whose diagnoses were unequivocal to me, if not to their previous physicians. I had spent many years ordering extensive, esoteric immunological lab tests that may have had minor glitches one could associate with neurosomatic disorders, but they never helped me with treatment decisions. I stopped doing them in early 1989. I was in a state of cognitive dissonance because I believed my standards were the correct standards, and to judge me by the standards of mediocrity and bean counting was a gross miscarriage of justice. Both patients who filed complaints had significant improvement while under my care. At least that's what the progress notes said.

The medical board sent copies of the charts to two physician reviewers at university medical schools. These two evaluators were incompetent to evaluate a CFS case, which is *really different* from Ms. Jones coming in with a cold. One should have recused himself, as he was a resident while I was teaching in his program, and the other should have been charged with gross negligence based on her review of my chart, but medical board physicians are held harmless from any litigation that should ensue from their evaluation. I think that no physician involved with the case from day one to day 2,000-something had any expertise whatever in chronic fatigue syndrome or neurosomatic disorders, and this ignorance caused the nine-year travesty that almost ruined my life and marriage. But once the wheels started grinding it was very hard to get them to stop.

If I had been wealthy, my options would have been different.

1. Should I say to hell with it and just retire and read and write and spend time with my family?
2. Should I take a six-month suspension, paying overhead along the way?
3. Should I be on probation, with some equally uneducated physician looking over my shoulder and telling me what I was doing right or wrong?
4. Should I hire Dr. Gans as my consligliere, or in-house counsel, as Robert Duvall was for the Godfather, since it seemed that every single move I made had a legal ramification?
5. Should I have a trial (which was almost a done deal) at a cost of about $100,000, money that I didn't have and couldn't borrow?

Besides which, I was asked to pay for all the costs incurred by the medical board in investigating me, $20,000 or so.

I lined up my witnesses for this hearing. They were all tenured professors or distinguished professors of medicine. My patients who were testifying had all achieved complete remission and were attorneys and physicians. Who did the medical board have? Some resident who went to a few lectures on CFS/FMS? It was the Scopes trial redux. During this entire nine years, no one from the board had (as far as I know) looked at my curriculum vitae, read any of my articles or books, or spoke with anyone in the CFS/FMS community.

Nevertheless, they proceeded with unswerving rectitude until the time for the trial date neared. Then we began to have settlement conferences at the state courthouse in Los Angeles. I believed that any settlement would have been an admission of guilt and that I was innocent. If I wasn't competent to diagnose and treat CFS, who was? Behind the scenes, Dr. Gans, who knew everyone, had been negotiating. He finally got an offer from the board that if I could pass an oral competency examination on CFS given by three experts, then all charges would be dismissed. "Who could they possibly get to examine you?" asked several of my colleagues. "I don't know," I said. Every expert knew me, and although they might not like me, they would have had to recuse themselves. I thought for a while that the oral competency exam would never take place.

Then I received the location of a doctor's office in West Los Angeles where I was supposed to meet the leader of the group and two other physicians. I had just spoken with two doctors who had experienced oral competency exams and said they were very low key and collegial, sort of a pro forma way for the board to exit a situation it no longer wanted to pursue.

Some of the questions I answered incorrectly. The questions were supposed to be restricted to CFS only, but instead they dealt with matters that I hadn't even thought about in 15 years. I did not enter the room in a cognitive mode to retrieve information from long ago, although once upon a time I had the answers to all these questions right in my working memory. When I left I felt paradoxically exhilarated—it was the first time since 1975 that anyone had questioned my knowledge of any subject in medicine.

Passing score was a 70, and I was sure I had done that well. I received the failing grade of 69.5—no rounding off. I was found guilty of incompetence and gross negligence in the management of chronic fatigue syndrome.

. . . who shall judge the judges?

Samuel Johnson (1747)

The Plan of an English Dictionary

We had the competency exam rescored, erasures and all, by two independent eminent authorities. Both of them gave me a score of 85 percent. We sent the tape and the rescoring to the judge in charge of this case, and shortly thereafter, we were back in his court. He was displeased. He invalidated the examination and ordered a new one, specifying that the questions be restricted to CFS and that the examiners be experts in CFS. The deputy attorney general prosecuting me stipulated that I abide by the results of this new exam no matter what, but the objection that this precondition was arbitrary and unconstitutional was upheld. The position of the board was that I must be examined with a nationally recognized testing procedure that would establish that I was competent to practice medicine and manage CFS.

They suggested the ECFMG, a computerized test given to graduates of foreign medical schools. We responded that I had just again been recertified as a diplomate of the American Board of Family Practice by taking an all-day examination. I scored in the upper 20 percent, despite fading knowledge about obstetrics and newborn care. Scores on such examinations have been demonstrated to directly relate to competence and quality of primary care. "Serious and widespread quality problems exist throughout American medicine" (Chasin MR, Galvin RW, 1998), but apparently not in my practice if, indeed, "[t]he quality of health care can be precisely defined and measured with a degree of scientific accuracy comparable to that of most measures used in clinical medicine" (Chasin MR, Galvin RW, 1998). Thus I was well qualified to practice primary care, which I was not doing. Despite vigorous efforts by the judiciary, instruments to measure my competence in neurosomatic medicine have not been devised as yet.

The position of the medical board was that the family practice board exam was not nationally recognized. We elected to take our chances on a second oral competency exam, partly because I naively believed that the judge's orders would be obeyed and that no CFS expert could be found whom I did not know personally or who would think that such an examination of me was ludicrous.

An important fact that took a while to sink in was that the medical board was an extralegal entity. No extrinsic laws regulated its behavior; in other words, it could make up its own rules as it went along. Judicial orders were advisory only and could not compel the board to do anything. My professional career was in the hands of omnipotent functionaries who did not necessarily have any expertise in regulating how the wheels were grinding me. I began to suspect that no one involved in my case at the administrative level even knew what CFS was. I was a square peg being jammed into a round hole, which they weren't about to reconfigure just for me.

It was still mildly surprising to me that three experts had been found in CFS to administer the second oral competency exam. I knew they could not be experts, but I did not think a court order could be ignored by them with such blithe impunity. At 7:00 a.m. one morning I walked into a nearby hospital and met three family physicians I did not know, or even know of. We sat down at a table, and I informed them that very specific orders had been issued that all questions be about CFS. "No one told us that," replied the titular head of the triumvirate. I was offered the opportunity to refuse to take the exam, but nine years of living under a sword of Damocles was too much. I agreed to take the exam, reasoning that if they tried to screw me again, then the test could always be invalidated with another court hearing.

For this occasion, however, I had taken the precaution of leafing through *Harrison's Textbook of Internal Medicine* for two days, dredging up old memories. Even if they had been trying to fail me on purpose, which these doctors weren't, it would have been hard to do so. I believe I answered every question correctly except for describing the contents of the anterior, middle, and posterior mediastinum, areas of the middle chest, the anatomy of which I had neglected to rememorize. Shortly thereafter I was informed that I had passed the examination and that all charges were dismissed, although there was a postscript to the effect of "we'll be watching you." Nine years of agony that threatened to destroy my marriage, family, and career were erased— or were they?

Several months later I was testifying as an expert witness in a disability case. The head attorney for the insurance company, who looked like a combination of Demi Moore and Ally McBeal, casually asked, "You were found to be incompetent to treat chronic fatigue syndrome by the medical board, weren't you?" I realized that the goblins will always be lying in wait to grab me. This information will apparently be available to anyone who inquires for the rest of my life, although the fact that the accusation against me was dismissed accompanies the reply.

In retrospect, I really don't see how my problems with the medical board could have been avoided, and I expect I shall have more in the future. A host of physicians believe that deviation from textbook medicine is completely inappropriate in a nonresearch setting. Those who were employed to evaluate me did not understand, or made no attempt to understand, my mode of practice. The lack of knowledge about pharmacology among many physicians could encourage them to regard my methods as "dangerous." Anyone who attempts to treat the most difficult cases ("patients from hell") who have been dumped by tertiary-care medical centers will of necessity be using "nonstandard" treatment. As I found to my chagrin, the fact that the treatments have a sound scientific rationale does not offer protection if a doctor's practice is being evaluated by a physician who does not possess the database to understand the reasoning behind the treatment decisions.

A practice that attracts desperate people will inevitably include some who will dislike the physician or think he or she is a charlatan, no matter how caring and pleasant the physician is, no matter how much time is spent with them, and no matter how much information is supplied about what the physician is doing and why. The number and types of informed consent forms they sign prior to seeing them will not prevent their initiating a lawsuit or reporting the physician to a regulatory agency.

One cannot make a good living in neurosomatic medicine unless he or she has a wealthy clientele who can afford to pay fees commensurate with the time devoted to them or engages in what I consider to be dubious practices. Most medical insurance today is managed health care in which cost control is the primary motive, and even traditional medical insurance does not provide for caring for one's patients in the office for six to eight hours a day. There is no reimbursement for telephone consultations, which are essential in a practice that attracts patients from all over the world.

There are many more critical situations in neurosomatic medicine than any other type of office-based practice and no guidelines about how to deal with them, as there are, for example, in emergency medicine. If I am putting my career on the line with every patient encounter as it is, I am placing it in dire jeopardy when I attempt to deal with a crisis, which often occurs with a patient from 2,000 miles away whose family, friends, and physicians (if he or she has any) think that I am a loose cannon at best.

Why, then, would I, or anyone else, practice neurosomatic medicine? I can restate only three reasons, which thus far have countervailed (at times only barely) over all of the negative ones.

1. There is a tremendous ability to (often very rapidly) alleviate human suffering and help people to lead normal lives.
2. This realm is largely unexplored and offers a wonderful outlet for intellectual creativity, problem solving, and integrative thinking.
3. Because it is virtually impossible to practice my brand of neurosomatic medicine in the context of the presently constructed managed health care system, I operate outside this system. Thus, I can treat patients the way I have always preferred, knowing them intimately, not stinting on options, and relating to them as complete individuals, not as defective organ systems to be processed along a conveyor belt as rapidly as possible. I am familiar with the arguments of managed-care proponents (prudent allocation of resources, outcome-based practice, cost to benefit ratios, yada, yada, yada), but it would kill me if I had to practice that way.

Chapter 4

Treatment Case Examples

INSTANTANEOUS NEURAL NETWORK RECONFIGURATION BY PHARMACOLOGIC MODULATION OF AFFERENT CRANIAL NERVE INPUT

"Oh, no!" as Mr. Bill might say. "Please don't hit me with that gibberish again." Even though for many this title may as well have been written in Sanskrit, I'm going to translate this section's title as simply as I can.

From what I have written in previous chapters, most readers should have an inkling that a medication does not necessarily have to reach the brain itself in order to change the way the brain handles information ("reconfiguring a neural network" or "switching a nerve circuit"). Many, if not most, nerves may be acted upon outside the brain ("peripherally") in order to affect brain ("central") function. The nerve impulses from the peripheral to the central nervous system are termed "afferent," as opposed to "efferent." Efferent, in this context means *from* the brain (and spinal cord, also part of the central nervous system [CNS]) to the peripheral nervous system (PNS).

Well-known examples of this process, although not always understood in this manner by their practitioners, are acupuncture, chiropractic, trigger-point injections, and transcutaneous electrical nerve stimulation (TENS) to treat pain. As far as I can tell, no one (except those physicians who use my treatment protocol), knows how to change the nature of afferent neural transmission pharmacologically.

Most fibers in nerves connecting the CNS and the PNS are afferent, i.e., from the PNS to the CNS. In the vagus nerve, for example, 90 percent of information goes from the viscera and other organs to the CNS. The brain needs to know what is going on so that it can respond appropriately by neural regulation, e.g., using the 10 percent of vagal fibers remaining to travel the CNS to direct the internal organs.

There are twelve cranial nerves (nerves coming out of the head). They are designated by Roman numerals I through XII. Cranial nerve I is nearest to the brain, and cranial nerve XII is furthest or lowest down in the brainstem, just above the top of the spinal cord. For example, the olfactory nerve (smell) is I, the trigeminal nerve is V, and the vagus nerve is X. As the name implies, the trigeminal nerve, which primarily conveys sensation from the face, is divided into three divisions: VI supplying the forehead and the eyes, V2 innervating the nose and upper jaw, and V3 supplying the lower jaw.

As I have explained to some extent in previous articles, these nerves have receptors for neurotransmitters on them. V enters the brainstem and forms tracts, or pathways, that go down the spinal cord and up to the switchboard of the brain, the thalamus, in the trigeminothalamic tract. Such a thick nerve tract contacts many other structures on its way up that are involved in neural regulation and integration of information so that just the most relevant, or "salient," bits of information will be given sufficient weight so that they will pass through neural gates to enter networks and be processed. The gates are synapses, the spaces between which one neuron communicates with another. The weighting of neural input for gating is partly done by *attention,* an extremely important function that does not operate properly in neurosomatic disorders. I shall write about attention and salience in subsequent chapters. The discipline that studies salience and attention, as well as learning and memory, object and face recognition, language and communication, spatial relationships, and thinking and problem solving is *cognitive science.* It is crucial that any neurosomatic researcher or health care provider have a good working knowledge of this subject. In particular, understanding how salience and attention are focused is critical if neurosomatic illnesses are to be properly conceptualized.

Until quite recently, I have not been able to pharmacologically access receptors on the X nerve (the vagus). Its input function can be electrically modulated by implanting a nerve stimulator in the upper chest, which activates vagal input in epileptic patients when they are about to have a seizure, thus preventing its occurrence. The mode of action of the vagal stimulator almost certainly involves *chaos theory,* a fascinating digression I shall not permit myself to make here. The same kind of vagal stimulation also increases memory in normal human subjects.

In reading an article about the sensory transduction mechanisms of taste, I learned that the taste buds are innervated by VII, IX, and X. The neurobiology of taste transduction is complex and mostly irrelevant to this discussion. Taste transduction is performed by the taste bud. Most of the neurotransmitters have not been identified, but the primary transmitter from the tongue to the brain stem is *glutamate,* the major excitatory neurotransmitter. Substance P (SP) and gamma aminobutyric acid (GABA) have also been identified. Perhaps I could access the vagus nerve via the taste buds.

The nerve from the taste bud to the brainstem is called a first-order neuron. It synapses with another neuron called a second-order neuron, analogous to twisting two wires together when making a circuit. All of the many branches of the vagus nerve join in a brainstem nerve bundle called the solitary tract, which has an integrative function like the trigeminothalamic tract. The two tracts join together, along with the upper-cervical (neck) neurons high in the brainstem. Chiropractic cranial manipulation probably modulates the activity of these neurons mechanically in this region. These impulses reach the cerebral cortex via fourth- or fifth-order neurons. The primary transmitter in the solitary tract is also glutamate.

Thus, it would make sense to decrease glutamate neurotransmission in a patient who has a disorder of synaptic gating, those who do poorly in high-stimulus environments, such as malls, and those who are overly sensitive to many sensory inputs as is frequently seen in CFS, FMS, IBS, multiple-chemical sensitivity (MCS), PMS, and too many other "esses" than I care to mention.

Furthermore, a fact that I neglected to mention in previous articles is that when I prescribe very diluted pharmacologic nasal sprays, receptors on cranial nerve I, the olfactory nerve, are affected, as well as those of V2. Again, odorant transduction in the ciliary cells of the lining of the nose is very complicated. The two best-studied transmitter systems from the olfactory bulb to the second-order neuron and thence directly to the pyriform cortex in the limbic system involve the glutamate and dopamine D_2 receptors. NMDA attaches to the NMDA receptor for glutamate (there are several other glutamate receptors) with ten times the affinity of glutamate. Thus, there is a rationale for using NMDA-receptor antagonists (there are no liquid pharmacologic "agonists," or stimulators except glutamate itself), as well as dopamine and dopamine D_2-receptor antagonists, of which haloperidol (Haldol) is a prime example. To complicate matters, humans may (or may not) have a vomeronasal organ (VNO) that senses pheromones (proteins or peptides secreted by animals that have behavioral effects on other members of their species). If we do have a functional VNO, agents that stimulate the production of cyclic adenosine monophosphate (cAMP) could activate it. Lest I confuse the reader, I shall not further discuss the possible neuropharmacology of the cranial nerves in this section.

To test my hypothesis, I applied two drops of very diluted ketamine to the top of a patient's tongue, had him swirl it around in his mouth, and swallow it. When I had done the same thing to myself, I felt no different. In a few seconds, the patient felt much better. He had previously responded to ketamine eyedrops and nasal spray, but he said his response was more robust and somehow qualitatively different. I thought the effect was enhanced because more (and different) nerve fibers were being recruited.

Without packing someone's mouth with gauze and isolating just the tongue, I was unsure whether V2 and V3 were also involved. Before I had a chance to do this experiment, serendipity intervened. A CFS patient told me that her teeth always hurt, especially when she drank cold water. Her dentist ascribed this problem to her enamel being too thin. I had her swirl two drops of a 1:10 ketamine solution, about 0.15 mg, far too little to have a systemic effect by absorption under the tongue or through the lining of the cheek.

She had a biphasic response. She reported that her tooth pain disappeared instantaneously, as I would expect if neural modulation went up to the trigeminal ganglion, where the three divisions branch, a neural nexus that would modulate sensory input a very short distance away from her teeth. Several seconds later she noted that all of her other symptoms had been relieved, to a greater degree than using nasal sprays or eyedrops, which she found inconvenient anyway. I assume this effect occurred via VII, IX, and X. Of course, it may still have primarily involved the trigeminothalamic tract, so I may have to do the packing experiment sometime soon. Preliminary results suggest that only a few patients respond to medication by the taste buds alone. I have them protrude their tongues through a slit in plastic wrap, rather than use packing.

The V_1 nerves on the cornea appear to be the most sensitive but have the least effect in most people (but the most effect in a few), perhaps because other cranial nerves are not involved in the response. I consult a professor of neuroophthalmology when preparing eyedrops because I do not want to damage the eye. He believes in general that almost any parenteral solution can be safely instilled into the lining of the lower eyelid if it is diluted one to ten. I have had no problems following this advice.

Nasal sprays are more effective than eyedrops for most people. Perhaps there is more surface area inside the nose, or, more probably, it is because receptors on the olfactory nerve are involved as well.

In general, the taste bud-oral cavity route is the most effective. The same receptors seem to occur in all three areas. People who are made worse by dopamine are virtually always made better by its D_2-receptor antagonist, haloperidol. Those who are made worse by agents that stimulate cyclic AMP production (e.g., milrinone) are made better by agents that decrease cAMP (e.g., adenosine). The thyrotropin-releasing hormone (TRH) receptor is antagonized by midazolam, a benzodiazepine (BDZ), so these two agents usually have opposite effects, as well.

The medications I currently employ are nafarelin, aminophylline, lorazepam, glutamate, oxytocin, naphazoline, TRH, ketamine, dopamine, haloperidol, adenosine, midazolam, milrinone, and prostaglandin agonists and antagonists, the latter only as eyedrops so far. Sumatriptan (Imitrex) eyedrops work fairly well for headaches, and for some people, to feel better in general, but their duration of action is too short. I have tried every other eyedrop in the *Physician's Desk Reference [PDR]* for Ophthalmology (a separate book), but they don't work much better than naphazoline, an alpha-adrenergic stimulator. I thought that alpha$_2$ agonists (such as clonidine) or cholinergic agonists (such as Mestinon) or antagonists (such as Levsin) might work like their systemic counterparts, but so far they don't. Pilocarpine (a cholinergic agonist) has some effect in a few people. I shall be modifying numerous other parenteral agents for use on the tongue (probably the safest route) in the near future. Because there is considerable variability in patient response, however, it is best to try eyedrops, nasal spray, and two or three drops of a more-concentrated solution to swirl (the medical word for "swish around") in the mouth.

THE PATHOPHYSIOLOGY OF CFS
AND RELATED NEUROSOMATIC DISORDERS

Although I believe that the neurosomatic disorders are caused basically by a misperception of information salience with resultant inappropriate allocation of attentional resources by the brain, the number of pharmacologic agents I need to employ in an attempt to correct this malfunction is currently about 140 and climbing rapidly. When physicians visit my office to experience a hands-on sample of my treatment process, which involves administering medications in rapid succession, they are often bewildered and depart with a feeling of hopelessness, even though they witness one or more miraculous recoveries each day.

After the first treatment to which the patient has a good (or bad) response, subsequent medication selections are based upon the pharmacologic mechanism of the previous response. I have created an algorithm, or a "decision tree" as a rough guide to treating the brain (See Appendix). Each branch has a fairly opposite mode of action. For example, if drug A lessens symptoms, use drug B. If drug A increases symptoms, then use drug C, and so forth, down to drugs X, Y, and Z. Such a reductionistic approach to modulating the function of the most complex object in the known universe (the human brain) is obviously often wrong or unsuccessful. Still, it is a better approach than trying my treatments in numerical order or randomly "spinning the wheel of fortune," as I describe it sometimes to patients.

The ultimate goal increasingly appears to be (for most patients) to reduce the sensitivity of the NMDA receptor, one of the primary receptors for the excitatory amino acid (EAA) neurotransmitter glutamate. Many other receptors are, of course, dysregulated and contribute to misperception of salience, but I am singling out the NMDA receptor as the most important.

Certain patients, usually with a numerically reduced constellation of symptoms, commonly not including diffuse pain, seem to require *activation* of the NMDA receptor instead. Stimulating the NMDA receptor is involved in making new memories while concomitantly determining whether the information received is novel enough to be worth "encoding," or making a new memory out of it. This determination is termed "salience" in cognitive neuroscience and is the Holy Grail of neurosomatic medicine.

One may thus metaphorically view attentional outlay as the volume of wine that is poured from the cup. If this process works properly, specific neural network activity patterns selectively alter input to active synapses. There are corresponding modifications in what is termed "synaptic strength" or how tightly the neural connections have been chemically formed. The degree to which the NMDA receptor is activated determines the expanse of the "receptive field" or the breadth of the interoceptive (inside the body), exteroceptive (outside the body), and cognitive (inside the brain itself) information pool from which to extract a stimulus and compare it to past experience. This process, termed "attention," has been rather simplistically compared to a spotlight.

The attentional beam markedly increases the synaptic weight of a stimulus, enabling it to activate neural networks more readily. If receptive fields are too wide, irrelevant stimuli will be scanned. If the salience selecting system is too sensitive, i.e., if an individual is hypervigilant, too many stimuli will be interpreted as novel and must be further evaluated for possible threat. This phenomenon results in a decreased signal-to-noise ratio (SNR).

Mice bred to have a genetic defect in the structure of the $GABA_A$ receptors have ". . . a bias for interpreting ambiguous scenarios as threatening . . ." (Crestani F et al., 1999). Perhaps some humans have a similar hereditary trait. GABA is the primary inhibitory neurotransmitter that regulates the sensitivity of the NMDA receptor, and it does so in a very complex manner (Crestani F et al., 1999). If an individual is temperamentally, developmentally, and/or environmentally predisposed to interpret too many stimuli as possibly threatening, then attentional resources, which require increased secretion of the neurotransmitters norepinephrine (NE) and dopamine (DA) (among others), will be consumed locally at too rapid a rate, and the brain will develop a deficit in them sooner or later. Then, an overt neurosomatic disorder will occur. This process usually occurs outside of a person's awareness, "implicitly" or "covertly" to use the neuroscientific terms.

The cellular volumes of the locus coeruleus (LC) and the ventral tegmental area (VTA) and associated ventral pallidum (VP), which supplies the mesolimbic and mesocortical tracts may decrease, or more likely, there will be an alteration in how the prefrontal cortex (PFC) regulates its own neurotransmitters. The prefrontal cortex is the only area of the brain able to regulate its input of neurotransmitters depending upon perceived stimulus salience. This function is probably dysregulated in neurosomatic disorders.

The physiology of much covert (automatic) attentional scouting does not necessarily have a locus in the prefrontal cortex. Normal shifts in visual attention, for example, occur in area V1 of the visual cortex, which is regulated by the ventral occipitotemporal cortex, where much of a certain type of visual information may enter other neural networks. Visual information about "what" is being seen traverses the "ventral stream," which ends in this area of the cortex (Brefczynski JA, De Voe EA, 1999). Information about the location of the object, or "where" is transmitted through the "dorsal stream" ending in the parietal cortex.

The interaction of the NMDA receptor with hundreds of other neurotransmitters and thousands of different receptors defies comprehension (Sanes JR, Lichtman JW, 1999). It is quite apparent, however, that there are numerous individual variations in how the NMDA receptor, and all other receptors for that matter, can be regulated. It is extremely common for me to administer the same medication to two or three different patients in the office at the same time and observe a positive, negative, or no response simultaneously. Strains of mice have been bred that are exactly the same except for how they respond to a certain medication, e.g., serotonin-reuptake inhibitors (SRIs) such as Prozac. Interestingly, one of the leading candidates for the mechanism of action of the antidepressants, often prescribed in mainstream medical treatment of neurosomatic disorders, is a reduction in sensitivity of the NMDA receptors.

GABAergic interneurons are almost certainly involved in this process (Paulsen O, Moser EI, 1998). They are widely distributed, modify synaptic weight in a complex manner, and may be those most affected by gabapentin (GBP, Neurontin). The mechanism of action of gabapentin may also involve modulating dopaminergic tone. Cognitive-behavioral therapy (CBT), when it works, probably does so in the same way. Aaron Beck, the progenitor of cognitive therapy, has just published a book about the neuropsychology of CBT with two of his colleagues (Clark DA et al., 1999). Neurotransmitter dysregulation is omitted in this volume, however.

The treatment decision tree is far from infallible. Patients may have adverse reactions to selective administration of two medications that as far as I know are agonists (stimulators) and antagonists (blockers) of the same receptor. This phenomenon can occur because multiple competing systems might regulate the neurotransmitter in question. For example, both glutamate agonists and antagonists can increase dopamine levels in a region of the brain called the striatum, which is involved with motor behavior and motivation. The function of the striatum is impaired in patients with Parkinson's disease.

It is also impossible for me to factor in positive expectancy (the placebo effect, or "my charisma," as I blushingly refer to it), or negative expectancy (a negative placebo, or "nocebo"). These expectancies are regulated by a network that includes the prefrontal cortex, which I consider the "leader of the band," nucleus accumbens (NAc), anterior cingulate cortex (ACC), hippocampus, and "extended amygdala," which includes parts of the thalamus and the basal ganglia. These areas are also affected by NMDA-receptor sensitivity as described previously. I alluded to this process in *Betrayal by the Brain* (p. 92).

I do not intend to glibly dismiss the role of the extended amygdala, or the nucleus accumbens, for that matter, in neurosomatic disorders. This topic has been well reviewed for the reader with some neuroscience background (Heimer L et al., 1997). I shall more fully describe the actual treatment of neurosomatic disorders in my next book, *Brain Static: Case Studies in Neurosomatic Medicine.*

Although many neurosomatic patients have felt unsafe for long periods of time, and some have had one or more extremely traumatic episodes, the amygdala does not appear to be as reactive as in patients with post-traumatic stress disorder (PTSD) (Shin LM et al., 1997). When patients describe their memories to me, there is no change in their symptoms, either at the time or subsequently. Thus, I have not done functional brain imaging while patients generate mental images of such events to investigate whether amygdala activation occurs. They also do not relate intrusive thoughts or recurrent dreams of the event, or other DSM-IV symptoms in the "B" and "C" categories of the diagnostic criteria for PTSD. The function of the amygdala in neurosomatic disorders has been extensively discussed in my previous books, especially in regard to its relationship to the hippocampus. I noted that hippocampal volumes were normal as calculated by MRI in twelve neurosomatic patients who were diagnosed with CFS.

Salience and attention have been investigated in a different context by Mircea Steriade and his colleagues in Quebec at the University of Laval (Steriade M, 1999). Steriade and his research on the electrophysiology of thalamocortical oscillations has influenced my thinking greatly over the last 15 years. The neurophysiology of memory has been discussed from a somewhat different perspective by Chun and Phelps in the September 1999 issue of *Nature Neuroscience* (Chun MM, Phelps EA, 1999). The implication of their work is that conscious memory occurs because the information solely about the experienced event is stored along with other information ("contextually") that enables the associational combination to form a neural network, which makes the conscious remembrance of the experience accessible to an individual's awareness. In this experiment, the process occurred in the hippocampus, but similar events can apparently occur in the anterior cingulate cortex, in thalamocortical loops, or simultaneously in all these areas (and more), thus forming a widely distributed neural network in which various regions are activated instantaneously.

Steriade's work is too complex to summarize here but is characterized by integrative thinking, a rather unusual tendency in the research community. Relevant to this chapter is his recent work on the *augmenting response,* whereby after mild increases in the activity of excitatory neurons (excitatory postsynaptic potentials, or EPSPs), subsequent responses are increased in amplitude.

> Augmenting responses are associated with short-term plasticity processes, that is, persistent and progressive increase in depolarizing synaptic responses and decrease in inhibitory responses. Such changes can lead to self-sustained oscillations, owing to resonant activities in closed loops, as in memory processes. . . . The repeated circulation of impulses in reverberating circuits, especially when considering those corticothalamic and thalamic bursting neurons that are able to discharge rhythmic spike-bursts, could lead to synaptic modifications in target structures, which favor alterations required for memory processes. (Steriade M, 1999)

Such a system deals with information rapidly and appropriately.

However, "augmenting responses are blocked during brain stem reticular stimulation, which stimulates strong behavioral arousal" (Steriade M, 1999). If the activation is too weak, too much behavioral synchronization could arise that would not be constrained by inhibitory processes. Too much synchronization in the brain can cause epileptic seizures, an event that occurs with less-than-average frequency in neurosomatic patients. Almost all who have an alleged history of seizures have pseudoseizures, which are quite different both in pathophysiology and treatment. Pseudoseizures appear superficially to be epileptic seizures, but no EEG abnormalities accompany them. They are currently viewed as dissociative disorders. True seizures and pseudoseizures can manifest in the same patient, making diagnosis problematic. Twenty-four-hour video-EEG monitoring is often used to distinguish the two. Several years ago I surveyed four physicians who specialized in CFS. Only one had a patient with epilepsy in his or her practice.

Thus, if there is overt or covert ("explicit" or "implicit") hypervigilance, the required augmenting responses processing the requisite synchronous oscillations to strengthen synaptic associations, such as those involved in making new memories, are not allowed to occur at their normal rate. A hypervigilant state is the usual disposition of most neurosomatic patients.

The implications of Steriade's work are fairly profound, but space and complexity does not permit further discussion.

It is beginning to appear that using my decision tree ("receptor profiling") works for most, if not all, disorders of how the brain deals with information from pervasive developmental disorder (autism) to allergies. The NMDA receptor is probably involved in all of these illnesses to varying degrees. The decision tree allows me to probe the function of many receptors. If I had more pharmacologic options, e.g., a $GABA_B$-receptor antagonist for people who get much worse after taking baclofen, which is a $GABA_B$ agonist, the efficacy of my therapeutic process would be greatly enhanced. Most of these unavailable agents have been synthesized and are in various stages of clinical or preclinical trials. The most effective medication would act one or two (or many) synapses away from the NMDA receptor and reconfigure the involved neural networks. Otherwise, almost everyone would respond to ketamine, an NMDA- receptor antagonist, and tolerance, or receptor desensitization, would never occur. Ketamine has its most profound effect at the lowest dose in the anterior cingulate cortex. I give ketamine by slow intravenous infusion in normal saline in a dose of 0.5 mg/kg (Schmid RL et al., 1999), transdermally 240 mg/Gm in pluronic lecithin organogel (Crowley KL et al., 1998), and 50 mg/ml diluted 1:10 in eyedrops and nasal sprays. The latter two routes antagonize NMDA receptors on the trigeminal nerve (Goldstein JA, 1999). Ketamine might also be given orally (Fisher K, Hagen NA, 1999). The human anterior cingulate cortex is involved with executive control of cognitive processes, response selection, conflict resolution, internal monitoring, anticipation and preparatory processes, and affective and motivational aspects of behavior. Decisions are computed in the lateral prefrontal areas and then channeled to the anterior cingulate cortex for translation into motor output, during which selection between alternative responses takes place (Turken AU, Swick D, 1998). The functions and malfunctions of neural networks, which include the anterior cingulate cortex, have been extensively explained in my previous books. Higher doses of ketamine have a negative effect in the medial prefrontal and premotor cortex. The medial prefrontal area, along with the amygdala, helps to determine when a stimulus should provoke fear and when this particular fear response is no longer appropriate (extinction). The same receptors are regulated differently in the various parts of the central nervous system, adding another level of complexity to the issue.

An additional approach to dealing with this situation would be discovering the relevant postreceptor events for each individual and modulating these. At present, we have a limited number of postreceptor interventional strategies, such as increasing AMP (directly with papaverine, indirectly with other agents) or injecting heparin, which blocks the inositol triphosphate (IP_3) receptor inside neurons and glial cells. The IP_3 receptor regulates intracellular release of calcium, an extremely important event. Most receptors have had some of their postreceptor mechanisms characterized. Response to various pharmacologic probes may also be interpreted by commonality in postreceptor events, particularly if relationships between receptors on the neuronal membrane do not adequately explain patient response. Future neuropharmacology will increasingly deal with postreceptor mechanisms, right down to altering function of DNA and the expression of gene products. Patients can, therefore, expect to get better and better in the new millennium.

(I apologize if it is necessary to read this section more than once. If I made it any simpler, the process would not be adequately explained. It has taken me twenty years of thinking to succinctly synthesize what is described here, i.e., improper selection of salience produces overuse of the "attentional spotlight," which raises signal-to-noise ratio by overly frequent secretion of dopamine and norepinephrine. At some time during a person's life, a neural network orchestrated by the prefrontal cortex may be unable to induce sufficient production of these transmitter substances. This inability may be sporadic or virtually constant, but the result will be neurosomatic symptoms. Background for this hypothesis will be found in my recent books, published by The Haworth Medical Press, Binghamton, New York. *Chronic Fatigue Syndromes: The Limbic Hypothesis* [1993] and *Betrayal by the Brain* [1996]).

I discuss whiplash injury extending in the diffuse pain of posttraumatic fibromyalgia in a summary I give to every attorney who wishes to depose me (see Chapter 3). Even a minor painful extension-flexion injury of the cervical spinal muscles can augment activation of muscle spindles and nociceptive groups III and IV afferent fibers causing a facilitation of the trigeminal motor nucleus by an activation of the lateral reticular system. The connections of the upper cervical dorsal roots are considered an afferent pathway of the trigemino-trigeminal circuit modulating the exteroceptive (ES2) of the voluntary contracted temporalis muscle. ES2 is much shorter in the whiplash patient than in normals. Thus, the inhibitory temporalis reflex (ITR) is deranged and impairs the descending inhibitory pain-control system. NE and 5-HT (serotonin) projections to the trigeminal motor nucleus are considerably attenuated in this situation. Decreased NE, in particular, can decrease the activation of the inhibitory neurons mediating the ES2 response. A dysfunctional anterior pretectal-periaqueductal gray (PAG)-nucleus raphe magnus (NRM) circuit has been shown to converge on wide-dynamic range neurons in the trigeminal nuclear complex. These WDR neurons are under direct descending control of the PAG and NRM. ES2 shortening of the inhibitory temporalis reflex should provide objective diagnostic evidence of whiplash (posttraumatic fibromyalgia) and might provide insights about remediation directed at restoring normal trigeminal nerve function. The functional neuroanatomy and modulation of the trigeminal nerve is discussed extensively in this book.

THYROID FUNCTION IN NEUROSOMATIC DISORDERS: STIMULATION OF TRIGEMINAL NERVE ACTIVITY WITH THYROTROPIN-RELEASING HORMONE (TRH)

I use thyrotropin-releasing hormone nasal spray to treat people with what I term neurosomatic disorders. These illnesses include FMS, CFS, IBS, PMS, and a host of other disorders in which information is not handled properly by the brain, resulting in inappropriate regulation of the body by the brain. TRH has a number of properties that would make it valuable to treat disorders such as FMS. I have been using it for several years, intravenously injecting 500 mcg with moderate success. At this dose, it primarily affects mood disorders and alertness, but it can affect all symptoms. Some transient signs of arousal of the autonomic nervous system (ANS), which can be produced by TRH, are nausea, change in blood pressure, and an urge to urinate. The effects of intravenous TRH usually last a week or two when the medication is effective.

TRH enhances norepinephrine, dopamine, and serotonin secretion. Norepinephrine is a major brain neurotransmitter that increases signal-to-noise ratio, i.e., the ability to filter out relevant from irrelevant stimuli. Many patients with neurosomatic disorders are highly distractible and function poorly in environments of stimulus overload. Their performance also deteriorates in neuropsychological testing situations when the amount of information presented is increased, even if the information is in the form of helpful cues. Dopamine also increases signal-to-noise ratio even more than norepinephrine and is implicated in anticipation of reward. Dopamine, acting at the level of the nucleus accumbens, a structure near the basal ganglia of the brain, makes people feel considerably better in general and increases their activity and sensations of pleasure and motivation. The interaction of dopamine with other neurotransmitters in the nucleus accumbens is too complex to discuss here. Serotonin, which stabilizes information flow in neural networks in the brain, thus constraining behavioral, affective, and cognitive output, has been found to be decreased in FMS cerebrospinal fluid, as have norepinephrine and dopamine metabolites. TRH has nerve endings on structures in the brainstem called the dorsal raphe nuclei (DRN), which secrete serotonin. TRH is a string of three amino acids. When amino acids are strung together they are called peptides. When peptides act in the nervous system they are called neuropeptides. TRH is a neuropeptide in addition to its role in stimulating the release of thyroid-stimulating hormone (TSH), which I shall discuss shortly.

A physician can buy TRH in 500 microgram (mcg) ampules of 1 ml. Five hundred micrograms is the usual amount that is administered during a TRH stimulation test, which is performed to measure the amount of TSH the pituitary gland will secrete in response to TRH. The neurons that secrete TRH are in the hypothalamus, right above the pituitary gland in the paraventricular nucleus (PVN), which also contains other regulatory peptides such as corticotropin-releasing hormone (CRH) and gonadotropin-releasing hormone (GnRH).

I make a dilution of 500 mcg or 1 ml of TRH in 9 ml of normal saline and put it in a nasal spray bottle. Each spray delivers approximately 3 mcg of TRH, an amount that one would not think would have a physiologic effect if injected intravenously. However, receptors for TRH must be somewhere in the nasopharynx or in adjacent ganglia such as the sphenopalatine ganglion, because patients who respond to one spray of TRH solution in each nostril report that they feel much more alert and much more energized in less than one minute.

I have written extensively about simulating two of the three branches of the trigeminal nerve, which conveys sensory input from the face, with pharmacologic agents. This mode of administration has an effect on brain function because the tract of the trigeminal nerve in the brainstem is an important integrator of sensory information. The solitary tract of the vagus nerve performs a similar function but is much more difficult to access for external modulation (Clark KB et al., 1999). It can only be stimulated electrically with various wave-form intensities and rates. The trigeminal nerve synapses with almost all of the relevant nuclei that would be involved in having a desirable physiologic response in FMS. These include the locus coeruleus, the periaqueductal gray, the parabrachial nucleus, the dorsal raphe nucleus, and the ventral tegmental area, which secretes dopamine to the nucleus accumbens. Other important modulatory structures are involved, but I do not want to make this discussion too technical. Because trigeminal nerve function can be altered pharmacologically, electrically, and mechanically, this route allows the use of a wide range of modalities to tune brain function.

One bottle of TRH nasal spray lasts for about 45 days, and patients usually give themselves one spray in each nostril three times per day. There has not yet been a side effect in my experience, except for an occasional mild allergy. I have also been using TRH ophthalmic solution, again in a 1:10 dilution with artificial tears. This product works quite well, but perhaps not quite as well as TRH nasal spray. Some patients use both of them. The eyedrops act instantly when they are effective. TRH and NMDA receptors appear to be on the cornea, as has been demonstrated for substance P (Nakamura M et al., 1997).

In general, I do not think that dysfunction of the thyroid or the hypothalamic-pituitary-thyroid axis plays very much of a role in FMS. However, it has been found that many patients with FMS have autoimmune thyroiditis, as determined by detectable anti-microsomal thyroid antibodies. In one study (Aarflot T, Bruusgaard D, 1996), 16 percent of patients with widespread musculoskeletal complaints had detectable thyroid antimicrosomal antibodies. Some patients with FMS and thyroid auto antibodies have lab tests indicating borderline hypothyroidism, determined by a high normal thyroid-stimulating hormone level, as well as a low normal level of free thyroxin index, a measure of T_4, one of the two types of thyroid hormone. Such individuals should probably receive a therapeutic trial of thyroid hormone in the range of 75 to 88 micrograms a day.

Thyroid hormone is made by the thyroid gland in two forms, T_4, a tyrosine molecule that has four iodides attached to it, and T_3, a tyrosine molecule that has three iodides attached to it. The active form of thyroid hormone is T_3. In peripheral tissues, T_4 has an iodide molecule removed to convert it to T_3 so that it can be metabolically active. However, if one wishes to increase thyroid hormone levels in the brain, administering T_3 or Cytomel is not a good idea because the mitochondria, the energy producing organelles in the neurons of the brain, are unable to use T_3. Instead, they take up T_4 and deiodinate the T_4 to T_3. T_3 decreases intraneuronal thyroid function and suppresses TRH levels in the brain, although there are T_3 receptors on neuronal membranes. Therefore, it may be a useful agent to augment antidepressants, but only for those patients who are subclinically hyperthyroid.

Most neurosomatic patients are not, but many patients with major depression are hypothyroid (Joffe RT, 1998). Interestingly, several antidepressants such as desipramine and fluoxetine, as well as lithium and carbamazepine, enhance the activity of the enzyme that removes the iodine from T_4 to increase the tissue concentration of T_3. This information is relevant when using thyroid hormone to enhance the effects of antidepressants when treating depression, but it has little value when discussing FMS. Antidepressants have little role in this disorder except for cyclic antidepressants, which have an inherent analgesic and sedative effect. Lithium and carbamazepine (Tegretol) have no role at all.

Certainly, thyroid hormones are important. They influence cell respiration and total energy expenditure and the turnover of all metabolically active substances. The mode of action of thyroid hormone intracellularly is too complex to discuss in this space. In clinical practice, if a person does not have Hashimoto's thyroiditis and lab tests do not indicate hypothyroidism (a low T_4 and a high TSH), there would be no reason to give thyroid hormone to patients with fibromyalgia.

The symptoms of hypothyroidism are learned by every physician in medical school. Common signs include an enlarged thyroid, cold intolerance, lethargy, fatigue, weight gain, hair loss (particularly in the lateral third of the eyebrows), coarse dry hair, brittle nails, dry scaly skin, low heart rate, high blood pressure, constipation, menstrual irregularities, elevated cholesterol, depression, poor concentration, decreased speech, difficulty thinking, and a family history of possible autoimmune thyroid disease. This history may include other types of autoimmune diseases as well, such as type I diabetes, premature graying, pernicious anemia, vitiligo, and rheumatoid arthritis. Measuring TSH and T_4 with a free thyroxin index should be part of every workup of a person with a neurosomatic disorder, since many of the symptoms of hypothyroidism can mimic those of neurosomatic disorders. Even when hypothyroidism is corrected, however, it is very common for neurosomatic symptoms to persist. There should be a high index of suspicion for a thyroid disorder in the patient population with fibromyalgia because of the significant incidence of autoimmune thyroiditis.

The preferred treatment for hypothyroidism today is thyroid replacement in the form of L-thyroxin. It is not recommended to administer "natural" preparations such as Armour thyroid, which might contain too much T_3. Such agents might overstimulate noradrenergic function in a susceptible individual, causing numerous symptoms, including a rapid heart rate. In an elderly person or a person with heart disease, cardiac function could be compromised because of a sudden increase in metabolic rate. Dose titration of thyroid hormone should be gradual. One should begin with 25 mcg of L-thyroxin, which may be increased by 25 to 50 mcg increments at four-week intervals until a normal metabolic state is obtained. Some articles in the literature have described making treatment-resistant patients with depression or rapid-cycling bipolar disorder hyperthyroid on purpose (Bauer M, 1997). The best results of this type of therapy have been reported in bipolar patients, but some physicians find the benefit to be transient. All patients with neurosomatic disorders who I have rendered iatrogenically hyperthyroid have not felt any better. They have had no adverse reactions, which would coincide with the reports from the literature about the safety of this approach. However, it should be done slowly.

Patients with FMS have a blunted TRH test. When a fibromyalgia patient receives 400 or 500 units of TRH, he or she responds with a lower secretion of TSH and thyroid hormone than expected and also a higher increase of prolactin (PRL), another hormone that is regulated by TRH. This abnormality is also seen sometimes in depression. The meaning of this finding is somewhat unclear, although it may imply a down-regulation of receptors for

TRH in the area of the anterior pituitary gland where TSH is secreted. In contrast, the TRH receptors in the neuronal bodies that secrete prolactin might be up-regulated. The primary inhibitory factor for prolactin is dopamine, which is decreased in the brain of patients with neurosomatic disorders, although not necessarily in the region that regulates prolactin secretion (the "tuberoinfundibular region"). Abnormal TRH tests are difficult to explain in general in the absence of hypo- or hyperthyroidism.

Two other neuropeptides, neurotensin and somatostatin (SS), may inhibit TSH secretion and may be possible factors in the blunted TRH responses that are seen in neurosomatic patients. There may also be enhanced endogenous TRH secretion causing down-regulation of TRH receptors.

As far as I know, none of these explanations is sufficient to explain the blunted TRH response. I would prefer the simple reason that there is not enough TRH secreted. The secretion of TRH is mediated not just by dopamine but also by norepinephrine, and both neurotransmitters are low in neurosomatic patients. A certain strain of rat, the Wistar Kyoto rat, has been bred for anxiety and depression. These rats have low levels of TRH precursors. TRH has antidepressant properties in rats and humans. Somatostatin levels are not reduced in my neurosomatic patients because their symptoms are not improved by somatostatin injections. Spinal-fluid levels of somatostatin and neurotensin have not been measured in neurosomatic patients to my knowledge. Excess somatostatin suppresses growth-hormone release.

As is clear from this section, the issue of thyroid dysfunction, particularly low thyroid function, or hypothyroidism, in patients with neurosomatic disorders can become extremely complicated. Practically, though, I treat only patients who are demonstrably hypothyroid by low T_4 and high TSH measurements or those that have autoimmune (Hashimoto's) thyroiditis with borderline T_4 and TSH levels. I find antidepressants in general to be of little value in treating the entire symptom complex of neurosomatic disorders, although they treat depression well. Serotonin-reuptake inhibitors may actually increase the intensity of a peripheral painful stimulus (Dirksen R et al., 1998). Thyroid augmentation of antidepressants in the neurosomatic patient has not proven to be beneficial even when raised to hyperthyroid levels, at least in my practice.

Chapter 5

Case Reports

MY SO-CALLED ILLNESS: IS IT REAL OR ALL IN MY HEAD?

Aside from my lower back problem, I have enjoyed excellent health all my life. Since 1983, for example, I have not missed a day of work except for meetings or going to the library. About fifteen years ago, I was involved in a chain-reaction motor vehicle accident on the Santa Ana Freeway in Los Angeles. My neck hurt a little, and it never had before, so I got an X ray and an MRI scan of my cervical spine. Both showed moderate *cervical spondylosis,* an osteoarthritic and degenerative disc condition found in most middle-aged men. My spinal canal was narrowed, although my spinal cord was not compressed. The nerves exited from the spinal canal through holes called neural foramina, which were encroached upon by this process as well. My neck pain resolved rapidly, and I gave no further thought to the matter. Cervical spondylosis is often, perhaps even usually, asymptomatic.

My son, Jordan, and I used to enjoy playfully wrestling together (he's eleven). Sometimes he would pretend that he was Kato and that I was Inspector Clouseau from the "Pink Panther" movies with Peter Sellers. In this role, he would sometimes make a sneak attack on me as I entered a "rheum." About four months before writing this chapter he tackled me around the neck as I was walking into the family room. Suddenly my arms and legs felt like they were full of electricity, and I couldn't stand up or walk very well because my legs were weak. My arms and hands were weak also, and it was difficult for me to grasp a pen to write. I experienced urinary hesitancy, i.e., difficulty in starting to urinate, that same evening. My larynx, jaw, and tongue felt like "pins and needles."

I realized that one or more cervical discs had been further herniated and were protruding into the spinal canal and compressing my spinal cord, a process termed "myelopathy." There was no treatment for this process I knew of except for drugs such as Advil, a soft cervical collar, or surgery. Advil and a soft cervical collar did nothing. My neck pain, radiating into my shoulder muscles (trapezii), was excruciating.

The next day I saw one of my anesthesiologist friends who was a pain specialist. He relieved the pain in my trapezii with trigger-point injections but had nothing else to offer except injections of cortisone around my spinal cord (epidural steroids), which he said usually didn't work very well. He told me to get an MRI scan, which I had already scheduled. I would have the procedure at an imaging center to which I had previously referred at least a thousand patients over the years. He agreed to prescribe trial medications for me.

As I filled out the MRI information form (with some difficulty), I wrote in large capital letters that I had an acute compressive myelopathy superimposed on chronic cervical spondylosis, and that I wanted to know what the diameter of my spinal canal was at various levels and how much spinal cord compression there was. I was in considerable discomfort and did not know how, when, or if I would get relief.

The radiologist who interpreted the scan was new and did not know me. She completely ignored the history or what information I wanted and dictated a report indicating degenerative disc disease and neural foraminal encroachment at several levels. Such carelessness is quite common in medicine today. She issued a new report that addressed the relevant issues after I spoke with her. I had significant cord compression, which is what I expected.

By this time I had been to the local hospital library (there was no way I could have gotten to UCLA, much less stayed there very long) and copied the chapters in two current neurosurgery textbooks about cervical spondylosis. I also did a MEDLINE search. I thought there must be some microsurgical approach to the cervical spine as there is to the lumbar spine, although I had not heard of it.

The results were not encouraging. I had expected the standard procedure to be a posterior decompression laminectomy as is done by Michael Rosner, a neurosurgeon who treats patients with fibromyalgia who were born with narrow spinal canals ("congenital cervical spinal stenosis"). He usually chose patients who had "hard signs" on a neurologic exam, such as evidence of spasticity. I had performed a neurologic examination on myself that was fairly normal except for mild weakness, most of which resolved in the ensuing weeks. I decided to get an expert opinion from a neurosurgeon about a course of action, because my electric-shock feelings (paresthesias) were so severe I didn't know if I could continue practicing medicine, or do anything at all, for that matter. I had tried single doses of other sorts of analgesic medicines, which, as is often the case with neuropathic pain, did no good whatsoever. Strangely, I had no pain at all when I awoke in the mornings, but it gradually returned in 30 to 60 minutes. It occurred to me that some aspect of sleep neurochemistry was modulating my neural transmission, but I didn't know what it was. Recumbency while awake had no effect at all. Cervical traction, or pulling my head to lengthen my neck, hopefully to relieve pressure on nerves, made my symptoms much worse almost immediately.

I asked some of my physician friends if they knew a competent neurosurgeon who wasn't crazy. This request might seem bizarre to the lay reader, but in medical circles, neurosurgeons, even more than psychiatrists, are known to be quite eccentric, although the reason for this trait is speculative. I certainly did not know of such an individual. I had assisted in craniotomies and spinal operations with several neurosurgeons, all of whom seemed to have an idiosyncratic world view, and two of whom were so drunk I could barely tolerate being across the table from them. Because most of these cases were emergencies, when I got the neurosurgeon on call for my patient, I was in no position to ask for a replacement.

Some of my surgical friends flatly stated they did not know of even one "sane" neurosurgeon, and would not know whom to consult if they or a family member needed neurosurgical care. Two of them suggested the same person, whom they had not met but had heard good things about. He was young and a rapidly rising star. I had heard of him also and had referred a patient with a difficult type of brain tumor to him. Both the patient and his wife liked him and said he was thorough and compassionate. Let's pseudonymously call him Dr. Green.

I brought my MRI scan with me to the appointment. I saw Dr. Green with a (I assume) neurosurgery resident in one of the examining rooms. I succinctly related my history in about two minutes and handed him the MRI scan. He left the room while the resident performed a much less thorough neurologic exam than I had performed on myself. After a while, Dr. Green came back in and said that he wasn't going to do surgery on me yet and that I should wear a soft cervical collar. I could return if I couldn't walk anymore. Then he left. I was in his presence for a total of three minutes, four at the most. I had no chance to ask him any questions, and he behaved as if there were none to be asked. I was too stunned to run after him, because I had gone to see him with worries and fears that I thought would be addressed. I called back the next day, but he refused to speak with me. His nurse called while I was seeing patients, but when I called back, she was unavailable and did not return my call.

The books said that the best results for cervical spondylosis with compression myelopathy were obtained if the surgery was performed within six months after the onset of symptoms. Posterior multilevel cervical decompression laminectomy, or removing the back part of all the involved vertebrae to open the canal, was falling out of favor. There was a high rate of postoperative spinal instability, and sometimes the operation did not work because the spinal cord, as a result of inflammation, was stuck to (by adhesions, or scar tissue) the front part ("body," or "corpus") of the vertebrae. The currently favored procedure, therefore, was a multilevel corpectomy, or removing several entire vertebral bodies and filling in the space with a large iliac (pelvic bone) graft. It took one to three years to recover from this operation, and it usually didn't relieve all the symptoms, just some of them. Statistics varied depending upon the medical center reporting and how much experience the surgical team had with this procedure, which was fairly new. There were no microsurgical options, and I couldn't find out from Dr. Green what he thought of cervical epidural steroids for my kind of problem. I was angry that he just "blew me off" like that. I have requested my records and MRI scan several times with no response. After I made further inquiries, another physician friend came up with the name of a neurosurgeon that he heard wasn't crazy and who specialized in spinal disorders.

One of the interesting aspects about the clinical presentation of cervical spondylosis is that unless the degree of spinal cord compression is very severe, the patient's symptoms bear little correlation to the MRI findings. This observation implies that the spinal cord itself and descending regulatory neurons from the brain modulate myelopathic nociception, an important determinant of the clinical presentation. Although I had never seen a patient in my practice who I thought had symptoms of a cervical myelopathy, I had examined many patients with supposed carpal tunnel syndrome, thoracic outlet syndrome, peripheral neuropathy, and reflex sympathetic dystrophy that were comorbid with the primary problem for which they were consulting me (usually fibromyalgia). These nerve entrapment or autonomic dysfunction syndromes often greatly improve as the fibromyalgia pain is relieved. Reflex sympathetic dystrophy (RSD) has been renamed. It is now "complex regional pain syndrome." This type of pain is called neuropathic and is most commonly exemplified by diabetic peripheral neuropathy. Although my pain is "central," from the brain and/or spinal cord, as I have discussed in previous books, all pain is central to some degree.

Complex regional pain syndrome was successfully treated by sodium amytal interview and hypnosis according to one case report (Simon EP, Dahl LF, 1999). My experience with this approach has been entirely negative. I attempted this therapy numerous times when I began to specialize. One of my wheelchair-bound patients subsequently had a dissociative episode and found herself in her bathroom, not knowing how she got there.

When discussing this phenomenon with patients, and when I used to lecture to physicians, I gave the very concrete example of hitting one's thumb with a hammer. Nerves in the thumb are injured and send messages to this effect to the spinal cord and brain, the central nervous system. The projections by which neurons communicate with other neurons, axons and dendrites, rearrange themselves, and the area of the sensory cortex devoted to the thumb gets much larger. In the course of time, the thumb nerves heal, and neuronal connections in the brain return to their pre-injury state, but not quite. The brain retains a memory of the pain, particularly in the thalamus. Some people, including those with fibromyalgia, seem less able to restore normal functional connections and experience pain in old scars or injuries when their illness flares up. A similar situation exists with the autonomic nervous system, which has only been separated from the CNS by anatomical convention. The CNS and the ANS work together as one functional unit (Blessing WW, 1997).

A considerable amount of research has focused on neuropathic pain and how to treat it pharmacologically in the last fifteen years or so. One of my favorite journals, *Pain,* has published an article on this topic in almost every issue lately. An experimental model of neuropathic pain has been devised and standardized by constricting a rat sciatic nerve with sutures. Unfortunately, no work of a similar nature (that I was able to find) has been done on spinal cord pain, except for compression of the emerging nerve roots by neural foraminal encroachment, which would be a neuropathic pain. As far as I can tell, I don't have much of that.

I subsequently consulted another neurosurgeon, who told me I needed immediate surgery and that I was at risk of quadriparesis. "You'll be as good as new in three months," he cheerfully informed me. Going for the best two out of three, I was examined physically and electrophysiologically by a neurologist whom I did not know personally. I did not want to contaminate his evaluation by prior experience. He said I didn't need an operation. I asked him if he knew a "reliable" neurosurgeon, but he did not. A cardiologist friend of mine had just come up with the name of someone he trusted. "I'd let him operate on me," he said. Let's call him Dr. Brown. I asked the neurologist whether he knew Dr. Brown. "Oh, yes!" he exclaimed. "He's an excellent surgeon, is very conservative, and has very good judgment. I forgot about him."

So I went to see Dr. Brown. By this time, by working with the pain specialist and the neurologist, we found that Neurontin diminished my discomfort considerably and had no adverse reactions. I still take it three times a day. Coincidentally, a case report was published soon thereafter about the efficacy of Neurontin (gabapentin) for intractable pain in a paraplegic patient (Ness TJ et al., 1998).

Dr. Brown was quite courteous and raised his eyebrows ever so slightly when I informed him of my two previous interactions with neurosurgeons. He advised me that I did not need surgery and never would. "Almost every cervical spine in a person your age looks like that," he commented after looking at my MRI.

My myelopathic and nerve-root symptoms are much better now, about nine months after their onset. My improvement is due, at least in part, to altering the perception of sensory input by a neural network including the anterior cingulate cortex, parts of the thalamus, the caudate nucleus, and the somatosensory cortex. Sometimes my symptoms are almost undetectable, and at other times they are mild to moderate. I am fairly stoic about somatic discomfort and now have to lie down for only 30 minutes about once a month. I'm glad I followed the advice I have always given to my patients: Never have spinal surgery unless there is no other choice. I have treated a multitude of patients with symptoms from failed spinal surgery, and the large majority of them have improved significantly without reoperation.

ONE-SECOND EPIPHANIES

"Plunk your magic twanger, Froggy." *(puff of smoke)*
(Guttural) "Hiya kids, hiya, hiya!"

Smilin' Ed summoning Froggy the Gremlin (1950)

Sometimes I feel like Froggy the Gremlin, from Smilin' Ed's Gang, but never more so than when I make someone suffering for years feel better in a few seconds. I can sometimes hear the "thrummm" of *my* magic twanger resonating in my office.

Neurobiologists now realize that neural networks can be instantaneously reconfigured, a process that occurs continually as we change tasks. They can also be "bistable" (stable in two different configurations) and shift when one network reaches certain strength through homeostatic mechanisms. A familiar example to all is the sleep-wake cycle. Although I have been therapeutically rapidly reconfiguring neural networks for many years, the idea does not seem to have seeped into the mainstream of medicine yet.

Patients sick for years have gotten better in one second on numerous occasions. I shall restrict the initial case reports to eyedrops, since they work in about a second (the speed of neural conduction is 250 miles per hour).

A 26-year-old runner had been unable to compete due to CFS for two years. He came to see me from Paris. One second after the first eyedrop, he said, "I feel fine." I suggested, as I usually do in such situations, that he run around the block and come back and tell me how he felt. He was gone for an hour. He returned perspiring, after having run several miles. He said he felt well. I gave him a bottle of eyedrops with instructions about how to use them and asked him how long he would be in the United States. "About a month," he said. I told him to come back if he felt worse or to call me before he left for France. He called about a month later to thank me and said he was still doing well.

Not everyone appreciates such a rapid improvement. A 24-year-old woman, who seemed somewhat bewildered by my hypothesis, became asymptomatic in one second, an uncommon but not rare experience. She got a stunned look on her face, which I'll never forget, like a deer caught in headlights. After incredulously telling me all her symptoms were gone, she got up and ran out of the office. I never heard from her again. I guess some people can't tell the difference between white and black magic.

A 48-year-old woman with bright red hair (that's how I remember her) had been ill for twenty years. All her symptoms resolved after eyedrops. Her gratitude was underwhelming. "My appointment with you was supposed to be two hours. You've made me better in five minutes." (I talked to her first and had reviewed her medical records at length.) She demanded to have the fee for her initial patient visit prorated so that she would only pay 1/24 of it (5 minutes), thinking that I was somehow ripping her off. I never saw her again either.

Just last week, I saw a 28-year-old attorney who was facing the closing of his practice because of fatigue and neurocognitive dysfunction. The eyedrops didn't help him, but the first nose drop (adenosine) did. In fact, he felt normal in ten seconds (nose drops take longer). I suggested that he leave the office and engage in an activity that would usually cause a relapse. He never came back either. We called him the next day. (It's hard to meet your payroll when too many patients skip.) He said that he still felt fine but didn't think he should pay the full fee. This time we negotiated a better recompense than 1/24, however.

I have seen about 20,000 CFS patients. One of my most memorable consulted me about three years ago, accompanied by his wife. He was a middle-aged businessman, Mr. Smith, who had been apparently well until six months previously when he developed the symptoms of CFS and then depression. His medical records disclosed that he had seen the usual West Los Angeles mavens (experts) in a fruitless quest for an esoteric disorder. The eventual consensus was that he had CFS.

Many patients tell me that if I can't help them then they are going to kill themselves. No one has yet. This man informed me, while slumped in his chair looking like a bassett hound with myasthenia gravis, that "if you can't help me *today,* I'm going to kill myself *tonight!*"

Usually, in cases like this, I perform what I term a "resurrection." Mrs. Jones arrives by ambulance in a hospital bed where she has been confined for months or years (take your pick). That day will be, I'm sure, my only crack at her. I can usually get Mrs. Jones ambulatory, often with intravenous medications, by the end of the day, so that she can walk into my office on her next visit.

Just before I told my nurse to set up for a resurrection, I instilled naphazoline 0.1 percent ophthalmic solution, one drop in each eye. In one to two seconds, Mr. Smith's entire demeanor changed. He sat upright, became animated, and then began to run around my office flapping his arms like a chicken while telling nonstop jokes. Mr. Smith assured me that he had no desire to end his life and cackled out the door with his wife and a sample bottle of eyedrops. I asked him to call me in the next day or two. There being no contact, I called him on postconsultation day number three. When he came to the phone, he spoke to me in a rational, composed manner. He said that he felt fine and was still using the eyedrops. He would contact me if any change occurred. I never heard from him again.

Events like these occur in my office almost every day, and usually with multiple patients. Many times, the "miracles" take place in patients I have been seeing for many years when I happen to hit the magic button with the 101st medication. Even though my nurse tells new patients what to possibly expect ("Don't be surprised if you feel better in thirty seconds." "Yeah, right, after I've seen over twenty-five doctors and spent my life savings"), they are understandably flabbergasted when his prediction comes true.

A different sort of "miracle" occurs when I diagnose and treat piriform muscle syndrome. The piriform muscle is located in the pelvis. If it is in spasm, or contains trigger points, sciatica can be produced, because the piriform muscle can compress the sciatic nerve. Many patients with this problem have had failed back surgery, since piriform muscle syndrome is thought to be rare or nonexistent by most physicians, if they have ever even heard of it. My belief is that most do not know how to properly examine a patient to detect it and do not know how to treat it (fairly easily, actually) if they detect it.

My nurse, Mario, still remembers the middle-aged lady who came to see me for CFS. When he ushered her into my office, she was dragging one leg and walking in an unusual posture, one that I had seen many times before. "What's wrong with your leg?" I inquired. "Doc, I've had if for fifteen years and no one knows what's wrong."

I nodded to Mario, and he prepared the patient for a manual pelvic examination. In ten seconds she almost hit the ceiling twice as I palpated both piriform muscles. After they were injected with lidocaine under fluoroscopy (to avoid perforating the colon), she got up and stood up straight and then walked without pain for the first time in many years. Because I diagnose and treat this condition frequently, hundreds of thousands of sciatic patients in the world must be doomed to a life of chronic pain. To read more about piriform muscle syndrome and hundreds of other obscure musculoskeletal conditions, consult *Myofascial Pain and Dysfunction: The Trigger Point Manual,* by David Simons and Janet Travell (Simons DG et al., 1999).

MY MOST UNUSUAL CASE

Every day in my office is phantasmagoric and has been for the past 20 years. Previously normal people have somehow been transmogrified into patients labeled as having CFS, a system complex that can be extremely elastic. I encounter so many unusual case presentations that when I asked Mario and my receptionist, Martha, to think of the most bizarre patient who wasn't psychotic, they felt incapable of sorting through the thousands of candidates. Just as we were having the discussion, Rachel B.'s husband called. "She's the one!" we exclaimed simultaneously.

Rachel B. was a 47-year-old woman who tripped over a forklift in a market three years before I first evaluated her in 1997. Two days after the accident she developed various kinds of abnormal sensations all over her body. She had seen many physicians prior to seeing me, with the consensus diagnosis being fibromyalgia.

In 1995 she was advised by a neurologist to stay in bed for two months. During this period, she began to experience panic attacks. She also described frequent headaches and constant neurocognitive dysfunction. Physical examination revealed 18 out of 18 fibromyalgia tender points and bilateral piriform muscle tenderness. She was unable to lie on her back due to pain and came to the office in a wheelchair.

She had a fairly good initial response to several medications. Her pain, energy, and cognition were improved. Piriform muscle injections were not beneficial. Many patients with fibromyalgia do not respond to trigger-point injections.

Subsequently her symptoms waxed and waned but were always relieved by infusions of lidocaine and ketamine, which had a duration of action of several weeks. She continued trials of other medications and had just begun Effexor when she entered a very stressful period in her life. She was going through bankruptcy, and her panic attacks began to recur. She became unable to perform independent activities of daily living (shopping, cleaning, cooking, etc.).

Fourteen weeks after her first office visit we had another consultation. On this occasion she spoke *entirely in rhyme,* in a singsong voice (dysprosody), eliding some verbs, and exhibiting numerous other syntactical irregularities. Her rhyming was effortless; she was unable to speak without rhyming. Her eccentric speech was consistently improved with intravenous lidocaine and ketamine. When not rhyming, she was often dysarthric point of speech arrest. Over the next year, she required less frequent infusions and had a higher baseline when they wore off. Rhyming occurred on only one more occasion and was present for about a month in its most active phase.

Prosody refers to paralinguistic elements of speech, including intonation, melody, cadence, loudness, timbre, accent, and timing of pauses. It is learned in the preverbal stage of development. Rachel's "hyperprosody" did not reflect a lack of vocabulary, as is seen in Broca's aphasia, and may have involved a hyperfunction of the nonclassic language areas in the left temporal cortex. Unfortunately, she was not able to afford brain imaging to demonstrate an anatomic or functional lesion. At the present time, Rachel is able to function as a homemaker and is active as a leader in her church group. I have not been able to find a similar case in the medical literature except as anecdotally reported by V.S. Ramachandran and S. Blakeslee (1998) in their book, *Phantoms in the Brain.* The patient was a sixty-year-old professor with right temporal lobe epilepsy who began to *think* in rhyme, but not to speak that way.

BUG-OF-THE-MONTH CLUB

One use for antibiotics may involve an antimicrobial action. Some cases of IBS are apparently caused by small intestinal bacterial overgrowth. Eradication of this overgrowth can cause reduction of symptoms in a subset of IBS patients (Pimental M et al., 2000).

Because this experimental demonstration of this concept is not in accord with standard concepts, I shall describe it in more detail than usual. Two hundred two IBS patients met Rome I criteria (gastroenterologists met in Rome a few years ago to decide these). They were referred from the West Los Angeles community (not the most compliant group of patients) for a lactulose hydrogen breath test (LHBT). Patients drink 10 gm of lactulose and perform a breath test first at baseline and then every 15 minutes for three hours. The breath test measures the concentration of hydrogen in PPM (parts per million). Elevated hydrogen production at times when the lactulose should have been in the small intestine and then should have been in the colon were evaluated. Eradication of small intestinal bacterial overgrowth (SIBO) was assumed to have occurred when breath hydrogen at various times was below certain criteria. Neomycin, ciprofloxacin, metronidazole, or doxycycline were used for ten days to eradicate SIBO.

Of 202 subjects, 188 were treated with antibiotics. Of these, 47 were further evaluated to confirm eradication of their SIBO, 25 achieved complete eradication as determined by LHBT, and 22 had incomplete eradication.

Antibiotic treatment reduced hydrogen production from 68.0+/–35.5 PPM to 35.0+/–29.1 PPM in the 47 patients, a highly significant change. Greater reduction in hydrogen was seen in those whose SIBO was completely eradicated.

Successful eradication of SIBO reduced the number of subjects complaining of diarrhea and abdominal pain, but the noneradicated group experienced no significant difference. Two previous experiments demonstrated similar results. The glaring limitation of this study (and the subsequent one) is the small number of subjects returning for follow-up LHBT. What response did the other 155 patients have (two-thirds of the entire sample)? Also, the diagnosis of SIBO was made entirely by LHBT. SIBO is thought to be caused by proximal migration of colonic flora. Cultures, therefore, are difficult to do and are potentially hazardous to patient and physician (particularly in West Los Angeles).

One of the cardinal rules in academic medicine is that researchers publish as many papers from an experiment as possible. Thus, we are presented with the possibility that SIBO may be associated with fibromyalgia (Pimental M et al., 2001).

One hundred twenty-three subjects of (I assume) the same experimental group had FMS. Of these, 96 (78 percent) had SIBO. Returning subjects reported a 57+/–29 percent overall improvement in symptoms with significant improvement in bloating, gas, abdominal pain, diarrhea, joint pains, and fatigue [P = <0.05] ("the magic number" for statistical significance). It is well known that many patients (about two-thirds) overlap between CFS, FMS, and IBS. Most improvement was in IBS symptoms. This sounds pretty darn good until one reads that only 25 (about one-fourth) returned for a LHBT. Eleven achieved complete eradication. Despite this number, 22 of the 25 returning participants reported the 57+/–29 percent improvement.

The authors conclude that no bacterial pathogen has been clearly implicated in the pathogenesis of IBS. They report that SIBO causes bacterial migration to mesenteric lymph nodes and can produce systemic effects believed to be mediated by gram-negative endotoxemia causing soft tissue hyperalgesia.

As a postscript, I have seen as patients in my office some of those who underwent SIBO eradication. They reported that their symptoms returned shortly after they stopped taking antibiotics. I do SIBO eradication only after many other treatments have been tried, and even then, only at the patient's request. It seems to me that a more vigorous attempt at follow-up could have been made, as is done in most community-based studies. These are excellent as a first step.

Chapter 6

Married to a Doctor Who Is Married to His Practice

(as might be written by Gail Coplin Goldstein
if she were willing to air the dirty linen)

Give me your tired, your poor, your huddled masses yearning to breathe free . . .

Emma Lazarus (1883)
The New Colossus: Inscription
for the Statue of Liberty, New York Harbor

This altruistic quotation was suitable for a large young nation with an expanding frontier but is unfortunately inappropriate for a solo medical practice with no external source of funding. When I married Jay 24 years ago we were very much in love. I knew that his practice management style was chaotic, or even nonexistent, and that he did not have the knowledge, ability, or inclination to run his office so that he could support himself, much less a family. I thought that we had formed a partnership so that I could help him to make a decent living while fulfilling his dream. His almost delusional pursuit of his sense of ideal medical practice proved to be stronger than my most vigorous intentions and efforts. His method of medical practice and a few of his patients have harmed our marriage, in spite of our love.

Jay is very accomplished, even brilliant, in his self-invented specialty of neurosomatic medicine. He is a likeable, caring person and a wonderful father to our son, Jordan. His intellectual attainments and database of knowledge are prodigious, and his predilection for bantering is often hilarious but can be quite irritating and distracting when interposed into serious conversation. These qualities are so accentuated in his personality that he is at times almost like an idiot savant. He is so inept at any task requiring manual dexterity that he must have a congenital learning disorder. Early in our marriage I gave him a pair of pliers to fix something and he returned sheepishly with the tool in two parts, a feat that I have been unable to duplicate even when I try. I had the pieces framed.

Jay literally "did not have a pot to piss in" when I married him. He did not have the money to pay support to his first wife, and for the first year of our marriage my entire salary as a supervisory school psychologist for a school district went to this end. Prior to meeting me he had invested in a coal mine venture with a four-to-one tax write-off that was disallowed by the IRS, and he could not afford to pay his taxes. He had been verbally advised (nothing in writing, of course) by a prestigious Los Angeles tax-law firm that the investment was valid and legal, and therefore kept tossing letters from the IRS saying that he owed them money, into the wastebasket. The day of reckoning arrived in 1980 when I had to withdraw all the money in my pension fund to pay his back taxes and fund his pension plan.

His insurance agents churned his various policies every year or two so they could get new commissions. He had no idea how to charge anyone for anything and believed it was unethical to do unnecessary tests. His idealism about medicine was like a religious calling. He refused to treat anyone or perform any procedure if he thought that another physician nearby, or in some cases, anywhere, could do it better than he could. He was afraid to change any of his office procedures, because even though he knew they weren't very efficient, he thought that the evil that he knew (but didn't understand) was better than the evil that he didn't know. If something unpopular had to be done, he would blame me, reasoning that it didn't matter if staff and patients disliked me. It was very important to him to be considered a good guy. He didn't understand that it is possible to set limits and still be liked.

Because I had worked as an administrator for some years, I thought that his office procedures could be vastly improved and actually was appalled at the way things ran. Jay was very resistant to my efforts to change things because he didn't know what would happen as a consequence. He worked six days a week to make ends meet since his charges and collections (an incredible mess of ignored bills) were so low, even though he had an enormous practice volume and his patients (for the most part) seemed to love him. The ones not paying *especially* loved him, and in his naïveté, he actually believed their blandishments. He was on call every night because some of his patients had such complicated problems that if they had an emergency, no other doctor in the area would understand how they were being treated.

He had a magical way of thinking about money. He seemed to believe that even though he wasn't making very much (about what an elementary school teacher did), that some day, somehow, the world would realize what a good doctor he was and he would be showered with rewards. When I met him, he was spending money that he didn't have in such an expectation. Although he is no longer extravagant, he continues to believe money will magically come his way.

He asked me to make changes, but found it was difficult to implement those we agreed upon. Jay gradually let me make some changes in his practice, but with considerable passive-aggressive resistance. I felt sabotaged by him and his staff. His revulsion for physicians who took gross advantage of the laissez-faire medical insurance system of the day was so great that my valid legal and ethical suggestions were followed only grudgingly, and so did not work very well. In the meantime, all the doctors we knew were making small fortunes.

There has always been a great disparity in income between physicians who did "procedures" and those who practiced cognitive medicine, which consisted primarily of examining and talking to patients. Jay would do procedures, but only when he thought they were necessary for patient care. He would not perform procedures that were in the gray zone, those that would provide additional information and might benefit the patient a little but would increase his income closer to what other physicians at the time were making. As a result, we had a hand-to-mouth existence, and I, who paid the bills, was always borrowing from Peter to pay Paul. Sometimes checks bounced. Because I did not marry for money, having a high income was unimportant to me, but paying bills was extremely important to me, with my corn-fed midwestern value system. Jay, nevertheless, kept seeing patients for free when they would give him a hard-luck story, or he would make "side deals" with them, so they would hardly have to pay anything, and not tell me about it. This proclivity of his used to drive me crazy and engendered ill will among patients when we would attempt to collect from them. He is such a "soft touch," putting optimal patient care over every other conceivable consideration, even paying for patients' medications with money we did not have, that I eventually had to put a sign on his desk saying he would not discuss finances with anyone. To this day, that sign is ignored. It eventually disappeared. For many years, Jay lived in a world as he thought it should be, somewhat like Don Quixote, rather than as it was.

Jay was always reading medical books and journals in his spare time when I first met him. He absolutely felt that it was his obligation to provide the best possible medical care to every patient who saw him, so he had to learn everything relevant to his profession—which I think he did.

I always wanted Jay to follow his star, and I helped him as much as I could and as much as he would let me. I did the grunt work of managing his office as it grew larger, as well as organizing five international conferences on chronic fatigue syndrome and fibromyalgia for him. I've always thought he was a special individual and wanted to help him realize his potential as a person as well as a doctor. I was a first-class enabler who thought for years I was a partner but was, in reality, only thought of as a secretary by the doctor.

During the incredible confusion of the late 1980s when we had 25 employees and no money coming in, I had to stop working as a psychologist in the practice to devote all of my attention to management and to keeping us afloat. This period was extremely stressful for me, and when Jay's imbroglio with the medical board began, I almost decompensated. But I hung in, still thinking we were life partners, sharing the ups and down of life.

I was pregnant with Jordan at the time, and we were also dealing with Jay's one malpractice suit that went to arbitration (during which I went into labor). The suit was filed by a patient of Jay's who was angry at me because I had been seeing his wife for counseling after she had filed for divorce. "I'll get you!" he threatened, after I wouldn't give him his wife's records. He sought revenge by suing my husband, a case the patient lost; however, the situation was still personally and emotionally damaging for me.

Being pregnant, almost going bankrupt, dealing with a husband who was killing himself with unremunerative work on patients, each of whom I had begun to regard as potentially dangerous, almost drove me over the edge. The medical board fiasco was added on in the same year, for which I can't help blaming Jay because of his misguided priorities and seemingly heedless refusal to protect himself from the depredations and reprisals of unstable and possibly borderline patients because he was unflinchingly devoted to helping them. I consider him to be addicted to his patients. I can see now why there is such a high divorce rate among CFS specialists, although none of them I've met seems to be very much like Jay. Significant others end in second place to the practice and usually won't accept this.

We have lost hundreds of thousands of dollars that could have gone toward our retirement and a less-suicidal schedule for Jay, if he had only listened to reasonable suggestions from me, his colleagues, his friends and advisors. I'm bitter, angry, and resentful, and think I shall always be so to some degree. He could have been more careful and wiser and taken better care of his family. We are worth at least as much as his patients and should be worth more. When Jay shambles into the house at 9:00 p.m., exhausted and spent by having to work at top speed for one entire day ("burn," as he calls it), too little is left for me and Jordan. Thankfully, he has stopped seeing patients on Saturday and is now beginning to have a life. Jordan and I continue to wait and tune out his excuses for not participating in a family life.

As a result of Jay's "problems," as I generically refer to the various financial, regulatory, and institutional situations that have bedeviled us, I became hypervigilant over the years. I needed a change. I went back to school to become a registered nurse in large part so I could care for him, my parents, and my child physically should they become ill. As a former teacher, administrator, and school psychologist, I became employed as a school nurse. This position enabled me to help children in many ways while providing a regular income with good health benefits. Because Jay seems intent on pursuing his current mode of practice, at least we could enjoy a modest lifestyle and have medical and dental insurance, which we could not afford for several years. Unfortunately, I had surgery, was hospitalized with sepsis, and had to quit my job.

Almost every time Jay calls me or initiates a conversation with me now I expect some sort of bad news or a crisis with which to deal. Although such is usually not the case anymore, it is difficult to break old habits. I feel that I've been running behind him our entire marriage with a "pooper scooper," since he appears singularly unable to deal with ordinary events of daily life. He reminds me of one of those wavy men floating through a surrealistic Chagall painting, or a "luftmensch," an apt German term Jay has thoughtfully provided.

Although I have worked hard to help Jay realize his personal goals and "actualize" himself, including urging him to write his articles and helping to edit his books, I think now that I have functioned somewhat as an enabler of his single-mindedness. I have almost stopped wishing for a life with Jay apart from his patients, his research, and his books. The shared happiness that we have with our darling Jordan is wonderful, but at times I think that the continued stressors of our marriage make me short-tempered and peevish with even him. It wounds me to think that I am not as good a mother as I ought to be, although Jordan is as loving, smart, handsome, and self-confident as a thirteen-year-old boy could be. I don't trust Jay to do his share emotionally in the family. He knows that he could have modified his life to make more room for us, but he chose not to, using any number of rationalizations.

Jay has told me about how family doctors and general practitioners used to make money. He did locum tenens (substitute) work for them early in his career while they were on vacation. They made sure that (and this was over 20 years ago) no patient left the office with a bill of less than $100, no matter what the diagnosis. One doctor had a rule that every patient received an injection on every visit, sometimes two or three times a week. Many had their own X-ray machines, which may have dated from the 1930s, and they usually took films of minimum quality and maximum radiation exposure. X rays could still be used to rule out pneumonia on everyone with a cough, to rule out a fracture on everyone with a sprain or strain, and to rule out an "acute abdomen" or bowel obstruction on everyone with a stomachache. X ray alone could double a physician's income. Most used physical therapy "modalities" such as ultrasound, diathermy, and intermittent traction, as well as machines that gave mechanical massages with moving rollers, all of which were prescribed freely, perhaps because they could be administered by a medical assistant and insurance would pay for them. The patients thought they were being treated, and the "modalities" didn't hurt them, except those who drove 20 to 30 miles to receive this therapy and left feeling worse than when they had come. Many doctors had laboratories in their offices, as well as electrocardiograph machines, treadmill test machines, ultrasound machines (used routinely on every pregnant woman), and almost every other device that could invade orifices or image organs. It was vastly more lucrative to do such procedures, and often took much less time, than to sit and talk to a patient for 15 or 20 minutes.

Physicians often sold medications they prescribed for their patients, and some recommended an array of nutritional supplements that they provided. Such a practice is ethical if the doctor can provide a scientific rationale for their use and if the contents of the products have been verified by the physicians. It is important that a physician not use his or her position of authority to profit from direct sales to patients. Jay recalls one physician for whom he did a locum tenens who sold patients a special cough syrup with gold in it ("auric chloride") for $100 a bottle. On the other hand, because patients purchase nutritional supplements frequently, often on the advice of a store clerk, products of reliable composition and potency may be sold by a physician acting in the best interests of his or her patients. The abuse of this fiduciary responsibility in the past has contributed to mismanaged health care in the present.

The financial incentives for high-tech medicine, which Jay spurns, were dramatically illustrated to me recently. One of Jay's friends, a cardiologist, did almost exclusively high-tech medicine and until recently had a yearly income that greatly exceeded our net worth. The incursions of managed health care and burn-out caused him to forsake his cardiology practice (except for one day a week) for a general internal medicine practice in a well-to-do California beach community. He returned to full-time cardiology after three years. "I was very busy," he related, "but I couldn't make a living examining and talking to people all day, and I refuse to run a 'mill.'"

Well, perhaps it is harder to make a high income as a doctor today, but when Jay could have done it, and done it ethically, he wouldn't (or didn't). I didn't marry him for his money (he had none), and I never wanted him to do excessive tests or procedures to bleed patients and insurance companies. I did, however, resent seeing every dime I worked for get pissed away by his inability to tell when he was being conned by a deadbeat patient, or his indifference to the hard economic realities of life. A children's book about a Mr. Toad, careening heedlessly down a dangerous road, comes to mind. Mr. Toad was always being bailed out by concerned friends but never learned his lesson and never changed.

Postscript Actually Written by Gail

I don't think our life and problems are the business of anyone but ourselves. I am a private person and dislike the spotlight. When Jay asked me to write this chapter I refused, so he decided to write it for me, without my permission. His ability to view the past through my eyes rather surprised me. I did edit it to a minor extent. I made a choice to stand by him come hell or high water. At any time during our marriage I could have given up, walked away, walked out, or divorced him. As maddening, annoying, insensitive, sabotaging, ego-driven, and consuming as he is, I haven't walked away yet—because I love him and he loves Jordan.

Being the wife of a famous man at times brings unwanted attention. Although anyone is vulnerable to threats or stalking, the danger is increased when one's spouse is in a visible position. Although I have asked him not to talk about our family, he seems to cross that boundary often. He shares information about me and our son that is personal and gives out our home phone number to some patients, without regard to their mental stability or our safety. Some patients become fixated on him and very possessive. They fabricate a relationship that does not exist and become jealous of his family. Rebuffed, some of them become threatening to us. These individuals at times are not even patients of my husband, have never met him in person, and know of him only through his books and articles. He will chat briefly with a person who admires his work and then give out personal information about our son and me because they ask.

One patient who has attempted to harm my husband through legal action and complaints has destroyed the life's work and reputation of another researcher. This person told a staff member of ours that she made her living suing physicians. I was only informed of this comment after her baseless accusations were dismissed, again at great financial and psychological cost to us. There is no protection for physicians against frivolous claims, and no controls or punishment for evil people of this kind when accusations are dismissed. One day my husband will quit his practice, driven out by those motivated by greed and malice. I understand that insurance companies are now, without patient permission, filing complaints against physicians who do not follow their rigid treatment protocols. This trend will hamstring innovative medical care even further than it is at present.

Recently a woman who knew him only as a speaker and author called him. He chatted with her and then the flood of letters and faxes began. He did not respond. The faxes and letters became angry and threatening. She described me as an evil person who did not, to put it mildly, have my husband's best interests at heart. She described in detail the sounds of animals in their death agonies and rambled on about dying Palestinian boys. Law enforcement in her state and in California agreed that she could be charged with terrorist threats, but she would have to be brought to California to face charges and would be free on bail, and therefore closer to my son and me. What a choice! I had to notify my son's school and explain the situation, so they could monitor him more carefully. I had to explain the danger to my son. I had to ask neighbors to watch our property. I decided that since the police and county social services in her state promised to monitor her, that I couldn't risk her being brought here to be closer to our son. All the while, Jay was blasé and indifferent to the situation, never believing anyone could ever hurt us. He "blew off" all my concerns and fears.

This is one of the downsides of my life. Although this is the worst of the threats, it is not over and never will be. I never know when another person will develop a fatal attraction to my husband and attempt to destroy our lives. I have become hypervigilant, attempting to protect my husband from himself, from vengeful patients, and from jealous or contemptuous so-called professionals in the field of CFS and fibromyalgia. It used to be a puzzle to me why fellow doctors and researchers would defame him and his work. Now, I just accept that their insecurities, pettiness, and/or blindness simply make them behave that way.

For 24 years I have stood by this man. I have shared in the chaos and miseries and successes of his practice. I worried about him and nursed him. When I read this chapter, I come across as self-pitying, with a bit of a martyr complex. Although we have problems, it is my choice to stay and support him as best I can.

While going through old correspondence, I came across a letter written to me by one of my husband's patients in 1993. It touched me, and was one of the few acknowledgments I received.

April 10, 1993
Dear Gail,
After our conversation this afternoon, I wanted to sit down and write a letter which I think you not only deserve, but quite frankly, perhaps need at this point.

I'm not a doctor's wife, but I have a good imagination and I also have a very good "sense" about people—good people. When we spoke today, I could feel your frustration, I could hear your unspoken anger, and most of all, I could almost *taste* your heart-breaking fatigue. I think perhaps it's been a very long time since someone from "our group" stopped to say to you, "Thanks . . . we don't know what we'd do without you." Oh, I'm sure they do—I'm sure you hear it all the time in passing—on the fly. But I bet most of the thanks you hear are for your husband. And we are thankful to him, of course. But it's usually the wife—the one behind the scenes—talking to patients (as well as your own)—quieting the nerves—softening the edges—who is left with all the phone calls, such as the one I made to you today. I'm not apologizing for that particular call, because I felt it had to be made, sorry as I was to make it—but I am sorry for the crazy calls you have no doubt received, no doubt will continue to receive, as long as you deal with CFIDS patients. And perhaps that's what I'm writing this letter to say. I am sorry for all the problems we create, not always due to this disease.

You have given ceaselessly to our cause. You have joined us in the enormous battle of disbelief, humiliation, and above all, financial insecurity. There are not many wives who would have "put up with us," let alone join us in our struggle. I just need to tell you how much we appreciate all that you have done—that we love both you and your husband, and that we are better people because you have touched our lives.

I'm sure people have thanked you many times, Gail—but today, while the sun spent its light and warmth on this beautiful holiday weekend, you spent your time and energy reassuring me, and I just want to say:

Thanks. I don't know what I'd do without you.

In summary, Jay is a good man who has given his life to his patients for little reward. I truly hope that the contributions he has made to better the lives of patients will not be forgotten once he has gone.

FIGURES

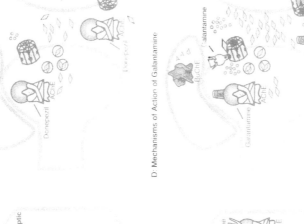

A: Normal Cholinergic Neuron Functioning

B: Mechanisms of Action of Donepezil

C: Mechanisms of Action of Rivastigmine

D: Mechanisms of Action of Galantamine

FIGURE 1. Inhibition of AchE causes Ach levels to increase. All three cholinesterase inhibitors block this enzyme (2B-D). Donepezil blocks only AchE (2B), thus improving cognition and possibly helping to reduce disruptive behavior common to Alzheimer patients. (*Source:* SM Stahl, The new cholinesterase inhibitors for Alzheimer's disease. Part 2. Illustrating their mechanisms of action. *The Journal of Clinical Psychiatry.* 61, 814. 2000. Copyright 2000, Physicians Postgraduate Press. Reprinted by permission.)

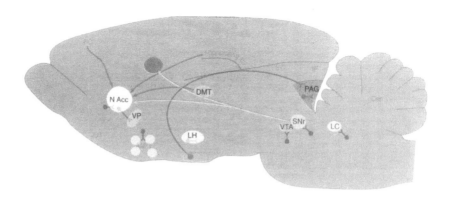

FIGURE 2. Sagittal section through the brain of a rat depicting the neurochemical systems implicated in the reinforcing effects of drugs of abuse. Yellow indicates limbic afferents to the nucleus accumbens (N. Acc). Orange represents efferents from the nucleus accumbens thought to be involved in psychomotor stimulant reward. Red indicates the projection of the mesocorticolimbic dopamine system thought to be a critical substrate for psychomotor stimulant reward. This system originates in the A10 cell group of the ventral tegmental area (VTA) and projects to the N. Acc., olfactory tubercle, and ventral striatal domains of the caudate-putamen (CP). (*Source:* Reprinted from *Fundamental Neuroscience,* 49, GF Koob, Drug reward and addiction, 1268, Copyright 1999, with permission from Elsevier.)

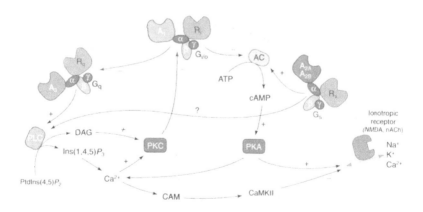

FIGURE 3. Schematic diagram of some of the mechanisms that might be involved in the interactions between adenosine receptors (A_1, A_2, and A_3) and other neurotransmitter or neuromodulator receptors in neurons. (*Source:* Reprinted from *Trends in Pharmacological Science,* 21, AM Sebastiao and JA Ribeiro, Fine-tuning neuromodulation by adenosine, 344, Copyright 2000, with permission from Elsevier.

FIGURE 4. Proposed role of the ATP-sensitive K^+ (K_{ATP}) channel on glucose-responsive (GR) neurons. GR neurons contain K_{ATP} channels composed of the Kir6.2 pore-forming unit and a sulfonylurea receptor (SUR). Glucose is transported into the cell body and terminal by a glucose transporter, possibly Glut2. The rate

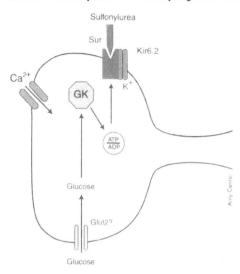

of glycolysis is regulated by glucokinase (GK). Glycolytic and oxidative (mitochondrial) metabolism of glucose raises the ATP/ADP ratio, causing ATP to bind to the K_{ATP} channel complex. This inactivates (closes) the channel, producing accumulation of intracellular K^+, membrane depolarization, influx of Ca^{2+} through a voltage-gated Ca^{2+} channel, and increased neuronal firing. Nerve terminal K_{ATP} channels can also lead to transmitter (glutamate and γ-aminobutyric acid, GABA) release. (*Source:* BE Levin et al., 2001, Brain glucosensing and the K-ATP channel. In *Nature Neuroscience,* 4(5), p. 459. Reprinted with permission.)

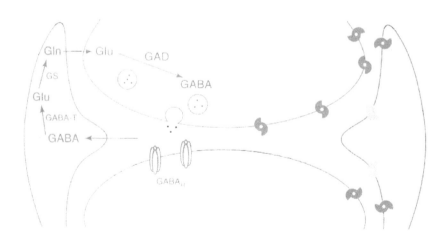

FIGURE 5. Factors influencing GABA transient in the cleft: plasma membrane transporters. Fate of GABA released from the axon terminal (left) and the location of different GABA transporters (GATs) (right). (*Source:* Reprinted from *Trends in Neurosciences,* 24, E Cherubini and F Conti, Generating diversity at GABAergic synapses, 157, Copyright 2001, with permission from Elsevier.)

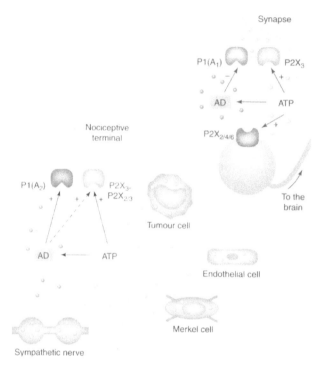

FIGURE 6. The roles of purine nucleotides and nucleosides in pain pathways. At sensory nerve terminals in the periphery, the $P2X_3$ receptor has been identified as the principal P2X receptor present. The $P2X_3$ receptor is found predominantly in sensory ganglia, and it might work in heteromultimeric combination with other P2X receptors, such as $P2X_2$. Other known P2X receptor subtypes are also expressed at low levels in dorsal root ganglia. Although less potent than ATP, adenosine (AD) also appears to act on sensory terminals, probably directly via adenosine A_2 receptors; however, it might also act (broken arrow) to potentiate $P2X_3$ or $P2X_{2/3}$ activation. At synapses in sensory pathways in the CNS, ATP appears to act both presynaptically via $P2X_3$ receptors to enhance glutamate release and postsynaptically via $P2X_2$ and/or $P2X_4$ and $P2X_6$ receptor subtypes, and after breakdown to adenosine, it acts as a prejunctional inhibitor of transmission via adenosine A_1 receptors. Sources of ATP acting on $P2X_{2/3}$ sensory terminals include sympathetic nerves and endothelial, Merkel, and tumour cells. Molecules of ATP area represented by green circles, and molecules of adenosine are represented by red circles. (*Source:* Reprinted from *Trends in Pharmacological Sciences,* 22, G Burnstock, Purine-mediated signaling in pain and visceral perception, 185, Copyright 2001, with permission from Elsevier.)

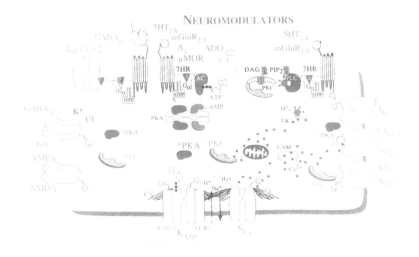

NEUROMODULATORS

FIGURE 7. Schematic illustration of receptor-activated intracellular signaling pathways and modulation of ion channels. Metabolism and voltage-controlled are the channels that are sensitive to cytosolic ATP (K_{ATP}), which in respiratory neurons are homomeric Kir6.2 channels binding to sulfonylurea-sensitive SUR receptors, and a group of voltage- and calcium-activated K^+ channels K_{Ca}. (*Source:* DW Richter et al., *The Neuroscientist* 6(3), p. 187, copyright © 2000 by Sage Publications. Reprinted by permission of Sage Publications.)

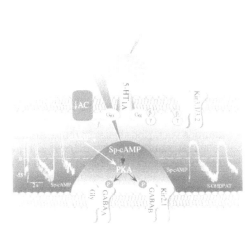

FIGURE 8. 5-HT$_{1A}$ receptor agonists depress excitability of respiratory neurons by inhibition of PKA. The intracellular signal pathways activated by 5-HT$_{1A}$ receptors are indicated by scheme that is also a frame for insets of original measurements in the anesthetized cat. The scheme indicates that activation of 5-HT$_{1A}$ receptors may activate two divergent pathways: A, inhibition of adenylylcyclase (AC) through an inhibitory $G_{i\alpha}$ protein reduces (cAMP); and decreases PKA-mediated phosphorylation of voltage- and ligand-controlled channels. Glycine and GABA$_{AB}$ as well as inwardly rectifying Kir2.1 K^+ channels are listed as the predominant targets. (*Source:* DW Richter et al., *The Neuroscientist* 6(3), p. 189, copyright ©2000 by Sage Publications. Reprinted by permission of Sage Publications.)

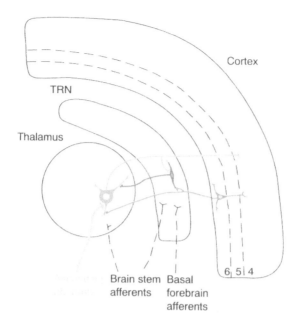

FIGURE 9. The major connections between thalamic relay cells (blue), cells of the thalamic reticular nucleus (TRN; red) and the cerebral cortex (orange). Cortical layers 4, 5, and 6 are indicated by numbers. (*Source:* Reprinted from *Trends in Neurosciences,* 21, RW Guillery et al., Paying attention to the thalamic reticular nucleus, 29, Copyright 1998, with permission from Elsevier.)

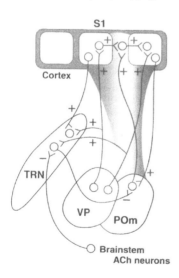

FIGURE 10. A possible role for intrathalamic inhibition in regulating cortical plasticity. VP projects to the barrel domains in layer IV of S1 cortex, and POm axons project to the septa around the barrels, where they promote intracortical spread of activity. The TRN normally inhibits POm neurons via an intrathalamic route. Arousal activates neurons that inhibit the TRN, thereby reducing its inhibition of POm neurons, which increases cortical plasticity. (*Source:* J Kaas, Ebner F, 1998, Intrathalamic connections: A new way to modulate cortical plasticity? In *Nature Neuroscience,* 1(5), p. 342. Reprinted with permission.)

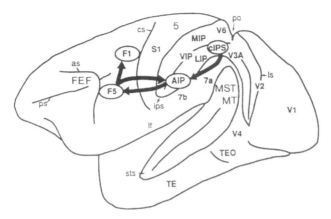

FIGURE 11. The location of cortical areas related to spatial attention in the macaque brain. Modified from Sakata et al. Abbreviations: as = arcuate sulcus; cIPS = caudal intraparietal sulcus; cs = central sulcus; FEF = frontal eye field; F1 = primary motor area; F5 = hand region of ventral premotor cortex; ips = intraparietal sulcus; lf = lateral (sylvian) fissure; LIP = lateral intraparietal area; ls = lunate sulcus; MIP = medial intraparietal area; po = parieto-occipital sulcus; MT (V5), MST = motion-sensitive visual areas of the superior temporal sulcus; ps = principal sulcus; sts = superior temporal sulcus; S1 = primary somatosensory area; TE and TEO = inferotemporal visual association areas; VIP = ventral intraparietal area; V1-4, V6 = the primary, secondary, third, fourth, and sixth visual areas; 5, 7a, 7b = Brodmann areas. (*Source:* M-M Mesulam, 2000, p. 222. From *Principles of behavioral and cognitive neurology* by Marek-Marsel Mesulam, copyright— 2000 by Oxford University Press, Inc. Used by permission of Oxford University Press, Inc.)

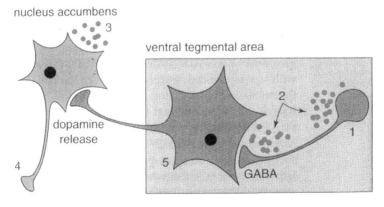

FIGURE 12. A tonic GABA inhibitory neuron (1) is inhibitd by a mu opioid (2), which binds to heteroreceptors on the neuron. Release of dopamine from the nucleus accumbens (3,4) occurs because the ventral tegmental area neurons (5) are disinhibited. This process in part accounts for the stimulatory effects of opioids in some patients. (*Source:* Koob GF, 1992)

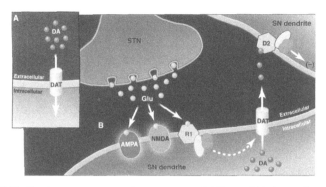

FIGURE 13. Putting transporters into reverse. DATs on SN dopaminergic neurons export as well as import DA. (A) DATs are thought to be involved in the elimination of extracellular DA after its release at synapses between neurons. (B) However, the finding that there is modulated efflux of DA from the dendrites of SN dopaminergic neurons suggests that DATs may be able to export as well as import DA. (*Source:* Reprinted with permission from RD Blakely, 2001, Dopamine's reversal of fortune. *Science* 293(5539), p. 2408. Copyright 2001 American Association for the Advancement of Science.)

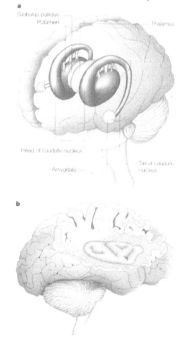

FIGURE 14. The human amygdala, basal ganglia, and insula. (*Source:* Reprinted by permission from *Nature Reviews Neuroscience,* AJ Calder et al., Neuropsychology of fear and loathing, p. 353. Copyright 2001 Macmillan Magazines Ltd.)

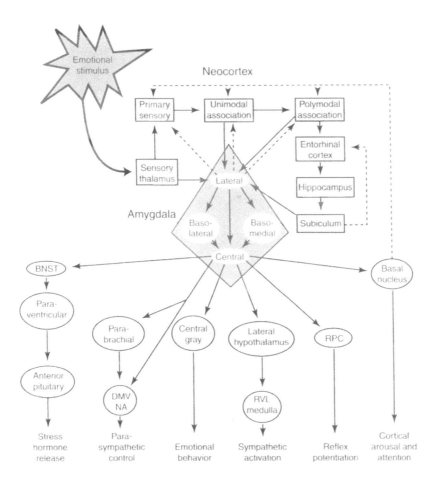

FIGURE 15. A model of the neural circuit involved in conditioned fear. A hierarchy of incoming sensory information converges on the lateral nucleus of the amygdala. Through intra-amygdala circuitry, the output of the lateral nucleus is transmitted to the central nucleus, which serves to activate various effector systems involved in the expression of emotional responses. Feedforward projections are indicated by solid lines, and feedback projections are indicated by dashed lines. BNST, bed nucleus of the stria terminalis; DMV, dorsal motor nucleus of the vagus; NA, nucleus ambiguus; RPC, nucleus reticularis pontis caudalis; RVL Medulla, rostral ventrolateral nuclei of the medulla. (*Source:* Reprinted from *Fundamental Neuroscience*, 55, JM Beggs et al., Learning and memory: Basic mechanisms, 1435, Copyright 1999, with permission from Elsevier.)

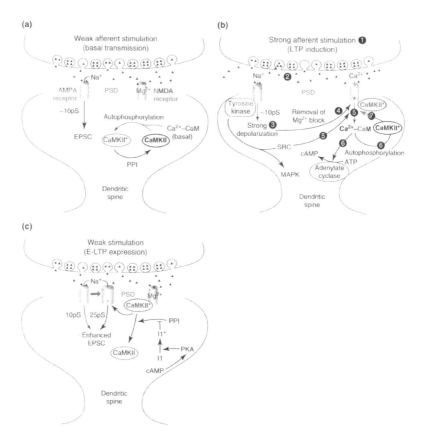

FIGURE 16. Postsynaptic protein phosphorylation mechanisms during LTP in the CA1 region of hippocampus. (a) Basal synaptic transmission via glutamate (triangles) is mediated largely by low-conductance state (~10pS) AMPA receptors that give rise to an EPSC. NMDA receptors are inactive because of voltage-dependent block of their channels by Mg^{2+}. (b) LTP induction by tetanic afferent stimulation (1) elicits enhanced glutamate exocytosis (2) and strong post-synaptic depolarization via AMPA receptors (3) to remove the Mg^{2+} block of the NMDA receptor (4) AMPA-receptor stimulation also activates associated SRC-family tyrosine kinases that phosphorylate (*) and further enhance conductance of the NMDA-receptor channel, which is permeable to Ca^{2+} (5) The elevated levels of the Ca^{2+}-CaM complex stimulate type-1 adenylate cyclase and also stimulates autophosphorylation (*) of CaMKII (6) This constitutively active CaMKII translocates to the postsynaptic density (PSD), in part through interaction with the NMDA receptor (7) (c) Early-phase LTP (E-LTP) expression is due, in part, to CaMKII-mediated phosphorylation of the AMPA receptor GluR1 subunit (*), which converts it largely to higher conductance states (~25 pS). (*Source:* Reprinted from *Trends in Neurosciences,* 23, TR Soderling and VA Derkach, Postsynaptic protein phosphorylation and LTP, 76, Copyright © 2000, with permission from Elsevier.)

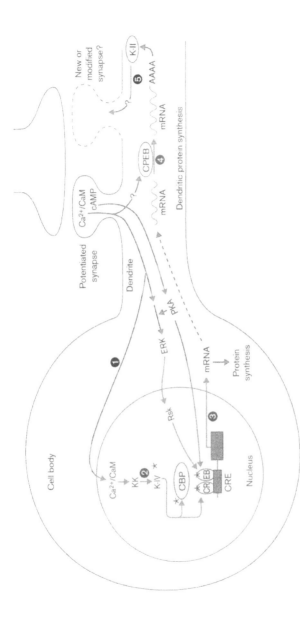

FIGURE 17. Putative roles of CaM-kinases in late-phase synaptic plasticity. Synaptic potentiation can cause translocation of Ca²⁺/CaM from the potentiated spine to the nucleus (reaction 1) with resulting activation of CaM-KIV (reaction 2) and CREB-mediated transcription (reaction 3). Other potential CREB kinases and activation pathways stimulated by LTP are shown for reference. mRNA for CaM-KII, and selected other proteins required for L-LTP, are transported out into dendrites (dotted line). Localized protein synthesis from mRNAs, such as CaM-KII, in the dendrite can be stimulated by activation of CEPB (reaction 4). The increased CaM-KII (and other proteins) may be involved in remodeling or formation of new synapses at potentiated sites (reaction 5). KK, CaM-KK; K-IV, CaM-KIV; *, phosphorylation. (*Source:* Reprinted from *Current Opinion in Neurobiology*, 10, TR Soderling, CaM-kinases: Modulators of synaptic plasticity, 377, Copyright 2000, with permission from Elsevier.)

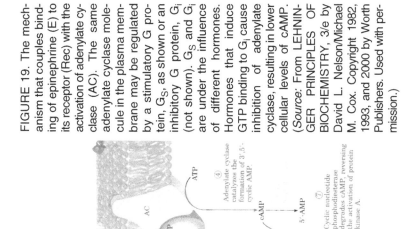

FIGURE 19. The mechanism that couples binding of epinephrine (E) to its receptor (Rec) with the activation of adenylate cyclase (AC). The same adenylate cyclase molecule in the plasma membrane may be regulated by a stimulatory G protein, G_S, as shown or an inhibitory G protein, G_i (not shown). G_S and G_i are under the influence of different hormones. Hormones that induce GTP binding to G_i cause inhibition of adenylate cyclase, resulting in lower cellular levels of cAMP. (*Source:* From LEHNINGER PRINCIPLES OF BIOCHEMISTRY, 3/e by David L. Nelson/Michael M. Cox. Copyright 1982, 1993, and 2000 by Worth Publishers. Used with permission.)

① Epinephrine binds to a specific receptor.

② The occupied receptor causes replacement of the GDP bound to G_s by GTP, activating $G_{s\alpha}$.

③ G_s (α subunit) moves to adenylate cyclase and activates it.

④ Adenylate cyclase catalyzes the formation of 3',5'-cyclic AMP.

⑤ cAMP-dependent protein kinase (protein kinase A) is activated by cAMP.

⑥ Phosphorylation of cellular proteins by protein kinase causes the cellular response to epinephrine.

⑦ Cyclic nucleotide phosphodiesterase degrades cAMP, reversing the activation of protein kinase A.

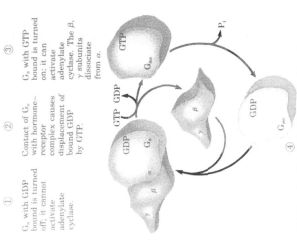

① G_s with GDP bound is turned off; it cannot activate adenylate cyclase.

② Contact of G_s with hormone–receptor complex causes displacement of bound GDP by GTP.

③ G_s with GTP bound is turned on; it can activate adenylate cyclase. The β, γ subunits dissociate from α.

④ GTP bound to G_s is hydrolyzed by the intrinsic GTPase at $G_{s\alpha}$; $G_{s\alpha}$ thereby turns itself "off." The inactive α subunit reassociates with the β, γ subunits.

FIGURE 18. The protein G_S acts as a self-inactivating switch. (*Source:* From LEHNINGER PRINCIPLES OF BIOCHEMISTRY, 3/e by David L. Nelson/Michael M. Cox. Copyright 1982, 1993, and 2000 by Worth Publishers. Used with permission.)

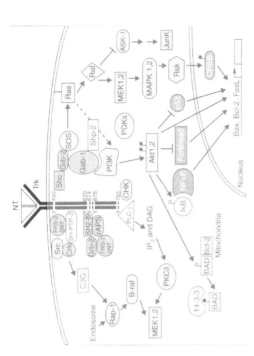

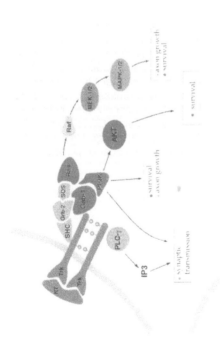

FIGURE 20. Neurotrophins bind to and stimulate the activity of their receptors, the Trk tyrosine kinases. The activated Trk receptors in turn activate multiple signal transduction pathways that mediate cell survival, axonal growth, and synaptic transmission. Both PI-3 kinase and PLC regulated synaptic transmission, through the generation of their respective second messenger molecules, PIP3 and IP3. (*Source:* DR Kaplan, E Cooper, 2001, PI-3 kinase and IP3: Partners in NT3-induced synaptic transmission. In *Nature Neuroscience*, 4(1), p. 6. Reprinted with permission.)

FIGURE 21. Diagram of neurotrophin signal transduction pathways mediated by Trk receptors. The nomenclature for tyrosine residues of Trk receptors is based on the sequence of human TrkA. In the diagram, adapter proteins are colored orange, kinases pink, small G proteins green, and transcription factors blue. APS, adaptor molecule containing PH and SH2 domains; CHK, Csk homologue kinase; MEK, MAPK/ERK; P, serine/threonine (filled, phosphorylated); SNT, suc-1-associated neurotrophic factor target. (*Source:* Reprinted from *Current Opinion in Neurobiology*, 11, A Patapoutian and LF Reichardt, TRK receptors: Mediators of neurotrophin action, p. 274, Copyright 2000, with permission from Elsevier.)

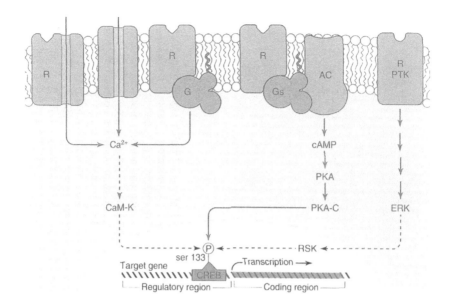

FIGURE 22. Schematic illustration of the mechanism by which diverse types of first messengers converge on the phosphorylation of serine 133 of cAMP response element-binding protein (CREB). Some first messengers do this by increasing cAMP concentrations by activation of G protein-coupled receptors (R), G_S, adenylyl cyclase (AC) and cAMP-dependent protein kinase (PKA), which then phosphorylates CREB on ser 133. Others do so by increasing Ca^{2+} concentrations by activation of ionotropic receptors (R) that flux Ca^{2+}, by activation of voltage-gated Ca2+ channels through membrane depolarization or by activation of G protein-coupled receptors that elevate intracellular Ca^{2+} concentrations, for example, via the phospholipase C pathway. Increased concentrations of Ca^{2+} then lead to activation of Ca^{2+}/calmodulin-dependent protein kinases (type IV and, possibly, I) (CaM-K), which also phosphorylate CREB on ser 133. (*Source:* EJ Nestler and P Greengard, in *Basic neurochemistry: Molecular, cellular, and medical aspects, Sixth Edition,* GJ Siegel et al., eds. Lippincott, 1999. Used with permission.)

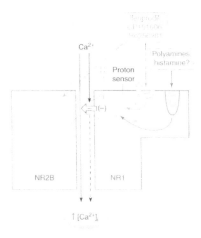

FIGURE 23. Interactions between endogenous modulators and ifenprodil-like selective antagonists of NR2B-containing NMDA receptors. By modulating the proton sensor, polyamines selectively potentiate this subtype of NMDA receptor, whereas ifenprodil-like compounds selectively inhibit this receptor subtype. (*Source:* Reprinted from *Trends in Pharmacological Sciences,* 22, BA Chizh et al., NMDA receptor antagonists as analgesics: Focus on the NR2B subtype, 637, Copyright 2001, with permission from Elsevier.)

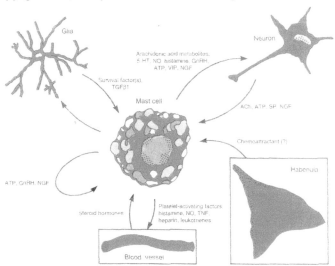

FIGURE 24. This schematic shows a composite mast cell in relation to other elements of the brain. It is presented so as to emphasize the potential range of components of the CNS that might be influenced—and that in turn might influence—mast cells. (*Source:* Reprinted from *Trends in Neurosciences,* 19, R Silver et al., Mast cells in the brain: Evidence and functional significance, 30, Copyright 1996, with permission from Elsevier.)

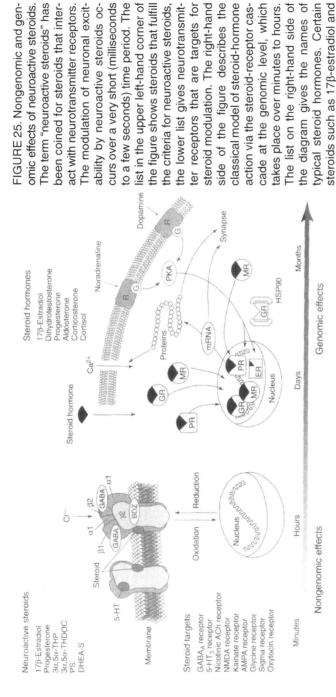

FIGURE 25. Nongenomic and genomic effects of neuroactive steroids. The term "neuroactive steroids" has been coined for steroids that interact with neurotransmitter receptors. The modulation of neuronal excitability by neuroactive steroids occurs over a very short (milliseconds to a few seconds) time period. The list in the upper left-hand corner of the figure shows steroids that fulfill the criteria for neuroactive steroids, the lower list gives neurotransmitter receptors that are targets for steroid modulation. The right-hand side of the figure describes the classical model of steroid-hormone action via the steroid-receptor cascade at the genomic level, which takes place over minutes to hours. The list on the right-hand side of the diagram gives the names of typical steroid hormones. Certain steroids such as 17β-estradiol and progesterone have to be defined both as steroid hormones and as neuroactive steroids. Abbreviations: BDZ, benzodiazepines; DHEA-S, dehydroepiandrosterone sulfate; ER, estrogen receptor; G, G-protein; GR, glucocorticoid receptor; HSP90, heat-shock protein 90; MR, mineralocorticoid receptor; PKA, protein kinase A; PR, progesterone receptor; PS, pregnenolone sulfate; R, receptor; THDOC, tetrahydrodeoxycorticosterone; THP, tetrahydroprogesterone. (*Source:* Reprinted from *Trends in Neurosciences,* 22, R Rupprecht and F Holsboer, Neuroactive steroids: Mechanism of action and neuropsychopharmacological perspectives, 414, Copyright 1999, with permission from Elsevier.)

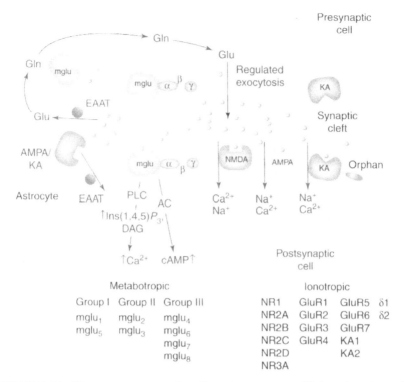

Metabotropic			Ionotropic			
Group I	Group II	Group III	NR1	GluR1	GluR5	δ1
mglu$_1$	mglu$_2$	mglu$_4$	NR2A	GluR2	GluR6	δ2
mglu$_5$	mglu$_3$	mglu$_6$	NR2B	GluR3	GluR7	
		mglu$_7$	NR2C	GluR4	KA1	
		mglu$_8$	NR2D		KA2	
			NR3A			

FIGURE 26. Glutamate receptor function at a synapse. Glutamate released from presynaptic neurons diffuses across the synaptic cleft to bind to receptors on the postsynaptic cell membrane (although presynaptic receptors have been identified, their function is not well understood). G-protein-coupled metabotropic glutamate (mglu) receptors are divided into three groups: Group I receptors (mglu$_1$ and mglu$_5$) are coupled to phospholipase C (PLC), and Groups II and III receptors initiate the inhibitory cAMP pathway. Ionotropic receptors (NMDA, AMPA, and kainate receptors) are ligand-gated ion channels with permeability primarily for Na^+ and Ca^{2+}. The function of the orphan receptors (δ1 and δ2) is not known. Released glutamate is removed predominantly by specific excitatory amino acid transporters (EAAT1-5) expressed by neighboring astrocytes, although neuronal cells also express glutamate transporters. Within the astrocytes, accumulated glutamate is converted to glutamine and delivered to the presynaptic cell, which via mitochondrial glutaminase forms glutamate for re-release. Astrocytes have also been shown to express AMPA and kainate ionotropic receptors as well as metabotropic receptors, providing evidence for bidirectional glutamate signalling between neurones and astrocytes. Abbreviations: AC, adenylyl cyclase; DAG, diacylglycerol; Gln, glutamine; Glu, glutamate; Ins(1,4,5)P_3, inositol (1,4,5)-trisphosphate; KA, kainate. (*Source:* Reprinted from *Trends in Pharmacological Sciences*, 2, TM Skerry and PG Genever, Glutamate signaling in non-neuronal tissues, 175, Copyright 2001, with permission from Elsevier.)

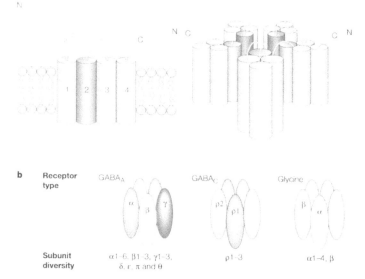

FIGURE 27. Proposed pentameric structures of GAGA_A, GABA_C, and glycine receptor subtypes. Most GABA_A receptors are believed to be composed of α, β, and γ subunits in the ratio of 2:2:1. The δ, ε, and θ subunits can replace the δ subunit in some receptor subtypes. (*Source:* Reprinted by permission from *Nature Reviews Neuroscience,* SJ Moss and TG Smart, Constructing inhibitory synapses, p. 241. Copyright 2001 Macmillan Magazines Ltd.)

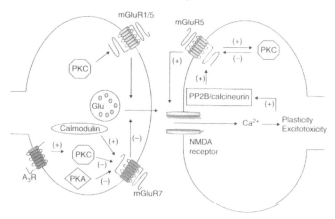

FIGURE 28. Diagram of synaptic regulation of metabotropic glutamate receptors (mGluRs). A_3R_1, adenosine receptor; Glu, glutamate; PP2B, phosphatase 2B. (*Source:* Reprinted from *Current Opinion in Neurobiology,* 11, S Alagarsamy et al., Coordinate regulation of metabotropic glutamate receptors, 359, Copyright 2001, with permission from Elsevier.)

a Homosynaptic (activity-dependent)
plastic change

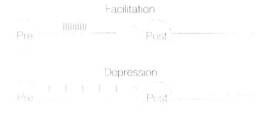

b Heterosynaptic (modulatory input-dependent)
plastic change

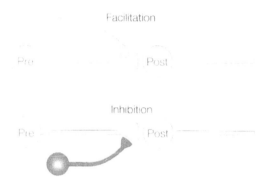

FIGURE 29. Homosynaptic and heterosynaptic mechanisms for long-term plasticity. (a) The plastic changes that underlie long-term memory follow a homosynaptic rule, that is, the events responsible for triggering synaptic strengthening occur at the same synapse as is being strengthened. These changes can result in an increase in synaptic strength (for example, homosynaptic facilitation), or a decrease in synaptic strength (for example, homosynaptic depression). (b) Synaptic strengthening between a presynaptic and a postsynaptic cell can occur as a result of the firing of a third neuron, a modulatory interneuron, whose terminals end on and regulate the strength of the specific synapse. These changes can result in an increase (heterosynaptic, modulatory facilitation) or in a decrease (heterosynaptic inhibition) in synaptic strength. (*Source:* Reprinted by permission from *Nature Reviews Neuroscience,* CH Bailey et al., Is heterosynaptic modulation essential for stabilizing hebbian plasticity and memory?, p. 12. Copyright 2000 Macmillan Magazines Ltd.)

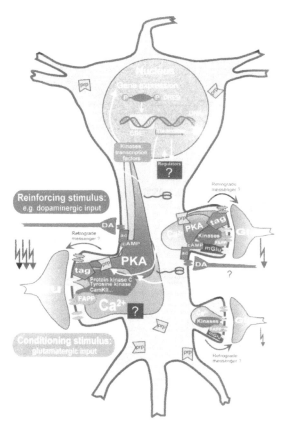

FIGURE 30. A model of the cellular processes specifically required for the induction of late LTP in the hippocampal CA1 region. Late LTP involves mRNA and protein synthesis at extrasynaptic but intracellular sites. Induction of early LTP involves mechanisms restricted to the activated synapse. High-frequency stimulation of fibers in the stratum radiatum leads to the associative and co-operative activation of the glutamatergic NMDA receptor. Influx of CA^{2+} activates intracellular processes necessary for early LTP (activation of "fast-acting plasticity processors" [FAPPS]). During the early period immediately after LTP induction, a synaptic tag is set. Anatomical changes and phosphorylation of receptors and kinases are possible tag candidates. In addition to glutamatergic activation, a separate signal, activation of dopaminergic receptors, must arrive to activate the cAMP/PKA-pathway. This leads to gene activation and, in turn, to the synthesis and distribution of plasticity-related-proteins (prp) that can be captured by synaptic tags to reveal or stabilize new effector mechanisms (such as new receptors or ion channels). At this stage of LTP consolidation, the FAPPs will be reset, allowing additional change at these synapses. (*Source:* Reprinted from *Trends in Neurosciences,* 21, U Frey and RGM Morris, Synaptic tagging: Implications for late maintenance of hippocampal long-term potentiation, 185, Copyright 1998, with permission from Elsevier.)

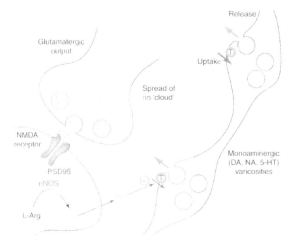

FIGURE 31. Activation of neuronal nitric oxide synthase (nNOS) in the CNS. Release of glutamate stimulates NMDA receptors, and the concomitant influx of Ca^{2+} (not shown) activates nNOS coupled to the receptor via PSD95. NO synthesized by the enzyme spreads over in a sphere and reaches monoaminergic varicosities in the environment of activated synapses. The actual extracellular concentration of monoamines depends on the balance of release and uptake processes. The nonsynaptic signal, that is, the appearance of NO, inhibits the function of transporters (T), which increases the extracellular concentration of monoamines in a local volume around the activated glutamatergic synapse, even if the amount of released monoamines is unchanged. (*Source:* Reprinted from *Trends in Neurosciences,* 24, JP Kiss and ES Vizi, Nitric oxide: A novel link between synaptic and nonsynaptic transmission, 213, 214, Copyright 2000, with permission from Elsevier.)

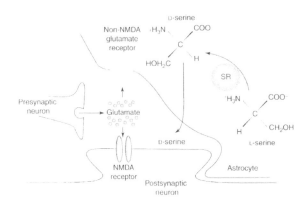

FIGURE 32. D-serine is a co-agonist at the NMDA receptor. Type II astrocytes ensheath synapses containing NMDA receptors. In these astrocytes, D-serine is synthesized from L-serine, by a cytosolic enzyme, serine racemase (SR). When the presynaptic neuron releases glutamate, it acts not only on the postsynaptic neuron, but also on the surrounding astrocyte. Activation of the astrocytes non-NMDA glutamate receptors releases D-serine, which binds to the NMDA receptor at the same site as glycine. The concerted binding of D-serine and glutamate results in opening of the NMDA receptor channel. (*Source:* Reprinted from *Trends in Neurosciences,* 24, DE Barañano et al., Atypical neural messengers, 103, Copyright 2001, with permission from Elsevier.)

(a)

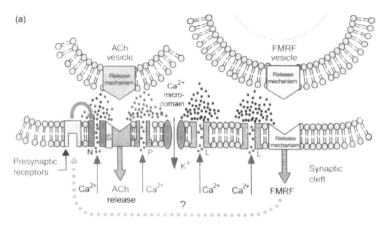

FIGURE 33a. The role of the different types of presynaptic Ca²⁺ channels. The Ca²⁺ influx is also modulated by syntaxin *S*. (*Source:* Reprinted from *Trends in Neurosciences,* 22, P Fossier et al., Calcium transients and neurotransmitter release at an identified synapse, 162, Copyright 1999, with permission from Elsevier.)

(b)

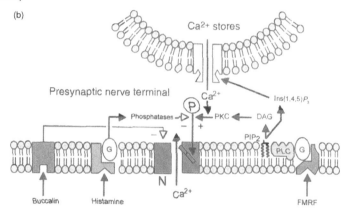

FIGURE 33b. Modulation of Ca²⁺ influx through N-type channels by presynaptic receptors. The stimulation of Phe-Met-Arg-Phe (FMRF) receptors, activates a G protein (G) and phospholipase C (PLC), which leads to the synthesis of diacylglycerol (DAG) and Ins(1,4,5)P₃. Diacylglycerol activates protein kinase C (PKC), which phosphorylates N-type Ca²⁺ channels thus increasing their voltage sensitivity. Ca²⁺ released from presynaptic Ca²⁺ stores by Ins(1,4,5)P₃ could either participate in the triggering of ACh release or act as a cofactor in the phosphorylation of N-type Ca²⁺ channels. Conversely, histamine induces a dephosphorylation of N-type Ca²⁺ channels through the activation of a G protein and a phosphatase. Buccalin reduces Ca²⁺ influx by another mechanism that does not involve a G protein or affect the threshold of activation of N-type channels. (*Source:* Reprinted from *Trends in Neurosciences,* 22, P Fossier et al., Calcium transients and neurotransmitter release at an identified synapse, 163, Copyright 1999, with permission from Elsevier.)

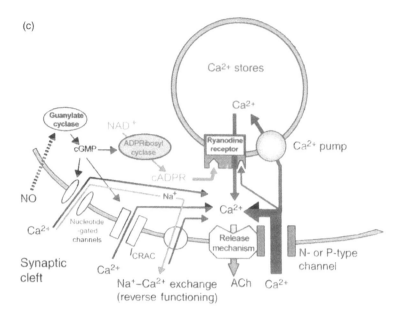

(c)

FIGURE 33c. Some of the Ca^{2+} entering the nerve terminal through N- and P-type channels activates the ryanodine receptor. Ca^{2+} released from Ca^{2+} stores participates in the triggering of ACh release. The ryanodine receptor is sensitized by cADPR produced from NAD^+ by ADPRibosyl cyclase (ADPR cyclase). This enzyme can be activated by cGMP via the nitric oxide (NO)-cGMP pathway. cGMP can also open cyclic-nucleotide-gated channels, which allow Ca^{2+} or Na^+ influx into the nerve terminal. The induced increase in intracellular Ca^{2+} concentration, which has been detected by Ca^{2+} imaging following cGMP injection, could result either from direct Ca^{2+} influx or from a massive influx of Na+ that leads to a reverse functioning of the Na^+-Ca^{2+} exchanger, similar to the mechanisms proposed to underlie ciguatera disease. cGMP has also been described to be a regulator of store-operated Ca^{2+} influxes of which Ca^{2+} release-activated Ca^{2+} current (I_{CRAC}) is the best characterized. (*Source:* Reprinted from *Trends in Neurosciences,* 22, P Fossier et al., Calcium transients and neurotransmitter release at an identified synapse, 165, Copyright 1999, with permission from Elsevier.)

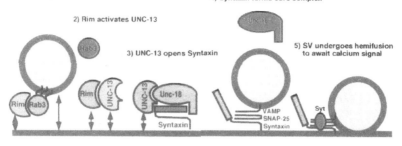

FIGURE 34. Model for priming of synaptic vesicles. Green, on; yellow, neutral; red, off. Double arrows, proteins localizing to the active zone are unknown. (*Source:* TE Lloyd, JH Bellen, 2001, pRIMing synaptic vesicles for fusion. In *Nature Neuroscience,* 4(10), p. 966. Reprinted with permission.)

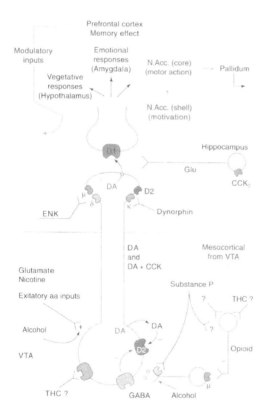

FIGURE 35. Schematic representation of the different substances able to produce rewarding responses by stimulation of the activity of dopamine-containing neurons located in the ventral tegmental area (VTA). Deletions of genes encoding mu (μ), D2, NK_1, or THC receptors or administration of naloxone have shown that the firing of dopamine-containing neurons seems crucially dependent on regulation by endogenous opioids of the dopamine mesolimbic pathway. A very simplified hypothesis to explain these data could be that the threshold to reach strong opioid-related rewarding responses is modulated by the local concentrations of the various neurotransmitters and neuropeptides released at the level of dopamine-containing neurons. This provides some support to the theory of an imbalance in the endogenous opioid system in vulnerability to drug dependence. (*Source:* Reprinted from *Trends in Pharmacological Sciences,* 21, BP Roques, Novel approaches to targeting neuropeptide systems, 481, Copyright 2000, with permission from Elsevier.)

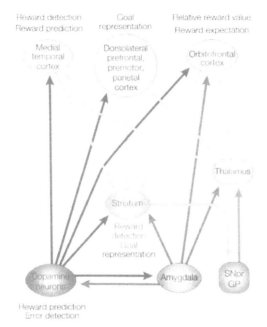

FIGURE 36. Reward processing and the brain. Many reward signals are processed by the brain, including those that are responsible for the detection of past rewards, the prediction and expectation of future rewards, and the use of information about future rewards to control goal-directed behavior. (SNpr, substantia nigra pars reticulata; GP, globus pallidus.) (*Source:* Reprinted by permission from *Nature Reviews Neuroscience,* W Schultz, Multiple reward signals in the brain, p. 200. Copyright 2000 Macmillan Magazines Ltd.)

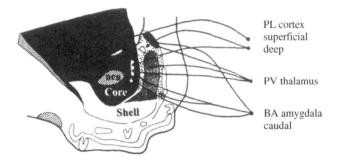

FIGURE 37. Convergence and segregation of accumbens afferents. Schematic representation of the relationships of three fiber systems of the medial part of the accumbens: the prelimbic area (PL) of the prefrontal cortex, the midline paraventricular thalamic nucleus (PV), and the caudal part of the basal amygdaloid complex (BA). (*Source: Journal of Neuropsychiatry and Clinical Neuroscience,* 9, 364, 1997, Copyright 1997, the American Psychiatric Association; http://JNCN. psychiatryonline.org. Reprinted by permission.)

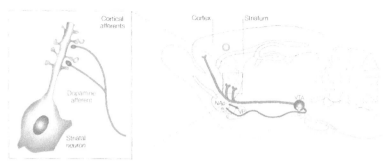

FIGURE 38. Dopamine-glutamate interactions in the striatum. Approximately 95 percent of neurons in the dorsal striatum and nucleus accumbens (NAc) are medium-sized spiny projection neurons, which use GABA (γ-aminobutyric acid) as their main neurotransmitter. These neurons receive glutamatergic projections from the cerebral cortex, which form well-defined synapses on the heads of dendritic spines. Dopaminergic axons from the midbrain pass by the necks of spines, where they release neurotransmitter; however, dopamine receptors are widely distributed on the cell membrane, including the soma. (*Source:* Reprinted by permission from *Nature Reviews Neuroscience,* SE Hyman and RC Malenka, Addiction and the brain: The neurobiology of compulsion and its persistence, p. 699. Copyright 2001 Macmillan Magazines Ltd.)

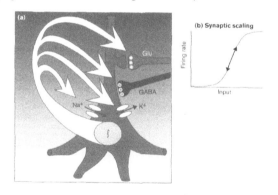

FIGURE 39. (a) Homeostatic plasticity uses some measure of activity (such as integrating average firing rate over some long time scale, indicated by the integral sign) to adjust excitatory and inhibitory synaptic strengths, as well as the voltage-dependent conductances (Na+ and K+) that control neuronal firing properties. These two forms of homeostatic plasticity are likely to have different functions in cortical networks. (b) By scaling the strength of all of a neuron's inputs up or down ("synaptic scaling"), a neuron's properties can be shifted up or down its input/output curve; this determines how fast the neuron fires for a given amount of synaptic drive. Excitatory and inhibitory inputs can be regulated independently, which allows neurons (and circuits) to adjust the balance of excitation and inhibition in an activity-dependent way. (*Source:* Reprinted from *Current Opinion in Neurobiology,* 10, GG Turrigiano and SB Nelson, Hebb and homeostasis in neuronal plasticity, 359, Copyright 2000, with permission from Elsevier.)

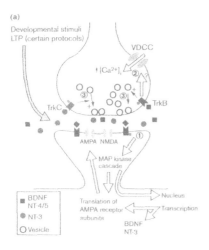

(a)
Developmental stimuli
LTP (certain protocols)

VDCC

↑[Ca²⁺]ᵢ

TrkC

TrkB

AMPA NMDA

MAP kinase cascade

Nucleus

Translation of AMPA receptor subunits

Transcription

BDNF NT-3

■ BDNF NT-4/5
● NT-3
○ Vesicle

FIGURE 40. Neurotrophins and local protein synthesis: involvement in synaptic plasticity and maturation. (a) Schematic diagram of neurotrophin's involvement in synaptic plasticity during development and after LTP stimulation. Neurotrophins have strong short- and long-term effects on synaptic transmission and intrinsic excitability of target neurons. Binding of neurotrophins (BDNF, NT-4/5, and, in some cases, NGF) to Trk receptors triggers the Ras-MAP kinase cascade (1) thereby influencing gene expression and translation activation (including AMPA receptor subunit synthesis). Activation (phosphorylation) or TrkB and TrkC receptors results in increased intracellular Ca²⁺ concentration (2) through voltage-dependent Ca²⁺ channels (VDCCs). Their ligands, BDNF and NT-3, strengthen glutamatergic transmission. The presence of Trk receptors at the synapse is essential for its maturation and vesicle clustering at presynaptic membrane (3), as well as for vesicle exocytosis and neurotransmitter release. (*Source:* Reprinted from *Current Opinion in Neurobiology,* 9, AY Klintsova and W Greenough, Synaptic plasticity in cortical systems, 204, Copyright 1999, with permission from Elsevier.)

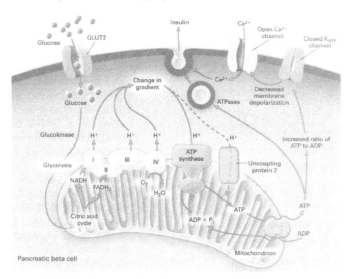

FIGURE 41. Opening the K_{ATP} channel decreases Ca⁺⁺ influx and neurotransmitter secretion. (*Source:* D Langin, 2001, Diabetes, insulin secretion, and the pancreatic beta-cell mitochondrion. *The New England Journal of Medicine* 345(24), p. 1773. Copyright © 2001 Massachusetts Medical Society. All rights reserved.)

FIGURE 42. The circuitry mediating the perception of reward and the initiation of adaptive behavioral responding to reward. Three major transmitter systems used in the circuit are indicated, although other transmitters, such as enkephalin, serotonin, and acetylcholine, are also present in the circuit. The nucleus accumbens is viewed as a primary anatomical locus for integrating GABAergic, glutamatergic, and dopaminergic input, and the ventral pallidum is viewed as the primary output nucleus communicating with classic motor systems. (*Source:* Reprinted from *Current Opinion in Neurobiology,* 9, PW Kalivas and M Nakamura, Neural systems for behavioral activation and reward, 223, Copyright 1999, with permission from Elsevier.)

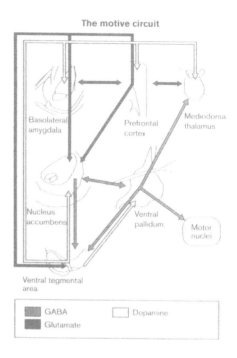

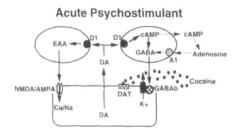

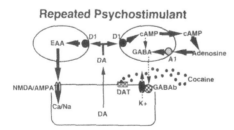

FIGURE 43. Changes in the VTA associated with the expression of behavioral sensitization to psychostimulants. There is a long-term increase in glutamate transmission and a decrease in D_1-stimulated GABA transmission in the VTA following repeated injections of cocaine. Bold lines represent increases, while dotted lines indicate decreases in neurotransmission. (*Source:* Reprinted from *Brain Research Reviews,* 25, RC Pierce and PW Kalivas, A circuitry model of the expression of behavioral sensitization to amphetamine-like psychostimulants, 204, Copyright 1997, with permission from Elsevier.)

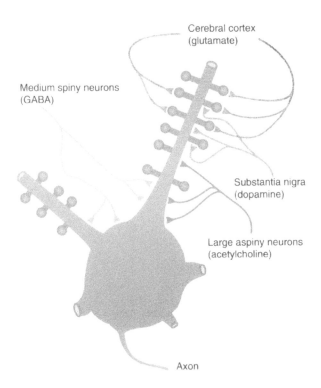

Cerebral cortex
(glutamate)

Medium spiny neurons
(GABA)

Substantia nigra
(dopamine)

Large aspiny neurons
(acetylcholine)

Axon

FIGURE 44. Pattern of termination of afferents on a medium spiny neuron. Shown here are the soma and the proximal section of two dendrites with their spines. Modifed from Smith and Bolam, 1990. (*Source:* Reprinted from *Fundamental Neuroscience,* 34, JW Mink, Basal ganglia, 955, Copyright 1999, with permission from Elsevier.)

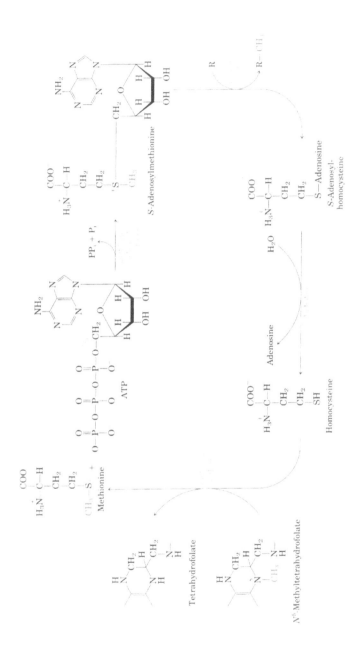

FIGURE 45. Transmethylation synthesis of methionine and *S*-adenosylmethionine as part of an activated methyl cycle. The methyl group donor in the methionine synthase reaction is methylcobalamin in some organisms. *S*-adenosylmethionine, which has a positively charged sulfur (and is thus a sulfonium ion), is a powerful methylating agent in a number of biosynthetic reactions. The methyl group acceptor is designated R. (*Source:* From LEHNINGER PRINCIPLES OF BIOCHEMISTRY, 3/e by David L. Nelson/Michael M. Cox. Copyright 1982, 1993, and 2000 by Worth Publishers. Used with permission.)

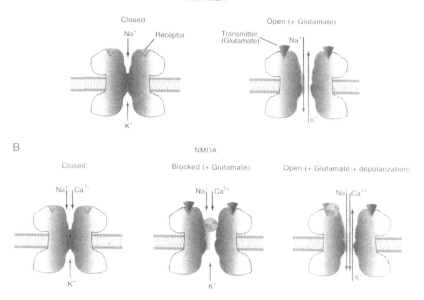

FIGURE 46. Features of non-NMDA and NMDA glutamate receptors. (A) Non-NMDA receptors: (left) in the absence of agonist, the channel is closed; (right) glutamate binding leads to channel opening and an increase in Na^+ and K^+ permeability. (B) NMDA receptors: (left) in the absence of agonist, the channel is closed; (middle) the presence of agonist leads to a conformational change and channel opening, but no ionic flux occurs, because the pore of the channel is blocked by Mg^{2+}; (right) in the presence of depolarization, the Mg^{2+} block is removed and the agonist-induced opening of the channel leads to changes in ion flux (including Ca^{2+} influx into the cell). (*Source:* Reprinted from *Fundamental Neuroscience,* 12, JH Byrne, Postsynaptic potentials and synaptic integration, 354, Copyright 1999, with permission from Elsevier.)

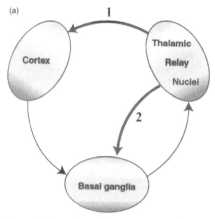

(a)

1

Cortex

Thalamic
Relay
Nuclei

2

Basal ganglia

FIGURE 47. (a) Diagram of the dual role of thalamic relay nuclei in basal ganglia circuitry. (1) Thalamic relay nuclei transmit basal ganglia output to the frontal cortex, and (2) thalamic relays provide a direct input to the striatum. Colored gradient in cortex, thalamus, and basal ganglia indicates functionally related regions in each of these areas. (b) Hypothetical parallel segregated circuits connecting the basal ganglia, thalamus, and cerebral cortex. The five circuits are named according to the primary cortical target of the output from the basal ganglia: motor, oculomotor, dorsolateral prefrontal, lateral orbito-frontal, and anterior cingulate. Abbreviations: ACA, anterior cingulate area; APA, arcuate premotor area; CAUD, caudate; (b) body; (h) head; DLC, dorsolateral prefrontal cortex; EC, entorhinal cortex; FEF, frontal eye fields; GPi, internal segment of globus pallidus; HC, hippocampal cortex; ITG, inferior temporal gyrus; LOF, lateral orbitofrontal cortex; MC, motor cortex; MDpl, mediulis dorsalis pars paralamellaris; MDme, medialis dorsalis pars magnocellularis; MDpc, medialis dorsalis pars parvocellularis; PPC, posterior parietal cortex; PUT, putamen; SC, somatosensory cortex; SMA, supplementary motor area; SNr, substantia nigra pars reticulata; STG, superior temporal gyrus; VAmc, ventralis anterior pars magnocellularis; Vapc, ventralis anterior pars parvocellularis; VLm, ventralis lateralis pars medialis; VLo, ventralis lateralis pars oralis; VP, ventral pallidum; VS, ventral striatum; cl, caudolateral; cdm, caudal dorsomedial; dl, dorsolateral; l, lateral; ldm, lateral dorsomedial; m, medial; mdm, medial dorsomedial; pm, posteromedial; rd, rostrodorsal; rl, rostrolateral; rm, rostromedial; vm, ventromedial; vl, ventrolateral. (*Source:* [a] S Haber and NR McFarland, *The Neuroscientist* 7(4), p. 323. Copyright ©2001 by Sage Publications. Reprinted by permission of Sage Publications; [b] Reprinted from *Fundamental Neuroscience,* 34, JW Mink, Basal ganglia, 956, Copyright 1999, with permission from Elsevier.)

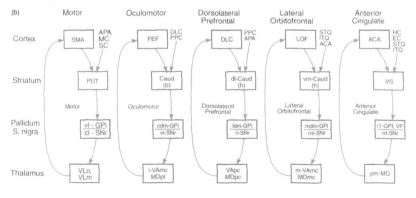

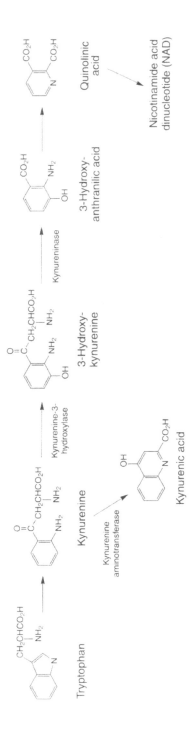

FIGURE 48. The major components of the kynurenine pathway that possess neurobiological activity are shown. The pathway, which accounts for the majority of nonprotein tryptophan metabolism in most tissues, includes quinolinic acid (an agonist at NMDA receptors), 3-hydroxykynurenine (a radical-generating neurotoxin), and kynurenic acid (a glutamate receptor antagonist with differences in potency at the various receptor subtypes). The conversion of tryptophan to kynurenine is catalysed by tryptophan-2,3-dioxygenase in the liver and by the less selective indoleamine-2,3-dioxygenase in most other tissues. In most cases, this is the rate-limiting step in the pathway. (*Source:* Reprinted from *Trends in Pharmacological Sciences,* 21, TW Stone, Development and therapeutic potential of kynurenic acid and kynurenine derivatives for neuroprotection, 150, Copyright 2000, with permission from Elsevier.)

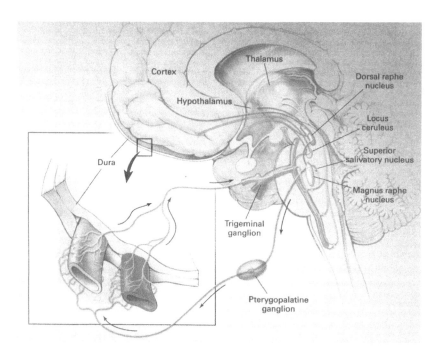

FIGURE 49. Pathophysiology of migraine. Migraine involves dysfunction of brainstem pathways that normally modulate sensory input. The key pathways for the pain are the trigeminovascular input from the meningeal vessels, which passes through the trigeminal ganglion and synapses on second-order neurons in the trigeminocervical complex. These neurons, in turn, project through the quintothalamic tract, and after decussating in the brainstem, form synapses with neurons in the thalamus. (*Source:* PJ Goadsby et al., 2002, Migraine—Current understanding and treatment. *The New England Journal of Medicine* 346(4), p. 259. Copyright 2002 Massachusetts Medical Society. All rights reserved.)

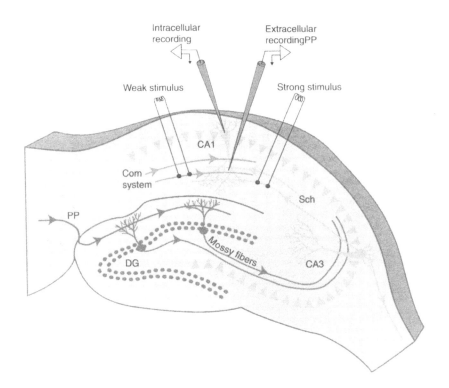

FIGURE 50. Schematic of a transverse hippocampal brain slice preparation from the rat. Two extracellular stimulating electrodes are used to activate two nonoverlapping inputs to pyramidal neurons of the CA1 region of the hippocampus. Both inputs consisted of axons of the Schaffer collateral/commissural (Sch/com) system. By suitably adjusting the current intensity delivered to the stimulating electrodes, different numbers of Sch/com axons can be activated. In this way, one stimulating electrode was made to produce a weak postsynaptic response and the other to produce a strong postsynaptic response. Sometimes three or more stimulating electrodes are used. Also illustrated is an extracellular recording electrode placed in the stratum radiatum (the projection zone of the Sch/com inputs) and an intracellular recording electrode in the stratum pyramidal (the cell body layer). Also indicated is the mossy-fiber projection from the granule cells of the dentate gyrus (DG) to the pyramidal neurons of the CA3 region. (*Source:* Reprinted from *Fundamental Neuroscience,* 55, JM Beggs et al., Learning and memory: Basic mechanisms, 1439, Copyright 1999, with permission from Elsevier.)

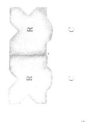

Inactive

Regulatory subunits:
empty cAMP sites

Catalytic subunits:
substrate binding
sites blocked by
autoinhibitory
domains of R subunits

4 cAMP ⇌ 4 cAMP

Active

Regulatory subunits:
autoinhibitory
domains buried

Catalytic subunits:
open substrate
binding sites

C   +   C

FIGURE 51a. Activation of cAMP-dependent protein kinase. Cyclic AMP activates the protein kinase by causing dissociation of the catalytic (C) subunits from the inhibitory regulatory (R) subunits. This allows phosphorylation and activation of phosphorylase b kinase, which in turn phosphorylates and activates glycogen phosphorylase. (*Source:* From LEHNINGER PRINCIPLES OF BIOCHEMISTRY, 3/e by David L. Nelson/Michael M. Cox. Copyright 1982, 1993, and 2000 by Worth Publishers. Used with permission.)

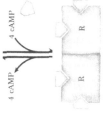

Phospho-Ser

Phospho-Thr

Phospho-Tyr

FIGURE 51b. The reactions catalyzed by protein kinases involve phosphate group transfer to the hydroxyl in the side chain of a Ser, Thr, or Tyr residue. One large class of protein kinases, typified by cAMP-dependent protein kinase, phosphorylate only Ser or Thr residues and thus are called serine-threonine kinases. Another class of protein kinases, typified by the insulin receptor, act only on Tyr residues. In each case, the addition of the highly charged and bulky phosphate group alters the conformation of the phosphorylated protein, bringing about a change in its activity or in its kinetic properties. (*Source:* From LEHNINGER PRINCIPLES OF BIOCHEMISTRY, 3/e by David L. Nelson/Michael M. Cox. Copyright 1982, 1993, and 2000 by Worth Publishers. Used with permission.)

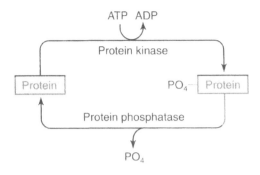

FIGURE 51c. Schematic diagram of the conversion of a dephosphoprotein to a phosphoprotein by a protein kinase and the reversal of this reaction by a protein phosphatase. (*Source:* EJ Nestler and P Greengard, in *Basic neurochemistry: Molecular, cellular, and medical aspects, Sixth Edition,* GJ Siegel et al., eds. Lippincott, 1999. Used with permission.)

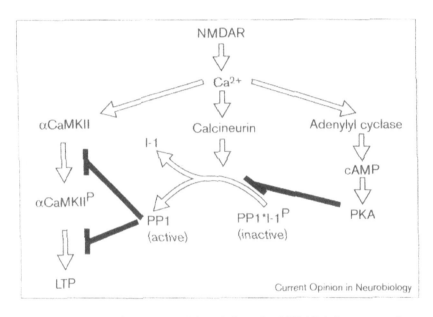

FIGURE 51d. Role of PKA and calcineurin in gating LTP. High-frequency stimulation causes the influx of Ca^{2+} through NMDARs. This influx results in the autophosphorylation of αCaMKII, and the subsequent phosphorylation of αCaMKII substrates required for LTP induction. The influx of Ca^{2+} also activates Ca^{2+}/CaM-dependent adenylyl cyclase, resulting in the production of cAMP, which is required for PKA activation. PKA phosphorylates the PP1 inhibitor I-1, thereby inactivating PP1 ("gate" open). In contrast, failure to activate the cAMP-dependent pathway results in the dephosphorylation (inactivation) of I-1 by calcineurin, and allows PP1 to dephosphorylate aCaMKII and its substrates ("gate" closed). (*Source:* Reprinted from *Current Opinion in Neurobiology,* 9, Y Elgersma and AJ Silva, Molecular mechanisms of synaptic plasticity and memory, 210, Copyright 1999, with permission from Elsevier.)

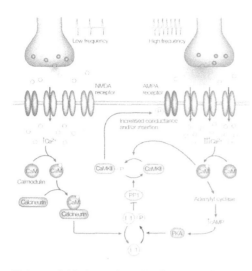

FIGURE 51e. How does the same initial stimulus—the activation of the NMDA (*N*-methyl-D-aspartate) receptor—elicit potentiation of synaptic transmission in some cases, but depression in others? This question was posed early on in the field of synaptic plasticity. John Lisman put forward the model illustrated here, proposing that the concentrations of intracellular Ca^{2+} achieved by the activation of NMDA receptors have a critical role in determining whether long-term potentiation (LTP) or long-term depression (LTD) is elicited. This model is based on the fact that, in vitro, calcineurin (PP2B) has a much higher affinity for Ca^{2+} than do calcium/ calmodulin-dependent protein kinase II (CaMKII) and protein kinase C. Weak activation of the NMDA receptor (depicted on the left) would elicit low-level increases in Ca^{2+}, resulting in the preferential activation of PP2B over CaMKII, and the dephosphorylation of substrates, leading to LTD. On the other hand, strong activation of the NMDA receptor (right) would give rises in Ca^{2+} sufficient to recruit CaMKII and PKC, resulting in the induction of LTP. (*Source:* Reprinted by permission from *Nature Reviews Neuroscience,* DG Winder and JD Sweatt, Roles of serine/threonine phosphates in hippocampal synaptic plasticity, p. 468. *Nature Reviews* 2(7). Copyright 2001 Macmillan Magazines Ltd.)

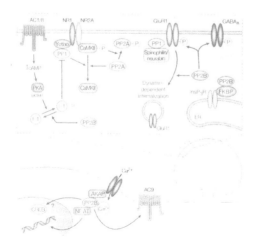

FIGURE 51f. Postsynaptic-biased model of phosphatase localization and function. A schematic illustration of a CA1 pyramid neuron, showing some of the potential targeting molecules of phosphatases in these cells, as well as potential substrates. (*Source:* Reprinted by permission from *Nature Reviews Neuroscience,* DG Winder and JD Sweatt, Roles of serine/threonine phosphates in hippocampal synaptic plasticity, p. 464. *Nature Reviews* 2(7). Copyright 2001 Macmillan Magazines Ltd.)

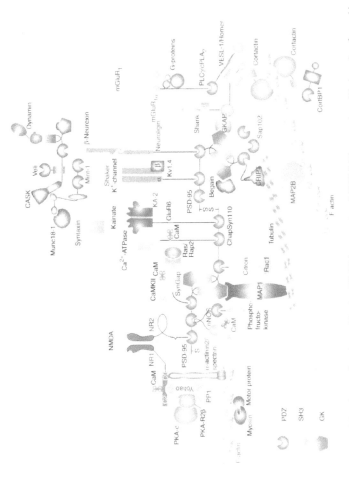

FIGURE 52. Putative assembly of proteins found in the NMDA receptor (NMDAR) complex. Molecules found in the analysis of the NMDAR complex are depicted and interactions based on published profiles. Many of the proteins could be neuropharmacologic targets. (*Source:* Reprinted from *Trends in Neurosciences*, 24, H Husi and SGN Grant, Proteomics of the nervous system, 262, Copyright 2001, with permission from Elsevier.)

(a)

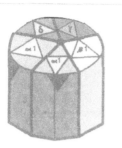

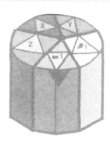

Location:
  Neuromuscular junction.
  Postsynaptic.
Function:
  Contracts skeletal tissue.

Location:
  Peripheral nervous system
  autonomic ganglia. Postsynaptic.
Function:
  Regulates the autonomic nervous
  system; releases catecholamines
  from the adrenal gland.

(b)

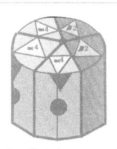

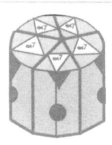

Location: Central nervous system.
  Presynaptic or postsynaptic.
Function: May be involved in
  neuronal migration during brain
  development; decreased in
  cerebral cortex in early
  Alzheimer's disease; up-
  regulated by nicotine for
  smoking.

Location: Central nervous system.
  Presynaptic.
Function: Regulates a calcium
  channel; rapidly desensitizes
  after stimulation by agonists;
  stimulates further acetylcholine
  release; stimulates release of
  glutamate, serotonin,
  norepinephrine, and other
  neurotransmitters; regulates
  auditory-gating deficit of
  schizophrenic patients; is the
  target of novel cognitive
  enhancers.

FIGURE 53. (a) Left: $\alpha\beta\delta\gamma$. Right: $\alpha\beta XYZ$. (b) Left: α_4-β_2. Right: α_7. (*Source:* SM Stahl, The function of nicotinic receptors, *The Journal of Clinical Psychiatry.* 61, 628, 628, 2000. Copyright 2000, Physicians Postgraduate Press. Reprinted by permission.)

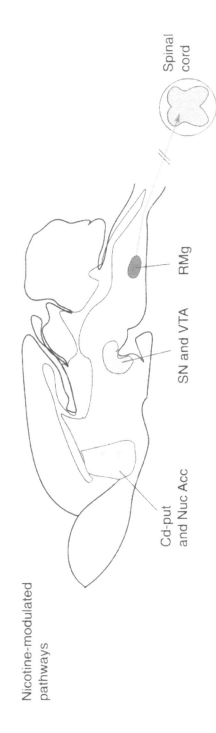

Nicotine-modulated pathways

Spinal cord

RMg

SN and VTA

Cd-put and Nuc Acc

FIGURE 54. Involvement of nicotinic acetylcholine receptors (nAChRs) in ascending dopamine-mediated and descending 5-HT-mediated pathways. Dopaminergic projections (green) from the substantia nigra (SN) and ventral tegmental area (VTA) to the caudate-putamen (Cd-Put) and nucleus accumbens (Nuc Acc), and 5-HT projections (red) from the raphe magnus (RMg) to the spinal cord are shown. (*Source:* Reprinted from *Trends in Pharmacological Sciences,* 21, M Cordero-Erausquin et al., Nicotinic receptor function: New perspectives from knockout mice, 215, Copyright 2000, with permission from Elsevier.)

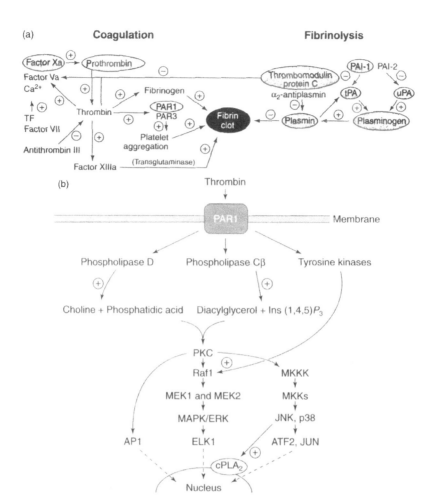

FIGURE 55. (a) Components of the coagulation and fibrinolysis pathways present in the CNS. Components for which protein or mRNA are produced in neurons or glia area highlighted in gray. (b) Signaling pathways coupled to the protease-activated receptor (PAR1). Thrombin initiates transmembrane signaling by cleaving the extracellular region of the receptor. This generates a new N terminus, which then functions as a tethered peptide ligand that binds intramolecularly to the body of the receptor, and initiates both transmembrane and nuclear signaling. Many of the signaling cascades are similar to those triggered by muscarinic ACh receptors, but nuclear responses are more prominent. (*Source:* [a] Reprinted from *Trends in Neurosciences,* 23, MB Gingrich and SF Traynelis, Serine proteases and brain damage—Is there a link?, 400, Copyright 2000, with permission from Elsevier; [b] Reprinted from *Trends in Neurosciences,* 23, M Hernandez et al., Cytosolic phospholipase A2 and the distinct transcriptional programs of astrocytoma cells, 262, Copyright 2000, with permission from Elsevier.)

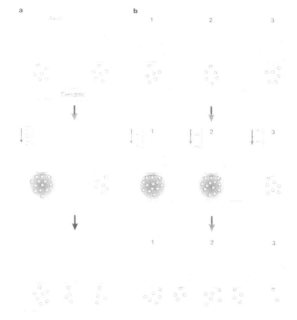

FIGURE 56. Neurotrophins as synaptic morphogens. (a) Top: Constitutive secretion of neurotrophins (NTs) from postsynaptic dendrites results in a low level of extracellular NTs at the synapse, which is required for maintenance of normal synaptic function, including the capability for the induction of long-term potentiation (LTP). Middle: Following intense synaptic activity, a transient high level of postsynaptic calcium (for example, accompanying the induction of LTP) results in a high level of NT secretion that raises the local extracellular NT concentration (possibly corresponding to early-phase LTP). Bottom: High NT levels locally trigger sprouting of nerve terminal arbors and dendritic spines, leading to the formation of new synapses (possibly corresponding to late-phase LTP). (b) The NT hypothesis for activity-dependent refinement of connections. Top: Synapses made by the terminals of different axons co-innervating the same postsynaptic dendrite are maintained in a normal functional state by the low-level constitutive secretion of NTs. Middle: Correlated activity in axon 1 and axon 2 causes large postsynaptic depolarization (and spiking) immediately following synaptic activation at axon 1 and axon 2, resulting in a transient high level of calcium and a high level of NT secretion. By contrast, uncorrelated activity in axon 3 does not experience postsynaptic spiking at the time of its synaptic activation, and therefore does not secrete high levels of NT. Bottom: Terminals of axon 1 and axon 2 sprout and new spines are formed in response to local high levels of NT. The synapse made by axon 3 may lose its postsynaptic supply of NT, owing to the directed transport of NT-containing granules toward adjacent synapses with correlated activity, leading to synaptic weakening and eventually withdrawal of the nerve terminal. (*Source:* Reprinted by permission from *Nature Reviews Neuroscience,* M Poo, Neurotrophins as synaptic modulators, p. 29. Copyright 2001 Macmillan Magazines Ltd.)

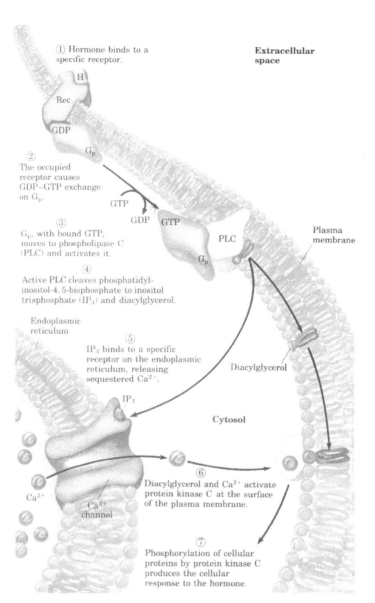

① Hormone binds to a specific receptor.

Extracellular space

H

Rec

GDP

② The occupied receptor causes GDP–GTP exchange on G_p.

G_p

GTP

③ G_p, with bound GTP, moves to phospholipase C (PLC) and activates it.

GDP GTP

PLC

G_p

Plasma membrane

④ Active PLC cleaves phosphatidyl-inositol-4,5-bisphosphate to inositol trisphosphate (IP_3) and diacylglycerol.

Endoplasmic reticulum

⑤ IP_3 binds to a specific receptor on the endoplasmic reticulum, releasing sequestered Ca^{2+}.

Diacylglycerol

IP_3

Cytosol

⑥ Diacylglycerol and Ca^{2+} activate protein kinase C at the surface of the plasma membrane.

Ca^{2+}

Ca^{2+} channel

⑦ Phosphorylation of cellular proteins by protein kinase C produces the cellular response to the hormone.

FIGURE 57a. Two intracellular second messengers are produced in the hormone-sensitive phosphatidylinositol system: inositol-1,4,5-trisphosphate (IP_3) and diacylglycerol. Both contribute to the activation of protein kinase C; IP_3, by raising cytosolic $[Ca^{2+}]$, also activates other Ca^{2+}-dependent enzymes. Thus Ca^{2+} also acts as a second messenger. (*Source:* From LEHNINGER PRINCIPLES OF BIOCHEMISTRY, 3/e by David L. Nelson/Michael M. Cox. Copyright 1982, 1993, and 2000 by Worth Publishers. Used with permission.)

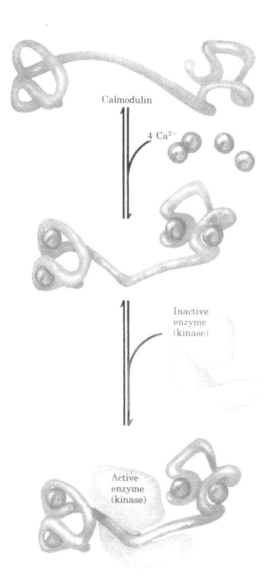

FIGURE 57b. Calmodulin, the protein mediator of many Ca^{2+}-stimulated enzymatic reactions, contains four high-affinity Ca^{2+}-binding sites. The binding of Ca^{2+} induces a conformational change in calmodulin, allowing it to interact productively with the proteins that it regulates. One of the many enzymes regulated by calmodulin and Ca^{2+} is Ca^{2+}/calmodulin-dependent protein kinase, which phosphorylates Ser and Thr residues in target proteins. (*Source:* From LEHNINGER PRINCIPLES OF BIOCHEMISTRY, 3/e by David L. Nelson/Michael M. Cox. Copyright 1982, 1993, and 2000 by Worth Publishers. Used with permission.)

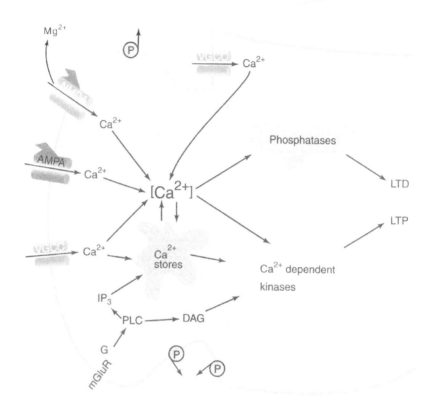

FIGURE 57c. Events leading to LTP or LTD. The schematic depicts a post-synaptic spine with various sources of Ca^{2+}. The NMDA receptor-channel complex admits Ca^{2+} only after depolarization removes the Mg^{2+} block. Calcium may also enter through the ligand-gated AMPA receptor channel or voltage-gated calcium channels (VGCC), which may be located on the spine head or dendritic shaft. Also, certain subtypes of metabotropic glutamate receptors (mGluRs) are coupled positively to phospholipase C (PLC), which cleaves membrane phospholipids into inositol triphosphate (IP_3) and diacylglycerol (DAG). Increased levels of IP_3 lead to the release of intracellular Ca^{2+} stores, whereas increases in DAG activate Ca^{2+}-dependent enzymes. Calcium pumps, located on the spine head, neck, and dendritic shaft, are hypothesized to help isolate Ca^{2+} concentration changes in the spine head from those in the dendritic shaft. (*Source:* Reprinted from *Fundamental Neuroscience,* 55, JM Beggs et al., Learning and memory: Basic mechanisms, 1444, Copyright 1999, with permission from Elsevier.)

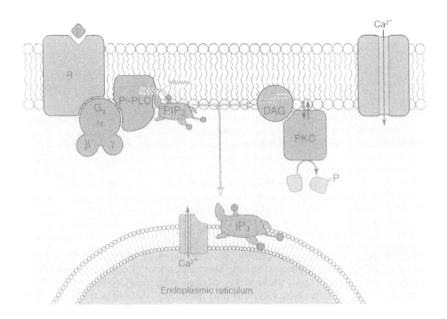

FIGURE 58. Linkage between receptor activation, phosphoinositide hydrolysis, Ca^{2+} signaling and activation of protein kinase C (PKC). Agonist occupancy of a cell-surface receptor results in the activation of phosphoinositide-specific phospholipase C (PI-PLC), which in this example is mediate through an intervening G protein, G_q. Phosphatidylinositol 4,5-bisphosphate (PIP_2) is phosphodiesteratically cleaved by PI-PLC to yield diacylglycerol (DAG) and inositol 1,4,5-tris-phosphate (IP_3). DAG activates PKC, following its translocation ($\downarrow\uparrow$) from cytosol to plasma membrane. Activation of PKC results in the phosphorylation of many cellular proteins, for example, the myristoylated, alanine-rich PKC substrate (MARCKS). When released, four molecules of IP_3 interact with a specific IP_3 receptor present in the endoplasmic reticulum and Ca^{2+} is liberated, raising its concentration in the cytosol. Depletion of the intracelular pool of Ca^{2+} results in the opening of a plasma membrane Ca^{2+} channel. (*Source:* SK Fisher and BW Agranoff, in *Basic neurochemistry: Molecular, cellular, and medical aspects, Sixth Edition,* GJ Siegel et al., eds. Lippincott, 1999. Used with permission.)

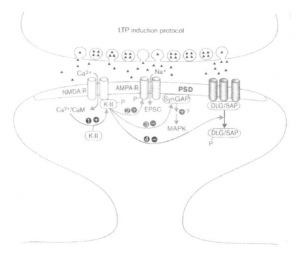

FIGURE 59. Putative roles of CaMKII in early-phase synaptic plasticity. Activation of CaMKII due to autophosphorylation (reaction 1) can cause its translocation to the PSD in part through interactions with the NMDAR. At the PSD, activated CaMKII can phosphorylate and potentiate AMPARs (reaction 2) to strengthen the excitatory postsynaptic current (EPSC), inhibit SynGAP (reaction 3) resulting in possible activation of MAP kinases, and phosphorylate a PDZ domain in the scaffold protein DLG/SAP family (reaction 4), causing disruption or remodeling of synaptic structure. (*Source:* Reprinted from *Current Opinion in Neurobiology,* 10, TR Soderling, CaM-kinases: Modulators of synaptic plasticity, 376, Copyright 2000, with permission from Elsevier.)

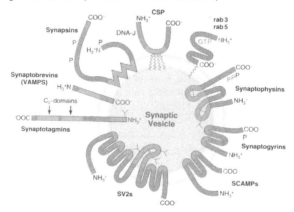

FIGURE 60. Trafficking proteins of synaptic vesicles. The structures of the major trafficking proteins of synaptic vesicles are shown schematically. Trafficking proteins are defined as those proteins with a likely function in the synaptic vesicle cycle and not in neurotransmitter uptake. Only proteins tightly associated with synaptic vesicles are pictured. (*Source:* TC Sudhof, in *Basic neurochemistry: Molecular, cellular, and medical aspects, Sixth Edition,* GJ Siegel et al., eds. Lippincott, 1999. Used with permission.)

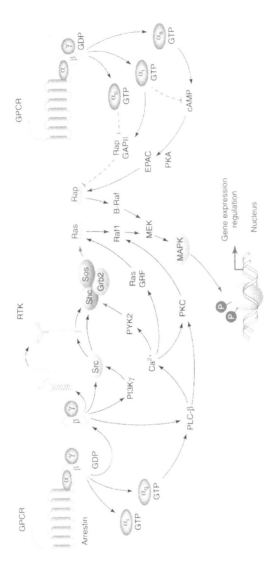

FIGURE 61. Multiple pathways link G-protein-coupled receptors (GPCRs) to mitogen-activated protein kinase (MAPK). Biochemical routes initiated by β-γ-subunits can stimulate Ras by the activation of receptor and non-receptor tyrosine kinases, which results in the recruitment of Sos to the membrane and the exchange of GDP for GTP bound to Ras. Activated Gα$_q$ can stimulate Raf1 through protein kinase C (PKC) or by stimulating Ras by the Ca^{2+}-dependent activation of RasGRF and tyrosine kinases acting on Sos, Gα$_i$, Gα$_o$ and Gα$_s$ can also use tissue-restricted pathways regulating Rap, which can stimulate B-Raf and lead to the activation of MAPK. Activated MAPK translocates to the nucleus and phosphorylates nuclear proteins, including transcription factors, thereby regulating gene expression. Arrows represent positive stimulation and broken lines represent inhibition. Abbreviations: EPAC, exchange protein activated by cAMP; GAP, GTPase-activating protein; GRF, guanine-nucleotide releasing factor; MEK, MAPK kinase; PI3K, phosphoinositide 3-kinase; PKA, protein kinase A; PLC, phospholipase C; RTK, receptor tyrosine kinase. (*Source:* Reprinted from *Trends in Pharmacological Sciences,* 22, MJ Marinissen and JS Gutkind, G-protein coupled receptors and signaling networks: Emerging paradigms, 372, Copyright 2001, with permission from Elsevier.)

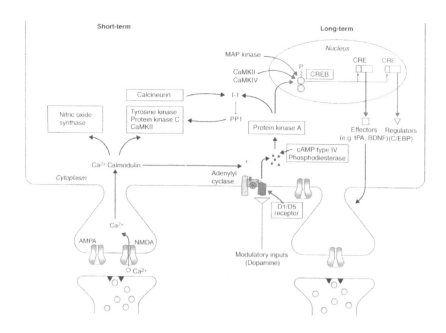

FIGURE 62. Molecular events that underlie the early and late phases of long-term potentiation. Stimulation of NMDA-type glutamate receptors, as a result of postsynaptic depolarization through AMPA receptors and the binding of glutamate, allows Ca^{2+} to enter the postsynaptic neuron. Among the immediate effects of Ca^{2+} are the activation of CaMKII, PKC, and calcineurin. Long-lasting LTP occurs when adenylyl cyclase is activated by Ca^{2+} or by modulatory inputs, which stimulate adenylyl cyclase through G-protein-coupled receptors. This leads to increases in cAMP levels, which activate PKA, which then translocates into the nucleus where it phosphorylates CREB. Other protein kinases, such as CaMKII, CaMKIV, and MAP kinase, also regulate gene expression, and it is now understood that there is extensive crosstalk among these different kinase pathways. (*Source:* Reprinted from *Current Opinion in Neurobiology,* 11, T Abel and KM Lattal, Molecular mechanism of memory acquisition, consolidation, and retrieval, 181, Copyright 2001, with permission from Elsevier.)

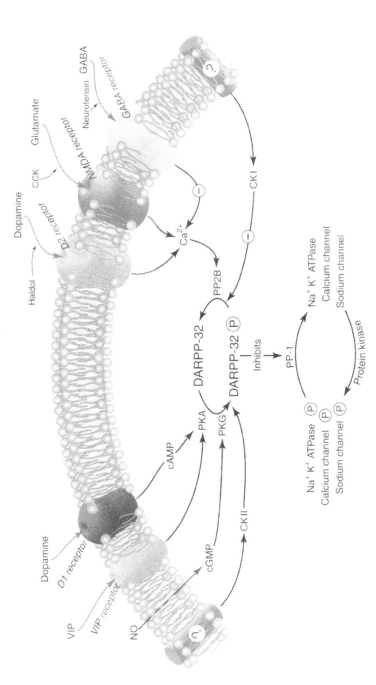

FIGURE 63. Neurotransmitter signaling in a medium spiny neuron. DARPP-32 coordinates the actions of a large number of neurotransmitters. (*Source*: Reprinted from *Fundamental Neuroscience*, 10, H Schilman and SE Hyman, Intracellular signaling, 298, Copyright 1999, with permission from Elsevier.)

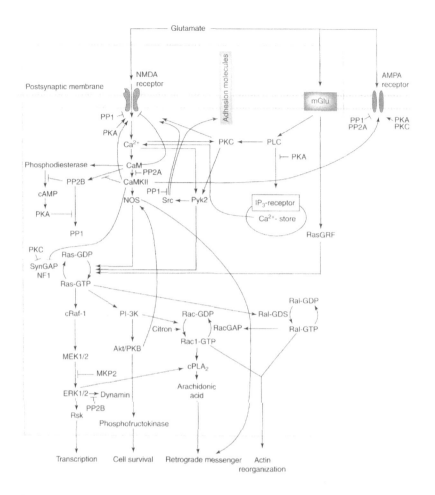

FIGURE 64. Putative signaling pathways in NMDA receptor complexes. (*Source:* Reprinted from *Trends in Neurosciences,* 24, H Husi and SGN Grant, Proteomics of the nervous system, 263, Copyright 2001, with permission from Elsevier.)

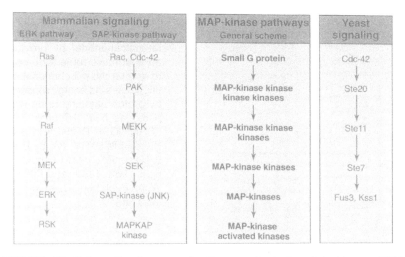

| Mammalian signaling | | MAP-kinase pathways | Yeast |
ERK pathway	SAP-kinase pathway	General scheme	signaling
Ras	Rac, Cdc-42	Small G protein	Cdc-42
	↓	↓	↓
	PAK	MAP-kinase kinase kinase kinases	Ste20
↓	↓	↓	↓
Raf	MEKK	MAP-kinase kinase kinases	Ste11
↓	↓	↓	↓
MEK	SEK	MAP-kinase kinases	Ste7
↓	↓	↓	↓
ERK	SAP-kinase (JNK)	MAP-kinases	Fus3, Kss1
↓	↓	↓	
RSK	MAPKAP kinase	MAP-kinase activated kinases	

FIGURE 65. Schematic diagram of mitogen-activated protein kinase (MAP kinase) pathways. To the right is shown the original pathway delineated in yeast. To the left are shown the homologous pathways more recently identified in mammalian cells, including brain. MEKK, MEK kinase; MEK, MAPK, and ERK kinase; ERK, extracellular signal-regulated kinase; RSK, ribosomal S6 kinase; SEK, SAP-kinase kinase; SAP-kinase, stress-activated protein kinase; JNK, Jun kinase; MAPKAP kinase, MAP-kinase-activated protein kinase; PAK, p21-activated kinase. (*Source:* EJ Nestler and P Greengard, in *Basic neurochemistry: Molecular, cellular, and medical aspects, Sixth Edition,* GJ Siegel et al., eds. Lippincott, 1999. Used with permission.)

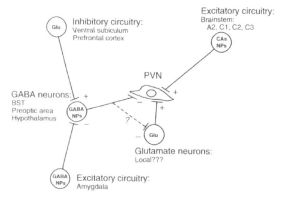

FIGURE 66. Schematic representation of central stress circuitry. According to this scenario, stimuli integrated by way of the "processive" stress pathway project to GABA-containing neurons in the bed nucleus of the stria terminalis (BST), preoptic area, and hypothalamus. Inhibitory circuits present excitatory output to GABA-containing neurons, resulting in an increase in inhibition at the paraventricular nucleus (PVN). Excitatory circuits present inhibitory input to GABA-containing neurons, attenuating inhibition at the PVN. (*Source:* Reprinted from *Trends in Neurosciences,* 20, JP Herman and WE Cullinan, Neurocircuitry of stress: Central control of the hypothalamo-pituitary-adrenocortical axis, 82, Copyright 1997, with permission from Elsevier.)

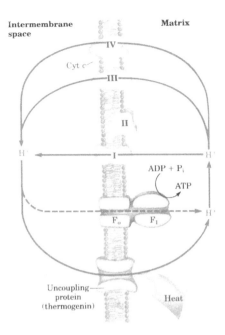

FIGURE 67. The uncoupling protein (thermogenin) of brown fat mitochondria, by providing an alternative route for protons to reenter the mit chondrial matrix, causes the energy conserved by proton pumping to be dissipated as heat. (*Source:* From LEHNINGER PRINCIPLES OF BIOCHEMISTRY, 3/e by David L. Nelson/Michael M. Cox. Copyright 1982, 1993, and 2000 by Worth Publishers. Used with permission.)

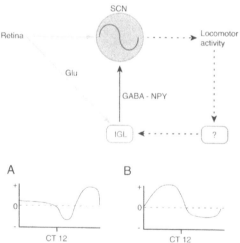

FIGURE 68. The actions of two entrainment pathways. The RHT projects to the SCN and IGL. The SCN controls the rest-activity cycle, and locomotor activity feeds back through the IGL projection to the SCN to affect SCN pacemaker function. The effect of RHT activation is shown by the light phase response curve (PRC) (A), and the effect of IGL-RHT activation is shown by the nonphotic PRC (B). (*Source:* Reprinted from *Fundamental Neuroscience,* 45, RY Moore, Circadian Timing, 1196, Copyright 1999, with permission from Elsevier.)

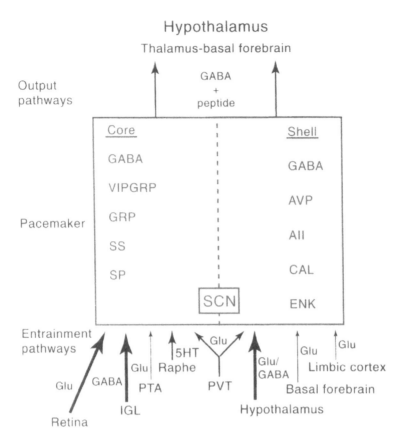

FIGURE 69. Organization of the SCN in mammals. The SCN has two subdivisions: a core, which contains neurons in which vasoactive intestinal polypeptide (VIP), gastrin-releasing peptide (GRP), calretinin (CAL), somatostatin (SS), or substance P (SP) is colocalized with GABA, and a shell, in which arginine vasopressin (AVP), angiotensin II (AII), or enkephalin (ENK) is colocalized with GABA. (*Source:* Reprinted from *Fundamental Neuroscience,* 45, RY Moore, Circadian Timing, 1193, Copyright 1999, with permission from Elsevier.)

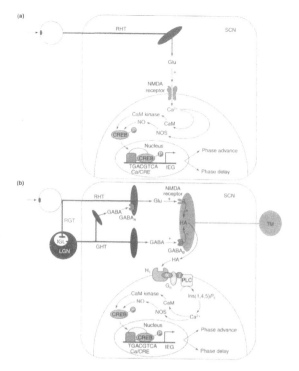

FIGURE 70. Models for the entrainment of circadian rhythms by photic input during the subjective dark period (SDP). (a) The currently accepted model suggests that glutamate (Glu), released from neurons of the retinohypothalamic tract (RHT), acts on NMDA receptors in the suprachiasmatic nucleus (SCN) to cause an influx of Ca^{2+} that activates the calmodulin (CaM) kinase pathway. This results in phosphorylation of cAMP responsive element-binding protein (CREB) and induction of the transcription of immediate early genes (IEGs) such as *Fos* and *Jun-B*. Nitric oxide synthase (NOS) is also thought to promote phosphorylation of CREB. Regulation of the transcription of IEGs is thought to be responsible for phase shifts in circadian rhythms. (b) The proposed model suggests that histamine (HA) is the final mediator in the entrainment of circadian rhythms. Release of HA from neurons of the tuberomammillary nucleus (TM) that terminate in the SCN is thought to be regulated by both Glu, released from RHT neurons, and GABA, released from neurons of the geniculohypothalamic tract (GHT). By activating $GABA_B$ receptors, GABA can inhibit the release of Glu by neurons of the RHT and thus inhibit HA release indirectly. Furthermore, by activating $GABA_A$ receptors on histaminergic neurons in the SCN, GABA can inhibit HA release directly. Abbreviations: Ca/CRE, Ca^{2+}/cAMP-responsive element; G_q, G protein coupled to PLC; IGL, intergeniculate leaflet; Ins(1,4,5)P_3, inositol (1,4,5)- trisphosphate; LGN, lateral geniculate thalamic nucleus; NO, nitric oxide; PLC, phospholipase C. (*Source:* Reprinted from *Trends in Pharmacological Sciences,* 21, EH Jacobs et al., Is histamine the final neurotransmitter in the entrainment of circadian rhythms in mammals?, 295, Copyright 2000, with permission from Elsevier.)

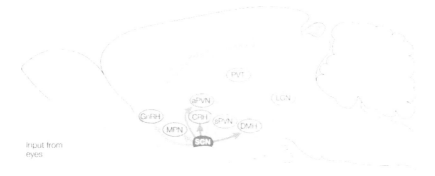

Input from
eyes

FIGURE 71. Targets of the SCN. The hypothalamic structures through which the suprachiasmatic nucleus (SCN) signal is translated into a hormonal pattern are shown. We propose that the SCN uses four important means to organize hormonal secretion: first, by direct contact with neuroendocrine neurons, for example, those containing gonadotropin-releasing hormone (GnRH) or corticotropin-releasing hormone (CRH); second, by contact with neuroendocrine neurons via intermediate neurons, for example, those of the medial preoptic nucleus (MPN), the dorsomedial hypothalamic nucleus (DMH), or the sub-paraventricular nucleus (sPVN); third, by projections to the autonomic PVN (aPVN) to influence the autonomic nervous system, preparing the endocrine organs for the arrival of hormones; and fourth, by influencing its own feedback. (*Source:* Reprinted by permission from *Nature Reviews Cancer,* RM Buijs and A Kalsheek, Hypothalamic integration of central and peripheral clocks, p. 523. *Nature Reviews* 2(7). Copyright Macmillan Magazines Ltd.)

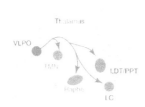

FIGURE 72. The projections from the ventrolateral preoptic nucleus (VLPO) to the main components of the ascending arousal system. Axons from the VLPO directly innervate the cell bodies and proximal dendrites of neurons in the major monoamine arousal groups. Within the major cholinergic groups, axons from the VLPO mainly innervate interneurons, rather than the principal cholinergic cells. Abbreviations: LC, locus coeruleus; LDT, laterodorsal tegmental nuclei; PPT, pedunculopontine tegmental nuclei; TMN, tuberomammillary nucleus; VLPO, ventrolateral preoptic nucleus. The blue circle indicates neurons of the LDT and PPT; green circles indicate aminergic nuclei; and the red circle indicates the VLPO. (*Source:* Reprinted from *Trends in Neurosciences,* 24, CB Saper et al., The sleep switch: Hypothalamic control of sleep and wakefulness, 728, Copyright 2001, with permission from Elsevier.)

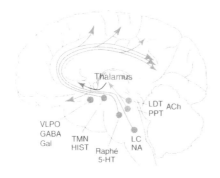

FIGURE 73. The ascending arousal system sends projections from the brainstem and posterior hypothalamus throughout the forebrain. Neurons of the laterodorsal tegmental nuclei and pedunulopontine tegmental nuclei (LDT and PPT) (blue circles) send cholinergic fibers (Ach) to many forebrain targets, including the thalamus, which then regulate cortical activity. Aminergic nuclei (green circles) diffusely project throughout much of the forebrain, regulating the activity of cortical and hypothalamic targets directly. Neurons of the tuberomammillary nucleus (TMN) contain histamine (HIST), neurons of the raphe nuclei contain 5-HT and neurons of the locus coeruleus (LC) contain noradrenaline (NA). Sleep-promoting neurons of the ventrolateral preoptic nucleus (VLPO, red circle) contain GABA and gelanin (Gal). (*Source:* Reprinted from *Trends in Neurosciences,* 24, CB Saper et al., The sleep switch: Hypothalamic control of sleep and wakefulness, 727, Copyright 2001, with permission from Elsevier.)

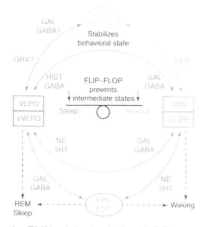

FIGURE 74. A model for reciprocal interactions between sleep- and wake-promoting brain regions, which produces a flip-flop switch. Inhibitory pathways are shown in red, and the excitatory pathways in green. The blue circle indicates neurons of the LDT and PPT; green boxes indicate aminergic nuclei; and the red box indicates the VLPO. Aminergic regions such as the TMN, LC, and DR promote wakefulness by direct excitatory effects on the cortex and by inhibition of sleep-promoting neurons of the VLPO. During sleep, the VLPO inhibits amine-mediated arousal regions through GABAergic and galaninergic (GAL) projections. Most innervation of the TMN originates in the VLPO core, and input to the LC and DR predominantly comes from the extended VLPO. This inhibition of the amine-mediated arousal system disinhibits VLPO neurons, further stabilizing the production of sleep. The PPT and LDT also contain REM-promoting cholinergic neurons. The extended VLPO (eVLPO) might promote REM sleep by disinhibiting the PPT-LDT; its axons innervate interneurons within the PPT-LDT, as well as aminergic neurons that normally inhibit REM-promoting cells in the PPT-LDT. Orexin/hypocretin neurons (ORX) in the lateral hypothalamic area (LHA) might further stabilize behavioral state by increasing the activity of aminergic neurons, thus maintaining consistent inhibition of sleep-promoting neurons in the VLPO and REM-promoting neurons in the PPT-LDT. (*Source:* Reprinted from *Trends in Neurosciences,* 24, CB Saper et al., The sleep switch: Hypothalamic control of sleep and wakefulness, 729, Copyright 2001, with permission from Elsevier.)

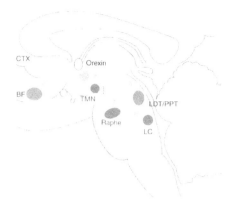

FIGURE 75. Orexin neurons in the lateral hypothalamic area innervate all of the components of the ascending arousal system, as well as the cerebral cortex (CTX) itself. Blue circles indicate cholinergic neurons of the BF, LDT, and PPT; green circles indicate monoaminergic nuclei. (*Source:* Reprinted from *Trends in Neurosciences,* 24, CB Saper et al., The sleep switch: Hypothalamic control of sleep and wakefulness, 730, Copyright 2001, with permission from Elsevier.)

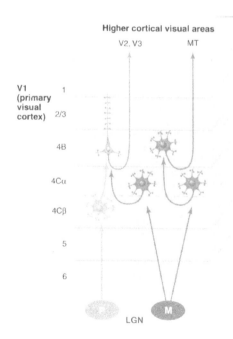

FIGURE 76. Information relays in the visual cortex. Distinct types of visual signals (M and P) are relayed from the retina through separate divisions of the lateral geniculate nucleus of the thalamus (LGN) to different portions of primary input layer 4C of the primary visual cortex (V1). A further relay conveys these signals to layer 4B, which provides a major output from V1 to higher visual areas (V2, V3, MT). Spiny stellate cells in layer 4B (orange), which project to area MT (V5), receive a strong M input but no P input. Pyramidal cells (purple), which project to areas V2 and V3, receive both M and P inputs. (*Source:* Reprinted with permission from JB Levitt, 2001, Function following form. *Science* 292(13), p. 232. Copyright 2001 American Association for the Advancement of Science.)

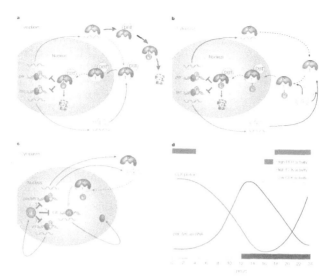

FIGURE 77. The *Drosophilia* circadian clock. The parts of this figure emphasize different aspects of the clock. Dashed lines are used to indicate steps at which significant delays can occur, and question marks indicate uncertainties in the pathways. (a) Model for DBT- and TIM-dependent accumulation, function, and degradation of PER in the *Drosophilia* clock. Although *per* and *tim* are coordinately activated by E-box binding of the transcription factors CLK (C) and CYC (B), the PER (P) and TIM (T) proteins do not accumulate with the same kinetics. PER is intially phosphorylated by DBT, a CK1ε orthologue, and then degraded. Cytoplasmic PER eventually accumulates and binds to TIM, which blocks DBT-dependent phosphorylation. Association of PER and TIM also allows their transfer to the nucleus. TIM is later eliminated from nuclear PER/TIM/DBT complexes allowing strong repression of *per* and *tim* transcription. DBT-dependent phosphorylation of nuclear PER promotes its degradation and restarts the cycle. (b) Role for SGG. The timing of PER/TIM nuclear translocation is determined by the level of SGG (S) activity. SGG seems to control this step by phosphorylating TIM. (c) Additional autoregulatory loops in the fly clock. The clock proteins CLK and VRI are rhythmically produced. Nuclear PER, or PER/TIM, somehow promotes transcription of *Clk*. *vri* is activated by CLK/CYC and suppressed by nuclear PER. High levels of VRI block *per* and *tim* expression. Although the basis for the effects of VRI on *per* and *tim* expression is unknown, VRI might directly block *per/tim* transcription, suppress activity of CLK/CYC proteins, or influence cycling *Clk* expression. X, hypothesized activator of *Clk* expression. (d) Two-step autoregulation in the fly clock. During the day, *Clk* RNA and protein levels decline, whereas *vri* RNA and protein accumulate. This could cause *per*, *tim,* and *vri* transcription to stall by early evening (VRI is abundant and CLK is at its lowest level). After a delay (a), nuclear transfer of PER/TIM complexes stimulates the next cycle of *Clk* RNA synthesis and suppresses the activity of newly accumulating CLK/CYC, CLK, Clock; CYC, Cycle; DBT, Double-time; PER, Period; Ph, phosphate; SGG, Shaggy; TM, Timeless; VRI, Vrille. (*Source:* Reprinted by permission from *Nature Reviews Genetics,* MW Young and SA Kay, Time zones: A comparative genetics of circadian clocks, p. 704. *Nature Reviews* 2(9). Copyright 2001 Macmillan Magazines Ltd.)

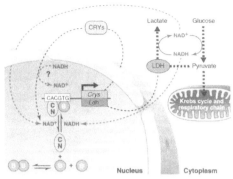

FIGURE 78. Metabolic states and circadian oscillators. The mammalian circadian feedback loop in gene expression is established by the BMAL1 (B) and Clock (C) transcriptional activator proteins and by the CRY transcriptional repressor proteins. In some brain regions, NPAS2 (N) substitutes for Clock, BMAL1 can bind to Clock or NPAS2, and these heterodimers activate transcription. Alternatively, BMAL1 can form homodimers with itself that do not activate transcription. The formation of the Clock:BMAL1 and NPAS2:BMAL1 teterodimers and their binding to DNA is stimulated by reduced NADH and inhibited by oxidized NAD. These heterodimers enhance the expression of the clock genes Cry and Per (not shown) and the clock output gene Ldh. CRY proteins repress Clock:NPAS2-mediated gene activation, possibly by oxidizing the NAD^+ cofactors associated with these proteins. Conceivably, the negative action of CRY proteins on Clock-NPAS2 could be reinforced by lactate dehydrogenase (LDH), which may increase the cellular concentration of NAD^+. (Only unphosphorylated NAD electron carriers are shown.) (Source: Reprinted with permission from U Schibler et al., 2001, Chronobiology—Reducing time. Science 293(7), p. 437. Copyright 2001 American Association for the Advancement of Science.)

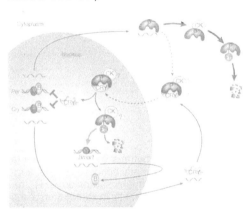

FIGURE 79. Regulatory interactions in the mammalian clock. Casein kinase 1ε (CK1ε) seems to affect PER stability and nuclear localization. For some PER proteins, phosphorylation by CK1ε could mask a PER nuclear localization signal. Formation of PER/CRY complexes promotes nuclear translocation in cultured cells and in vivo. Nuclear PER2 and CRY might have different targets in the nucleus: PER2 up-regulates expression of Bmal1, whereas CRY1 and CRY2 negatively regulated Per and Cry transcription. This separation of functions is illustrated schematically, but CRY and PER might act in association with each other and/or other proteins in the nucleus. B, BMAL1; CK, cassein kinase 1ε; C, CLOCK; CRY, CRY1/2; P, PER1-3; Y, PER2 might enhance the acitivity of a positive regulator or suppress a negative Bmal1 regulator; Ph, phosphate. Dashed arrows, possible delays. (Source: Reprinted by permission from Nature Reviews Genetics, MW Young and SA Kay, Time zones: A comparative genetics of circadian clocks, p. 707. Nature Reviews 2(9). Copyright 2001 Macmillan Magazines Ltd.)

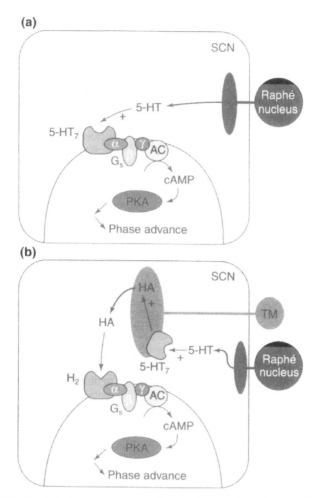

FIGURE 80. Models for entrainment of circadian rhythms by nonphotic input during the subjective light period (SLP). (a) The currently accepted model suggests that 5-HT, released from neurons of the raphe nucleus, acts on 5-HT$_7$ receptors in the suprachiasmatic nucleus (SCN), which results in stimulation of the cAMP-PKA (protein kinase A) pathway and induction of phase advances in circadian rhythms. (b) The proposed model suggests that histamine (HA) is the final mediator of phase advances induced by nonphotic input. Thus, activation of 5-HT$_7$ receptors on terminals of histaminergic neurons of the tuberomammillary nucleus (TM) leads to release of HA, which in turn activates HA H$_2$ receptors on neurones of the SCN and leads to stimulation of the cAMP-PKA pathway and induction of phase advances. Abbreviations: AC, adenylate cyclase; G$_S$, G protein positively coupled to AC. (*Source:* Reprinted from *Trends in Pharmacological Sciences,* 21, EH Jacobs et al., Is histamine the final neurotransmitter in the entrainment of circadian rhythms in mammals?, 297, Copyright 2000, with permission from Elsevier.)

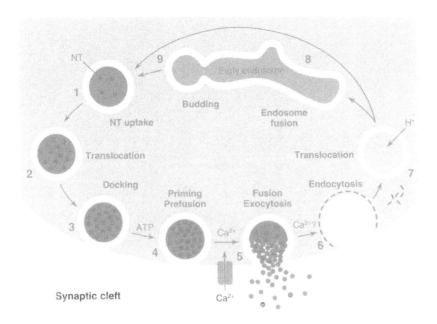

FIGURE 81a. The synaptic vesicle cycle. The pathway of synaptic vesicles in the nerve terminal is divided into nine stages. (1) Empty synaptic vesicles take up neurotransmitters by active transport into their lumen using an electrochemical gradient that is established by a proton pump activity. (2) Filled synaptic vesicles are translocated to the active zone. (3) Synaptic vesicles attach to the active zone of the presynaptic plasma membrane, but to no other component of the presynaptic plasma membrane, in a targeted reaction (docking). (4) Synaptic vesicles are primed for fusion in order to be able to respond rapidly to a Ca^{2+} signal later. Priming probably is a complicated, multicomponent reaction that can be subdivided further into multiple steps. (5) Ca^{2+} influx through voltage-gated channels triggers neurotransmitter release in less than 1 msec. Ca^{2+} stimulates completion of a partial fusion reaction initiated during priming. (6) Empty synaptic vesicles are coated by clathrin and associated proteins in preparation for endocytosis. Ca^{2+} may be involved in this process. (7) Empty synaptic vesicles shed their clathrin coat, acidify via proton pump activity, and retranslocate into the backfield of the nerve terminal. (8) Synaptic vesicles fuse with early endosomes as an intermediate sorting compartment to eliminate aged or mis-sorted proteins. (9) Synaptic vesicles are freshly generated by budding from endosomes. Although some synaptic vesicles may recycle via endosomes (steps eight and nine), it is likely that the endosomal intermediate is not obligatory for recycling and that synaptic vesicles can go directly from step seven to step one. (*Source:* TC Sudhof, in *Basic neurochemistry: Molecular, cellular, and medical aspects, Sixth Edition,* GJ Siegel et al., eds. Lippincott, 1999. Used with permission.)

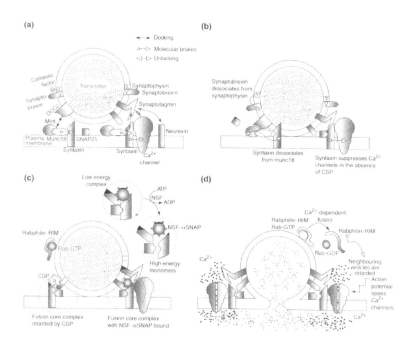

FIGURE 81b. The basic components of the transmitter release machinery. This simplified scheme aims to capture the essential components. It is not intended to be a complete description of the mechanisms involved. (a) Docking involves interactions between proteins (and phospholipids) in the vesicular membrane and proteins in the plasma membrane at an active zone. The "molecular brakes" restrict entry of the fusion-core proteins (SNAREs or SNAP receptors) into the fusion-core complex. These brakes include synaptobrevin or vesicle-associated membrane protein (VAMP) in the vesicular membrane, which binds to synaptophysin, an interaction that is promoted by a cytosolic factor (in adults). Syntaxin in the plasma membrane binds to munc 18, which prevents its entry into the fusion-core complex. Without a docked vesicle (and its associated cystein string proteins—CSPs), Ca^{2+} channels in the plasma membrane are suppressed by an interaction with syntaxin. (b) As vesicles dock, SNARE proteins are "unlocked" by, for example, an interaction between munc 18 and mint, which combines with DOC2 in the vesicular membrane and unlocks syntaxin, so that it can bind SNAP25. (c) The fusion-core complex forms (synaptobrevin, syntaxin, and SNAP25) and becomes a high-affinity binding site for αSNAP, which then binds the ATPase, NSF. (d) Fusion occurs when a fully release-competent vesicle receives an adequate influx of Ca^{2+} through the voltage-gated channels that form an integral part of the release machinery and the contents of the vesicle are discharged into the synaptic cleft. After, or during, Ca^{2+}-triggered fusion, RAB proteins in the vesicular membrane hydrolyse their bound GTP, and RAB-GDP and its bound effector protein (rabphilin or RIM) dissociate from the vesicle. This action in some way retards activation of neighboring vesicles. Abbreviations: NSF, N-ethylmaleimide-sensitive factor; RIM, RAB3-interacting molecule; SNAP, soluble NSF attachment protein; SNARE, SNAP receptor; SNAP25, 25 kD synaptosomal-associated protein. (*Source:* Reprinted from *Trends in Neurosciences,* 23, AM Thomson, Facilitation, augmentation and potentiation at central synapses, 311, Copyright 2000, with permission from Elsevier.)

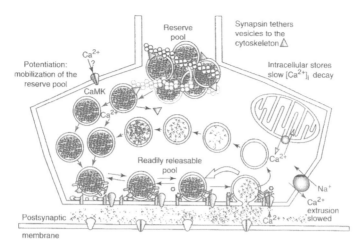

FIGURE 81c. Facilitation, augmentation, and potentiation. Facilitation, augmentation, and potentiation contribute to the responses of low probability connections to repetitive bursts of presynaptic APs. Augmentation is proposed to result from a gradual loading of the presynaptic terminal with Ca^{2+} as the Na^+-Ca^{2+} exchange slows down, and as intracellular buffers and stores enter an equilibrium with cytoplasmic Ca^{2+}. Potentiation results from the release of additional vesicles from the reserve pool, as synapsin, a vesicular membrane phosphoprotein that tethers vesicles to each other and to the cytoskeleton, dissociates from vesicles under the influence of Ca^{2+} and Ca^{2+}-dependent protein kinase I or II. This dissociation liberates vesicles from the reserve pool into the readily releasable pool. An increase in this population alters the equilibrium with docked vesicles, increasing occupancy of release sites. (*Source:* Reprinted from *Trends in Neurosciences,* 23, AM Thomson, Facilitation, augmentation and potentiation at central synapses, 311, Copyright 2000, with permission from Elsevier.)

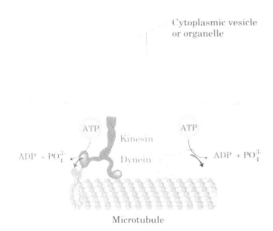

FIGURE 82. Kinesin and dynein are ATP-driven molecular engines that move along microtubular "rails." (*Source:* From LEHNINGER PRINCIPLES OF BIOCHEMISTRY, 3/e by David L. Nelson/Michael M. Cox. Copyright 1982, 1993, and 2000 by Worth Publishers. Used with permission.)

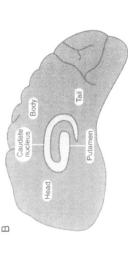

FIGURE 83b. Schematic drawing of the basal ganglia circuitry. Excitatory connections are indicated with red arrows and inhibitory connections with green arrows. The dopamine-containing connection from the substantia nigra pars compacta (SNpc) is both excitatory and inhibitory, depending on the postsynaptic receptor. Structural abbreviations: GPe, globus pallidus pars externa; GPi, globus pallidus pars interna; IL, intralaminar thalamic nuclei; MEA, midbrain extrapyramidal area; SC, superior colliculus; SNpc, substantia nigra pars compacta; SNpr, substantia nigra pars reticulata; STN, subthalamic nucleus. Neurotransmitter abbreviations: DA, dopamine; D1 and D2, dopamine receptor types 1 and 2; DYN, dynorphin; ENK, enkephalin; GABA, γ-aminobutyric acid; Glu, glutamate; SP, substance P; VA/VL, ventral anterior and ventral lateral nuclei of the thalamus. (*Source:* Reprinted from *Fundamental Neuroscience*, 34, JW Mink, Basal ganglia, 954, Copyright 1999, with permission from Elsevier.)

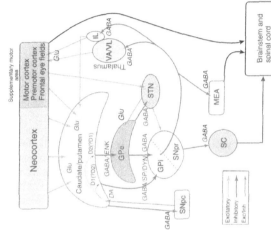

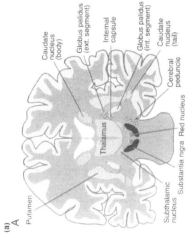

FIGURE 83a. The location of the basal ganglia in the human brain. (A) Coronal section. (B) Sagittal section. (*Source:* Reprinted from *Fundamental Neuroscience*, 34, JW Mink, Basal ganglia, 952, Copyright 1999, with permission from Elsevier.)

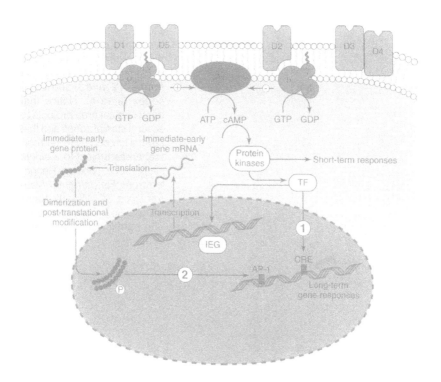

FIGURE 84. Effect of dopamine on intracellular signaling pathways. Stimulation of receptors by agonists can change enzyme activities as well as gene expression. Five subtypes of dopamine receptor have been identified. The D1 and D5 receptors are coupled to adenylyl cyclase (AC) via a stimulatory G protein (G_S). The D2 receptor inhibits cyclase activity via coupling to an inhibitory G protein (G_i). Activation of D3 and F4 receptors also inhibits cAMP production. Adenylyl cyclase catalyzes the conversion of ATP into cAMP, which in turn causes dissociation of the regulatory and catalytic subunits of protein kinase A. The activated catalytic subunit catalyzes conversion of protein substrates into phosphoproteins. This in turn can lead to a short-term response within the cell or activate transcription factors (TF) which enter the nucleus and alter gene expression. Long-term gene responses can be initiated by the action of constitutively expressed TFs either directly on DNA ① or via a mechanism involving transcription of an immediate-early gene (IEG) and cytoplasmic production of its protein. This protein can then act on DNA via an adaptor protein 1 (AP-1)-binding site ②. TF, constitutively expressed transcription factors, such as a cAMP-response element (CRE), *IEG*, immediate-early genes, such as c-*fos*, c-*jun*, and *knox*. (*Source:* MJ Kuhar et al., in *Basic neurochemistry: Molecular, cellular, and medical aspects, Sixth Edition,* GJ Siegel et al., eds. Lippincott, 1999. Used with permission.)

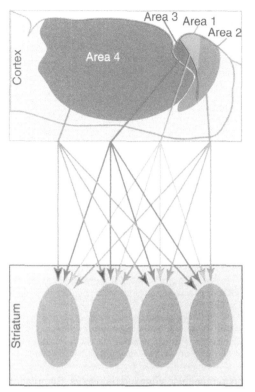

FIGURE 85. Schematic representation of projections to the striatum from arm areas in the somatosensory cortex (areas 1, 2, and 3) and motor cortex (area 4). Notice that each cortical area projects to several striatal zones and that several functionally related cortical areas project to a single striatal zone. (*Source:* Reprinted from *Fundamental Neuroscience,* 34, JW Mink, Basal ganglia, 957, Copyright 1999, with permission from Elsevier.)

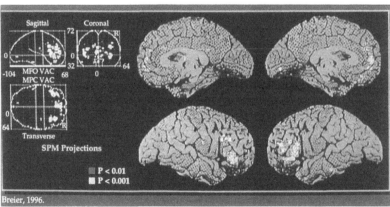

FIGURE 86. The effects of ketamine on cerebral metabolic rate in healthy controls. A FDG/PET study. Colored areas in the prefrontal cortex indicate increased metabolic activity. (*Source:* BS McEwen, 1999, in *Neurobiology of mental illness,* pp. 484, 485, DS Charney et al., eds. Reprinted with permission from the *American Journal of Psychiatry,* copyright 1997 American Psychiatric Association.)

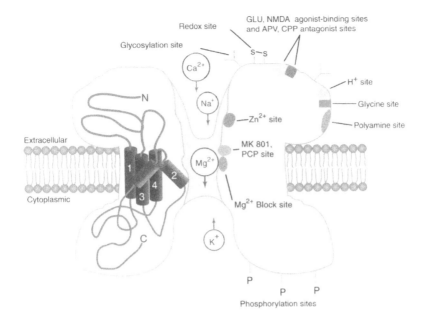

Redox site

Glycosylation site

GLU, NMDA agonist-binding sites
and APV, CPP antagonist sites

S~S

Ca²⁺

Na⁺

—Zn²⁺ site

H⁺ site

Glycine site

Polyamine site

Extracellular

Cytoplasmic

N

Mg²⁺

MK 801,
PCP site

Mg²⁺ Block site

C

K⁺

P

P   P

Phosphorylation sites

FIGURE 87. Diagram of NMDA receptor. Binding sites for numerous agonists, antagonists, and other regulatory molecules are identified. The locations of these bindings sites are approximate. Highlights include the Mg^{2+}-binding site that lies within the channel and produces the voltage-dependent block in ion permeation and the significant permeability to Ca^{2+}. (*Source:* Reprinted from *Fundamental Neuroscience,* 9, MN Waxham, Neurotransmitter receptors, 251, Copyright 1999, with permission from Elsevier.)

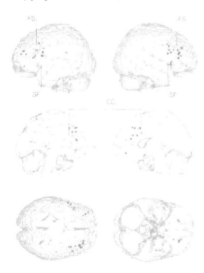

FIGURE 88. Prefrontal activations associated with five different cognitive demands. Green, response conflict; pink, task novelty; yellow, number of elements in working memory; red, working memory delay; blue, perceptual difficulty. Lateral (top) and medial (middle) views of each hemisphere, together with whole brain views from above (bottom left) and below (bottom right). CC, corpus callosum; IFS, inferior frontal sulcus; SF, Sylvian fissure. (*Source:* Reprinted by permission from *Nature Reviews Neuroscience,* J Duncan, An adaptive coding model of neural function in prefrontal cortex, p. 822. Copyright 2001 Macmillan Magazines Ltd.)

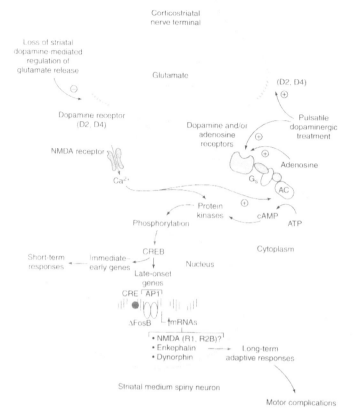

FIGURE 89a. Possible sequence of events in the striatum leading to L-dopa-induced dyskinesias. Heterodimers composed of a member of Fos family and a member of Jun family bind DNA at AP1 regulatory sites and generally function as transcriptional modulators. Chronic Fos-related antigens named ΔFosB are formed in striatal neurons in response to excessive glutamate-mediated activation of these neurons, or because of absent or abnormal dopamine-mediated modulation of these neurons. They form altered AP1 binding complexes that might possibly favor expression of subset of genes encoding NMDA receptors, dopamine D1 receptors, enkephalin, and dynorphin. Phosphorylation of CREB (cAMP-response-element-binding protein) and NMDA-receptor subunits might also play an important role. These modifications trigger a cascade of other interrelated changes, for example, in GABA- and glutamate-mediated transmission, which are responsible for the abnormal response to dopamine-like agents that, in primates and humans, translates into dyskinesias. Abbreviations: AC, adenylate cyclase; AP1, activator protein 1. (*Source:* Reprinted from *Trends in Neurosciences,* 23, F Calon et al., Dopamine-receptor stimulation: Biobehavioral and biochemical consequences, Suppl., Copyright 2000, with permission from Elsevier.)

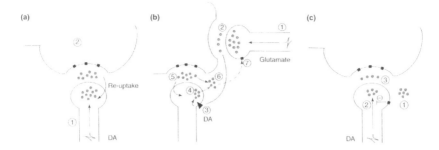

FIGURE 89b. The tonic-phasic model of dopamine system regulation can account for a number of phenomena related to dopamine (DA)-mediated modulation of motor control within the striatum. (a) Phasic stimulation. DAergic terminals in the striatum (1) synapse primarily on the side or the neck of dendritic spines (2) that arise from striatal medium spiny neurons. Action potentials generated by dopaminergic neuron discharges arrive into the axon terminal within the striatum (1) to cause spike-dependent DA release (red circles) into the synaptic cleft, where it stimulates postsynaptic DA receptors (squares). The DA released in this manner is high in amplitude (up to 1 mM) but very brief in duration, in that it is rapidly removed from the synaptic cleft by the DA transporter and accumulated in the presynaptic terminal before it can escape the synaptic cleft. This high-amplitude but brief-duration DA release is termed the phasic DA input, and is proposed to mediate behaviorally relevant events. (b) Tonic stimulation. Tonic DA release is proposed to be mediated by at least two events. Action potentials arising from glutamatergic afferents (1) cause the release of glutamate (blue circles) into the synaptic cleft (2) at the spine-head of the medium spiny neuron. The glutamate is of sufficient concentration to diffuse from the synaptic cleft and stimulate (either directly via presynaptic glutamate receptors (3) or indirectly via NO) the dopaminergic terminal to release DA. These presynaptic signals might trigger the release of DA from the terminal at sites distal to the synaptic cleft (4). Studies have shown that the DA that escapes reuptake (5) from the synaptic cleft after sustained spike activity also contributes to this tonic DA pool (6). This pool is constantly present in the extrasynaptic space, and is tightly regulated by multiple feedback systems. Tonic extrasynaptic DA levels are very much lower in concentration (that is, tens of nanomolar) compared with those found in the phasic DA response, and thus are not capable of effectively stimulating intrasynaptic DA receptors (squares). Tonic DA is also in dynamic equilibrium with glutamatergic afferents, as studies have shown that such levels of DA are sufficient to provide baseline stimulation of presynaptic D2 receptors (squares) on corticostriatal afferents (7), thereby limiting glutamate-stimulated DA release as well. (c) Tonic DA will presynaptically inhibit spike-dependent phasic DA release. Although the tonic levels of DA present in the extrasynaptic space (1) are very low in concentration, they are nonetheless sufficient to provide constant baseline stimulation of presynaptic D2 receptors. In particular, they provide stimulation of the synthesis- and release-modulating autoreceptors present on the dopaminergic terminal (squares). In this way, tonic DA provides a feedback inhibition of spike-dependent DA release (2), resulting in a lower concentration of DA released phasically in response to action potentials in the DA terminal (3). (*Source:* Reprinted from *Trends in Neurosciences,* 23, SP Onn et al., Dopamine-mediated regulation of striatal neuronal and network interactions, S49, Copyright 2000, with permission from Elsevier.)

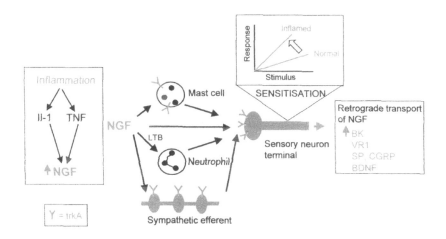

FIGURE 90. Diagrammatic illustration of the actions of NGF in inflammatory pain states. Nerve growth factor (NGF) has a number of acute actions involving the peripheral sensitization of nociceptors. These involve a direct action on those nococeptors that express the high-affinity NGF receptor trkA and indirect actions mediated by mast cells and sympathetic efferents that also express trkA. (*Source:* DL Bennett, *The Neuroscientist* 7(1), p. 15. Copyright © 2001 by Sage Publications. Reprinted by permission of Sage Publications.)

Chapter 7

This Is . . . Los Angeles

No, this is not the wraith of Edward R. Murrow reporting as if from the London Blitz, but this is Jay Goldstein reporting from the floor of the Los Angeles Convention Center after attending five days of the 28th Annual Meeting of the Society for Neuroscience, the largest and most important annual neuroscience conference in the world. I try to attend whenever I can, and on this occasion I definitely am reporting from the floor of the Convention Center, where I am lying after being blitzed by 12,000 experiments in five days. This averaged out to about 1,200 experiments every morning and another 1,200 experiments every afternoon. This meeting marks a watershed in my association with the study of neuroscience.

Back in the early 1980s, when the Society for Neuroscience was fairly small, I taught a course in medical neurobiology for psychiatry residents that I had to invent because no neuroscience textbooks existed at that time, at least none that I knew of, and now there are 12,000 experiments.

The last Society for Neuroscience conference that I had attended was two years ago, at which time about 5,000 experiments were explained in the same number of days. I was able to absorb this amount of information, although with great difficulty due to the time involved and the increasing complexity of the material. At the current conference, I realized that I could no longer encompass the totality of neuroscience, if indeed I ever was able. My previous confidence in my knowledge of neuroscience may have been somewhat delusional. I was encouraged, however, by the number of findings that were presented at this conference reflecting hypotheses that I had made in my earlier books about how the brain worked and how it malfunctioned in neurosomatic disorders, of which CFS is one.

Strangely enough, no members of the board of the American Association for Chronic Fatigue Syndrome (AACFS) were present at this 1998 meeting. One would think that these worthies had realized that in patients with CFS the brain didn't work right and that they might want to learn more about why this was so. However, they must have been staggered with the enormous information overload that they received at the AACFS meeting in Boston two weeks earlier, although at the moment I can't recall any information presented there that would overload circuitry. Reviewing the program and the abstracts, I was reminded of the refrain "Let's do the time warp again." If it had been played at the meeting, I might have been induced to attend, because at least I could have had a little bit of fun dancing.

The continued emphasis on cognitive-behavioral therapy as perhaps the only treatment aside from the checkered performance of Ampligen reminded me of an earlier song by Dr. Feelgood and the Interns called "You've Got the Right String, Baby (But the Wrong Yo-Yo)."

Cognitive therapy done pharmacologically is much more effective than cognitive-behavioral therapy done by psychologists. At one time, two psychologists were doing CBT with my patients. One psychologist was my wife, Gail. Both eventually left the practice as I became more adept at pharmacologically manipulating signal-to-noise ratio and perception of saliency of information so that it could be gated properly.

I would like to review what I consider to be the most important presentations related to neurosomatic disorders at this conference. I will, of necessity, omit the vast majority of the experiments presented, since I can hardly allude to 12,000 experiments in this chapter. I will be referring to the pages in the abstracts of the Society for Neuroscience of the 28th Annual Meeting when I discuss the experiments. If readers would like to obtain the abstracts, which are extremely technical but also very interesting, they can contact the Society for Neuroscience and request the Society for Neuroscience Abstracts Volume 24, Parts I and II, 1998.

I will start with Part I. Each part usually has five or six abstracts on each page. I will be mainly focusing on norepinephrine, dopamine, NMDA-receptor antagonism, GABA, and the regulation of these substances physiologically and pharmacologically. Norepinephrine is important in regulating sensory and cognitive gating, as is dopamine and the NMDA receptor, one of the receptors for the excitatory amino acid transmitter glutamate, which seems to have a central role in much of the pathophysiology. The inhibitory neurotransmitter GABA, which has a significant role in almost every neuronal activity, is also important. I will also be referring to some of the medications that I use in the treatment of neurosomatic disorders as they were discussed in the context of the neuroscience meeting. Remember that these experiments were primarily done by PhD or MD researchers, who rarely, if ever, see patients and who focus primarily on an extremely narrow aspect of neuroscience. One researcher, with whom I discussed my use of thyrotropin-releasing hormone in the form of nasal spray and eyedrops exuberantly exclaimed right there on the convention floor, "My whole life is TRH!" TRH is a very small polypeptide molecule that is cleaved from precursor polypeptides. This man's whole life was TRH, exemplifying the focus of those involved in research. No one that I spoke with at this meeting had a very clear vision of how to integrate his research with the health and illness of an entire person. The gulf between basic science and clinical practice is still fairly wide.

Page 353: Prolonged stress may decrease dopamine in the nucleus accumbens, an extremely important structure in neurosomatic disorders. It mediates reward and pleasure. Most of my treatments, when effective, increase dopamine and turn on norepinephrine, especially in the NAc, as well as the PFC where alpha$_2$ receptors are stimulated and alpha$_1$ receptors are inhibited.

Page 355: Very early life events can be extremely important in the predisposition to develop neurosomatic disorders. Newborn rats separated from their mothers for 180 minutes on days 2 to 14 had markedly elevated norepinephrine secretion from the locus coeruleus, the main nucleus in the brain for NE secretion. After a while, at least in humans, this elevated response can become fatigued, tire out, or be dysregulated by inappropriate perception of the salience of sensory or cognitive information. Synaptic fatigue may be one of the few indications for precursor therapy, e.g., taking large amounts of tyrosine to increase biosynthesis of DA and NE.

Page 357: Carbamazepine (Tegretol) and valproic acid (VPA, Depakote) do not increase dopamine levels in the NAc. They are also not very good treatments for neurosomatic disorders.

Page 357: The primary source of dopamine secretion in the areas of the brain involved in neurosomatic disorders is called the ventral tegmental area. Dopamine secretion from the VTA to the NAc and PFC is regulated in various ways. One of them is by muscarinic and nicotinic receptors for acetylcholine (Ach). That's how medications such as Cognex, Aricept, and nicotine patches can make some patients feel better, depending upon whether these circuits are working properly (no response), too much (worse), or too little (better).

Page 491: Rats that are bred to have too little GABA in their dorsomedial hypothalamus (DMH) appear to develop panic attacks, because almost everywhere glutamate, the excitatory amino acid, is present GABA is present to balance its effect by inhibiting it. In this case, infusion of an antagonist to the NMDA receptor for glutamate prevented panic attacks caused by the infusion of lactate. This medication helped to restore the balance. Fibromyalgia patients, but not normals, are much more likely to have a lactate-induced panic attack.

Page 504: Alpha$_1$ agonists (such as midodrine or ProAmatine) cause the secretion of oxytocin. NE is also an alpha$_1$ agonist. On the relatively few occasions when midodrine helps a patient to feel better, I suspect oxytocin (OXT) is somewhat involved because OXT therapy also improves the same symptoms.

Page 507: As measured by $H_2^{15}O$ PET (positron-emission tomography), which can be done rapidly, the right prefrontal cortex is critical in maintaining attention to a task when distractors are present. If the right PFC does not work correctly (see *Betrayal*) subjects will be easily distracted and their concentration will be poor.

Page 528: A brief injury to a neonatal rat can increase the rat's pain sensitivity for the rest of its life. There is a critical time window for this fairly mild injury to produce this effect.

Page 529: Emeran Mayer has become the leader in irritable bowel syndrome research. I got to know him and invited him to speak at one of my conferences when he was fairly new at this research and introduced him to the role of the brain in IBS. He presented PET-scan studies of IBS patients and normals. Patients fail to activate the anterior cingulate cortex (more about this later) and abnormally activate the left dorsolateral PFC when anticipating and receiving rectal distention with a balloon. He followed up this work at the society's meeting. Moderate nonnoxious rectal distention caused PFC activation in patients but not normals. After sensitization with repetitive painful balloon distention, the IBS patients activated the ACC following nonpainful stimulation, not seen in normals. Mayer suggested that normals inhibit pain better from an area of the brainstem called the periaqueductal gray, so they aren't sensitized (develop "hyperalgesia"). I'm not so sure this is the way it works (higher centers are involved in regulating the PAG and interpreting painful visceral stimuli), but his work is the closest to mine of any researcher.

Page 592: I have suggested that endothelin in excess can make neurosomatic patients feel sick. The effects of endothelin on sensory gating have not been studied, but activation of the endothelin A receptor (there are A and B receptors that work quite differently) caused reduction in a potassium K_{ATP} channel response produced by activation of the mu-opioid receptor (done also by morphine-like drugs, gabapentin, minoxidil, and clonidine). Because these agents are often beneficial for neurosomatic disorders, endothelin's blocking of K_{ATP} channels makes it even more implicated in neurosomatic pathophysiology. The effect of endothelin was mimicked by arachidonic acid (AA), produced by the enzyme phospholipase A_2 (PLA_2) which is the main constituent of honey bee venom, one of my treatments that works on a few people. The biochemistry is too complicated to discuss here, but AA is an indirect NMDA-receptor agonist/antagonist, as well as a stimulator of dopamine secretion. This experiment suggests that endothelin might be beneficial, at least in a very few people.

Page 601: Amerge (naratriptan) is a migraine headache medicine, similar to Imitrex (sumatriptan), Zomig (zolmitriptan), and Maxalt (rizatriptan). What makes Amerge different is that it has few side effects or drug interactions and has a higher affinity for the serotonin (5-HT_{1B}) receptor, which is related to the inhibitor's 5-HT_{1D} receptor, which all of these drugs stimulate. The triptans as a group block the release of substance P and calcitonin gene-related peptide (CGRP), and can decrease (I have found) the symptoms of cervical spinal stenosis, in which nerve roots and the spinal cord are being compressed, with the release of (particularly) CGRP. Amerge can help more than migraines and spinal cord problems. The 5-HT_{1B} receptor is crucial for the action of serotonin-reuptake inhibitor antidepressants. Hypothetically, if the 5-HT_{1B} receptor is blocked, SRIs should be less effective. Directly stimulating the 5-HT_{1B} receptor might be a good thing if lower serotonin levels are desired. Amerge sometimes alleviates fibromyalgia and helps CFS patients feel better in general. It also might be the best migraine medicine for them because it may specifically decrease 5-HT in the PFC, one of the places that the drug really needs to act.

Page 707: If neurosomatic patients are hypervigilant, they should be more easily stressed, particularly when they perceive the stressor to be uncontrollable, as is the case with many. Blocking the NMDA receptor in the dorsal raphe nucleus, where most of the serotonin in the brain is made, ameliorates this sort of stress in rats. If the NMDA antagonist had been infused elsewhere (numerous other places) the amelioration would have been greater, but the neurotransmitters all work together, like an orchestra. Some play louder and longer than the others in certain situations.

Page 708: When people are stressed, neuronal overactivation occurs in numerous areas of the brain. This overactivation is not good for the brain, and so it makes more *adenosine,* an inhibitory neurotransmitter like GABA, to decrease the activation. Adenosine can cause fatigue and sleepiness.

Page 709: Exercise decreases the amount of norepinephrine in the PFC of stressed rats (and perhaps people), one reason for exercise-induced relapse. There are others. The complexity of the brain is beyond imagination. Scalding rats (a stressor) releases endothelin-1 (there are three kinds) from the hypothalamus into the blood stream.

Page 711: NMDA receptors in the PFC constantly ("tonically") inhibit dopamine release. If dopamine levels in the PFC are too low, as they probably are in neurosomatic disorders, then blocking the NMDA receptors for glutamate in the PFC will increase PFC dopamine. Blocking NMDA receptors in the VTA, however, decreased PFC dopamine, suggesting that glutamate neurons in the brains of neurosomatic patients were *hypofunctioning,* because if their PFCs sent more glutamate to the VTA, they would get more dopamine back. Interestingly, schizophrenia has been postulated to be a *hyperglutamatergic* disorder, but one that increases dopamine secretion in the PFC, the opposite of what happens in neurosomatic disorders, which are more akin to Parkinson's disease, if anything.

Increasing dopamine in the PFC helps "working memory," the ability to organize multiple tasks and solve problems. I wish I knew an easy way to increase PFC dopamine.

Blocking the NMDA receptor with a systemic drug increased PFC dopamine, NE, and acetylcholine. Infusing this drug into the PFC increased DA and NE, but not Ach, which is independently regulated. All three are involved in increasing attention (focusing), a basic CFS problem, without using atypical neuroleptics.

Talwin (pentazocine) could be an antidepressant. The related drug igmesine is.

Page 712: Lamictal (lamotrigine, LTG), one of my favorite medications, inhibits the release of glutamate. Thus, it decreases glutamate's effect at all its receptors. Rilutek (riluzole) has this effect also.

Page 746: Repetitive transcranial magnetic stimulation (rTMS) has few side effects and might help some patients with CFS. Probes were implanted in the hypothalamic paraventricular nucleus and dorsal hippocampus of rats, who were then given rTMS. Increases in glutamate, taurine, aspartate, serine, and serotonin were noted.

Page 771: Marinol (delta-9-tetrahydrocannabinol) is a very useful agent in neurosomatic disorders. It stimulates AA release and inhibits glutamate reuptake, thereby increasing glutamate levels. Other experiments find different results, especially that cannabinoids are NMDA antagonists.

Page 854: Dopamine, acting at the D_1 receptor (there are at least five of them) acts on L-type calcium channels, the same ones that are blocked by drugs such as Nimotop (nimodipine). D_1-receptor activation can cause GABA release and can rapidly change neuron discharge, noise-to-signal ratio, and neural plasticity in the PFC. Calcium-channel blockers can "fine tune" these effects.

Page 861: Pindolol increases DA and NE, but not 5-HT, in the PFC of rats. This effect helps many CFS patients. I don't understand why it doesn't help more of them.

Page 892: Analgesia produced by TENS is blocked by the opioid antagonist naloxone in arthritic rats.

Page 893: Improgen, an H_2-receptor antagonist like Tagamet or Zantac, relieves pain by a nonopioid mechanism. It is an NMDA-receptor antagonist and a cholinesterase inhibitor, but these experimenters were apparently unaware of this fact.

Page 949: OXT increases enkephalin and hence dopamine levels in the NAc. Opioids increase DA in the NAc. That's why some patients have all of their symptoms relieved when they take a Vicodin. I don't know why OXT doesn't work in everybody, either.

Page 1021: The muscarinic Ach receptor couples to PLA_2 to release AA, which is an L-type calcium-channel blocker, like Nimotop.

Page 1109: Pindolol potentiates SRIs. It is known to be a 5-HT_{1A} antagonist, but its $5\text{-HT}_{1B/1D}$ antagonism might be more important in the potentiation. This result is almost the opposite of what I wrote about Amerge.

Page 1131: Many patients with FMS have temporomandibular dysfunction (TMD), manifested by jaw clenching and teeth grinding. Often, TMD is a precursor to FMS. As seen on PET, postclench jaw pain was associated with activation of the thalamus and cingulate gyrus, structures thought to mediate the increase in pain.

Page 1134: The amygdala is a structure crucial to producing fear and other defensive and aggressive emotions. It is also involved in the pain relief produced by morphine. Infusion of a cannabinoid (CB) into the amygdala of rats produces potent pain relief.

Page 1135: In a very complex way, patients with FMS pay more attention to stimuli they perceive as painful. When a person attends to something else, the same stimulus should be perceived as less painful, but FMS patients have difficulty switching attention due to their hypervigilant anxiety about impending pain and altered perception of salience of sensory and cognitive information. The main cortical region that processes painful input is called the primary somatosensory cortex (S1). When normal subjects studied with water PET attended to or did not attend to painful stimuli, the activation of S1 differed, decreasing when they did not pay as much attention to it.

Page 1160: NE can act as an NMDA-receptor antagonist by enhancing the effect of inhibitory interneurons.

Page 1172: AA increases NMDA-evoked brain blood flow. An agonist in some situations, an antagonist in others.

Page 1193: Brain alpha-1 receptor stimulation (by NE or ProAmatine) is a protective factor during stress but only at a low range, above which adverse effects predominate. Parnate and Nardil work better than Eldepryl or moclobemide in an animal model of anxiety. I've found this in people, too.

Page 1198: OXT injected into the PVN stimulates nitric oxide (NO) and causes penile erection. NMDA infused into the PVN also causes penile erection, but by a different mechanism.

Page 1245: Marinol, acting at the $cannabinoid_1$ receptor, increases PFC DA, probably useful in many neurosomatic patients.

Page 1252: The dorsolateral PFC selects, or *gates,* visual and spatial information, selecting salient stimuli from irrelevant ones, as shown by functional magnetic resonance imaging.

Page 1253: Cannabinoids inhibit *windup,* a centrally mediated increase in the response of spinal cord dorsal horn neurons to successive stimuli. Windup can be a precursor to chronic pain conditions.

Page 1319: Norepinephrine enhances $GABA_A$ receptor-mediated synaptic transmission in rat hypothalamic paraventricular neurons. Thus, norepinephrine can have an inhibitory effect by stimulating GABAergic interneurons as discussed previously. Norepinephrine also has a direct effect on the cell membranes by hyperpolarizing them and making them less apt to be depolarized and activated by weak stimuli. Thus, it can raise signal-to-noise ratio. This neurophysiologic effect translates in neural networks to a patient being less distractible and better able to concentrate.

Page 1392: For those patients who have cervical spinal stenosis, which could also compress spinal nerve roots exiting from the spinal canal, CGRP and substance P are secreted in excess in this situation and enhance pain. These substances can be inhibited by one of the triptan drugs that are used to treat migraine. CGRP and substance P are also inhibited by gabapentin, which acts as well on the thalamus and the anterior cingulate cortex as discussed in an article by Ness and colleagues in the journal *Pain* (Ness TJ et al., 1998).

Page 1438: Thyroid status differentially affects behavior of the depression-prone Wistar Kyoto rat. Wistar Kyoto rats show hyperresponsiveness to stress in depression and anxious behavior. They are more likely to become hypothyroid but are not helped by being given thyroid hormone.

Page 1430: A precursor to thyrotropin-releasing hormone has antidepressant behavioral responses in the rat. TRH itself also appears to have antidepressant and antineurosomatic properties in human beings when given intravenously in a dose of 500 units and also when given by nasal spray in a dose of three units in each nostril. It can also be given as an eyedrop.

Page 1491: An agent similar to Talwin, called igmesine, increases extracellular levels of NMDA but not 5-HT in the brain. Talwin and igmesine are sigma 1 stimulators or "ligands." Talwin is thought to have many neurobehavioral effects, not just as an antidepressant but also as a potential antipsychotic.

Page 1620: A pathway from the lumbosacral spinal cord to the penis can regulate penile erection in rats. It is originally stimulated by oxytocin at the level of the lumbosacral spinal cord which stimulates the secretion of nitric oxide which then releases cyclic GMP (guanosine monophosphate), a vasodilator that causes penile erections. Therefore, an oxytocin-nitric oxide-cyclic GMP pathway from the lumbosacral spinal cord to the veins of the penis can cause penile erection. Because oxytocin may be low in patients with CFS, giving oxytocin might be helpful.

Page 1628: When rats have pain caused by a nerve injury, it is called neuropathic pain. This sort of injury can be experimentally induced, and it is fairly well known that the effect of morphine on such injuries is somewhat limited, just as it is on central pain. Giving Marinol to rats with neuropathic pain decreased the pain significantly. This pain relief was independent of the NMDA and opioid systems. Furthermore, in a second experiment on the same page, researchers noted that cannabinoids suppressed pain processing at the level of the medial thalamus, the main switchboard of the brain. They acted there by a nonopioid and non-NMDA mechanism.

Page 1629: Neuropathic pain is relieved by clonidine, a medication that stimulates the alpha$_2$ adrenergic receptor. Clonidine increases the release of acetylcholine and nitric oxide at the level of the spinal cord. The acetylcholine attached to both nicotinic and muscarinic receptors to elicit nitric oxide production in pain relief. The inhibitory neurotransmitter adenosine acting at the A$_1$ adenosine receptor works as an NMDA-receptor antagonist. It therefore can be analgesic in this situation and also blocks the release of amino acids that occur secondarily to NMDA-receptor activation. Amino acids blocked include glutamate, aspartate, and taurine.

Page 1680: The activity of 130 neurons in the locus coeruleus of a monkey was recorded when the monkey had to make rapid choices between salient and nonsalient targets. When the monkey performed this task, enhanced activity occurred in the locus coeruleus. Because the locus coeruleus is the primary nucleus in the brain that secretes norepinephrine, I would expect that neurosomatic patients would perform rather poorly in such tasks.

Page 1681: Another experiment reports that locus coeruleus neurons are selectively activated by attentive stimuli suggesting reward availability, as well as other salient events such as loud noises. The part of this response that occurs early when the monkey is performing tasks rapidly which require discrimination between cues is thought to indicate enhanced attentiveness during this condition and may reflect sensory gating that would prime the locus coeruleus and many associated structures. Thus, events would be processed more rapidly. Obviously, performance on this kind of test would be impaired in neurosomatic patients.

Another experiment finds that the right PFC is necessary to inhibit unattended semantic information. These results support models suggesting right hemisphere dominance for human attention. We have found that there is usually right hemispheric impairment on brain SPECT (single photon emission computed tomography) when we examine patients with CFS.

Page 1682: Researchers examined the function of the human anterior cingulate cortex, which is involved with executive control of cognitive processes, response selection, conflict resolution, internal monitoring, anticipation and preparatory processes, and affective and motivational aspects of behavior. Although these terms sound rather technical, they are all aspects of behaviors that are often impaired in patients with neurosomatic disorders. These experimenters found that decisions are computed in the lateral prefrontal areas and then channeled to the anterior cingulate cortex for translation into motor output, during which selection between alternative responses takes place. Another experiment discusses the amygdala in the context of fear learning in previously fear-conditioned rats. This experiment would apply to neurosomatic patients who are hypervigilant due to either genetic or developmental factors. If the NMDA receptors in the amygdala are blocked, new fear learning disappears rapidly, i.e., *extinction* occurs rapidly when the NMDA receptors are blocked.

Page 1926: An experiment again looks at Wistar Kyoto rats and looks for precursors of TRH to understand underlying mechanisms of depression. In Wistar Kyoto rats, two regions that were examined, the paraventricular nucleus of the hypothalamus and the bed nucleus of the stria terminalis (BST), had a lower density of nerve fibers that manufactured precursors to TRH than did regular Wistar rats, which were not vulnerable to depression.

Page 1928: An important experiment shows that transforming growth factor (TGF)-beta released in the brain by physical exercise causes the sensation of fatigue. Rats that became fatigued were found to have elevated levels of this substance in their cerebrospinal fluid. Their fatigue was suppressed by injecting anti-TGF-beta antibody into their cerebrospinal fluid. Injecting TGF-beta into their spinal fluid suppressed their activity. These results suggest that either inhibiting the biosynthesis of TGF-beta or blocking its effects in humans might be an effective treatment for fatigue along with adenosine-receptor antagonists that do not cause jitteriness like caffeine does.

There is no published interaction between adenosine and TGF-beta. Substances that inhibit the action of TGF-beta are not particularly effective in alleviating fatigue in my patients. These include losartan, intravenous immunoglobulin, prolactin and substances that increase it (such as haloperidol), tamoxifen, and corticosteroids. Intravenous immunoglobulin is the only agent among these putative TGF-beta blockers that benefits neurosomatic patients, probably by an unrelated mechanism.

Many more experiments were presented at this meeting that I did not discuss due to constraints of space and also because of their complexity. Many of these relate to how different circuits or neural networks in the brain are regulated, an important concept for understanding neurosomatic disorders. Other complex work related to attentional mechanisms and the anatomy and function of the nucleus accumbens and its interactions with other structures. Absent from the presentations were detailed experiments on the neurophysiology of instantaneous reconfiguration of neural networks. Sadly, no experimenter was doing work remotely related to mine, i.e., how to pharmacologically modify information gating in the brain. These topics, which are vital to understanding the pathophysiology of neurosomatic disorders, will be addressed in this book.

Chapter 8

Neurosomatic Pearls

Another Society for Neuroscience conference has come and gone. The 29th annual meeting was held in Miami Beach, Florida, October 23 to 28, 1999, with over 13,000 experiments presented. I will attempt to summarize and annotate what I consider to be important presentations and also will later review articles written in the last three years or so, that I think are particularly relevant.

1. Much work has been done in understanding sounds called distress-like vocalizations in mouse pups, i.e., neonatal rodents. Pups emit ultrasonic vocalizations when they are separated from their mothers, which may indicate their distress and result in prompt retrieval by the mother. Pharmacologic agents to alleviate anxiety in humans reduce the emission of these calls by acting on $GABA_A$ and $5-HT_1$ receptor subtypes. Opioids also have this effect.
2. One way to inhibit glutamate secretion is by decreasing its production. A source of glutamate is the breakdown of a compound called N-acetyl-aspartate glutamate, also known as NAAG. The enzyme that breaks down NAAG can be inhibited, resulting in a decreased conversion of NAAG to glutamate. Such enzyme inhibition would have the same effect as inhibiting glutamate release, which is done by chlorzoxazone, Lamictal, and Rilutek among clinically available drugs.
3. Some of my patients feel stimulated by nicotinamide, which can be purchased in a health food store. This drug partially antagonizes the effects of phencyclidine (PCP) and almost totally antagonizes the effects of lysergic acid diethylamide (LSD). Nicotinamide is an adenosine diphosphate (ADP)-ribosyl cyclase inhibitor. Nicotinamide inhibits calcium release related to PCP and also to caffeine. The same effects can be obtained by inhibiting nitric oxide synthase.
4. You will be hearing much more in the near future in the medical and lay press about nicotine receptor agonists and antagonists, particularly for specific receptors. The nicotine alpha receptor seems to be the most promising. Agents that stimulate nicotine seem to have an effect on

Tourette's syndrome, i.e., affecting the stimulation of the $5\text{-HT}_{2A/C}$ receptor. $5\text{-HT}_{2A/2C}$ agonists are difficult to obtain in clinical medicine, should the need ever arise for one. LSD works as an agonist at these receptors. The two drugs that are available in clinical medicine for this purpose are Methergine and Sansert. Both of these are used for the treatment of migraine headaches and are 5-HT_2 antagonists with partial agonist effects.

5. NMDA-receptor antagonists and sigma agonists may have similar effects in several situations but usually antagonize each other.

6. Dopamine D_1-receptor agonists increase cognitive performance mediated by the prefrontal cortex. Unfortunately, at this time, no specific dopamine D_1-receptor agonists can be used in clinical medicine.

7. The combination of dopamine D_2-receptor antagonists, such as haloperidol, and 5-HT_1 agonist, such as buspirone, may have potent effects on fear-potentiated startle response and more generally on anticipatory anxiety.

8. Glucocorticoids such as cortisone interact with $alpha_1$ adrenoceptors in the basolateral nucleus of the amygdala in mediating memory storage via an activation of $alpha_1$ adrenoceptors. Therefore, it should theoretically be possible to improve memory by giving an $alpha_1$-adrenoceptor agonist, such as midodrine or ProAmantine, and combining it with cycloserine. $Alpha_1$ antagonists/$alpha_2$ agonists may prevent nightmares in people with PTSD. Another way to do the same thing is to give a selective noradrenergic-reuptake blocker. This would affect $alpha_1$ and $alpha_2$ receptors, but perhaps would preferentially affect $alpha_1$ receptors in the amygdala. The selective noradrenergic-reuptake blocker reboxetine is now available.

9. A class of cognitive enhancers called nootropics is not available in the United States but is available in many other countries. The prototypical nootropic is called piracetam. This agent causes an increase in GABA-ergic activity, an increase in nerve growth factor (NGF) activity, and an increase in an as-yet-unknown adrenal hormone, which is not a corticosteroid. It is also a cholinergic and AMPA (alpha-amino-3-hydroxy-5-methyl-4-isoxazolepropionic acid) agonist, as well as an NMDA antagonist. Other nootropics act by variations of this pharmacology. Numerous nootropics are in the developmental stage. The isomer of piracetam is now marketed as the antiepileptic drug (AED) levetiracetram, also known as Keppra. It is devoid of nootropic activity but is a good agent to treat myoclonus.

10. An NMDA-receptor antagonist decreases cortisone responses to stress. The NMDA receptor is one of the receptors for the excitatory neurotransmitter glutamate. Glutamate input to the periventricular nucleus of

the hypothalamus excites the hypothalamic-pituitary-adrenal axis (HPA axis). On the other hand, serotonin increases the secretion of cortisone. It does so by indirectly increasing the secretion of corticotropin-releasing hormone which stimulates adrenocorticotropin (ACTH), thereby stimulating adrenal corticosteroid levels.

11. Serotonin-reuptake inhibitors, such as Prozac, can control the expression of glucocorticoid receptors (for cortisone) in the hippocampus without the presence of serotonin at all. They can apparently do so directly due to an effect on receptor expression.

12. Prolactin, which is elevated if its secretion is not inhibited by dopamine and other factors, is an endogenous anxiolytic neuropeptide that reduces the HPA axis and oxytocin responses to stress at the brain level. Prolactin is increased after ejaculation in males and is partly responsible for their postcoital sexual refractory period by inhibiting mesocorticolimbic DA secretion. Male CFS patients often relapse after orgasm, because they often do not have enough dopamine and norepinephrine reserve to perform independent activities of daily living even prior to ejaculation, or because their catecholamine autoreceptors are hypersensitive.

13. Androgens such as testosterone increase the secretion of dopamine, probably by decreasing the activity of the dopamine transporter. Ritalin and cocaine also have this action. Androgens also increase DA by interacting with NO.

14. The amino acid taurine inhibits the dopamine transporter and may work somewhat like Ritalin. Taurine is an agent I have tried on several of my patients. It did not enhance dopamine effects but may augment lamotrigine in some individuals.

15. Nicotine induces a moderate level of norepinephrine release in the occipital cortex, as well as the cerebellum and the cervical section of the spinal cord. A much greater release has been found in the rat brain hippocampus and frontal cortex, as well as the locus coeruleus. The most important nicotinic cholinergic receptor as far as neurosomatic disorders are concerned is the alpha$_1$ receptor, which is involved in the stimulatory effects of nicotine on mesolimbocortical dopaminergic function. The doses of nicotine necessary to achieve this goal are rather high, but selected agonists at this receptor might be tolerated.

16. In numerous situations, nicotine can increase the secretion of dopamine. Nicotine can also increase the secretion of GABA. At least one method by which this may be accomplished is by activation of D_1 heteroreceptors on GABAergic nerve terminals. Nicotine agonists will soon be used as nonopioid analgesics.

17. It is important for the brain to detect deviance from the usual order of things, or "novelty." The anterior cingulate cortex is usually involved in this process, as is the right prefrontal cortex and bilateral temporo-parietal junction. Patients with functional lesions of the right prefrontal cortex, often seen in patients with neurosomatic disorders, may have a heightened response to novelty or deviance as a result of dysregulation of the right hemisphere.

18. In rats that are testosterone deficient, the density of tyrosine hydroxylase (TH)-immunopositive axons in the prefrontal cortex increases. Tyrosine hydroxylase converts tyrosine to dopa and is usually the rate-limiting enzyme in the biosynthesis of the catecholamines. The dysregulation of TH is attenuated by supplementing rats with testosterone. The effect is mainly on dopamine and not norepinephrine. Testosterone depletion produces a dopamine hyperinnervation in the prefrontal cortex in an attempt to compensate for decreased production of dopamine.

19. $GABA_A$-receptor levels are inversely related to hypothalamic oxytocin secretion. Many antibiotics and the loop diuretic furosemide (Lasix) are $GABA_A$-receptor antagonists. Oxytocin is also an $alpha_2$ adrenoceptor antagonist, as is buspirone, via 1-(2-pyramidinyl-piperazine) (1-PP), its metabolite.

20. Serotonin and norepinephrine induce a process termed CREB (CAMP-response element-binding protein) phosphorylation, i.e., adding a phosphate group to a nuclear substance called CREB which is induced by AMP. CREB participates in the transcriptional regulation by DNA of brain-derived neurotrophic factor, or BDNF, which has potent antidepressant properties. CREB phosphorylation may be one of the mechanisms by which antidepressants produce their behavioral effects and is an important regulator of the rebound period after opioid deprivation. CREB activity does not have a circadian role, and CREB activity does not trigger the onset of rest. CREB serves a restorative function of rest that permits prolonged wakefulness. Because restorative sleep is notably absent in patients with neurosomatic disorders, the classic cAMP-protein kinase A (PKA)-CREB signaling pathway, or a variation thereof, may be dysfunctional (Hendricks JC et al., 2001).

21. Tetrahydrobiopterin is a required cofactor for the synthesis of tryptophan, dopamine, and nitric oxide. The rate-limiting enzyme in the biosynthesis of tetrahydrobiopterin, or BH_4, is ultimately regulated by AMP. BH_4 is supposedly being sold now as a nutritional supplement, but I have yet to try it in any of my patients. I can't get it since it is not made by any source of which I am aware. It should theoretically be beneficial, but I can vaguely recall a Japanese study in the early 1980s that

studied the use of BH_4 as an agent to treat depression in monotherapy. BH_4 alone was ineffective.

22. Another substance available in health-food stores is called forskolin. Forskolin in a general activator of adenyl cyclase (AC), which increases AMP. Forskolin seems to work in a different manner than rolipram, an investigational antidepressant drug, that also stimulates the increase of AMP. Rolipram seems to act in a more specific manner than forskolin, by inhibiting phosphodiesterase-4.

23. If there is overexpression of glutamate transport, there might be dampening of the excitability changes resulting from neuromodulation by noradrenergic hyperinnervation.

24. Even though I certainly have not seen this effect clinically, one report explains that cyclooxygenase (COX) inhibitors such as indomethacin and acetylsalicylic acid potentiate the suppressive effects of opioids on presynaptic GABA neurotransmission in periaqueductal gray neurons. A COX pathway is also present in mesolimbic dopamine neurons. When COX inhibitors are given to rats together with morphine, mesolimbic dopamine secretion is further potentiated. Morphine enhances mesolimbic dopamine secretion by inhibiting tonic GABAergic suppression of dopamine release.

25. Some patients receive glutathione as a treatment. Glutathione is excitotoxic in rat cortical slices. The excitotoxicity is not affected by various glutamate antagonists or by ascorbic acid (vitamin C), which is a significant inhibitor of excitotoxicity.

26. In some situations, estrogen appears to be a serotonin (5-HT_2)-receptor agonist since it inhibits what are called *lordosis effects* in rats, which are produced by 5-HT_2-receptor antagonists. Estrogen reduces the effectiveness of 5-HT_{1A}-receptor agonists and is a monoamine oxidase inhibitor (MAOI). Progesterone modulates lordosis, tending to inhibit it, but only if the rat is primed with estrogen. Serotonin also inhibits lordosis. This inhibition can be attenuated by infusion of norepinephrine into the ventromedial hypothalamic nucleus of sexually receptive female rats. There appears to be a functional interaction between 5-HT_{1A} and alpha$_1$ noradrenergic receptors. The method by which serotonin is released in the prefrontal cortex has been the subject of some investigation. This release may be suppressed by mu-opioid agonists such as morphine. Serotonin, via neurons from the midline and intralaminar thalamic nuclei, releases glutamate in the medial prefrontal cortex. Serotonin, via 5-HT_{2A} receptors, modulates excitatory transmission in cortical circuits, which may account for fluctuations in mood, attentional state, and capacity for information processing. These

effects vary according to the density of 5-HT$_{2A}$ receptors in the six different layers of the cortex.

27. Clonidine, an alpha$_2$ agonist, inhibits serotonin firing from the dorsal raphe nucleus because there are alpha$_2$ heteroreceptors on the serotonergic neurons. However, the secretion of serotonin can be increased by a phosphodiesterase inhibitor (PDEI). Phosphodiesterase is the enzyme that degrades AMP. There are six or more subtypes of phosphodiesterase. Medications specific for different types of phosphodiesterase include Pletal (cilostazol), which is specific for phosphodiesterase-3, and Viagra (sildenafil), which is specific for phosphodiesterase-5, with some overlap into phosphodiesterase-6, which can cause alteration of color vision by its action in the retina.

For several years, I have wondered how the prefrontal cortex can regulate its own serotonergic innervation. Now it has been shown that the medial prefrontal cortex can modulate the activity of the majority of raphe serotonergic neurons. A reciprocal interaction seems to occur between these two regions. Serotonin via 2A and 2C receptors excites GABAergic interneurons in the dorsal raphe nucleus, and this mechanism has been adduced to explain suppression of firing of a subset of serotonergic neurons by certain types of hallucinogenic agents. Serotonin can also stimulate the release of acetylcholine. The mechanism of this process involves serotonin 1A and 2A receptors. Presynaptic glutamatergic heteroreceptors inhibit somatically evoked cortical acetylcholine secretion by acting at presynaptic NMDA autoreceptors but not at other receptors for glutamate. Adenosine or GABA$_B$ receptors are not involved. In other situations, however, cholinergic muscarinic and nicotinic receptors appear to evoke glutamate secretion.

For several years now a debate has ensued about whether the beta agonist pindolol, which has intrinsic sympathomimetic activity as a 5-HT$_{1A}$ antagonist, may be used as augmentation strategy when giving antidepressants. Pindolol does not appear to enter the brain well, although, as seen in previous work, crossing the blood-brain barrier (BBB) is not essential for action of a drug if it can stimulate receptors on extracranial nerves that affect gating. Stress also may make the blood-brain barrier more porous. A possible important synergistic action has been found between lidocaine and 5-HT$_{1D}$ agonists in relieving certain kinds of pain. 5-HT$_{1D}$ agonists are also known as *triptans* and are used in the treatment of migraine headaches. The combination does not seem to be harmful and could be productively used in treating migraine headache and other types of neuropathic pain.

28. Neurotensin, a 13-amino acid peptide that has neuroleptic properties, apparently confers resistance to the sedating effects of alcohol. Mice

bred to not express neurotensins are hypersensitive to the effects of alcohol. Neurotensin levels in people with CFS have not been determined to my knowledge. Alpha interferon, a substance that has been associated at times with CFS, decreases L-type calcium channels in the hippocampus. One might thus think that an alpha interferon deficiency is present in patients who responded to L-type calcium-channel blockers, such as nimodipine. Hypocretin (another term for orexin), a substance related to secretin, increases activity in the locus coeruleus, the main noradrenergic ganglion in the brain. Secretin has been associated with improvements in autism, although a double-blind experiment using secretin in autism did not show any benefit when performed recently. Orexins in general are increased in the locus coeruleus, and orexins also stimulate transmitter substances in the vagus nerve. The main transmitter substance in the vagus nerve is glutamate. Orexins are involved with appetite stimulation and are low or absent in CSF patients with familial narcolepsy. Some new analgesic peptides, nocistatin and nociceptin, cause hyperalgesia in the rat spinal cord after they are injected into the spinal fluid. These compounds may be involved in tuning the response of the organism to painful stimuli. Corticotropin-releasing hormone, thought to be low in patients with CFS, directly stimulates dopamine secretion by neurons in the ventral tegmental area. In my formulation of neurosomatic pathophysiology, ventral tegmental dopamine secretion is significantly reduced.

29. Gabapentin (Neurontin) has analgesic activities. It has been shown to bind to the $alpha_2$-delta subunit of voltage-dependent calcium channels, of which L-type calcium channels are an example. In animals that have neuropathic pain, the $alpha_2$-delta subunit protein levels in the spinal fluid are increased. This elevation is possibly related to the mode of action of Neurontin.

    Brain-derived neurotrophic factor appears to be increased by administration of all antidepressants after a lag period for biosynthesis. BDNF also increases glutamate by acting as a retrograde messenger, much in the manner of nitric oxide. If the synaptic connection between the pre- and postsynaptic neuron, however, is strong, BDNF has no effect.

    Many patients with CFS have dysphagia. FMRI has been done while people voluntarily swallow. Large increases can be seen in regional cerebral blood flow in the inferior precentral gyrus bilaterally as well as the right anterior insula and the left cerebellum. Other areas of the brain also exhibit blood flow increases, but not as distinctly as the previously mentioned areas. These areas may be part of a dysfunctional circuit in dysphagic patients. In 5-HT$_{1A}$ knock-out mice, i.e., mice who do not make the 5-HT$_{1A}$ receptor, anxiety is resistant to benzodiazepines. A significant number of patients with anxiety disorders are similarly resistant to benzodiazepines. A mechanistic link between the serotonergic and GABAergic systems may explain this phenomenon.

30. The experimental drug agmatine appears to be an endogenous NMDA-receptor antagonist and is made merely by decarboxylating arginine. Arginine is the precursor to nitric oxide, which would be an NMDA-receptor agonist indirectly via its role as a retrograde messenger in glutamatergic synapses.

Mice that lack the 5-HT$_{1B}$ receptor, a receptor stimulated by the anti-migraine triptan medications, have enhanced self-administration of cocaine. It appears that this receptor is related to cocaine administration and is blocked by infusion of glial-derived neurotrophic factor (GDNF) into the ventral tegmental area and the nucleus accumbens. Thus, GDNF knock-outs have increased sensitivity to cocaine as well. Much can be learned from the study of drugs of abuse. Group III metabotropic glutamate receptors in the nucleus acumbens suppress relapse to cocaine abuse. The nucleus acumbens is in close approximation to the ventral tegmental area, which secretes dopamine. Repeated cocaine treatment selectively increases tonic adenosine inhibition of metabotropic glutamate receptor (mGluR) inhibitory neurotransmission in the dopaminergic neurons of the VTA, suggesting that elevated adenosine-receptor sensitivity may preferentially increase glutamate secretion. Medications that increase adenosine levels, such as dipyridamole, are useful agents in neurosomatic disorders, primarily, I think, because of their inhibition of glutamatergic neurotransmission. By the same token, giving baclofen into the VTA attenuates cocaine reinforcement. Baclofen is a GABA$_B$ agonist and inhibits the secretion of all neurotransmitters except for acetylcholine and, sometimes, serotonin.

Tyrosine hydroxylase is the rate-limiting enzyme for norepinephrine synthesis in the locus coeruleus, which sends diffuse projections throughout the central nervous system. The activity of tyrosine hydroxylase is fairly resistant to change by medication but can be regulated both by agents that block the norepinephrine transporter and by tetrahydrobiopterin. Neurons in aged animals have a sustained calcium leak through somatic membrane channels that impairs regulated transmitter release at synapses. This may contribute to age-related cognitive decline and is one reason why it might be a good idea to take nimodipine as one ages. If a patient has a good response to lidocaine but has problems with neurotoxicity that are not relieved by dosage adjustment, this adverse reaction may sometimes be attenuated by administering lithium carbonate. Lithium influences lidocaine-induced interactions with voltage-gated sodium channels. Riluzole (Rilutek), besides inhibiting the secretion of glutamate, also inhibits sodium channels, thereby reducing calcium-channel gating and catecholamine secretion. This may be another way that Rilutek works in amyotrophic lateral sclerosis (ALS) and may be useful in neurosomatic disorders for the same reason.

Patients with fibromyalgia have been found to have elevated levels of nerve growth factor. If NGF levels are too high, a phenomenon called apoptosis occurs. Apoptosis is associated with cell death. Using zinc in fairly physiologic concentrations attenuates the apoptosis induced by NGF. BDNF can also cause apoptosis and may be amenable to the same modulation. In experimentally stressed female mice who exhibit fear behavior, the fear behavior is increased by administering estrogen. Anxiety seems to involve a circuit including the central nucleus of the amygdala, two out of four areas of the periaqueductal gray, the locus coeruleus, and the lateral parabrachial nucleus. Prenatally stressed rats are an animal model of human depression. The "forced swimming test" is used to check for depressive behavior. Melatonin improves performance in the forced swimming test, as does tianeptine, a dopamine-reuptake inhibitor. Melatonin should have antidepressant effects in human beings but has not appeared to exhibit this property thus far. One of the main cognitive problems of people with neurosomatic disorders is deficits in short-term memory, also called working memory. Cells that inhibit other neural activity must be active in order to avoid an impairment in working memory by distractors. This recurrent neural network inhibition is most noted in the prefrontal and inferior temporal cortices of the behaving monkey. The model assumes a predominance of synaptic inhibition in the excitatory recurrent synapses with a significant NMDA-receptor-mediated component. Therefore, working memory in the prefrontal cortex must be dominated by inhibitory neurotransmission in order to be efficient.

Forskolin activates adenyl cyclase and increases cAMP and PKA. Few other clinically available substances increase cAMP levels. It appears that forskolin is fairly free of adverse reactions. Relevant to neurosomatic disorders, increasing cAMP and PKA increases the synaptic input from the neocortex to the thalamus in a region that involves impairing a well-studied phenomenon called long-term potentiation, a process generally associated with making new memories.

When estrogen is given to healthy menopausal women, significant increases are found in glucose metabolism in the right frontal and temporal cortices and a decrease in glucose metabolism in the left frontal cortex. Estrogen has been thought by many to be protective against associated cognitive decline, although recently the validity of this postulate has been called into question.

Protein tyrosine kinases (TrK) are widely expressed in the central nervous system, and one of their major functions is to regulate ion channels such as the NMDA receptor. Genistein inhibits protein tyrosine kinases, thereby reducing levels of the NMDA-receptor subunit 1 in arthritic rats. It may, therefore, have analgesic properties. Genistein is available in some health food stores. I am not aware of any adverse reactions associated with this agent. I have taken it myself and used it on some patients. Results are, as yet, inconclusive.

Numerous agents block the 5-HT$_{2A}$ receptor, such as nefazodone and risperidone. Only a few are clinically available to activate the 5-HT$_{2A}$ receptor, which leads to stimulation of various signal-transduction pathways, including those involving phospholipase C (PLC), phospholipase D, and phospholipase A$_2$. Honey bee venom might activate this receptor.

Cannabinoids have been reported to attenuate GABAergic transmission in the rat globus pallidus. The globus pallidus is best known for modulating motor activity and malfunctions in patients with Parkinson's disease. However, the globus pallidus has also been implicated in diffuse pain. Activating cannabinoid-1 (CB$_1$) receptors in the globus pallidus depresses GABAergic neurotransmission by a presynaptic mechanism.

The CB$_1$ receptor also produces the lipid second messenger *ceramide,* a result of sphingomyelin hydrolysis and de novo generation (Guzman M et al., 2001). The relevant function of ceramide to neurosomatics is that it regulates energy metabolism, particularly by stimulating the use of glucose. The CB$_1$ receptor may process analgesic and other modulatory properties by virtue of its inhibiting P/Q-type voltage-sensitive Ca^{2+} channels (VSCC) and activating G-protein-activated inwardly rectifying K$^+$ channels (GIRKs—although there are many GIRKs, space limitations do not permit extensive discussion of them in this book). CB$_1$ receptor activation can *decrease* the K$^+$ M-current (non-GIRK) in hippocampal CA1 neurons (Schweitzer PJ, 2000). The bottom line is just like every other process being discussed, the net result of CB$_1$ receptor activation is a functional reconfiguration of neural networks.

Dopamine D$_2$/D$_3$ autoreceptors modulate dopamine release. Researchers have recently found that glutamate can be a cotransmitter with dopamine in cultured neurons, particularly in the ventral tegmental area. Some D$_2$/D$_3$-receptor agonists are fairly specific, one of which is marketed for Parkinson's disease under the trade name Requip. Specific D$_2$-receptor agonists decrease glutamate secretion from dopaminergic neurons by a direct modulation of the secretory process, so when a D$_2$-receptor agonist is administered to a patient and a beneficial result is obtained, it may not occur solely by a postsynaptic mechanism. A D$_2$/D$_3$-autoreceptor-specific antagonist might be a good treatment for neurosomatic disorders, in which DA deficiency may occur because of hypersensitive autoreceptors in the meso-accumbens dopaminergic tract.

Coenzyme Q10 plays a role in the regeneration of vitamin E within mito-chondria. Aged mice may have their memory deficits reversed by giving coenzyme Q10 alone or with vitamin E.

Antidepressants may exert their effects by influencing the AMP system at the postreceptor level. Repeated treatment with imipramine in rats signif-icantly attenuates the effects of forskolin on the rats' behavior. This effect is thought to be related to decreased excitatory activity of all the neuro-transmitters whose receptors were coupled to potassium channels via acti-vation of PKA. Paradoxically, a selective phosphodiesterase-4 inhibitor, rolipram, which blocks AMP hydrolysis, is effective as an antidepressant. This effect was thought to be related to down-regulation of the phospho-diesterase-4 receptor.

Oxytocin is an alpha$_2$ antagonist in the vagus nerve. Norepinephrine is able to gate calcium channels. Kava kava substitutes for alcohol to an extent in alcohol-dependent rats. Numerous medications are nicotinic cholinergic-receptor blockers, although the receptors that they block have not been well subtyped. These include amiloride, methadone, bupropion, cocaine, keta-mine, nimodipine, and mecamylamine.

Periodontal disease is quite common among patients with CFS and other neurosomatic disorders. There is a fairly strong genetic and early postnatal environmental contribution to the pathogenesis of periodontitis, which is caused, at least in part, by high HPA-axis sensitivity. One of my patients keeps her gingivitis in remission as long as she takes guaifenesin, a glycine/NMDA antagonist. Furthermore, early maternal deprivation has an effect on the susceptibility of adult rats to the dopamine agonist apomorphine. The anti-narcoleptic medication modafinil (Provigil) has been found to promote wake-fulness through activation of hypothalamic arousal pathways, unlike amphet-amines which activate striatal neurons. Modafinil may stimulate secretion of histamine from the tuberomammiliary nucleus. Most physicians know that histamine-1-receptor antagonists can make people sleepy as well as make them gain weight. It is not safe to give histamine-1-receptor agonists because of the risks of mast cell activation. However, histamine-3- receptor inverse agonist thioperamide has a significant wake-promoting effect on genetically narcoleptic Doberman pinschers. Modafinil may also have this mode of action. We should be looking for histamine-3-receptor inverse agonists to increase arousal as another potentially useful agent in fatiguing disorders.

Functional brain imaging demonstrates that distinct right- and left-brain systems exist for deductive and probabilistic reasoning. Probabilistic rea-soning is subserved by areas predominantly in the left brain, and deduction activates primarily right-brain areas. Very little overlap occurs between the areas activated by the two types of reasoning. Interestingly, the amygdala, which imparts emotional significance, is activated only during deduction and only on the right side, which is consistent with the occurrence of sudden insight in logical but not probablistic reasoning. The amygdala is involved in memory consolidation (McGaugh JL, 2002), salience and reward (Baxter MG, Murray EA, 2002), and fear conditioning.

Nicotinic cholinergic receptors can increase dopamine and norepinephrine by increasing the levels of tyrosine hydroxylase. This property illustrates the propensity for nicotine to have an acute alerting action but to lose this effect over time since increased levels of tyrosine hydroxylase in the locus coeruleus have been associated with anxiety and depression. Perhaps more significantly, in the absence of structural change, the mode in which norepinephrine is secreted in the locus coeruleus, be it tonic (continuous) or phasic (intermittent), is also associated with mood and anxiety disorders. Although structural abnormalities have been demonstrated in individuals with such disorders, the rapid remediation of neurosomatic disorders through neural network shifts may be explained by changes in rate of secretion of neurotransmitters. Reboxetine, a pure noradrenergic-receptor-uptake inhibitor, which will be marketed as an antidepressant, seems to stimulate $alpha_1$ adrenoreceptors, resulting in an increase in burst firing in ventral tegmental area dopamine neurons but not in their average firing rate. This stimulatory effect was attenuated by pretreatment with the $alpha_1$-adrenoreceptor antagonist prazosin. Further analysis of the experimental results revealed that "whereas the dopamine output in the medial prefrontal cortex was both dependently increased by acute administration of reboxetine . . . dopamine output in the nucleus accumbens remained unchanged, tentatively reflecting the relative absence of noradrenergic terminals in the nucleus acumbens." The authors (Enderg H et al., 1999) speculated that "[t]he reboxetine-induced augmentation of central dopaminergic activity, particularly in the medial prefrontal cortex, may facilitate cognitive functioning and learning of reward-predicted behavior." Thus, we should find reboxetine to be useful not only in depression but also in other types of cognitive disorders, perhaps even Alzheimer's disease.

Neural networks which change according to alterations in the environment undergo "state shifts." Numerous transmitter substances can modulate state shifts. A neural network model of interacting pyramidal neurons and GABAergic interneurons in layer five of the prefrontal cortex shows that this neural network could be switched to a new pattern via D_2-mediated effects and that the new pattern could be stabilized by a dopamine D_1-mediated process. This work from the laboratory of T. J. Sejnowski (Durstewitz D et al., 1999), one of the more creative workers in the field, suggests that "dopamine has state-dependent effects on network dynamics, and different levels of D_1 and/or D_2 receptor stimulation might set the right dynamics for different cognitive operations in the prefrontal cortex."

Several new antiepileptic medications, including gabapentin, lamotrigine, tiagabine, and topiramate have recently been introduced. Each of these medications has a wide use in neurosomatic disorders and each has a different mechanism of action. Topiramate, or Topamax, potentiates $GABA_A$-receptor-mediated chloride currents in cultured neurons by increasing the apparent binding affinity for GABA. Topiramate preferentially enhances currents in $GABA_A$ receptors expressing the $alpha_2$, $beta_2$, and $gamma_2$ subunit combination. Thus, the effects of topiramate may vary among neurons, and the drug would have its most potent effect on neurons expressing these receptor subunits. Such expression is both genetically and environmentally determined and would account for individual differences in response to this particular medication.

Topiramate blocks AMPA/kainate receptors. It may be useful when ketamine, an NMDA antagonist, makes a patient worse. Administering ketamine stimulates the AMPA/kainate and metabotropic glutamate receptors because of glutamate overflow. Topiramate is also a sodium-channel blocker.

Lamotrigine (Lamictal) decreases glutamate secretion, inhibits carbonic anhydrase, and blocks Na^+ channels. Lamotrigine antagonizes ketamine and often synergizes with, or substitutes for, lidocaine. It is useful as an antidepressant and a mood stabilizer.

Mirtazapine (Remeron) enhances dopaminergic and adrenergic but not serotonergic transmission in rats. This reflects its action as an antagonist at frontocortical dopaminergic and $alpha_2$ adrenergic receptors. It is an H_1 antagonist, causing sedation and weight gain, and blocks the $5\text{-}HT_2$ receptor to decrease depression, the $5\text{-}HT_3$ receptor to decrease nausea, and the glycine coagonist site of the NMDA receptor.

The drug riluzole (Rilutek), which I use primarily to decrease glutamate release, also inhibits protein kinase C (PKC), an important intracellular messenger, and Na^+ channels. The ramifications of PKC inhibition are too profound to discuss in this section.

There has been a controversy about whether estrogen is an antidepressant. The weight of the evidence appears to favor its being an antidepressant, particularly in persons with hypercortisolemia caused by adrenal hypertrophy. This situation is not usually found in neurosomatic disorders, but among its many other effects, estrogen decreases stress-induced adrenal hypertrophy.

In anticipating reward, the nucleus accumbens has been implicated, particularly in regard to its dopaminergic innervation from the ventral tegmental area in the brainstem. It also receives strong inputs from the medial prefrontal cortex and sends feedback to the frontal cortex via several pathways. This functional neuroanatomy suggests that neural information from the medial prefrontal cortex to the nucleus accumbens might play an important role in anticipating future events, especially rewards. In task events that produce a reward, the neurons in the nucleus accumbens fire continuously, while its connections in the medial prefrontal cortex fire intermittently. Firing rate and timing of neuronal firing are increasingly appearing to be just as important as type and quantity of neurotransmitter release in neural network function.

One of the unsolved problems in neuroscience is how different areas of the brain work simultaneously in a neural network when dealing with a certain function (the binding problem). Most cortical network models are based on the idea that neurons with similar response properties to sensory stimuli excite one another. Some researchers have suggested that neurons forming a cortical map or network are connected indirectly to one another via a small group of excitatory neurons, which have been termed *neuronal pointers*. The sensory input goes to the map or network neurons, while top-down attentional input goes to the pointer neurons. The pointer neurons have the role of reporting and modulating by allocation of attentional resources the activity profile of the map. This principle has been particularly noted in the visual system in which there is a competition for visual attention between different neurons called "winner take all." Neuron-glia signaling networks have a prominent role in binding (Bezzi P, Volterra A, 2001) and will be discussed later in the book.

The substance agmatine is decarboxylated arginine. It has been recently identified in the mammalian central nervous system. Agmatine is thought to be a novel neurotransmitter and has been used to rescue mice from experimentally induced persistent pain. L-arginine is the precursor of nitric oxide. Capsaicin is an agonist at vanilloid receptors (VR) and is the active component of the medication Zostrix. Capsaicin destroys substance P-containing neurons and is inhibited by angiotensin II (AII), bradykinin (BK), and guanosine 3,5-cyclic monophosphate (cGMP). This finding suggests that medications that mimic the action of these agents may be helpful in pain induced by stimulation of the VRs. A VR agonist, resferinatoxin, successfully treats interstitial cystitis after instillation into the bladder.

When patients have an infection in the abdomen, they feel ill. Infections induce the secretion of various cytokines, including interleukin-1. Interleukin-1 has been found to be secreted by immune cells within the vagus nerve, the primary nerve from the viscera to the brain. Interleukin-1-induced fever can be blocked by ligating the vagus nerve. The induction of interleukin-1 in the vagus nerve also seems to have a role in elevating serum corticosterone levels, since this response is not strictly dependent on corticotropin-releasing hormone.

One of the difficulties I have in treating patients by using a receptor-specific medication is finding an opposite-acting drug when someone has an adverse reaction. With baclofen, a $GABA_B$ agonist, there is no specific $GABA_B$ antagonist that I can administer to the patient to see whether it might reverse the effect, that is, to make the person feel better rather than worse. Estrogen has been found to oppose the action of $GABA_B$ agonists. Therefore, a trial of estradiol or a mixture of naturally occurring human estrogens might be an appropriate treatment in patients who have an adverse reaction to baclofen. Other potential antagonists include forskolin, oxytocin, mexiletine, and reboxetine. Estrogen has effects on numerous other neurotransmitters. It stimulates the secretion of some dopaminergic neurons, particularly group A15. Estrogen also potentiates the response to glutamate in an area of the hypothalamus called the preoptic region. The subtype of glutamate receptors in the preoptic region that are potentiated may be of the AMPA class.

Early adverse life events may predispose a person to the development of major depression by permanently altering corticotropin-releasing hormone neuronal systems. Women with a history of childhood abuse without depression showed increased ACTH responses to CRH stimulation, while women with a history of childhood abuse with current major depression showed blunted ACTH responses. Both groups of abused women exhibited relatively low basal and stimulated cortisol levels. Blunted pituitary responses in women with depression may reflect down-regulation of pituitary CRH receptors due to chronic CRH hypersecretion as a result of chronic stress. It appears that reported early childhood abuse often has lasting effects on brain function and regulation. Patients with neurosomatic disorders often report feeling unsafe during childhood. Thus, the hypoactivity of the HPA axis may have childhood hypervigilance as one of its causes. Child abuse may also put people at higher risk for PTSD. Dissociative disorders are fairly uncommon in neurosomatic patients but are still seen with increased frequency in this population as compared to controls. Dissociation is a defense used by victims of abuse when they must protect themselves psychologically in abusive situations. Such patients also have hypocortisolemia.

In recent years, increased emphasis has been placed on how maternal stress can alter fetal brain development, especially in the third trimester, and thus affect the lifetime behavior of the offspring. If the mother is stressed, she will have higher cortisol levels in her serum. The cortisol will enter the placenta and disturb the fetoplacental barrier, resulting in increased anxiety and suppression of effective coping mechanisms in stressful situations in the offspring. This behavior may be related to dysregulation of gluco-corticoid receptors in the amygdala, a structure known to mediate anxiety. There is a strong association between psychosocial stressors early in life and increased risk for depression, anxiety, and neurosomatic disorders. Animals who have been separated from their mothers were found to have upregulation of CRH in regions of the cortex, especially the hippocampus. This effect was attenuated to an extent for the CRH_2 receptor by administration of the tricyclic antidepressant desipramine.

A functional linkage between cannabinoid and opioid receptors is increasingly obvious. Mice have been bred without cannabinoid receptors; they are called cannabinoid CB_1 receptor "knock-out" mice. Such mice not only do not respond to administration of cannabinoids, but also do not self-administer morphine. However, the self-administration of cocaine and D-amphetamine is not affected. This apparent inconsistency may be related to the fact that morphine does not increase the release of dopamine from the nucleus accumbens in CB_1 knock-out mice. CB_1 knock-out mice also do not respond as well to the proclivity of norepinephrine to decrease calcium currents, an effect apparently mediated by G proteins, an almost ubiquitous postreceptor signal transduction mechanism.

Cannabinoids are also NMDA-receptor agonists in some situations, an important action because we have a relative paucity of agents that stimulate the NMDA receptor. Cannabinoids have been found to enhance NMDA-evoked calcium signals in cerebellar granular neurons via phospholipase C and to produce calcium release from IP_3-gated stores. This effect would theoretically be blocked by heparin, which is an IP_3-receptor antagonist. Dantrolene also blocks intracellular calcium release via the ryanodine receptor, which gates a different Ca^{2+}-containing compartment.

This calcium-releasing effect of cannabinoids cannot be generalized to all regions of the brain because in some areas cannabinoids modulate excitatory, and in other regions inhibitory, neurotransmission. They promote inhibitory transmission predominantly by promoting GABA release. If cannabinoids are injected into the globus pallidus, the uptake of GABA will be reduced and voluntary movement will be inhibited, thus producing Parkinson's disease-like symptoms. There are endogenous cannabinoids called anandamide and 2-arachidonylglycerol (2-AG). When Parkinson-like behavior is induced in rats injected with cannabinoids in the globus pallidus, and then the Parkinson-like symptoms are reduced by administration of the dopamine agonist quinpirole, the levels of endogenous cannabinoids in the globus pallidus are reduced. In addition, the administration of a cannabinoid receptor antagonist potentiates the locomotor stimulant effect of quinpirole.

Cannabinoids are also $5\text{-HT}_{2A/C}$ antagonists. Other 5-HT_2 antagonists are antipsychotic drugs, such as the atypical neuroleptics, or the antidepressant drugs nefazodone (Serzone) and mirtazapine (Remeron). Whether the exogenous cannabinoid Marinol acts as an antidepressant, sedative, or stimulant appears to depend on how the sensitivity of dopamine D_1 and D_2 receptors are regulated by other neurotransmitter substances.

Considerable controversy has ensued over the effect of pindolol as an antagonist for presynaptic and postsynaptic 5-HT_{1A} receptors, although there appears to be no difference in the affinity of pindolol for pre- or postsynaptic 5-HT_{1A} receptors. Pindolol is thought to increase serotonin release in the rat brain by interaction with both pre- and postsynaptic 5-HT_{1A} receptors, particularly when coadministered with an SSRI. Both SSRIs and norepinephrine-reuptake inhibitors (NRIs) facilitate 5-HT_{1A} receptor function. Both of them desensitize the 5-HT_{1A} receptor-mediated inhibition of forskolin-stimulated adenyl cyclase. The 5-HT_{1A} receptor is coupled to adenylyl cyclase. Many medications used in the treatment of neurosomatic disorders either increase or decrease the activity of adenyl cyclase.

Estrogen appears to act in a similar manner to antidepressants in regard to desensitization of hypothalamic 5-HT_{1A} receptors. Physiologic levels of estrogen tonically suppress 5-HT_{1A}-receptor signaling, a result that is dose dependent, suggesting that estrogen may augment the effects of SSRIs in women. The hypothalamic 5-HT_1 receptors can also be desensitized by activation of the 5-HT_{2A} receptors. We do not have a medication that directly activates 5-HT_2 receptors, although 5-HT_2 receptors via phospholipase C do activate PKC.

We can expect in the future to see medications that are specific for the dopamine D_3 autoreceptor subtype, which has been recently targeted as a potential neurochemical modulator of the behavioral actions of psychomotor stimulants such as cocaine.

The ventral tegmental area supplies dopaminergic innervation to the nucleus accumbens. The NAc sends a negative feedback projection to the VTA. This feedback appears to be modulated by increasing the synaptic levels of dopamine in the NAc and activation of both D_1 and D_2 receptors within the NAc. The dopamine D_2 receptors, which are autoreceptors within the NAc, and the D_1 receptors, apparently function as interneurons. 5-HT_{2C} receptor agonists inhibit dopaminergic neurons in the ventral tegmental area by activating GABAergic interneurons. The VTA is innervated by 5-HT-containing neurons originating from the raphe nuclei. Thus, it appears that phasic stimulation of 5-HT_{2C} receptors activates nondopaminergic (presumably GABAergic) interneurons, which in turn inhibit the activity of dopamine neurons in the ventral tegmental area.

Pentazocine (Talwin) is in a class of drugs called sigma$_1$ receptor ligands. Neuroactive neurosteroids, which modulate several neurotransmitter systems in the brain, have been reported to interact with sigma$_1$ receptors. The effects of sigma$_1$ agonists can be enhanced by the neurosteroid DHEA, which has an anti-GABA effect and could be blocked by progesterone. Thus, progesterone might be an antidote for patients that have an adverse reaction to Talwin. As a neurosteroid itself, progesterone may have a beneficial effect. If a female patient responds to Talwin, its effect may be enhanced by pregnenolone and decreased by finasteride, a 5-alpha reductase inhibitor that blocks the conversion of progesterone to other substances. Finasteride leads to an accumulation of progesterone, which can attenuate the action of sigma$_1$ receptor ligands. Thus, the effect of Talwin can be enhanced by dehydroepiandrosterone (DHEA) and pregnenolone and can be antagonized by progesterone and finasteride, which is also known as Proscar.

Because Talwin acts somewhat like the dopamine D$_2$ antagonist haloperidol by inhibiting potassium-stimulated dopamine release, it is possible that neurosteroids, particularly progesterone, may enhance the action of haloperidol as a sigma$_1$-receptor agonist. Talwin enhances amphetamine-stimulated release of dopamine from certain brain slices. This amphetamine release can be augmented by agents that block the L-type calcium channel and may, therefore, modulate dopamine-transporter activities. Talwin is also an NMDA-receptor antagonist.

Clinically available GABA$_B$ receptor antagonists include valproate (Depakote) and ethosuximide (Zarontin). Both of these medications are antiepileptic compounds. Some work indicates that baclofen may be converted into gamma hydroxybutyrate (GHB), a substance which when taken in excess may cause epileptic seizures and has been banned by the FDA, although it was approved for limited use in 2002. Peripheral benzodiazepine receptors such as those that bind to zolpidem (Ambien) are abundant in endocrine tissues and help regulate the production of steroid hormones. This fact may account for unusual reactions that might not be attributed to such compounds. Zolpidem is an effective analgesic in some patients and is even activating in a few.

Certain metabolites of arachidonic acid inhibit GABA$_A$ receptor function. Prostaglandin E2 and thromboxane A2 have both been found to have this property in the solitary tract, the area of the brainstem that carries messages from the vagus nerve to the brain. Many antibiotics, especially penicillins and furosemide (Lasix), the loop diuretic, are also GABA$_A$ antagonists.

The dopamine receptors are divided into two families. The D$_1$-like receptor family includes D$_1$ and D$_5$. The D$_5$ receptor has been found to downregulate benzodiazepine receptors. The postreceptor events of these two compounds are structurally different but intercommunicate, a phenomenon that is found increasingly in molecular pharmacology. One receptor is

G-protein coupled and the other is *ligand gated.* The anterior cingulate cortex has a glutamatergic projection to the caudate nucleus, which is modulated by the NMDA receptor. This receptor is thought to play a major role in acquisition of new behaviors and reward-related processes. The caudate nucleus is specifically involved with cued learning and memory.

Inositol polyphosphates are ubiquitous compounds in most cells. I have referred to the use of inositol in a previous volume *(Betrayal by the Brain)* and have alluded to it in this chapter, describing the action of heparin in blocking the intracellular IP_3 receptor (inositol 1, 4, 5,-triphosphate), thus attenuating the release of intracellular calcium. There are many other inositol polyphosphates. IP_6 selectively interacts with subunits of AMPA receptors, probably contributing to their internalization, a method of desensitization. IP_6, however, has no effect on NMDA receptors. Methods of increasing IP_6 could, in the future, be a potentially nontoxic way to decrease AMPA-receptor sensitivity as topiramate does now. Glutathione has been used by some physicians as a treatment for CFS. If this treatment is effective, one way that it might work is by reacting with nitric oxide to form S-nitrosoglutathione (GSNO) which interacts with binding sites for glutamate and also binding sites for some NMDA and AMPA antagonists. It does not affect the binding of AMPA agonists. Other forms of glutathione are also effective in blocking the binding of glutamate receptors. Oxidized glutathione (GSSG) stimulates the binding of dizocilpine, an NMDA-receptor antagonist.

Acetylcholinesterases such as tacrine (Cognex) and donepezil (Aricept) are thought to increase the effect of acetylcholine at the muscarinic cholinergic receptors. One would think that since they increase acetylcholine levels that they would also increase the action of acetylcholine at the nicotinic cholinergic receptor like galantamine (Reminyl) does. Paradoxically, however, they have been found to directly block the neuronal nicotinic cholinergic receptor, suggesting that these compounds might be administered to patients who have an adverse reaction to nicotine patches and act like the nonspecific nicotinic cholinergic-receptor antagonist mecamylamine. Amiloride, which inhibits salty taste in the mouth, is also a nicotinic cholinergic-receptor antagonist. Anticholinesterases are often effective treatments for patients who have adverse reactions to NMDA antagonists and may improve mental clarity in such individuals.

Amphetamine is thought to act by increasing levels of dopamine and norepinephrine. However, it has also been found to increase levels of glutamate in the nucleus accumbens immediately after injection and to raise levels of GABA in the nucleus accumbens about 15 minutes later. Methamphetamine (Desoxyn) causes neuronal damage, predominantly by neurotoxicity at the level of the dopamine transporter. This effect may be attenuated by the medication mazindol (Sanorex), which hypothetically could be used to treat patients who have been methamphetamine abusers but are no longer using the drug. Unfortunately, mazindol is no longer being manufactured.

I had previously associated ibogaine with substances such as mescaline; however, it appears that ibogaine has antiaddiction properties. Ibogaine and its active metabolite, noribogaine, cause mood elevation and drug-craving reduction, and also block the symptoms of opioid withdrawal. It has the capacity to reset multiple opioid receptors and has affinity for the serotonin transporter. Ibogaine trials have been done on human subjects and have demonstrated considerable efficacy in small samples.

Another apparently effective anticraving drug useful in alcoholics is the experimental agent acamprosate. This substance blocks the polyamine site of the NMDA receptor. Two available medications that also have this property are nylidrin and isoxuprine, very effective medications for some neurosomatic patients, whether they have a history of alcohol abuse or not. They may synergize with other NMDA antagonists.

There has been some discussion about the mechanism of action of the atypical neuroleptics olanzapine (Zyprexa), ziprasidone (Geodon), risperidone (Risperdal), and quetiapine (Seroquel). These drugs are 5-HT_2-receptor antagonists. Olanzapine and risperidone bind to dopamine D_2 and D_4 receptors and, therefore, elevate the levels of D_2 receptors, particularly in the basal ganglia. This finding is consistent with the ability of olanzapine and risperidone to induce extrapyramidal side effects. Even after long-term administration of quetiapine, however, there is no change in the density of dopamine D_2 and D_4 receptors, suggesting that quetiapine may be the agent of choice when using an atypical neuroleptic in treating patients who may be prone to develop extrapyramidal syndrome and subsequently tardive dyskinesia (TD). Quetiapine has been recently introduced to the American market, and there is little information about the special aspects of its neuropharmacology. Ziprasidone apparently does not cause TD, either, and has the highest affinity for the 5-HT_{1A} receptor of any clinically available agent.

One of the theories of sleep promotion is that during wakefulness the levels of the neuromodulator adenosine increase. I have discussed this theory in *Betrayal by the Brain.* Extracellular adenosine levels are also increased by glutamate and its subtype agonist NMDA. Levels of adenosine are not affected by cholinergic agonists. These results suggest that activation of NMDA receptors by glutamate may be one mechanism by which extracellular levels of adenosine increase during wakefulness and that NMDA receptor antagonists might be useful in narcolepsy. A relatively new agent, modafinil (Provigil) is marketed as an antinarcoleptic medication and has some utility in the treatment of neurosomatic disorders. Modafinil also decreases adenosine accumulation in a complex manner. The levels of adenosine do not increase uniformly in all areas of the brain during wakefulness but seem to increase primarily in an area called the basal forebrain, where many cholinergic neurons are located. It has been found that high levels of adenosine in the basal forebrain acting at adenosine-1 receptors on cholinergic neurons promote drowsiness and the transition from wakefulness to sleep. However, the sleep-inducing area is not in the basal forebrain but in projection areas of the basal forebrain. When a cholinesterase inhibitor, which increases acetylcholine, is injected into the basal forebrain, it induces an increase in wakefulness and a decrease in slow wave sleep and rapid eye movement (REM) sleep.

It is tempting to speculate that modafinil is a hypocretin (orexin) analog. There are two hypocretin peptides (Hcrt-1 and Hcrt-2) and individual receptors for each of them in the tuberal region of the hypothalamus. Human narcolepsy is associated with low to absent levels of Hcrt in the cerebrospinal fluid (CSF). Hcrt administration to a rat induces wakefulness. Canine narcolepsy is associated with a mutation in Hcrt-2. Hcrt was undetectable in the hypothalamus, pons, and cerebral cortex of narcoleptic human subjects. Hcrt neurons project to the locus coeruleus, which secretes NE, and the ventral tegmental area, which secretes DA. Both neurotransmitters are wake promoting (Peyron C et al., 2000).

Modafinil and atypical neuroleptics, especially clozapine and olanzapine, antagonize each other (Sebban C et al., 1999). Alpha$_1$ antagonists make narcolepsy worse, and modafinil activates hypocretin neurons (Chemilli RM et al., 1999). Clonidine can antagonize the effect of modafinil. Perhaps the primary action of modafinil, however, is to increase secretion of the activating neurotransmitter histamine from the tuberomammiliary nucleus in the hypothalamus.

Augmentation of antidepressant treatment is another possible use for modafinil (Menza MA et al., 2000). Its mode of action is unlike other stimulant drugs, and its antidepressant effect can occur immediately, or within one to two weeks. It is particularly useful in fatigued patients or those with bipolar disorder. Induction of mania with modafinil is quite uncommon.

It has been demonstrated that paying attention to an object increases the activity of the neurons involved in perceiving this object. In monkeys and humans, spatial attention is able to enhance spatial visual resolution by a mechanism that is independent of perceptual learning.

One of the more effective treatments for neurosomatic disorders is thyrotropin-releasing hormone. TRH secretion is regulated by numerous transmitter substances including leptin, neuropeptide 1 (NPY), and agouti-related peptide (AgRP). These are contained in synaptic terminals that heavily innervate TRH neurons in the rat brain. It has been hypothesized that these peptides may contribute to the altered set point of the hypotha-lamic-pituitary-thyroid (HPT) axis during fasting. Dysregulation of this neural network may contribute to the weight gain and occasional weight loss often seen in patients with neurosomatic disorders. TRH neurons are strongly regulated by norepinephrine. The noradrenergic receptor subtypes that predominate on TRH neurons are alpha$_{1A}$ and alpha$_{1D}$. Because we have no specific ligands for these receptors, it would be interesting to see whether the alpha$_1$ agonist midodrine (ProAmatine) can cause weight loss. It has already been found to have an antidepressant effect, and alpha$_1$-recep-tor antagonists can block the action of certain antidepressants. One of the actions of NMDA-receptor antagonists is a complex disinhibition mecha-nism in which they abolish GABAergic inhibition of converging excitatory projections resulting in simultaneous excessive release of at least two neurotransmitters, acetylcholine at M$_3$ cholinergic receptors and glutamate at non-NMDA receptors. This excessive stimulation can be modulated by alpha$_2$ adrenergic, 5-HT$_1$, and sigma receptors. Olanzapine (Zyprexa) is a potent inhibitor of NMDA-receptor antagonists. It has been found that olanzapine may exert its effect by decreasing the sensitivity of acetylcholine M$_3$ receptors, since the cholinergic agonist pilocarpine can eliminate the protective effect of olanzapine in cases of NMDA toxicity.

Synaptic temporal dynamics are increasingly of interest in neuropharma-cology. The globus pallidus contains neurons that have variations, or "oscil-lations," in their firing rates. The firing rates are significantly and similarly increased by application of dopamine or stimulants such as amphetamine, methylphenidate, and cocaine. Thus, stimulants increase globus pallidus neuronal oscillations by increasing dopamine levels.

TRH is a ligand for a G-protein-coupled receptor that stimulates adenyl cyclase and also activates phospholipase C (PLC) to increase IP$_3$, thereby releasing Ca^{2+} from intracellular stores. PLC also produces diacylglycerol (DAG) which activates another important signal transduction pathway through PKC. Estrogens and glucocorticoids up-regulate TRH receptors. All three catecholamines, DA, NE, and epinephrine, densely innervate TRH neurons. NE is known to stimulate TRH release, and the two transmitters synergize their effects. Fasting results in decreased pro-TRH mRNA levels in hypothalamic paraventricular neurons, but this decrease is blunted by leptin. TRH is manufactured in the paraventricular nucleus and interacts with other substances produced there to be transported to the median emi-nence. These neuropeptides include CRH, neurotensin, galanin, enkephalin, and vasoactive intestinal peptide (VIP) (Toni T, Lechan RM, 1993). TRH is also a benzodiazepine antagonist and is one of the several (furosemide, aminophylline, some antibiotics, acyclovir) that can be used if flumazenil is not available.

Drops are typically used t.i.d., and subcutaneous injections are used daily. Intravenous injections have a highly variable duration of action. One patient feels completely normal as long as she receives 500mg of TRH intravenously every three months. Females have a lower CSF TRH level than males. The difference is most pronounced in the bipolar population (Frye MA et al., 1999).

P. J. Fletcher and A. Azampanah (1999) investigated how the stimulation of 5-HT_{1B} receptors in the nucleus accumbens reduces amphetamine self-administration. They accomplished this end by inhibiting dopamine-dependent reward-related behavior. Thus, one would expect medications such as the triptans, all of which are $5\text{-HT}_{1B/1D}$ agonists, to decrease the rewarding properties of drugs of abuse, all of which are dependent on dopaminergic mechanisms to some extent. I use this property clinically in the office when I wish to reverse the effects of delta-9 THC (Marinol), which has a dopaminergic effect as one of its properties. Should an individual have an adverse reaction to Marinol, I usually administer naritriptan (Amerge), and almost always the effects of the Marinol are attenuated if not completely eliminated. Verapamil also inhibits the effects of cannabinoids, as does the cAMP agonist forskolin. It is of interest that the effects of baclofen may also be inhibited by Amerge and verapamil. Patients have had similar adverse reactions to both baclofen and Marinol. If both medications are effective, they can synergize. Marinol has its primary use in my practice as an antinociceptive agent and seems to augment opioids and NMDA-receptor antagonists. The antinociceptive effects of the cannabinoids can be attenuated by kappa-opioid-receptor antagonists, which do not affect other commonly observed cannabinoid actions, including hypothermia, hypoactivity, and catalepsy. Cannabinoids are capable of inhibiting presynaptic release of glutamate in rat hippocampal cultures, whereas they fail to alter GABAergic synaptic transmission.

Tolerance can develop to most pharmacologic effects of delta-9-THC. There are two cannabinoid receptors, 1 and 2, and the CB_1 receptors are found predominantly in the brain, with the highest density in the hippocampus, cerebellum, and striatum. The CB_2 receptor is found predominantly in the spleen and haemopoietic cells and provides the molecular basis for the immunosuppressive actions of marijuana.

In the past ten years, endogenous cannabinoid-receptor ligands, including anandamide and 2-arachidonylglycerol have been described. It has been noted that the psychoactive cannabinoids increase the activity of dopaminergic neurons in the ventral tegmental area/mesolimbic pathway, producing facilitation of this system.

This topic has recently been reviewed by Angela Ameri (Ameri A, 1999). There are probable interactions with the CB_1 and other G-protein-coupled receptors such as opioid receptors, dopamine D_2 receptors, and $GABA_B$ receptors. Each receptor stimulates its own pool of G proteins, but they share adenylate cyclase. This mechanism provides a rationale for reversal of the effect of baclofen, a $GABA_B$ agonist, with agents that reverse the effects of Marinol. At high concentrations, cannabinoid agonists stimulate the release of arachidonic acid in vitro, but probably do not do so in vivo because nonsteroidal anti-inflammatory drugs generally have no effect on the action of Marinol except to inhibit the enzyme that degrades it, amidohydrolase. The nonsteroidal anti-inflammatory compound pravadoline is one of a group of compounds named aminoalkylindoles that have analgesic opioid receptor-independent activities, perhaps due to their cannabinomimetic activity.

The alpha nuclei of the basal ganglia, i.e., the globus pallidus and substantia nigra pars reticulata, exhibit extremely high levels of cannabinoid receptors which are predominantly localized on presynaptic terminals of the GABAergic striatonigral and striatopallidal terminals. They also coexist with D_1 and D_2 receptors. CB_1 receptor activation inhibits a D_1-mediated increase in cAMP accumulation and also decreases D_2-mediated inhibition of cAMP accumulation. Cannabinoids decrease locomotor activity by inhibiting GABA uptake or presynaptic GABA release. They also inhibit dopamine uptake in the striatum or stimulate its release. Cannabinoids decrease glutamate secretion from the terminals of the subthalamic nucleus, thereby inhibiting the firing of the substantia nigra. The cannabinoids may increase or decrease dopamine effects in the striatum depending upon the relative expression of D_1 and D_2 receptors. If this effect is unbalanced, cannabinoids may make an individual feel anxious and paranoid or lethargic and sleepy. Cannabinoids are useful in treating Parkinson's disease because glutamate release in the basal ganglia is inhibited and dyskinesias are decreased. Most researchers agree that cannabinoids decrease GABA and glutamate and increase DA.

In recent years it has become more apparent that cannabinoids may cause dependence and addiction, particularly since delta-9-THC increases the extracellular dopamine concentration preferentially in the shell of the nucleus accumbens but not in the core, similar to the action of heroin. This dopamine increase is prevented by mu_1-opioid-receptor antagonists. Chronic cannabinoid administration increases opioid gene expression in the nucleus accumbens and suggests an interaction between the cannabinoid and enkephalinergic system. Besides inhibiting glutamate release, cannabinoids can also inhibit norepinephrine and acetylcholine secretion in hippocampal slices. Delta-9-THC is neurotoxic to many hippocampal neurons, an effect that can be blocked by inhibitors of transcription, such as actinomycin D, as well as by vitamin E and inhibitors of phospholipase A_2 and cyclooxygenase. CB_1 activation may thereby generate free radicals.

Nevertheless, cannabinoids, when used appropriately, can have significant benefits. CB_1-receptor agonists can be antiemetic and analgesic, and can potentiate kappa- and delta-opioids which then potentiate mu-opioids. They can decrease glutamate release, which would be helpful in neurosomatic disorders as well as Parkinson's disease. Although CB_1 agonists can decrease DA in some areas of the brain, they usually increase it in the NAc shell, an important property in neurosomatic medicine. CB_1 agonists generally decrease the release of Ach and NE. CB_1 receptors are among the most abundantly expressed of the neuronal receptors, and CB_1 mRNA is up-regulated by the NMDA receptor. CB_2 agonists would have little use in neurosomatic medicine at present except as immunosuppresants. CB_1 agonists may have adverse effects such as tolerance, sedation, and lethargy. Some of these could be minimized by developing partial CB_1 agonists similar to arvanil (Izzo AA et al., 2000). Although Marinol is usually associated with impaired memory and cognitive impairment, in a similar manner to the NMDA antagonists, it can decrease attention in neurosomatic patients allowing for better stimulus selection. In some patients, as might be hypothetically suspected, Marinol improves all symptoms. My impression is that it is particularly efficacious in atypical facial pain. Doses below 10 mg usually do not impair cognition.

Dynorphin A is a nociceptive opioid with an NMDA binding site. Marinol decreases dynorphin release after a painful stimulus in the rat at the level of the spinal cord dorsal horn. It has a critical kappa-opioid receptor component (Mason DJ et al., 1999). There seems to be no consensus about the action of cannabinoids on the NMDA receptor. Some think that a CB_1 site on the NMDA receptor is antagonistic, and others find that cannabinoids enhance intracellular Ca^{2+} in NMDA neurons by increasing the release of Ca^{2+} from IP_3-regulated intracellular stores (Netzeband JG et al., 1999). The trend, however, is toward decreased GABA and glutamate release by presynaptic CB_1 receptors. The endogenous cannabinoids anandamide and 2-arachidonylglycerol are constitutively active. 2-AG is converted from DAG by DAG lipase (Piomelli D et al., 2000). Activating the NMDA receptor increases intracellular Ca^{2+}, which activates PLC to form DAG. 2-AG can then bind to the presynaptic CB_1 (and possibly the $mGlu_5$) receptor and decrease glutamate release. Activating the $mGlu_5$ receptor in the antinociceptive midbrain periaqueductal gray intensifies its analgesic properties (Izzo AA et al., 2000). Recent studies suggest that cannabinoids might increase the synthesis or release of endogenous opioids or both

(Manzanares J et al., 1999). CB_1 receptors inhibit small neurons that express tyrosine kinase A (trkA) and secrete SP and CGRP when stimulated, an analgesic action of cannabinoids accomplished by inhibiting inflammatory neuropeptide release.

Lamotrigine is a sodium-channel blocker as well as an inhibitor of glutamate release. Gabapentin is a potassium$_{ATP}$-channel opener. Both of these agents are calcium-channel blockers. Glyburide, a sulfonylurea (SUR) oral hypoglycemic agent, has an effect which is the opposite of gabapentin in that it is a potassium$_{ATP}$-channel antagonist. Glyburide as well as glipizide and glibenclamide would increase the secretion of norepinephrine and should be safe in low doses when used in normoglycemic patients in whom one would wish to increase norepinephrine levels. Sulfonylureas sometimes markedly increase alertness in patients who have adverse reations to gabapentin. Perhaps by the time this book is published, an agent called pregabalin will have been released. It is a novel anticonvulsant and antihyperalgesic agent that has been found to bind to the alpha$_2$-delta subunit of voltage-dependent calcium channels, as does gabapentin. Pregabalin also inhibits potassium-evoked norepinephrine and dopamine release from rat neocortical and striatal slices.

Another antiepileptic drug, vigabatrin (Sabril) increases total GABA levels in rat optic nerve, while gabapentin and pregabalin do not. Some of my patients have taken vigabatrin. It has made each of them depressed. Even though the number of people who have taken it is quite small, it is not an agent that I would eagerly use, when released, on the basis of these observations.

An addition to the sudden profusion of AEDs is tiagabine (Gabitril), a GABA-reuptake inhibitor that produces its effect by increasing the synaptic levels of GABA. Gabitril is surprisingly ineffective in most patients with neurosomatic disorders. Although it has been suggested that the drug may be effective in neuropathic pain, I have not found it to be so in neurosomatic pain. The main problem I have had with the drug is increasing the dose too rapidly. If the manufacturer's recommendations for upward dosage titration are not scrupulously followed, delirium or mania can be precipitated. Adverse reactions respond to furosemide or flumazenil, the latter often via nasal spray.

Felbamate (Felbatol) is an AED that is little used because it has rare bone marrow toxicity. It is a weak NMDA-receptor antagonist and probably has its anticonvulsant effect on that basis, as well as by substantially increasing GABA levels, a property shared by most AEDs. It is also a glycine/NMDA antagonist.

Rats were trained to discriminate other drugs from cocaine. The only drug that substituted completely for cocaine was D-amphetamine, but other dopaminergic compounds including methylphenidate (Ritalin), apomorphine (APO), and lisuride also had significant cocaine-like properties as far as the responsive rats were concerned. Drugs that did not appear to have cocaine-like properties included buspirone (BuSpar), fluoxetine (Prozac), yohimbine, and lidocaine.

The agent amperozide is a potent 5-HT$_2$ receptor antagonist. It also has a moderate affinity for alpha$_1$ adrenoceptors and a low to moderate affinity for D$_1$, D$_2$, D$_3$, and D$_4$ receptors. Amperozide increases social contact, promotes affiliation, inhibits aggression, and reduces craving for cocaine and alcohol without interfering with motor coordination or causing sedation (Rademacher DJ et al., 1999). Amperozide increases extracellular dopamine concentration in mesocorticolimbic structures but has limited abuse potential, suggesting that it may be useful as a cocaine and alcohol anti-abuse pharmacotherapy. This agent appears to be distinct from acamprosate, nylidrin, and isoxsuprine, all of which seem to have similar anticraving effects. They are antagonists at the polyamine site of the NMDA receptor. Nylidrin also antagonizes the NR1/NR2B receptors. Ifenprodil antagonizes NR2B subunits and may be useful in neurosomatic medicine.

MMAI (5-methoxy-6-methyl-2 aminoindan) is a nonneurotoxic and highly selective serotonin-releasing agent that possesses a behavioral profile similar to the anorectic drug fenfluramine. Combining MMAI with amphetamine markedly and significantly reduces body weight compared to MMAI alone (Marona-Lewicka D et al., 1999).

High doses of ascorbic acid have been shown to attenuate the behavioral activation induced by amphetamine in rodents, and considerably lower doses have been reported to have the opposite effect. Wang and Rebec (1999) reported that high and low concentrations of ascorbic acid may have opposing effects on neostriatal neurons, which play a critical role in amphetamine-induced behavioral effects. The neuropharmacology of ascorbic acid is important, and some other discoveries have been made in the past few years which I shall discuss in Chapter 10.

Amphetamine and cocaine decrease appetite, but the mechanism of action of these agents on the central noradrenergic system has not been well described. An abstract by Galeotti, Ghelardini, Morrachi, and colleagues (1999), found that this anorexic effect is mediated by the alpha$_{2AD}$ adrenergic receptor. There is an alpha$_{2BC}$ receptor, too. Interestingly, the alpha$_2$ agonists clonidine and guanabenz are also reported to have an anorectic effect, a finding that seems to be little known in the medical community (with which I do not agree).

Some recent work has examined the mechanism of action of electroconvulsive therapy. ECT appears to increase the levels of most neurotransmitters but also elevates thyrotropin-releasing hormone levels. Pekary and colleagues (1999) believe that ECT enhances the conversion of TRH prohormones to TRH in the anterior cingulate as well in the hypothalamus and lateral cerebellum. TRH is one of the more useful treatments in patients with neurosomatic disorders.

Bradykinin antagonists are sometimes useful in neurosomatic disorders. The prototypical small molecule bradykinin antagonist is kutapressin, which has a role in raising blood pressure and possibly decreasing bradykinin-induced pain. It is quite common for me to use kutapressin to reverse angiotensin-converting enzyme inhibitors such as enalapril and to administer enalapril to attenuate the effects of kutapressin.

An antidepressant that was unfortunately withdrawn from the market about ten years ago because of adverse reactions was nomifensine (Merital). No drug marketed in the United States since that time has a similar mode of action. Nomifensine has a marked dopaminergic effect and can produce analgesia which is partially caused by activation of dopaminergic systems. Until recently, the antidepressant tianeptine, a dopamine-reuptake inhibitor, was available in France. Insufficient numbers of my patients have obtained this agent of their own volition for me to make a judgment about its efficacy. However, one individual who had had an excellent response to nomifensine in the late 1980s had no response at all to tianeptine. There has been an ongoing debate about whether gabapentin (Neurontin) has an effect on brain GABA concentrations. Wu, Wang, and Richerson (1999) find that gabapentin increases GABA concentrations by an unknown mechanism, perhaps by increasing free cytosolic GABA concentrations, thus increasing the driving force for reversal of the GABA transporter. This mechanism has been termed *nonvesicular GABA release,* a novel form of activity-dependent inhibition.

Lithium has been found to have a neuroprotective action in NMDA-receptor-dependent excitotoxicity. Its mode of action was thought to be an inhibition of the densitization of the NMDA receptor by glycine, an NMDA coagonist. Lithium is helpful in an individual having an adverse reaction to parenteral lidocaine. It is difficult to potentiate the NMDA receptor pharmacologically. NMDA is not available to administer as a medication, and stimulating the NMDA receptor otherwise is fairly difficult and must be done indirectly. Compounds such as cycloserine, which acts like a potent form of glycine, and honey bee venom are two agents by which an NMDA receptor may be stimulated. Honey bee venom appears to do so by increasing the release of glutamate and would stimulate all glutamate receptors, not specifically the NMDA receptor.

Skifter and colleagues (1999) describe that insulin potentiates NMDA receptor activity. It may function by signaling through colony-stimulating factor 1 receptors, insulin transmembrane receptors, and pathways that are downstream of these receptors such as triiodothyronine-3' (TI3') kinase. Other modulators having these signaling pathways have the potential to modulate NMDA-receptor activity. As shown by Jorge and colleagues (1999), the serine proteases plasmin and thrombin, which participate in the blood coagulation and thrombolysis pathway, are also signaling molecules in the central nervous system. Both plasmin and thrombin significantly potentiate NMDA-evoked currents in rat hippocampal slices. The similar effect of the two proteases may be a common end point of different intracellular phosphate pathways. Thus, an agent which would inhibit the production of thrombin, e.g., heparin or coumadin, could have NMDA-receptor antagonist function. I shall discuss the CNS role of the coagulation cascade in Chapter 10. A procoagulant milieu may exist in an individual who is chronically stressed. The pathophysiology of this process is unknown.

In the future more and more nicotine-like drugs will be used in neuropharmacology. The $alpha_7$ nicotine receptor seems to be important for neurosomatic illnesses. Activation of this receptor induces tyrosine hydroxylase, the enzyme that converts tyrosine to dopa, and dopamine beta-hydroxylase, the enzyme that converts dopamine to norepinephrine. Some individuals are made anxious by nicotine. The anxiogenic effect of nicotine appears to be mediated by stimulation of the 5-HT_{2A} receptor. Nicotinic cholinergic agonists have been demonstrated to reduce distractability in working memory tasks and offer a potential therapeutic benefit in patients affected with cognitive disorders where attentional deficits and susceptibility to distraction are present. Tolerance to this effect of nicotine frequently develops in patients with neurosomatic disorders.

NMDA-receptor antagonists sometimes increase energy and activity in neurosomatic patients. The locomotor stimulatory effects of such compounds at the level of the ventral tegmental area in the brainstem are dependent upon ascending mesoaccumbens dopaminergic pathways. For the most part, NMDA-receptor antagonists increase dopamine levels rather than decreasing them or having no effect. However, when the NMDA-receptor antagonist ketamine is coadministered with heroin, mesolimbic dopamine release is decreased. Ketamine has been found to antagonize heroin reinforcement by inhibiting mesolimbic dopamine transmission.

Dopamine can be neurotoxic. It is concentrated 45 times by mitochondria using a sodium gradient as a source of energy for dopamine uptake. Therefore, a possible mechanism of dopamine neurotoxicity would be a dopaminergic interaction with mitochondrial respiration.

Malonate, a reversible inhibitor of succinate dehydrogenase, may damage dopaminergic or GABAergic neurons. Depletion of striatal dopamine stores as well as inhibition of the dopamine transporter may protect against malonate-induced damage. However, malonate, or malic acid, when administered in lower doses, could probably induce dopamine secretion at non-toxic levels and might be responsible for the beneficial effects of malic acid as a nutritional supplement. This action might not be related to its role in the Krebs cycle.

Methamphetamine toxicity is sometimes a comorbid problem in treating patients with neurosomatic disorders. It has been shown by Yu and Liao (1999, 2000) that "estrogen specifically protects the dopaminergic terminals from the toxicity of methamphetamine, whereas progesterone is prone to modulate serotoninergic function in response to methamphetamine treatment."

Serotonin-induced platelet calcium mobilization is enhanced in depression, whereas forskolin-stimulated platelet cAMP production is decreased in patients with depression. It is thought that there are alterations in post-receptor cross talk between cAMP and IP_3-mediated calcium mobilization in the platelets of depressed patients. In general, patients with depression have decreased cAMP signaling, and agents that increase cAMP may be useful in their treatment.

Dopamine D_1-receptor agonists and $5-HT_{1A}$-receptor agonists such as buspirone produce a marked enhancement of the acoustic startle response in rats. This result is the opposite of what would be desired in a neurosomatic patient, who generally has an overly active startle response to begin with. Certain neurosomatic patients, however, do seem to operate at a very low level of activation, and such agents may be of benefit to them.

Learned helplessness in rats is a model of depression. Unlike the observations with my patients, a chronic four-week treatment with nicotine produced a significant reversal of learned helplessness but not an acute treatment. This work needs to be validated in human subjects, although a considerable amount of work by now strongly suggests that nicotinic agonists of some sort should be valuable in the behavioral pharmacology of anxiety and depression, as well as neurosomatic symptoms. It has certainly been observed that both patients with schizophrenia and those with major depression are more likely to smoke cigarettes than other individuals. Investigators believe that cigarette smoking is a type of self-medication. Nicotine reduces the amount of monoamine oxidase-A, $alpha_2$ adrenoreceptors, and tyrosine hydroxylase in the locus coeruleus, the primary noradrenergic ganglion of the brain. It is increasingly recognized that all selective serotonin-reuptake inhibitors are not the same. For example, fluoxetine (Prozac) desensitizes the $5-HT_{1A}$ receptors with chronic treatment and decreases radioligand binding to the serotonin transporter. Sertraline (Zoloft) and paroxetine (Paxil) have neither of these effects. Sertraline is a sigma-receptor ligand. In patients susceptible to panic attacks, intravenous infusions of yohimbine and fenfluramine can induce panic-like responses just as an intravenous infusion of sodium lactate can. Rats that have a chronically low level of GABA in the dorsomedial hypothalamus also have lactate-induced panic attacks. The panicogenic effects of yohimbine are blocked by $alpha_1$-adrenoceptor antagonists but not by propranolol, a beta-receptor antagonist. The panicogenic effect of fenfluramine is partially blocked by both 5-HT_2 and 5-HT_3 antagonists in the dorsomedial hypothalamus of GABA-deficient rats. However, in some experimental situations, yohimbine, which usually induces anxiety, may attenuate anxiety elicited by stress. Certainly yohimbine is almost always anxiogenic in patients with post-traumatic stress disorder, although treatment of rats with yohimbine prevented the anxiogenic influence of restraint stress in one experimental paradigm.

The drug rolipram is a selective inhibitor of cAMP-specific phosphodiesterase-4. Rolipram has been investigated for many years as an antidepressant and seems to be effective. It also can attenuate the amnesic effects of scopolamine, an anticholinergic agent, but this effect is not mimicked by forskolin, an agent that activates adenyl cyclase. Inhibiting phosphodiesterase-4 also increases cAMP but by a specific signal transduction pathway rather than by a generalized increase. In the P/Q type of channel, the inhibition of norepinephrine release by gabapentin can be blocked by omega conotoxin. Omega conotoxin does not have this effect on L-type or N-type voltage-sensitive calcium channels.

Dooley and colleagues (1999) considered inhibition of potassium-induced release in synaptosomal calcium and potassium-evoked glutamate release from slices of rat neocortex by gabapentin. They thought that gabapentin may normalize excessive glutamate release associated with certain CNS disorders. In this experiment, too, the effect of gabapentin was inhibited by omega conotoxin. The researchers thought that modulation of these channels by gabapentin was a subtle way that neurotransmitter release could be inhibited.

One of the properties of human behavior is our skill at recognizing and making use of the orderly nature of the environment. Hester and colleagues (1999) discussed the way that the brain was able to recognize high order conditional regularities. This group believed that "the brain's basic mechanism for discovering such complex regularities is implemented at the level of individual pyramidal cells in the cerebral cortex" (p. 2258). The pyramidal cells have five to eight principal dendrites that teach one another to respond to their separate inputs with matching outputs. Thus, when "exposed to different but related information about the sensory environment, principal dendrites of the same cell tune to different nonlinear combinations of environmental conditions that are *predictably related*. As a result, the cell as a whole tunes to a set of related combinations of environment conditions that define an orderly feature of the environment" (p. 2258). When single pyramidal cells are organized into feed forward/feedback networks "they can build their discoveries on the discoveries of other cells, thus cooperatively unraveling nature's more and more complex regularities" (p. 2258). This type of contextual tuning is deficient in patients with neurosomatic disorders.

One of the longstanding issues in psychopharmacology has to do with the mechanism of action of mood-stabilizing agents, i.e., the agents that are used in manic-depressive disorders. These medications are often anticonvulsants and are useful in other illnesses as well, particularly those affecting pain control. The second generation of anticonvulsants, i.e., those excluding Dilantin, Depakote, phenobarbital, Mysoline, and ethosuximide, are more useful in neurosomatic disorders than the first-generation agents. It has been reported that both lithium and valproate (Depakote) reduce the levels of frontal cortex membrane-associated protein kinase B (PKB). Both drugs may function by inositol depletion (Williams RSB et al., 2002).

Protein kinases are essential agents in intracellular metabolism for transferring high energy phosphate groups. Lithium has also been found to regulate mitogen-activated protein (MAP) kinases. The three distinct MAP kinase signal transduction pathways in mammalian cells serve many functions. MAP kinases are abundantly present in the brain and are activated by growth factors in neurotrophin receptors, G-protein-coupled receptors, and ion channels. Chronic lithium treatment increases the level of certain MAP kinases, which are known to exert major neurotrophic effects. These processes may be related to some of lithium's long-term actions such as decreasing cortical atrophy. As a corollary, it may be concluded that MAP kinases are not particularly involved in neurosomatic disorders, for which lithium is notably ineffective. The laboratory of H. K. Manji, now at the Wayne State University School of Medicine in Detroit, Michigan, has been very active over the years in dissecting out the mechanism of action of lithium from G-protein-postreceptor events into cell nuclear neurotranscription.

Ascorbate, or vitamin C, keeps being mentioned more prominently in the neuroscience literature. One of the primary workers in this field is G. V. Rebec of Indiana University. Teagarden and Rebec (1999, p. 2210) note that "striatal infusion of glutamate yielded a significant increase in ascorbate in all drug-naive and saline-treated animals." This effect can be blocked for a week or so by the D_2 dopamine-receptor antagonist haloperidol, but it eventually returns despite the presence of haloperidol. Thus, it appears that glutamate and ascorbate can exchange for each other in the intracellular and extracellular compartments and that this exchange is partially modulated by D_2 receptors. Ascorbate has one of its main pharmacologic actions at the redox site of the NMDA receptor, which has a disulfide bond. Thus, ascorbate, at least in some situations, appears to be an NMDA-receptor antagonist, as do many other compounds that are useful in the treatment of neurosomatic disorders. Ascorbate is also required for the biosynthesis of several neuropeptides. I shall return to ascorbate in Chapter 10.

Perhaps the most important neurosteroid in neurosomatic disorders is allopregnanolone. After intracerebroventricular (ICV) injection of allopregnanolone, extracellular dopamine levels increase somewhat. Allopregnanolone also enhances the release of dopamine by opioids. This action may account in part for both the rewarding potential of opioids and their stimulatory effect in certain patients, perhaps about one-fourth of those in my practice.

There is a significant difference in the release of dopamine in the nucleus accumbens between high responders and low responders to novelty. This finding can perhaps translate into human beings. Persons who seek excitement in their lives would be analogous to low responders, and people who do not would be like high responders. Excitement produces more dopamine than would mere novelty. The release of dopamine from storage pools appears to be under different receptor regulation in both groups. The high responders have dopaminergic pools that are under inhibitory control of norepinephrine acting at alpha receptors, and low responders are under stimulatory control of norepinephrine acting at beta receptors. Therefore, high responders to novelty, which would include many patients with neurosomatic disorders, should release dopamine when given an alpha-receptor antagonist. This effect occurs only when such individuals are exposed to novelty and not during resting conditions. When both high and low responders are exposed to novelty, newly synthesized dopamine in the nucleus accumbens is under stimulatory control of norepinephrine acting at beta receptors in both high and low responders to novelty. Thus, beta agonists should have some utility in the treatment of neurosomatic patients. In practice, however, this is not the case. Almost no neurosomatic patients respond well to beta agonists.

GABA dysregulation is present in premenstrual syndrome, also known as late-luteal phase dysphoric disorder (LLPDD) or premenstrual dysphoric disorder (PMDD). Healthy subjects and women with LLPDD both have menstrual-cycle fluctuations in cortical GABA levels. However, the patients with LLPDD are 180 degrees out of phase with the healthy subjects. This abnormality is thought to relate to deficits in allopregnanolone in LLPDD, because allopregnanolone modulates GABA-receptor function. The GABA receptor composed of $alpha_4$-$beta_2$-delta subunits appears to be the most involved.

As mentioned previously, patients with schizophrenia and those with major depressive disorder have a much higher rate of smoking cigarettes than does the general population. Both of these groups of patients have certain cognitive deficits that can be alleviated by smoking or transdermally administered nicotine, presumably by altering prefrontal cortical neurochemistry. Drew and colleagues (1999) found that nicotine enhances amphetamine-stimulated (dopamine transporter-mediated) dopamine release from slices of rat prefrontal cortex but not from slices of striatum or nucleus accumbens. Higher levels of nicotine produce more enhancement of amphetamine-stimulated dopamine release. Other nicotinic agents also enhance amphetamine-stimulated dopamine release. This enhancement is reversed by the nicotinic cholinergic antagonist mecamylamine, which is again on the market in the United States. Mecamylamine is a potentially useful agent in those patients that have adverse reactions to transdermal nicotine patches. The findings of the abstract by Drew and colleagues "suggests that nicotine is acting via a high affinity nicotinic receptor which regulates outward flow of dopamine via the dopamine transporter" (p. 2239).

Insulin-like growth factor 1 (IGF-1) stimulates a tyrosine kinase when it binds to its receptor. This tyrosine kinase potentiates the activity of L-type calcium channels. There is increased phosphorylation of the $alpha_1$ subunit of the L-type calcium channel in response to IGF-1. This mode of action is somewhat similar to that of gabapentin, which acts at the $alpha_2$ subunit of the L-type calcium channel. The calcium-channel blocker nimodipine, which I have used extensively in my practice for many years, decreases 5-HT_{2A} receptor hyperactivity induced by glucocorticoids at a postreceptor level when used chronically. This result may explain the antidepressant effect of nimodipine when given over a several-week period but would not explain the rapid results that I see in my patient population. Nimodipine, however, is a useful alternative in the patient with treatment-resistant depression.

Gabapentin, by its action on the $alpha_2$-delta subunit of neuronal voltage-sensitive calcium channels, inhibits high-threshold calcium currents and neurotransmitter release. In particular, norepinephrine release is inhibited. Some non-dihydropyridine L-type calcium-channel blockers enhance norepinephrine release, an effect that is reversed by dihydropyridine calcium-channel blockers but not by gabapentin. Gabapentin also inhibits norepinephrine release by blocking N-type VSCCs and has the same effect in P/Q-type voltage-sensitive calcium channels. In the P/Q-type VSCCs, omega conotoxin blocks the inhibition of norepinephrine release by gabapentin, suggesting that GBP selectively modulates P/Q-type VSCCs, which have been implicated in GBP-responsive disorders such as epilepsy, migraine, and pain (Mieske CA et al., 1999). GBP also opens K^+_{ATP} channels, along with clonidine, minoxidil, morphine, cromakalim, galanin, diazoxide, atropine, and possibly baclofen.

ELDRITCH LORE ABOUT NEUROSOMATIC THERAPY

The apparent deficiency in mesocorticolimbic DA and NE can be explained by

1. a regional insufficiency of catecholamines caused by excessive utilization and resultant synaptic fatigue;
2. down-regulation of DA and NE receptors on a regional basis, since NE overactivity appears to be present in some regions at some times;
3. an abnormality in postreceptor events that has been elusive;
4. a dysregulation of the ratios of one or more DA receptors to another, e.g., D_3 and D_5; and
5. hypersensitivity of DA and/or NE autoreceptors.

PFC receptors stimulate BDNF, which acts on tyrosine kinase B (TrkB) in the striatum to increase D_3 receptors there, especially in the NAc (White FJ, 2001; Guillin O et al., 2001).

Considerable evidence supports catecholamine deficiency or dysregulation in CFS. We found abnormal pupillometric responses to noradrenergic eyedrops (dilatation) in most of the patients we tested. The cardiorespiratory perturbations are well known, if poorly understood, by non-neurobiologists and reflect, at least, noradrenergic inconsistency from the much vaunted and considerably overhyped tilt table test. This procedure is 1,000 times more expensive than pupillometry and proves less than a history of chills and sweats and the demonstrable acrocyanosis of Raynaud's disease.

Panic disorder is more frequency encountered in CFS patients than in the general population and is difficult to explain in an individual with purportedly low CRH and low catecholamines. Up-regulation of GABA receptors is found in the brain and on peripheral lymphocytes of such individuals, but the paroxysmal nature of the episodes is not well explained by this finding, unless GABA concentration is maintained in an unstable and precarious balance between the A and B receptors. Neurosteroids, especially allopregnanolone and the Cl^- channel opening metabolites of DHEA and pregnenolone are probably involved in the neurologic manifestations of PMS, and decrease in their activity could cause anxiety and depression in the luteal phase at other times. I suppose that minor falls in the transmitters or changes in their receptor density, affinity, or subunit composition could be held accountable, but I have never read a convincing explanation of the neurobiology of panic disorder in patients with atypical depression, a diagnosis into which many neurosomatic patients could be shoehorned. Perhaps the kindling hypothesis of Post could be modified to fit this situation.

Excessive secretion of SP and CGRP, plus a selection from the plethora of growth factors, could be algogenic by directly increasing glutamate secretion. Other transmitters, neuropeptides, and neurohormones are certainly involved, but their roles appear to be more specialized and perhaps permissive rather than causal.

Alpha-melanocyte-stimulating hormone (MSH), melanocortin-4, and uncoupling proteins must be primarily involved in obesity; they have secondary effects on other functions, cognitions, and behaviors. NPY has a larger role to play, but its primary functions thus far are orexigenic and anxiolytic. The orexins, or hypocretins, increase food intake but not weight gain and are deficient in narcolepsy and in some primary disorders of vigilance. TRH and oxytocin are obviously key: TRH in alertness and mood, as well as catecholamine synergy, and oxytocin in a litany of functions in the very important medial preoptic area (MPOA) and elsewhere. A typical response would be to increase mood and affiliation while decreasing pain somewhat and increasing energy and cognition.

The role of melanocortins in relation to obesity has recently been reviewed (Wisse BE, Schwartz MW, 2001). A dominant hypothesis is that transmitter substances generated in proportion to body fat/mass regulate hypothalamic nuclei involved in energy intake and expenditure. Melanocortins, segments of propopiomelanocortin (POMC) such as MSH, are secreted by affected hypothalamic nuclei to reduce food intake while increasing energy expenditure. This valuable property depends primarily on activation of the neuronal Mc4r melanocortin-receptor subtype. There is, of course, an endogenous Mc4r antagonist, agouti-related peptide (see Wisse BE, Schwartz MW, 2001, figure on p. 858).

Melanocortins participate in normal energy homeostasis and are secreted when rats are tube fed nutrients in excess of their daily caloric requirements. Caloric restriction has the opposite effect. Changes in body fat/mass index are accompanied by changes in leptin secretion. Leptin has not panned out as a weight-loss medication, since downstream tolerance develops to its continued administration. Leptin increases melanocortins and decreases AgRP.

The current consensus is that the hypothalamic melanocortin system plays a predominant role among the several circuits involved in response to body fat/mass index. A single-gene mutation in the Mc4r is present in 4 percent of severely obese people. Cachectic anorexia is no longer just the province of tumor necrosis factor-alpha (TNFα); melanocortins are even more involved.

Because there are several melanocortin receptors, it is important to target only the Mc4r receptor with a highly specific congener that would not have the other neuroendocrine actions of a Mc4r agonist on the HPA and HPT axis, erectile function, and immunomodulation.

Other regulatory systems in the hypothalamus can be potentially targeted in obesity treatment. These include cocaine- and amphetamine-regulated transcript (CART), melanin-concentrating hormone (MCH), and urocortin, which all act downstream of leptin. A gastric orexigen, ghrelin, could be antagonized. The results of such an intervention have not yet been published. The best results may be obtained with a combination of medically proven active ingredients. I don't expect that the general community will wait for four out of five Madison Avenue doctors to prescribe them, either.

Other candidates are beta$_3$ agonists with bearable adverse reactions, a derivative of the ciliary neurotrophic factor (CNTF), a hormone that regulates body weight by leptin-like mechanisms, and a synthetic form of a small region of human growth hormone. This latter drug, Advanced Obesity Drug 9604, speeds up the use of stored fat cells, increasing energy expenditure. There is even a cleaved product of a natural hormone produced by adipocytes. When administered to mice, they ate as much high-calorie, high-fat food as they could. The compound stimulates muscle oxidation of free fatty acids (Bonetta L, 2001).

Other suggested techniques of obesity reduction include using insulin analogs that occupy the receptor but do not activate it, and increasing the ratio of POMC to NPY. Because maintenance of adequate caloric stores is so essential to survival of the organism, numerous redundant mechanisms keep weight stable or to increase it. Multiple blocking agents may be required, and, as usual, the treatment should be tailored to the patient because of neurochemical individuality.

Histamine (HA) is involved in alertness but may already be secreted in excess peripherally because of the ubiquity of allergic rhinitis in neurosomatic disorders. It has an important role in the entrainment of circadian rhythms in mammals (Jacobs EH et al., 2000). How to best modulate HA in circadian circuits has proven problematic for me, and phase delay is too often intractable, despite modafinil. Acetylcholine function should be impaired more than is obvious, if only to counterbalance episodes of catecholaminergic hyperactivity. Its effect at the nicotinic acetylcholine receptor (nAchR), while occasionally beneficial, is too transient in most patients to be clinically valuable.

Stimulants are effective in only a minority of patients, particularly those who have had an adverse drug reaction (ADR) to ketamine and other direct or indirect NMDA antagonists. Some patients are unable to function without them.

Opioids are valuable in a manner analogous to stimulants. They enable about two-fifths of my patients to have less pain and one-fifth to have more energy, but since there are about 12 descending antinociceptive pathways, they are no longer the only game in town and haven't been for some time.

Triptans are not only antimigraine drugs; they can be effective for central pain, particularly in the patient who gets worse with SRIs. SRIs antagonize the 5-HT_{1B} receptor, which is stimulated by triptans. In the patient with ADRs to all SRIs, I want to block, one at a time, all the serotonin receptors I can, without doing a chemical serotonectomy. Thus, I would try triptans (maybe all five of them sequentially). They stimulate the $5\text{-HT}_{1B/1D}$ receptors, which are inhibitory. Next, I would probably try ziprasidone, the most potent 5-HT_{1A} agonist. The 5-HT_{1A} receptor is an autoreceptor and decreases serotonin release. Then I would try 5-HT blockers, the most encompassing of which is mirtazapine (Remeron), antagonizing the 5-HT_2 and 5-HT_3 receptors. It is very helpful as a sleep aid, but weight gain is a limiting problem.

The orexigenic action of Remeron appears to be, at least in part, a result of delayed satiety. I instruct patients taking Remeron to eat a normal portion and stop eating whether they feel full or not. I advise them that satiety will occur in 10 to 15 minutes if they can tolerate the hunger for that period of time. This strategy has proven to be remarkably successful during the six months or so that I have been suggesting it and has enabled me to prescribe Remeron for already overweight patients. If Remeron is out, I would try a combination of Seroquel (5-HT_2 antagonist) and Zofran (ondansetron), a 5-HT_3 blocker. I can't think of any $5\text{-HT}_4\text{-}5\text{-HT}_5$ antagonists, but a partial 5-HT_4 blocker is available to treat IBS (tegaserod). Narcotics and stimulants are a relatively minor part of my armamentarium.

Most of the medications I prescribe inhibit synaptic activity of one or more transmitters, although by doing so, they may stimulate the release of another. Adenocard spray often works better than dipyridamole, an adenosine-reuptake inhibitor and weak PDE_5 (phosphodiesterase) inhibitor. Adenosine has several subtypes; most are inhibitory, but some are excitatory, particularly for DA. It is not unusual for adenosine 1:10 or 1:1 nasal spray to reduce anxiety and/or increase energy. Anxiety reduction can liberate a patient from chronic tension and allow the wasted energy to go where it should: to improve mood, increase alertness, produce pain relief, and enhance stamina.

Amantadine is an excellent drug. It is like ketamine with fewer side effects. The intravenous form is spectacularly more successful than p.o. or pluronic oranogel (PLO) formulations. The effects last longer, and it is sometimes the only medication to which a patient responds. It is wise to premedicate with a BZD or clonidine. Some people get jittery during the infusion. Adenosine nasal spray is virtually unknown in its ability to ameliorate anxiety; it is safe and works immediately.

Ativan nasal spray 1:10 and 1:1 is the best treatment for panic attacks. It relieves them in 10 seconds, and its degree of effectiveness may be a signal to pursue GABAergic alternatives. Adenosine and GABA are fairly similar in their clinical effects. Baclofen is even better. It may be mixed in PLO, and its effect or lack thereof is apparent in two to four minutes. Baclofen is a good analgesic and anxiolytic. It sometimes increases mood and energy. It does not usually cause depression in my patients. I am using it in eyedrops and nose drops now.

Clonidine is a very versatile agent. It also may be prepared in a gel and is quite well tolerated. It is a very good anxiolytic but does not cross-react with GABAergic agents. The literature states that tolerance rapidly develops, but tolerance has not been a problem in my practice. It has the same general effects as baclofen and GBP. Clonidine, even more so than baclofen, can give people energy while keeping them, with luck, somewhat alert. Clonidine is an alpha$_{2ABC}$ agonist. This property may make some patients sleepy, but the alpha$_{2BC}$ effect makes it a delta opioid agonist, the only one available for clinical use. If the oral form does not work as well as the gel, consider a Catapres TTS patch, graduated from 1 to 4. They last a week. Clonidine is an effective analgesic.

Chlorzoxazone is the generic name for Parafon Forte, which has more or less been relegated to the dustbin of medicine. Its major action is to inhibit the presynaptic release of glutamate. It is not as useful as LTG, which has many other effects, but is probably more so than Rilutek (riluzole), which is very expensive.

Dopamine nasal spray and eyedrops are primarily of use to estimate who will respond to dopamine-agonist therapy. Some people like the spray well enough to use it on an ongoing basis. It occasionally causes jaw clenching.

Ergoloid mesylates, or Hydergine, is another diamond in the rough. It is a DA and Ach agonist (mainly DA), is well tolerated, and two 1 mg tablets either work or not in 30 minutes. When they do, the patient usually feels more energetic and has less pain with more mental clarity. They are effective in selected patients two-thirds of the time. Many patients have dry eyes and mouth. These disabilities can be relieved most of the time with Evoxac t.i.d. or Salagen t.i.d., peripheral cholinesterase inhibitors with few ADRs. I use them frequently. I have written enough about GBP, or Neurontin. It is the best oral medication, works better in a gel, and may be an NMDA antagonist along with its other actions. Its effect can be reversed by cycloserine, a NMDA/glycine agonist, which occasionally has a therapeutic effect of its own, usually in combination with LTG, lidocaine, hydergine, and tolcapone (a great drug when it works, which is not too often). Amantadine, pindolol, pramipexole, Modafinil, oxytocin, bupropion, and Talwin could be added to this list.

Isoxsuprine is available in a 4 percent gel and a 20 mg tablet t.i.d. It is sometimes effective for all symptoms. It is an antagonist at the polyamine site of the NMDA receptor. It slightly blocks the NR1/NR2B receptor as well, but nylidrin is more effective in this regard. Onset of action is immediate.

Indomethacin 10 percent PLO is the treatment of choice, along with the triptans, for acute migraine headache. It is best to use it as a 10 percent gel, since there is gastric stasis during migraine and it may not be absorbed for two to three hours. Vaginal or rectal suppositories are a less esthetic alternative. It relieves other types of pain also, particularly inflammatory or osteoarthritic. Some say Vioxx works as well. I'm not so sure. Other common agents for migraine prophylaxis include Depakote, GBP, propranolol, and tricyclic antidepressants. I like Depakote the best, but GBP is a close second right now. An ADR of GBP is headache.

I am omitting esoterica about LTG and lidocaine since I have discussed them extensively.

The anticholinesterases have occasional value in the patient who has an ADR to ketamine. They have an indirect NMDA agonist effect. I would be careful about galantamine (Reminyl), because a patient that has had an ADR to the nicotine patch may not like Reminyl because it has a nicotinic effect. Reminyl is, overall, the best cholinesterase inhibitor. I rarely prescribe Mestinon (pyridostigmine) anymore and have seen no advantage thus far to rivastagmine (Exelon). At least they can be reversed in minutes by 1mg of Artane (trihexyphenidyl). Cholinesterase inhibitors are being increasingly used to treat attention-deficit hyperactivity disorder (ADHD). They reverse Marinol.

Human growth hormone is just too expensive for my patients. If it works, it only gives 50 percent improvement in six months. I'm seeking a 100 percent improvement in three to four days.

Naphazoline, nitroglycerin, and nimodipine are still heavy hitters. Naphazoline .01 percent ophthalmic solution is the first medication I try. The drops are postsynaptic alpha$_2$ agonists, somewhat like clonidine. As is usual with eyedrops, the response is evident in one second. They are exactly like concentrated Clear-Eyes, and the only problem occurs when using them more than three times per day. As a vasoconstrictor, naphazoline can make people's eyes burn when used excessively.

I have stopped using nitroglycerin as much. Too many patients have migraine headaches, and nitric oxide has been found to cause this disorder. With no history of severe headaches, I can opt to try it (one-half of a 0.3 mg tablet). It either works or not. It sometimes acts as an NMDA agonist since it is a retrograde messenger. Those that respond to nitroglycerin will often benefit from testosterone, oxytocin, and agonists of DA, NE, and glutamate, all of which act in the MPOA to produce arousal and orgasm.

Nimotop (nimodipine) 30 mg remains one of the premier treatments. It is a lipophilic dihydropyridine Ca^{2+} channel blocker worth trying if a patient has insurance that will pay for it. Other dihydropyridines usually don't work as well. It will be clear whether it is beneficial in 30 minutes.

Marinol and baclofen are antagonized by Amerge (naratriptan) and verapamil (probably in its role as a dopamine blocker). I start testosterone gel at 10 mg/ml, particularly in women with decreased libido if they fail on transdermal estrogen. Their testosterone levels are usually very low. Because BuSpar is metabolized to 1-PP, I use it to rescue patients from ADRs to alpha$_2$ agonists. I prefer it to yohimbine, which often makes people jittery even if they have no history of panic disorder. I like to use tacrine (Cognex) in the office because of its short duration of action. I've heard it is being discontinued. T.I.D. dosing and the requirement for liver function tests made it unattractive to physicians and patients.

I use Coumadin in a dose of 1 mg. An anticoagulant dose is unneccessary since there is no thrombosis. If it will be effective, it acts somewhat like ketamine, and the patient usually feels better in 30 minutes or so. DDAVP (des-amino-d-arginine vasopressin) is only good for enuresis and nocturia. It has never helped one patient to feel better, which would be expected if neurosomatic patients have a vasopressin excess (Altemus M et al., 2001).

The NMDA/glycine site antagonists are excellent agents for the treatment of dysmenorrhea. Diltiazem is the best of the group. All of them are also 5-HT$_3$ antagonists and should potentially improve nausea, anxiety, bulimia, central pain, tardive dyskinesia, IBS, and energy (potentiates cocaine). They also antagonize ketamine and really aren't that effective for pain (except dysmenorrhea), anxiety, or energy. Most patients report only the antiemetic property. 5-HT$_3$ antagonists decrease vagal transmission.

I have given glipizide to several patients who have had ADRs to Neurontin, usually sedation. It reverses the ADR, but given alone, it is sometimes a useful agent. Glipizide blocks the K_{ATP} channel via one of its sulfonylurea channels. K_{ATP} channel openers are cough suppressants.

Gotu kola is the only available cholecystokinin (CCK) antagonist. CCK is anxiogenic. Gotu kola has had no effect on any patient so far, but hope springs eternal, particularly since right now it's the only game in town for CCK-induced symptoms. Atrial natriuretic factor beta (ANB) blocks CCK and produces anxiolysis as well as natriuresis. ANB deficiency may cause idiopathic cyclic edema.

It is difficult to reverse guanfacine. I usually administer it to patients who have a good response to clonidine, because it is less sedating, is specific for the alpha$_{2A}$ receptor (where most of the action is), and requires only once-a-day dosing. Yohimbine is fairly ineffective. BuSpar, via 1-PP, works a little better. Guanfacine is greatly underused for attention deficit disorder (ADD),

ADHD (Seahill L et al., 2001), generalized anxiety disorder (GAD), chronic pain, tic disorders, and neurocognitive disorders. It helps the numerous neurosomatic patients (most of them) who manifest the autonomic components of arousal and anxiety. It is very constipating, but I believe it binds to the mu-opioid receptor with an affinity similar to clonidine. The constipation is usually well treated with low-dose (0.5 to 3 mg) naloxone, which works for almost every kind of constipation, opioid-induced or not.

I have human chorlonic gonadatropin (HCG) on my list of treatment options because of reports that it is a Na^+ channel blocker. It has not helped anyone to a great degree, but I have only tried it a few times. I use it as one of my last resorts. It has been reported to induce mania.

Heparin also works rapidly. A response to 1,000 units takes about 20 minutes. Two thousand units is the most I have given. I do an activated partial thromboplastin time (APTT) before I give it to rule out a hereditary hemorrhagic diathesis, and if it works in the office, I do platelet counts every three days for three weeks or so. It is a fairly effective treatment and is unique among agents I can use to block the IP_3 receptor. It has six or seven auxiliary actions. Although some researchers have suggested that all Ca^{2+} stores in the endoplasmic reticulum (ER) commingle, my rate of success with dantrolene, which I start in a dose of 12.5 mg, is nil. Dantrolene blocks the ryanodine receptor, which releases intracellular Ca^{2+} when stimulated. Caffeine is known for its ability to release ryanodine-sensitive receptor (RyR)-gated Ca^{2+} stores. The prevailing view at present is that some Ca^{2+} is sequestered in subcompartments of the ER that function fairly independently (Blaustein MP, Golovina VA, 2001).

Inositol is also greatly underused. Ten years' worth of published double-blind experiments show its utility in depression and anxiety (10 to 20 mg a day in divided doses for six to eight weeks). The number of 1,000 mg capsules one needs to swallow is high, but side effects are usually restricted to diarrhea. Inositol is also made in powdered form.

By the time one of my patients gets to inositol, he or she has tried at least 150 other treatments. The patient's motivation is high to complete the course of treatment, and he or she may be beginning to feel a little desperate. Still, the results are good, and some change may be reported after week one.

Even though they are both nonoverlapping NMDA polyamine site receptors, I usually try isoxsuprine gel before nylidrin gel. Both are vasodilators and can cause headaches. Patients test them one at a time. Nylidrin blocks the NR1/NR2B receptor, and some patients prefer it over isoxsuprine, which is still available by prescription at your local pharmacy. Nylidrin must be compounded, and 6 to 12 mg three times per day in divided doses is usually required. Both isoxsuprine and nylidrin may cause headaches which should respond to over-the-counter (OTC) meds (such as acetaminophen).

Patients who report that these agents worsen their symptoms should try S-adenosylmethionine (SAMe), which donates methyl groups via the transmethylation pathway for polyamine biosynthesis.

In a desperately acute situation 800 mg of SAMe should do the job. SAMe has a major role in the transmethylation pathway, which also involves B_{12} and folate. Neurosomatic physicians should have a passing acquaintance with transmethylation—its tentacles creep into many brain functions and disorders. Figure 45 provides a diagram of methyl group transfers.

Norflex (orphenadrine citrate) acts like a weak ketamine. It, too, is an NMDA antagonist. I try it first as a transdermal gel, usually on both arms. Responses are fairly good. The next step is Norflex 100 mg b.i.d. The oral form often makes patients sleepy, a side effect that is less pronounced with the transdermal preparation. The PLO preparation works in two minutes, and application to both arms is usually required.

Quite a few practicing psychiatrists have never prescribed a monoamine oxidase inhibitor and will not do so because they don't know how. Even when I was still teaching psychopharmacology, it was not unusual for me to encounter a senior psychiatry resident with no MAOI experience. Phenelzine (Nardil) and tranylcypromine (Parnate) often are effective when no other medication is. They are not dangerous if a few simple precautions are observed: no wine (actually no red wine, no wine eliminates ambiguity), no cheese (really no aged cheese, but it is difficult sometimes to tell), no aged foods (not hard to avoid—beef jerky, Marmite, sausage, and the like), no medications that increase serotonin, no Demerol, no dextromethorphan, no epinephrine, no pigging out on other supposedly prohibited foods containing tyramine, the forbidden molecule, and no mass quantities of beer and soy sauce. I've been prescribing MAOIs for thirty years, and only one patient has gone to the emergency department. Patients can buy an electronic sphygmomanometer and keep 10 mg nifedipine capsules on hand in case of a hypertensive crisis. Orthostatic hypotension is much more common and can be treated with midrodrine. Reality-based precautions with MAOIs were published in the *Journal of Clinical Psychiatry* several years ago (Gardner DM et al., 1996). Many "forbidden" medications can be safely prescribed with MAOIs, including tricyclic antidepressants (TCAs), stimulants, bupropion, antihistamines, and reboxetine (if somehow the patient has obtained it). Rational use of MAOIs, alone or in combination, has saved many lives over the years. I received a letter from a patient in Alabama taking Parnate, reboxetine, and Geodon that ended: "Thank you Dr. Goldstein, I would not be alive today without you." The hard part is when I must monitor the patient by long distance because there is apparently no physician in his or her town or any nearby city who will prescribe MAOIs. Actually, it is not so hard, since these drugs are fairly safe. I have given several home-town physicians a short course over the telephone on how to prescribe Nardil or Parnate. An entire generation of physicians is now practicing who have never prescribed an MAOI, don't know how, and are afraid to do so. "It can kill you," patients have been told when they ask for it. I jokingly inform them when they come to the office that I can get them a discount at the local mortuary: "They drop like flies around here. Every week one or two carcasses are hauled out." Reversible MAOIs (RIMAs), such as meclobemide, do not seem to work as well. Selegiline (Eldepryl) in a low dose is selective for one type of MAOI, and food restrictions are unnecessary. It's supposed to be much more effective transdermally and may be marketed as a patch. Selegiline in PLO gel has been a bust for me.

S-adenosylmethionine may be an effective antidepressant in a dose of 1,600 mg per day. It works through the transmethylation cycle. It can also cause psychosis.

I harken back to the teaching of William F. Bunney: "Any medicine that can cause mania can be used as an antidepressant." Although in symbolic logic, if A, then B does not mean if B, then A. Any antidepressant can cause mania in a given person.

The atypical neuroleptics are anxiolytic. I don't prescribe Risperdal (risperidone) very often because it can cause extrapyramidal syndrome and tardive dyskinesia. I don't like to prescribe Zyprexa (olanzapine) because of weight gain. The weight gain may be prevented by H_2 antagonists (Saechetti E et al., 2000). That leaves Geodon (ziprasidone) and Seroquel (quetiapine). Geodon is less sedating, but some people have adverse reactions to it, more than to Seroquel, which causes a little weight gain. I prescribe more Geodon than Seroquel because of its greater 5-HT_{1A} agonism and its much greater efficacy—unlike Seroquel, it is not effective in treatment-resultant anxiety disorders. Two patients have become manic taking Geodon.

If prescribing Synarel for PMS, it will work while the patient is in the office. It causes a chemical oophorectomy, so long-term users should take birth control pills. In female neurosomatic patients with decreased libido, oxytocin often helps, although not as much as making them asymptomatic. Transdermal estrogens are often effective. If they are not, physicians should measure free testosterone and supplement (I use testosterone gel) if the levels are low.

Chapter 9

Neurosomatic Neuroscience

Except perhaps for the annual update on swimwear fashion kindly provided by *Sports Illustrated,* my most enthralling literary experience of each year is reading the abstracts of the meeting of the Society for Neuroscience, held in the year 2000 in New Orleans. From the 15,000 presentations, I have culled a number that might advance the theory and practice of neurosomatic medicine. In this section, I shall discuss pertinent abstracts, going from the beginning, designated Abstract 18.4, to the end. Because the number of abstracts is so great, I shall not give citations unless a discovery is of exceptional merit or relevance.

18.4   Acidosis, local or systemic, increases pain by activating cation channels in sensory neurons. It also induces the expression of the neuropeptide FMRF (phenylalnine-methionine-arginine-phenylalnine [Phe-Met-Arg-Phe])-amide, which potentiates cation-channel activation.

19.4   Estradiol enhances the action of catecholamines in various ways, including the stimulation of dopamine beta-hydroxylase, which converts DA to NE.

19.11   All drugs of abuse stimulate DA output in the BST, the ventral part of which is continuous with the MPOA.

19.12   Stress-induced NE release in the lateral BST acts through alpha$_1$ receptors and is anxiogenic.

35.7   Presynaptic C (small, unmyelinated) nerve fibers in sympathetic ganglia release luteinizing hormone-releasing hormone (LHRH, also called GnRH). LHRH secretion by the C fibers occurs by mechanical coupling of the L-type Ca^{2+} channels to ryanodine receptors, which release Ca^{2+} from intracellular compartments. This action relates to the extremely rapid and beneficial effect of Synarel (nafarelin) and Lupron (leuprolide), LHRH agonists, on PMS (LLPDD, PMDD, etc.). I find no need to use Lupron.

35.13   Oxytocin acts in a retrograde manner on presynaptic glutamate terminals to inhibit secretion. OXT decreases Ca^{2+} flux through N and

P/Q-type Ca^{2+} channels but increases levels of intracellular Ca^{2+} by release from stores of $[Ca^{2+}]_i$.

38.9   Genistein, which can be purchased in a "natural" soy-based capsule, inhibits Trk and long-term potentiation (LTP). Genistein also inhibits extracellular signal-related kinase (ERK), glutamate release, and Ca^{2+} flux. The latter effect occurs by modulating the Ca^{2+} channel alpha$_1$ subunit. High doses of genistein can be neurotoxic. I have seen no adverse reactions.

39.7   The vanniloid receptor (VR1) is a nonselective cation channel that acts as a transducer of painful stimuli. VR1 is activated by capsaicin, acidosis, anandamide, heat, and eicosanoids, as well as NGF, increased in FMS.

40.20   Gabapentin, besides binding to the alpha$_2$-delta subunit of the L-type Ca^{2+} channel peripherally, also binds to the alpha$_2$-delta subunit in the CNS. Pregabalin ("son of Neurontin") inhibits this GBP binding, as does L-leucine, which I have never used therapeutically.

41.7   This topic is discussed more fully in the nicotine section in Chapter 11, but the alpha$_7$ nicotinic subunit of the nicotine receptor is probably the most important in neurosomatic medicine. Its activation stimulates TH in the LC and tryptophan hydroxylase (TrypH) in the dorsal raphe.

42.1   Lithium and Zn^{2+} facilitate NMDA action at low pH (not necessarily a good thing).

42.3   Spermine, which enhances the open time of the NMDA receptor, has a pervasive effect on 5-HT$_2$ agonists to do so as well. Sperminesite and 5-HT$_2$-receptor antagonists might synergize as NMDA-receptor antagonists (or not—nylidrin plus nefazodone is not anything special).

42.4   Acamprosate is an anticraving, antiaddiction compound. It is a weak NMDA antagonist but may be more potent at specific areas in the brain.

42.5   Memantine is a rather weak noncompetitive NMDA blocker with no effect at the polyamine site of the receptor.

42.8   The amino acid taurine, the growth factor BDNF (which is also an antidepressant), and beta fibroblast growth factor prevent glutamate excitotoxicity through regulation of $[Ca^{2+}]_i$ and mitochondrial function. Glutamate increases Ca^{2+} channel open time and causes a concomitant decrease in mitochondrial function, an important alteration in a hyperglutamatergic state. Protecting the mitochondria may prevent fatigue, if the simplistic reasoning of low adenosine triphosphate (ATP) equals low energy is actually true for some patients.

42.9 Minocycline blocks NMDA-induced elevation in Ca^{2+}. So does tetracycline. Doxycycline is ineffective, but it can kill *Mycoplasma fermentans,* chlamydia, borrelia, Babesia, ehrlichiosis, and other members of the "Bug-of-the-Month Club." Because each bug has its own club of true believers, to avoid the *meinungschaos* (confusion) and save money, I would not need to order $2,000 of low-yield, overly sensitive, potentially bogus lab tests. I could just give everyone tetracycline for six to 12 months. Funny though, when I tried this protocol in 1989 for a year or so, it did not help anybody! But I might be able to keep my malpractice insurance this time. I was once found to have "overly litigious patients." Fittingly, long-term antibiotic therapy is no better than placebo in late Lyme disease (Klempner MS et al., 2001). Screening the population with borrelia lab tests in the absence of clinical signs or history of primary and/or secondary Lyme disease is supposed to be bad medical practice (Steere AC, 2001).

43.6 NAAG is supposedly elevated in people who were abused as children. The enzyme *N*-acetylated alpha-linked acidic dipeptidase (NAALADase) converts NAAG into glutamate and *N*-acetyl-aspartate. NAAG can even be detected on magnetic resonance spectroscopy (MRS). NAALADase inhibitors are being developed. They are analgesic in neuropathic pain, so they might help neurosomatic pain as well. NAALADase works as well as, more quickly than, and has fewer side effects than gabapentin. *N*-acetyl-aspartate is also found in the ACC and orbitofrontal cortext (OFC) of such patients and may be a marker for anxiety (Grachev ID, Apkarian AV, 2000).

43.12 NAAG is a mixed agonist/antagonist at the NMDA receptor.

45.4 I was not too keen on the alpha$_1$ agonist midodrine at first, but after a while I found it could augment stimulants. It can also treat Alzheimer's disease if combined with cycloserine, an NMDA glycine-site agonist. Modafinil (Provigil) also stimulates alpha$_1$ receptors and enhances 5-HT and DA function. In mice, restraint stress and corticosteroids attenuate the response to alpha$_1$ agonists, while lipopolysaccharide (LPS), which stimulates cytokine production in the brain, almost nullifies them. Could constitutive cytokines cause depression, or even fatigue?

45.10 If a patient responds to an alpha$_2$ agonist such as clonidine, guanfacine, or tizanidine (Zanaflex), the doctor should not give the patient a beta agonist. It will desensitize the alpha$_2$ adrenoreceptor (AR). Physicians should never give a pure beta$_2$ agonist (except as an asthma inhaler) to any neurosomatic patient. It usually worsens symptoms. Isoxsuprine and nylidrin are okay.

46.10   Even though the 5-HT$_2$ receptor is associated with schizophrenia, stimulating the receptor increases inositol metabolism (helps anxiety and depression). In the arcuate nucleus of the hypothalamus, 5-HT$_{2C}$ neurons coexpress POMC, the precursor to (among others) alpha-MSH, an anorectic peptide. Caution should be used prescribing inositol with an MAOI. Although enhancing the activity of mitochondrial uncoupling mechanisms may be the way to go in treating obesity, alpha-MSH or MCH should be tried. Some tinkering with the molecule would be necessary. One reason why atypical neuroleptics cause weight gain may be by 5-HT$_{2C}$ blockade. LSD binds to the 5-HT$_{2A}$ and 5-HT$_{2C}$ receptors.

47.7   NK1 (neurokinin 1) receptor antagonists have antidepressant properties.

47.8   NK1 knock-out mice have desensitized 5-HT$_{1A}$ receptors. If neuronal nitric oxide synthase (nNOS) is knocked out, both the 5-HT$_{1A}$ and 5-HT$_{1B}$ receptors are subsensitive. Such mice are aggressive and impulsive.

48.4   Tyrosine phosphylation is widespread in the brain and is particularly associated with a growth factor (such as NGF) and NMDA activity. Genistein, a phytoestrogen available as a constituent of soy capsules, inhibits all tyrosine kinases. It is not known to have adverse reactions when administered to humans in a dose of 16 mg b.i.d. It might be particularly useful in FMS, although I am a little uncomfortable with the nonspecific inhibition by genistein of all tyrosine kinases.

48.7   Add IGF-1 to the list of substances involved in the preoptic area, emerging as a (or the) dysfunctional locus in neurosomatic disorders. IGF-1, its receptors, and its binding proteins are locally synthesized in POA glia. IGF-1 stimulates cAMP production via the alpha$_1$ noradrenergic receptor in the presence of gonadal steroids.

72.9   Amygdaloid NMDA receptors are involved in the learning of but not the expression of conditioned fear. Such learning is blocked by a mitogen-activated protein kinase (MAPK) inhibitor or an NMDA-receptor antagonist. An IEG, EGR-1 (early growth response gene 1), is involved in amygdala fear conditioning but is blocked by NMDA-receptor (NMDAR) antagonists. Chronic corticosterone enhances contextual fear conditioning and CRH levels in the amygdala. CREB, as might be expected, is involved also. So is NE, for a brief period, in the "flashbulb" model of learning via beta receptors.

96.4 Baclofen attenuates the symptoms of morphine withdrawal in male mice but has no effect in females.

96.20 Baclofen also inhibits morphine activation in the VTA and may be an anticraving compound for cocaine.

97.14 Atypical antipsychotic drugs, which antagonize the effects of ketamine, facilitate NMDA-evoked current-and-voltage responses in pyramidal cells of the PFC, perhaps accounting for improving negative symptoms and cognitive dysfunction in schizophrenia.

97.20 $Sigma_1$ ligands (such as Talwin, or pentazocine) are being developed as atypical neuroleptics, antidepressants, and antianxiety medications. I have been on the verge of using Talwin in treatment-refractory schizoaffective patients but have always chickened out (fear conditioning) because of several experiences 30 years ago with such patients having Talwin-induced visual hallucinations. It sometimes even makes "normal" people feel weird.

142.4 NMDA neurotransmission recruits D_1 receptors from the cytoplasm to the cell membrane, altering the D_1/D_2 balance. Thus, it is probable that $D_{2,3,4}$ receptors are implicated in decreasing hyperactive NMDA activity. Trait or state D_1-D_2 ratio may be important in causing neurosomatic symptoms.

143.9 Amantadine has long been considered to be dopaminergic.

143.14 Zonisamide (Zonegran), a new AED that I rarely use due to potential toxicity (it usually does not help my patients anyway), is a 5-HT_{1A} agonist and selectively increases DA in the medial prefrontal cortex (mPFC). This mode of action is shared by buspirone, atypical neuroleptics, valproate (Depakote), and carbamazepine. Zonisamide does not increase DA in the NAc. Lithium has no effect on PFC DA, and lowers NAc DA, showing differential effects on the mesocortical and mesolimbic dopaminergic tracts.

143.19 Intraperitoneal (IP) injection of amantadine does not increase levels of DA or its metabolites in Wistar rats and completely prevents the rise of DA induced by amphetamine. MK-801, an NMDA noncompetitive receptor antagonist, has the same effect. Chronic amantadine treatment increases DA in the striatum, perhaps by an effect of presynaptic glutamate heteroreceptors on DA neurons, or indirectly by presynaptic DA autoreceptors.

143.22 cAMP increases striatal DA secretion; cGMP decreases it. A modest increase in kynurenic acid significantly increases striatal DA.

144.2 Pindolol increases glutamate secretion. Buspirone decreases it.

144.4   These drugs have opposite effects on the 5-HT$_{1A}$ receptor. This receptor, postsynaptically in the PFC, can regulate 5-HT firing by a long feedback loop. Thus, the PFC has been shown to regulate secretion to itself.

144.5   Of all "classical" neurotransmitters, 5-HT is the last one to have this mechanism identified. GABA$_B$ receptors suppress this action, and antimuscarinic receptor agents enhance it. 5-HT$_{1A}$ agonists act in the dorsal raphe nucleus. 5-HT$_{1A}$ autoreceptors inhibit the firing of other raphe neurons, and this inhibition may be further inhibited by postsynaptic 5-HT$_{1A}$ receptors.

145.2   The 5-HT$_{1B}$ receptor is primarily an inhibitory autoreceptor. Overexpression of this receptor in the DRN increases stress reactivity.

145.4   Conceivably, triptans, which are 5-HT$_{1B/1D}$ agonists, could have the same property. By clinical observation, such an adverse reaction is uncommon. Paroxetine (Paxil) increases 5-HT substantially more in 5-HT$_{1B}$ knock-outs compared to controls. The 5-HT$_{1B}$ receptor is also located in the VTA and NAc. Agonists at this location increase DA. When I prescribe a triptan, I usually choose the one with the most potent 5-HT$_{1B}$ agonist effect, Amerge (naratriptan). It also has the longest duration of action. Each triptan is slightly different, so it may be worthwhile to try them all.

145.12 Sexual dysfunction among those taking SRIs approaches 50 percent. Among the many (usually ineffective) options to manage this problem are 5-HT$_{1A}$ agonists or 5-HT$_{1B}$ antagonists (or both). Triptans increase [Ca^{2+}]$_i$ and may inhibit release of CGRP by the trigeminal nerve by this mechanism. Oxytocin may be the best treatment for SRI-induced erectile dysfunction.

153.18 Despite the positive results of these abstracts, St. John's wort has been shown to be no better than placebo in a large double-blind study.

153.19 Kava kava has too many reported adverse reactions for me to sanction its use any longer.

157.13 C1 and trigeminal nucleus caudalis (Vc) neurons project directly to the hypothalamus in the trigeminohypothalamic tract (THT).

157.14 Some Vc neurons project to the lateral reticular formation (LRF) and then to the hypothalamus in the reticulohypothalamic tract. Reticulohypothalamic tract neurons have large and complex receptive fields. Thus, stimulation of receptors on V$_{1,2,3}$ can directly affect hypothalamic control of homeostatic mechanisms, rather than going up to the thalamus and the cortex and back down again. The reticulohypothalamic tract relays sensory signals from the entire body, including the head. Trigeminal axons project to many CNS areas, but most of them are compactly bundled in the supraoptic decussation (SOD) in the lateral hypothalamus. Fifty-seven percent cross the midline to reach the posterior hypothalamus on the other side (Burstein R, Malick A, 2000).

160.11   Visceral pain induced by unpleasant colonic distension activates central histamine H_1 receptors, most notably in the anterior cingulate cortex, which also demonstrates increased regional cerebral blood flow (rCBF). Administration of a centrally acting H_1 antagonist reduces pain and decreases rCBF. The decrease in pain is proportional to the decrease in rCBF. These bizarre results must be confirmed, but it would not hurt to have IBS patients try a few doses of Benadryl, which may act as an NMDA antagonist of sorts.

160.14   Chronic pain and anxiety are interrelated, and their networks, identified by in vivo proton magnetic resonance spectroscopy (^{1}H-MRS), overlap.

160.15   Pain is processed in the dorsolateral prefrontal cortex (DLPFC) and OFC, while anxiety is seen mainly in the OFC and ACC. ^{1}H-MRS shows the highest chemical signature for anxiety in the OFC of middle-aged males.

174.8 $5-HT_3$ antagonists, among their numerous other properties, can block the reinforcing effects of cocaine, which produces a mesolimbic DA increase and locomotor activation. Physicians should think twice about giving a $5-HT_3$ antagonist with a stimulant because the stimulant might not stimulate. Stimulants often make neurosomatic patients fatigued. This outcome often occurs in neurosomatic patients, whether they are taking $5-HT_3$ antagonists (which include nimodipine, verapamil, diltiazem, mirtazapine, or atropine) or not.

175.3   For the second year in a row, Yamazaki and colleagues (2000) have correlated central TGF-beta elevations with fatigue after exercise. I emphasized that elevated TGF-beta (Goldstein JA, 1990) was related to stress and possibly involved in CFS pathophysiology. TGF-beta has poorly characterized effects in the adult CNS but is a powerful immunosuppressant. It inhibits TNF-alpha, a cytokine elevated in inflammation and by antidepressants. TGF-beta is inhibited by suramin, an ATP blocker and reverse transcriptase inhibitor that is too toxic for clinical use. Perhaps TGF-beta affects Trk, as many other growth factors do, and could be inhibited by genistein. Among the many properties of TGF-beta that I listed in 1990, two stand out today: TGF-beta (1) regulates the gene and promotes the transcription of plasminogen activator and (2) is dramatically increased by phorbol esters. Plasminogen activator is indirectly inhibited by heparin and warfarin. The entire coagulation cascade has an NMDA-like function in the brain. Phorbol esters in tung oil, used as a sealer, may have precipitated some early cases of CFS because they strongly activate protein kinases and markedly reduce TGF-beta. TGF-beta is a powerful protectant against neurodegenerative disorders and eliminates purported excitotoxicity (Flanders KC et al., 1997) caused by angiotensin-converting enzyme (ACE) inhibitors, which I have administered to some neurosomatic patients. Perhaps two or three have reported reduced fatigue, and none have had signs of neurotoxicity. ACE inhibitors release bradykinin in order to vasodilate. Elevated BK could be neurotoxic.

TGF-beta is really a cytokine and not a neurotrophin. Virtually every cell in the body produces TGF-beta and has receptors for it. Increases, decreases, or mutations in TGF-beta have been related to several structural disorders, but not functional ones (Blobe GC et al., 2000). There are three isoforms of TGF-beta and three receptors for them, I, II, and III. Types I and II contain serine/threonine protein kinases in their intracellular domains and are similar to Trk receptors in this respect. TGF-beta resists cell proliferation in cancer but aids metastasis, angiogenesis, and immunosuppression. It can suppress tumor growth. Mutations of TGF-beta-associated proteins can aid tumor progression. TGF-beta is involved in hereditary hemorrhagic telangiectasia, fibrotic disease, atherosclerosis, and developmental defects, but not in brain functional deficits, at least so far.

206.8   Prenatal sound stress is a causative factor in depression in immature animals. In adult animals who are no longer depressed, hearing that same sound causes them to be depressed. Children prefer certain styles of music played during their third trimester to other types.

206.9   Premenopausal women with PTSD have elevated levels of DHEA, which may cause them to have a sleep disturbance. Stress-induced DHEA levels are much higher than controls. The bottom line for physicians is do not give DHEA to women with PTSD. Allopregnanolone, when and if it becomes available, would be the neurosteroid of choice in this population.

206.10   Child abuse with resultant PTSD causes defects in hippocampal structure (smaller) and function (immediate recall).

234.4   Gabapentin inhibits high-threshold currents in cultured rat dorsal ganglia neurons.

234.6   This effect was significantly reduced in the presence of nifedipine. Unfortunately, in live neurosomatic patients (in vivo), response to dihydropyridine Ca^{2+}-channel blockers does not predict a lack of response to Neurontin more than slightly. The lesson here is not to give a trial of Nimotop (the most potent CNS Ca^{2+}-channel blocker) and Neurontin on the same day. GBP inhibited the $[Ca^{2+}]_i$ increase in response to K^+ and decreased release of neurotransmitters. This effect was eliminated by omega-agatoxin, which blocks P/Q voltage-gated Ca^{2+} channels, and by an AMPA antagonist. The only AMPA antagonist clinically available is topiramate (Topamax), which combines quite nicely with Neurontin in the few patients who take both medications. GBP, L-lysine, and L-arginine have also been found to open K_{ATP} channels (Kontos HA, Wei EP, 1998). So has galanin, a neuropeptide widely distributed in the brain. It is regarded as an endogenous anticonvulsant (Mazarati A et al., 2001), is analgesic, anxiolytic, and affects feeding and sexual behavior. Galanin is intimately involved in sleep onset and maintenance through its actions at the ventrolateral preoptic area (VLPO) and the surrounding area (extended VLPO) (Saper CB et al., 2001). A synthetic peptide named galnon, a derivative of warfarin, penetrates the blood-brain barrier, which galanin does not do very well. It is also protease resistant.

234.18 I alkalinize some patients with citrate (Polycitra-K). Alkalinization should block the effects of baclofen, a very useful agent, or somatostatin, which I have extensively discussed in previous books and has never helped one patient. I am sure I have tried it on at least fifty. Alkalinization enhances the function of N-type Ca^{2+} channels, the most important for regulating transmitter release.

236.4 One of the problems with prescribing estrogen or progesterone for neurosomatic patients is that their responses are so unpredictable. For example, I would usually expect progesterone and its metabolites to cause sedation, anxiolysis, or depression, if there were any resultant behavioral state after administering it. Progesterone can increase $alpha_4$ $GABA_A$ receptor subunit levels. Receptors with $alpha_4$ subunits produce anxiety that is insensitive to BZDs.

237.7 Occasionally, a patient has a very good response to topiramate (Topamax). Usually I attribute this effect to AMPA receptor antagonism, and adverse reactions to topiramate are often reversible by piracetam, which includes AMPA agonism among its various properties. What I did not suspect was that if a patient had $GABA_A$ receptors with $alpha_4$-$beta_3$-$gamma_2$ subunits, the patient would be particularly sensitive to their activation by topiramate.

243.3 Clonidine is underused as an analgesic. It binds to the mu-opioid receptor, and its analgesic effects are reversed by naloxone. If a patient is able to tolerate clonidine, the patient can reduce the dose of most opioids or ketamine by almost half. If a patient has ADRs to ketamine, they can often be prevented by coadministration of clonidine (or a BZD). Clonidine is an alpha$_{2ABC}$ agonist. The alpha$_{2BC}$ binding sites also bind to the delta-opioid receptor and are additionally analgesic via delta-opioid agonism.

243.4   The ACC is involved in the affective component of pain. Increasing dopaminergic input to the ACC by electrically stimulating the VTA can inhibit 73 percent of the ACC neurons. Lesioning the ACC per se does not cause analgesia, but stimulation of the upper cervical spine at C1 and C2 should be helpful in treating neurosomatic disorders. How to accomplish such stimulation is problematic. I have wondered whether appropriate chiropractic manipulation might be of value, but an external resonance device would be vastly more precise. There are case reports of complete relief of trigeminal neuralgia, probably involving Vc, by manipulations of the upper cervical spine, often injured in "whiplash." Cervical whiplash injury is sometimes associated with new onset obstructive sleep apnea (OSA). Some of my patients have had complete resolution of this sort of sleep apnea with intermittent intravenous lidocaine infusion.

Alterations in late exteroceptive suppression (ES2), an electromyogram (EMG) finding, are found in the 80 percent of individuals who suffer acute posttraumatic headache after whiplash injury. This discovery was made while investigating the antinociceptive inhibitory temporalis reflex. Shortening of the duration of the ES2 of this inhibitory trigemino-trigeminal reflex was thought to represent a decrease in descending nociceptive inhibitory control (DNIC) (Keidel M et al., 2001). Among 82 patients studied with a matched control group of 82 volunteers, higher pain was related to a shorter ES2. The authors hypothesize that there is a "facilitation of the trigeminal motor nucleus by the activation of the lateral reticular system," as a consequence of group III and IV afferent nociceptive fiber transmission after cervical trauma. They speculate that ES2 shortening could be used as a biologic marker for posttraumatic headache.

247.6   Proglumide, a CCK antagonist, prevents and reverses tolerance to opioids injected into the PAG. It is the CCK$_B$ receptor that is probably blocked.

247.9   Natriuretic peptide is anxiolytic in CCK$_B$-induced panic attacks. A deficiency of natriuretic peptide may be related to neurosomatic idiopathic cyclic edema (Wiedemann K et al., 2001). Natriuretic peptide type-B (NP-B) is produced in the brain as well as in the cardiac atria. Its mode of action may be the inhibition of CRH. I have been waiting to prescribe this agent for fifteen years. It is now available. Called "nesiritide," a synthetic recombinant human B-type natriuretic peptide, it can be infused in cases of congestive heart failure, which can be diagnosed by elevated levels of NP-B (Baughman KL, 2002). The only CCK antagonist that can be purchased is gotu kola, as a nutraceutical. So far, I am not impressed with its efficacy.

247.12 Catechol-orthomethyl transferase (COMT) inhibitors such as tolcapone (Tasmar) attenuate spontaneous activity of wide-dynamic range neurons in the spinal cord dorsal horns. Tolcapone does not affect descending pain regulation from the rostral ventrolateral medulla (RVLM), which I discussed in *Limbic Hypothesis.*

271.3 There is distinct functional glutamatergic regulation of the meso-accumbens and mesocortical dopamine neurons. Projections from the VTA to the PFC are tonically excited by AMPA receptors, while those from the VTA to the NAc are tonically inhibited.

294 Learning is enhanced by stressful experiences in male rats but is impaired in females. This difference is associated with estrogen-mediated increases in the density of dendritic spines in the hippocampus.

338.14 Nicotine induces NE release in the cortex. Its site of action is presynaptic, and its secretion is enhanced by opening N-type Ca^{2+} channels. NE transporter blockers, such as desipramine and reboxetine, inhibit nicotinic NE release.

340.9 Lysine attenuates neural activity in the CNS and may be a glutamate-receptor blocker.

350.3 The spinal antiallodynic action of $alpha_2$ agonists acts via the $alpha_{2A}$ subtype.

350.4 Imidazoline agonists, such as dextomodine and possibly clonidine, are also analgesic.

350.8 $Alpha_{1A}$ noradrenergic agonists, such as midodrine (ProAmatine), are proalgesic.

355.5 Acid pH increases CGRP release from V_1 during migraine headache. Perhaps alkalinization could be used in migraine prophylaxis.

356.11 NGF up-regulates bradykinin B2 receptors in nociceptive neurons. If Kutapressin is a BK antagonist, it may have an antinociceptive action in FMS.

364.6 Stressed subjects show increased false memories (see Conclusion to Chapter 11). There may be overlap of memories for percieved and imagined events (Gonsalves B, Paller KA, 2002).

370.5 $5\text{-}HT_{1B}$ agonists may cause hypophagia.

370.6   AMPA-induced feeding is partially mediated by AMPA receptors in the lateral hypothalamus. Topiramate probably causes weight loss by inhibiting these receptors.

370.8   Gastric satiety activates vagal neurons that enter the brainstem. Ninety percent of these neurons have NMDA receptors, and 40 percent of them have AMPA receptors.

370.16   Adenosine induces anorexia. I have not observed this response in patients taking the adenosine reuptake inhibitor dipyridamole, or using adenosine nasal spray on a chronic basis.

373.8   Oxytocin knock-out mice fail to recognize other mice they have repeatedly encountered and with whom they should be familiar. OXT-mediated affiliation causes activation (c-fos) in the medial amygdala. This area transduces socially relevant olfactory stimuli. OXT knock-out mice activate several other regions of the brain compared to controls, apparently in an attempt to compensate for lack of medial amygdala function.

373.15   Evidence suggests that GBP modulates glutamatergic activity. TRH is sometimes a cotransmitter in glutamate neurons. The bottom line of a complicated experiment is that GBP tended to increase TRH in most brain regions examined. This result is somewhat surprising to me, since GBP is usually anxiolytic, and TRH is a BZD antagonist. Response to GBP is not particularly correlated to response to TRH in my patient population.

         Gu and Huang (2001) find that Neurontin works by being a glycine/NMDA antagonist, perhaps allosterically, and is not active until PKC levels are elevated so that the NMDA receptor is phosphorylated. Thus, Neurontin would only be effective on activated cells. Cycloserine sometimes antagonizes Neurontin, which does not always synergize with, or even substitute for, other glycine-site antagonists, e.g., ondansetron, diltiazem, guaifenesin, verapamil, nimodipine, felbamate, and, indirectly, probenecid. The abstract says nothing about effects on the K_{ATP} channel.

374.2   NMDA antagonists prevent tolerance to other dependence-inducing substances such as opioids, amphetamines, and nicotine. I have occasionally noted ketamine to have this effect on my patients.

374.6 D_2/D_3 agonists produce obsessive-compulsive disorder (OCD)-like behavior in animals that is significantly attenuated by nicotine. Have we not been using nicotine patches for OCD and Tourette's for about ten years?

374.9   Alcohol-induced aggression in mice is inhibited by a 5-HT_{1B} agonist.

387.2 Induction of CREB is a common action of antidepressants. Transporting CREB to the neuronal nucleus with a viral vector has an antidepressant effect in and of itself. Often forskolin with one or two other cAMP-inducing agents has an antidepressant effect. It may increase energy and alertness even in patients who are not depressed.

387.3 Direct infusion of BDNF and neurotrophin-3 (NT-3) into the hippocampus has an antidepressant effect.

387.5 TRH is increased by ECT. It is increased in the hippocampus (only) by the antidepressant desipramine.

433.12 Stress, by amplifying noradrenergic activation in the central amygdala, recruits local galanin release, which is anxiolytic in this situation. I have been waiting for years to see a practical use for galanin, and suddenly there is an abundance (see 234.6).

435.16 Pentazocine (Talwin) may potentiate the effect of bradykinin in producing Ca^{2+} efflux via the IP_3 receptor. Pentazocine plus enalapril hasn't worked so far. ACE inhibitors produce vasodilation by releasing BK.

435.17 Haloperidol and pentazocine are both sigma-receptor ligands. Neurosteroids, perhaps progesterone, have been proposed to be endogenous ligands at these receptors. I have never been able to detect any similarity in patient response to haloperidol and pentazocine. Haloperidol is a sigma antagonist, pentazocine an agonist.

436.18 Forskolin stimulates the activity of tyrosine hydroxylase. NMDA and quinpirole, a D_2/D_3 agonist, reduce the forskolin enhancement of TH activity, probably by feedback inhibition. Patients who respond to stimulants, other cAMP-increasing agents, and phosphodiesterase inhibitors often respond quite robustly to forskolin augmentation.

453.8 K_{ATP} channel openers such as GBP, morphine, clonidine, and minoxidil are antinociceptive. I have tried minoxidil gel and oral tablets numerous times with neurosomatic patients and have seen an excellent response in most of those who respond to GBP; sometimes the benefit exceeds that of GBP (see further discussion of this under Gabapentin in Chapter 11).

454.10 Baclofen, a $GABA_B$ agonist, inhibits substance P and calcitonin gene-related peptide.

468.12 The cAMP phosphodiesterase (PDE4) inhibitor rolipram reverses memory impairment caused by NMDA antagonists and subsequently activates the Ras/MEK/ERK signaling cascade.

501.12 Prolonged eating of sugar causes naloxone-precipitated withdrawal symptoms in rats.

502.11 A major drawback to using atypical neuroleptics is weight gain. Patients taking these drugs display more insulin resistance and increased beta-endorphin levels. These findings suggest the use of a drug to improve insulin sensitivity (metformin) or opioid antagonists (naltrexone, NTX). Ziprasidone (Geodon) does not cause weight gain. H_2 antagonists may prevent olanzapine-induced weight gain.

511.8   Troglitazone, and perhaps other members of its family, enhances motoneuron survival and could be a treatment for ALS.

511.13 IGF-1 mediates exercise-induced neurogenesis in the hippocampus. I would ask my doctor to prescribe its inducer, growth hormone, for me after appropriate testing, but I cannot afford it. Some of my friends who take growth hormone regularly report quite a salubrious effect. Growth hormone may have several adverse reactions, however.

511.17 GDNF increases somatostatin release manyfold. Unfortunately, giving SS to neurosomatic patients does not help any of them, and since it decreases GH secretion, it might even be harmful.

511.18 It might be less expensive to take IGF-1 nasal spray, which enters the brain through the trigeminal nerve and the olfactory bulb, like a few of my nasal sprays do. It is being investigated by Chiron Corporation in Emeryville, California.

516.5   Kynurenic acid, increased by probenecid, blocks alpha$_7$ homomeric nicotine receptors in rat hippocampal neurons in culture. Most NMDA antagonists may work in those who have adverse responses to a nicotine patch, even if they also have an adverse reaction to the nicotine antagonist mecamylamine.

524.8   Nicotine receptors on VTA DA neurons desensitize in seconds, yet people keep smoking. Presynaptic nAchRs are located on the NMDAR and alpha$_7$ nAchRs. Nicotine is thought to cause long-term potentiation (LTP), which maintains the addiction.

525.3   If a patient cannot afford the glutamate secretion inhibitor riluzole (Rilutek), the physician should see whether the muscle relaxant chlorzoxazone (Parafon Forte) works. They both open small conductance calcium-activated K^+ channels of the SK2 type in a Ca^{2+}-independent manner.

526.6   A patient who has an adverse drug reaction to a nicotine patch that exacerbates his or her neurosomatic symptoms should remove the patch and try mecamylamine, which blocks all nAchRs except those containing the alpha$_7$ subunit. If the patient is still not improved, the physician should give probenecid, which increases kynurenate levels. Kynurenate, besides blocking the glycine coagonist site of the NMDA receptor, blocks $alpha_7$-containing nAchRs.

526.11 Tacrine (Cognex) blocks nAchRs.

526.12 Galantamine (Reminyl) is a cholinesterase inhibitor that stimulates nAchRs (Figure 1). Galantamine appears to be the cholinergic agent of choice in neurosomatic patients. Nefiracetam, a congener of piracetam, potentiates neuronal nAchRs by G_s (stimulatory guanine nucleotide) stimulation.

Nefiracetam potentiates nAchRs by a mechanism independent of PKA and PKC. Nootropics generally increase Ach and GABA, are agonists at AMPA receptors, and are antagonists at the NMDA/ glycine site. This latter property is shared by igmesine, diltiazem, verapamil, guaifenesin, probenecid (indirectly), atropine, felbamate, pentazocine, and gabapentin.

526.14 Because the actions of ethanol (EtOH) in the brain are so complex, I have not been able to understand why most neurosomatic patients tolerate alcohol so poorly unless DA depletion is involved. Selective $alpha_7$ nicotine-receptor agonists protect against EtOH-induced cytotoxicity. A critical mitochondrial enzyme is cytochrome C, and this enzyme is released by toxic doses of EtOH. If some neurosomatic patients have decreased levels of $alpha_7$ subunits or cytochrome C, they may be exquisitely sensitive to symptomatic exacerbation by EtOH.

528.20 AMPA-receptor potentiators improve age- and alprazolam-related cognitive deficits. The AMPA agonist available to me is piracetam; it is made of "natural" substances and thus may be legally compounded.

529.7 We badly need mGluR agonists and antagonists. Group II mGluRs (2 and 3) decrease presynaptic excitatory neurotransmission, perhaps by direct inhibition of VSCCs. KC1 (potassium chloride) induces GABA release in cortical neurons. GABA release can be inhibited by the EAA NAAG. NAAG's effect on GABA release is inhibited by pretreatment with forskolin, suggesting that NAAG achieves its effect by decreasing presynaptic cAMP. L-type dihydropyridine Ca^{2+}-channel blockers also inhibit KC1-evoked GABA release. NAAG's effect is blocked by PKA inhibitors. To sum up, the inhibition of KC1-stimulated GABA release by NAAG is mediated via presynaptic mGluR3 on cortical neurons. This effect is obtained by decreasing cAMP with a consequent decrease in PKA activity and L-type Ca^{2+}-channel conductance.

NAAG is a selective mGluR3 agonist and inhibits the release of GABA that is induced by KC1 in rat cortical neurons. NAAG decreases cAMP with resultant decrease in PKA and L-type Ca^{2+}-channel activation. *N*-acetyl-aspartate concentrations in the anterior cingulate are decreased in maltreated children and adolescents with PTSD, suggestive of neuronal loss, as measured by magnetic resonance spectroscopy (DeBellis MD et al., 2000). I found no abnormalities in MRS of over 30 CFS patients with and without fibromyalgia, again suggesting these patients do not develop neuronal atrophy. Perhaps their hyperglutamatergic state does not reach excitotoxicity. They certainly do not have hypercortisolemia, another cause of neuronal (hippocampal) atrophy seen in major depressive disorder (MDD).

531.12 Activation of D_2 receptors depolarizes rat dorsal raphe serotonin neurons.

538.4 Histamine H_3-receptor activation inhibits glutamate release in corticostriatal projections.

540.6 Both oxytocin and NE synergize with GnRH to produce the preovulatory GnRH and luteinizing hormone (LH) surge. TGF-beta$_1$ decreases levels of GnRH by 28 percent, an example of how this cytokine may be involved in neurosomatic disorders. Neurokinin-B, however, increases LH by 25 percent.

540.7 TGF-beta$_1$ decreases GnRH. GnRH is found in most sympathetic ganglia, and GnRH analogs (Synarel, Lupron) are often beneficial in neurosomatic disorders. GnRH does not just ameliorate PMS, PMDD, or LLPDD but probably regulates autonomic function. Conceivably, excess TGF-beta could cause dysautonomia.

544.16 Taurine is a GABA-like amino acid that has a tonic inhibitory effect on vasopressin release from the supraoptic nucleus (SON) in the posterior hypothalamus. Taurine stimulates glycine release, which hyperpolarizes surrounding neurons. None of my patients thus far have reported any effect from taurine. I'm adding it now to lamotrigine.

549.15 The thalamic reticular nucleus (TRN) acts as an attentional gate and is activated during selective attention. The type of attended stimulus, e.g., light or sound, activates the section of the TRN associated with its perception.

563.10 Pregnenolone sulfate, a neurosteroid, is a negative allosteric modulator of the $GABA_A$ receptor. Because gabergic neurons tonically inhibit Ach secretion, pregnenolone has a cholinergic effect.

566.8 Some find fish oil to be helpful in neurosomatic disorders. Fish oil contains omega-3 and omega-6 essential fatty acids that are eventually converted into PGE_1 and PGE_2 (prostaglandin E_1 and E_2). Application of PGE_2 to the tuberomamillary nuclei increases wakefulness via enhancing histamine secretion, as does modafinil. In general, PGE_1 elevation, because of its noradrenergic modulation, would be preferable. Omega-3 fatty acids may act as membrane stabilizers. They inhibit PKC, PKA, MAPK, and calcium/calmodulin kinase II (CaMKII). They disrupt LTP, often a valuable property in neurosomatic disorders (there's too much of it).

566.19 Calcitonin causes a depression-like syndrome in rats. In humans, it may improve Raynaud's disease by its vasodilatory properties.

566.31 NMDA-receptor antagonists can attenuate phase-resetting effects of light and dark in hamsters by the suprachiasmatic nucleus (SCN). They certainly do not alter circadian rhythms in my patients who may have an undue influence from PFC circadian oscillators.

659.11 From what my patients tell me, zopiclone is the best sleeping pill. It is related to zolpidem (very good) and zaleplon (poor) but has a longer half-life than zolpidem. The demethylated form of zopiclone has anxiolytic properties. Some patients find low-dose zolpidem to be activating. One patient took zolpidem "to remove my mind from stress." She eventually was hospitalized for zolpidem addiction. Withdrawal seizures have been reported. (Further discussion of zolpidem can be found in Chapter 11.)

684.12 The jury is still out on whether ketamine increases striatal DA. I have read numerous experiments showing an increase or no effect.

717.15 PKC activation induces tyrosine phosphorylation of NR2A and NR2B (subunits of the NMDA receptor) by nonreceptor tyrosine kinases. One way to avoid contracting a neurosomatic disorder is to stay away from tung oil. Tung oil is a phorbol ester found in sealers that activates PKC. Too much $alpha_1$ noradrenergic receptor activation during stress can activate PKC via a G-protein-coupled mechanism. Decreasing the activation of one or more types of PKC should be therapeutic in neurosomatic disorders (Senior K, 2002).

761.14 Oxytocin knock-out mice behave similarly to controls.

761.17 Once in a while, patients will feel symptomatically improved after taking an ACE inhibitor or an AII antagonist. Lactate can induce panic attacks in panic-prone patients. Angiotensin II, when infused into the dorsomedial hypothalamus, has very similar effects. Injecting the $GABA_A$ agonist muscimol into the DMH blocks both lactate- and AII-induced panic attacks. It has recently been discovered that ACE inhibitors do not lower blood pressure by ACE inhibition and that AII blockade does not do so, either. As far as I know, their antihypertensive mode of action is unknown at present. An efferent projection of the DMH is the BST, which also transduces events occurring in the MPOA, an area of major importance in neurosomatic disorders.

783.9 Down-regulation of the mu-opioid receptor by agonist stimulation occurs via activation of the Src tyrosine kinase family and can be prevented by genistein.

802.1 GBP is a K_{ATP} channel opener and is one of the most effective neurosomatic treatments. The K_{ATP} channels consist of Kir6.1 and Kir6.2 subunits in combination with sulfonylurea receptor isoforms (SUR1, SUR2A, and SUR2B). DA neurons in the substantia nigra have K_{ATP} channels. These channels are octamers consisting of four pore-forming units (Kir6.1 and Kir6.2) and four copies of an SUR protein. K_{ATP} channels are also present on glial cells. Channel opening is inhibited when ATP is increased; channel function is regulated in part by metabolism, and the K_{ATP} channels are considered to be direct functional response elements to the metabolic state of a neuron. They are blocked by sulfonylureas, which I have found to be beneficial in some patients with primary disorders of vigilance. Kir6.1 immunoreactivity is found in only glial cells, while Kir6.2 is restricted to neurons. Kir channels are regulated by polyamines, ATP, and H^+. SUR1 switches K_{ATP} on or off, depending upon the concomitant binding of ATP and ADP. An increase in the ATP/ADP ratio closes the channel, which leads to the opening of the voltage-sensitive calcium channels, a result of neuronal depolarization.

806.5 D_1 receptors do not inhibit NMDA function; they are up-regulated by NMDA activation. D_2 receptors activate a platelet-derived growth factor receptor (PDGFR) $\rightarrow$ PLC gamma $\rightarrow$ PKC/Ca^{2+}-calmodulin signaling system that depresses NMDA activity. Thus, D_2 agonists which could access the mesocortical DA system reliably, should be beneficial in my patients. Unfortunately, none are available to me.

806.6 Zinc can block NMDA receptors acutely and can also induce a Src family-mediated (tyrosine kinase) up-regulation of NMDA-receptor function.

806.7 Postsynaptic density 95 (PSD-95) not only anchors NMDARs to the cytoskeleton but also couples them to intracellular signaling pathways. PSD-95 increases channel open time, thereby reducing PKC potentiation of NMDARs.

806.8 There are insulin receptors in the CNS.

806.10- They stimulate NMDA-induced activity to three times their basal
806.11 rate by recruitment of new NMDA-channel molecules to the cell surface, a property that PKC and mGluR1 also exhibit.

806.17 All NMDA site-specific receptor antagonists slow colonic transit time.

807.4 Many CRH_1-receptor antagonists have been developed as potential treatments for anxiety, depression, stress-related disorders, and HPA dysfunction. Thus far, they all have too many adverse reactions to warrant large Phase III trials (as far as I know). CRH_2 receptors are found primarily in the lateral septal area and could be useful for illness localized to this region. Stress-induced sleep disorders can be treated with CRH_1 antagonists. An open-label trial of the CRH_1 antagonist R121919 was performed on 22 inpatients with major depressive disorder. It was well tolerated, and the fall in depression score was correlated with increasing dose. Vagal nerve stimulation antagonizes PFC CRH.

808.8 NK-1/SP antagonists have broad antiemetic activity in the area postrema and the nucleus of the solitary tract (NTS).

809.13 Prochlorperazine (Compazine) alleviates headaches through a central amplification of muscarinic transmission induced by the block of the D_2 heteroreceptor located on cholinergic neurons.

809.14 As I discussed in *Betrayal,* selective lesions of striatal neurons cause hypoalgesia, probably mediated by D_2 mechanisms.

812.11 Cannabinoid tolerance is blocked by NMDA-receptor antagonists.

813.5 Topical cannabinoids reduce cornea-evoked V_2 activity. Cannabinoids suppress central sensitization, a mechanism for chronic inflammatory pain. The endogenous cannabinoid anandamide is metabolized by fatty acid amidohydrolase. The action of the enzyme is blocked by nonsteroidal anti-inflammatory drugs (NSAIDs). If NSAIDs are effective in a neurosomatic patient, they may act by this mechanism.

814.6 The CB_1 receptor modulates release of various neurotransmitters in multiple brain areas. CB_1 activation presynaptically inhibits the release of glutamate. Cannabinoids and baclofen have many of the same properties. Cannabinoids can be reversed by naratriptan (Amerge) and verapamil. Because cannabinoids inhibit adenyl cyclase, drugs that stimulate this enzyme (such as forskolin) might antagonize its effects. The $5\text{-HT}_{1B/1D}$ receptors are inhibitory. Cannabinoids increase serotonin and may be blocked by serotonin antagonists.

815.4 Cannabinoids inhibit capsaicin-sensitive primary sensory neurons at the CB_1 receptor, decreasing the release of SP and CGRP.

815.8 One mechanism by which cannabinoids may produce anxiety is that presynaptic CB_1 receptors reduce $GABA_A$- but not $GABA_B$- induced synaptic inhibition by inhibiting VSCCs located on hippocampal CA1 (cornu ammonis) pyramidal neurons. Delta-9-tetrahydrocannabinol (Marinol) is the most active ingredient of the 60 or so psychoactive compounds in marijuana. THC, similar to other possible drugs of abuse, increases brain DA and NE. DA increase produced by THC does not occur by increasing firing rate of DA neurons in the VTA, but rather (probably) those in the NAc (Gifford AN et al., 1997). The D_1 to D_2 ratio is also important. Because the D_1 receptor is stimulatory, overexpression of it would more likely lead to a paranoid response. THC also increases endogenous opioids with chronic use by increasing the expression of the pro-opiomelanocortin gene in the arcuate nucleus of the hypothalamus. THC itself inhibits binding of mu- and delta-, but not kappa-, opioid agonists. THC-induced analgesia is reversed, causing withdrawal, if naloxone is administered (Corchero J et al., 1998).

In the arcuate nucleus of the hypothalamus, POMC is primarily processed into beta-endorphin. As might be expected, therefore, THC-induced analgesia is potentiated by mu- and, somewhat unexpectedly (but not really), kappa-opioid receptors. Kappa receptors potentiate mu receptors. THC activates spinal dynorphin, an NMDA agonist and mu-opioid antagonist. Antiserum against dynorphin prevents THC-induced analgesia according to this experiment. When I think of the effects of dynorphin, dysphoria is the first that comes to mind. Perhaps this reaction is unjustified.

816.7	The histamine H_3 receptor is primarily an autoreceptor that increases histamine levels when a substance such as the H_3 antagonist thioperamide is applied. Thioperamide results in increased excitation, increased monoaminergic transmission, and decreased forskolin-stimulated cAMP accumulation.

816.13	A complete blockade of histamine in the DRN requires both H_1- and H_2-receptor antagonists. It is a good idea to prescribe both in a treatment-refractory patient with nasal allergy.

816.21	Sigma$_1$ receptors are unique 223 amino-acid proteins that mediate beneficial neuromodulatory effects on memory, stress, or depression.

816.22	Sigma$_1$ proteins localize around mitochondria and the endoplasmic reticulum. Sigma-1 receptor expression does not change between ligands, including (+)pentazocine (Talwin), haloperidol, sertraline (Zoloft), progesterone, and DHEA. Chronic treatment with (+)pentazocine has an antidepressant effect and increases 5-HT secretion from the DRN by 40 percent.

819.1	Electroconvulsive therapy is extremely effective in treating depression but not particularly helpful in neurosomatic disorders. When neurosomatic patients undergo ECT, it is typical to see depression respond for six to 12 months but fatigue and pain for only a week or two. Retrograde and anterograde amnesia occur for two months or so. This memory loss usually resolves but occasionally never does. The best work on the mechanism of action of ECT has ben done by Harold Sackheim's group, and I discussed it in *Betrayal*. Levels of 5-HT transporters reliably decrease after ECT, and this transporter decrease is thought to be related to the antidepressant effect of ECT in a manner not explained in this abstract. Cerebral blood flow decreases as it does after antidepressant therapy and every successful neurosomatic treatment, even with a vasodilator. I have attempted to explain this phenomenon in *Betrayal* and in this book (DA as a vasoconstrictor with NE, or decrease in nNOS because of NMDA antagonism). Repetitive transcranial magnetic stimulation is not a total failure in my practice. It completely resolved the fibromyalgia pain of one of my patients but affected no other symptoms. ECT decreases serotonin-transporter mRNA expression in rat raphe nucleus.

820.1 Cyclic adenosine diphosphate ribose (cADPR) may be an endogenous agonist that stimulates release of Ca^{2+} from ryanodine channel-sensitive stores. NO is needed to synthesize and activate cADPR. The release of Ca^{2+} by cADPR is inhibited by the L-type dihydropyridine Ca^{2+}-channel blocker nimodipine. It does not seem to be generally appreciated that nimodipine can inhibit intracellular Ca^{2+} release, but it may antagonize agents that increase $[Ca^{2+}]_i$ such as TRH, DDAVP, and oxytocin.

821.5 Adenosine is analgesic in many of my patients, as well as being anxiolytic, in the form of a nasal spray. Often, but not always, this response indicates that the patient will respond to an adenosine-reuptake inhibitor, such as dipyridamole. This agent may inhibit glutamatergic synaptic transmission by modulating the nucleoside transporter rENT1 from the rat, for which dipyridamole is a selective inhibitor, acting through the adenosine A_1 receptor. I have been using dipyridamole in this manner for many years, and I marvel that no other physicians do. I asked one of my academic colleagues why. "They don't know about it," he replied. Inhibition of adenosine uptake, as is done by dipyridamole, attenuates glutamatergic synaptic transmission in the rat spinal cord in vitro.

821.9 NAAG is a mixed agonist/antagonist at the NMDA receptor that is metabolized to *N*-acetyl-aspartate and glutamate by the enzyme NAALADase. Inhibitory spinal NAALADase may play a role in analgesia during the rat formalin test.

823.11 Kappa-opioid agonists work better in females. Oxycodone is a partial kappa-opioid agonist and the only one available. It synergizes with mu-opioid agonists.

823.14 Analgesic sensitivity has a hereditary basis. Responses in 12 inbred mouse strains were compared to the mu-opioid agonist morphine; the kappa-opioid agonist U50488; the nicotinic Ach agonist epibatidine; and the cannabinoid agonist WIN55, 212-2. Analgesic responses to each agent were highly intercorrelated and differed by as much as 27-fold. So when a patient says "I need a lot of painkillers, Doc," the patient may not always be engaging in drug-seeking behavior.

823.19 Emeran Mayer's group at UCLA is doing some of the best work on the pathophysiology of IBS. Neonatal separation of Long-Evans rats produces visceral hyperalgesia and somatic hypoalgesia following psychological stress. The visceral hyperalgesia (balloon distension of the colon) is worsened by naloxone administration, which does not affect control rats. One of my patients, an 18-year-old woman, came to me with visceral hyperalgesia to the point that she was homebound and had lost 20 pounds. She had been seen by a member of Mayer's UCLA group and was told nothing could be done for her until tegaserod was available. She had accepted a basketball scholarship to college but could not keep this commitment. Her life was going down the tubes, and total parenteral nutrition was in the offing. As do many patients, she had suicidal ideation but no plan or intent. Her depression existed because of her symptoms. IBS is usually not too difficult to treat, and she responded as patients usually do to a combination of medications, which did not include tegaserod, since it is just available at the time of this writing. Today she is going to college, has regained her weight, plays intramural basketball, and has an active social life. I ran into her UCLA doctor at a Lakers game. I forgot myself and began to tell her that her former patient was well and how I had treated her, hoping that she might want to learn new ways to manage IBS patients. But she began to look away and found someone else to whom she needed to speak. I never saw her again that afternoon. Physicians are increasingly being taught not to listen or read *any* "anecdotal" evidence. In my enthusiasm, I made the faux pas of trying to relate some. By the way, oral naloxone can be used in very low 0.5 to 3.0 mg doses to treat opioid-induced constipation. Although naloxone is not supposed to be absorbed through the gastrointestinal (GI) tract, too high of a dose will cause withdrawal symptoms. Ondansetron (Zofran) is the closest medication to tegaserod and works fairly well for IBS. Emeran Mayer's group reports on stress-induced visceral hypoalgesia that activates endogenous opioid systems. This activation is compromised in adults who were separated from their mothers as infants.

824.2 Intravenous lidocaine and IV ketamine are almost never used in hospitals for analgesia. The situation is similar to 25 years ago when I tried to introduce patient-controlled analgesia with morphine. NMDA receptor antagonists attenuate pain behavior in an experimental pancreatitis model in rats. Pancreatitis pain is notoriously difficult to treat.

Because I am talking about hospitals, I may as well discuss surgical anesthesia in the neurosomatic patient. The first rule is to always use preemptive analgesia, of which there are several types. The brain is still receiving pain signals even though the patient is asleep. Neurosomatic patients, particularly those with hyperalgesia, will still widen their receptive fields and be sensitized to nociceptive input while anesthetized. I always suggest isoflurane, because it has a rapid emergence time and inhibits synaptic vesicle release by enhancing the action of synaptotagmin with syntaxin, thus reducing the exocytic soluble *N*-sensitive factor attachment protein receptor (SNARE) complex.

Neurotransmitters are secreted by fusion of transmitter-filled vesicles with the presynaptic membrane. This is a tightly regulated process. One of the last steps is the formation of the SNARE complex. The SNARE proteins include some I have mentioned: synaptobrevin, syntaxin, and synaptosomal-associated protein 25 (SNAP-25). Formation of the SNARE complex is an absolute requirement for vesicle fusion (Bajjalieh S, 2001). SNARE has been found to be formed in stages, and each stage can be regulated separately.

Isoflurane has occasionally caused remissions in neurosomatic symptomatology and has been used in treatment-refractory depression in Germany by G. Langer. Anesthetic emergence consumes vast amounts of NE and DA, and I believe prolonged emergence is associated with postsurgical neurosomatic relapse. An anesthetic cocktail that will be accepted by most anesthesiologists is (1) isoflurane or a related agent, (2) propofol, (3) ketamine, (4) fentanyl, and (5) midazolam. Ketamine and fentanyl may be used, along with local anesthetic infiltration, regional block, or nerve block, for preemptive analgesia. The latter may be done with cryotherapy in thoracic procedures. Propofol may produce prolonged remission, perhaps by resetting the $GABA_A$ receptors.

824.10 Ketamine blocks Na$^+$ and NMDA channels. Lidocaine blocks Na$^+$ channels without affecting NMDA channels (as I had previously thought it did). Uptake through vesicular monoamine transporters is Na$^+$-dependent and is blocked by lidocaine, increasing levels of DA, NE, and 5-HT. When NMDA-receptor activation triggers a postsynaptic action potential, dendritic spine sodium signals are greatly increased (Rose CR, Konnerth A, 2001b). The mode of action of systemic lidocaine remains poorly understood. In neuropathic pain, Na$^+$ channels cluster around the site of injury. I doubt this clustering occurs in neurosomatic pain, yet ketamine and lidocaine are numbers one and two as effective treatments for neurosomatic disorders. Ketamine increases glutamatergic transmission via non-NMDA receptors, AMPA, and kainate. Type II mGluRs decrease glutamate release. It has been suggested (I think with some merit) that decreased function of NMDA receptors produces decreased excitation of GABA receptors which decrease inhibition of excitatory neurotransmitters in the brain. Increased EAAs could then hyperstimulate corticolimbic areas, leading to symptoms of schizophrenia. Agents that inhibit glutamate release should then include Na$^+$-channel blockers, Ca^{2+}-channel blockers, K$^+$-decreasing agents, and Type II mGluRs. (For further discussion, see Chapter 11.)

824.17 NMDA antagonists are perhaps the most effective treatment for IBS pain, since glutamate is the primary afferent vagus neurotransmitter, and the NMDA receptor is densely expressed in the vagus nerve. Intravenous lidocaine is a close second. It was news to the neuroscience community, however, that the NMDA-receptor antagonist MK-801 inhibited the responses of both noxious or nonnoxious colonic distention (usually done with a balloon) at the level of the spinal cord. Maybe in five or ten years physicians will start treating patients with NMDA antagonists, but the patients must suffer until the appearance of evidence-based medicine. How scientifically rational and safe the treatment might be is apparently completely irrelevant.

827.2   Gonadotropin-releasing hormone modulates rodent chemosensory neuron responses to odors. This peptide has been underutilized in neurosomatic medicine. It is the best treatment for PMS, given either as an injection (leuprolide acetate, Lupron) or a nasal spray (nafarelin, Synarel). The injectable form is used as a treatment for endometriosis. GnRH is manufactured in the medial preoptic area of the hypothalamus, one of the most important sites for dysregulation in neurosomatic patients. The MPOA is just caudal to the suprachiasmatic nucleus, which controls circadian rhythms. One of the many functions of the MPOA is to secrete natriuretic peptide-B, a peptide that causes diuresis and excretion of Na$^+$. Deficient NP-B secretion may explain idiopathic cyclic edema in neurosomatic patients. NP-B may also be anxiolytic. (See Gonadotropin-Releasing Hormone in Chapter 11.)

827.5   GnRH is secreted in low concentrations in a chronic pulsatile fashion. Just prior to ovulation in women, the follicle secretes a large amount of 17-beta-estradiol that causes a massive secretion of luteinizing hormone from a pituitary primed by estrogen and GnRH during the follicular phase of the menstrual cycle. Transmitters that stimulate the GnRH surge include 5-HT, glutamate, NPY, and galanin. GnRH is inhibited by GABA, CRH, and endogenous opioids. NE stimulates the GnRH surge but inhibits its pulsatile secretion. GnRH analogs such as Lupron and Synarel down-regulate GnRH receptors and turn off gonadotropin secretion, so that less PKC and MAP kinase will be made in cells that express GnRH receptors. PKC and MAP kinase are increased by NMDA receptor activation. Receptors for GnRH are located in the hypothalamus, with their highest density in the MPOA and SCN, but are also numerous in the arcuate and ventromedial nuclei. The latter two nuclei secrete GnRH in a pulsatile manner in the basal state. The MPOA is responsible for the GnRH-LH "surge."

827.7   The nervus terminalis, a nerve containing GnRH in the nasal cavity, has been hypothesized to mediate olfaction. The nasal mucosa and vomeronasal organs of rodents express GnRH receptors. GnRH modulates the activity of this chemosensory neuron, usually inhibiting the response to odorant mixtures. GnRH analogs as nasal sprays are sometimes beneficial to patients with multiple chemical sensitivity. Fitting nicely into the emerging neurosomatic schema, sensory input from olfactory and vomeronasal chemoreceptors can activate neurons in the MPOA via pathways through the amygdala and BST. This activation is enhanced by intraventricular injections of GnRH, producing Fos expression in the medial MPOA. Another etiologic mechanism for MCS is NE depletion, which up-regulates NE receptors and lowers olfactory thresholds.

835.6   The BST projects to most areas involved with stress and is regulated, in part, by the MPOA. The primary function of the BST is to relay amygdala signals to the hypothalamus. Some BST fibers from the paraventricular nucleus of the hypothalamus terminate in the amygdala. The BST terminates in the preoptic area in the lateral hypothalamus. A hypothalamic structure that has input from the interfascicular nucleus of the BST is the dorsal pre-mammillary nucleus (PMd) in the posterior hypothalamus. It also receives projections from the VTA. The reason I mention the PMd is that it is involved in fear conditioning. I have searched in vain for some brain-imaging evidence of amygdala involvement (e.g., hypermetabolism) in neurosomatic disorders; such a finding would make the functional neuroanatomy much more comprehensible. The amygdala could contribute the hypervigilant template which the PFC could use to organize information (Drevets WC, 2001), although the PFC eventually transfers fear learning to other parts of the brain and deactivates. I do not know whether the PMd has this capacity, either singly or by recruiting other structures, but this finding opens up alternative possibilities, one of them being that the PMd is part of the BST relay into the "computer" composed of hypothalamic nuclei. Most hypothalamic nuclei communicate with one another.

846.22 Application of AMPA and SP to the SCN in vitro can produce phase shifts. Blocking Na^+ channels does not cause phase shifts, so lidocaine would not be an effective treatment for this disorder. Both SP and AMPA cause phase delays. SP antagonists or topiramate, which blocks AMPA receptors, could cause phase advance. I have not observed this treatment effect in my patients. (See also Dysregulation of Circadian Rhythms in Chapter 11.)

846.6 The dorsomedial hypothalamic nucleus (DMH) links the SCN and the LC. The LC has circadian rhythms to its NE secretion. The SCN→DMH→LC pathway is probably dysfunctional in neurosomatic disorders. In rats, tract-tracing studies have shown that the DMH is also connected to the rostral ventrolateral medulla (RVLM), the NTS, the pontine parabrachial nucleus (PPN), the hypothalamic PVN, ventromedial hypothalamus (VMH), and lateral hypothalamic area (LHA). The LHA secretes orexins, and its fibers also project to the LC. The VMH is massively innervated by amygdala CRH neurons. The PVN and VMH, as well as the DMH are part of a CNS noradrenergic circuit regulating food intake. The PVN receives NE projections from the NTS and RVLM, as well as from the LC. (See also Dysregulation of Circadian Rhythms in Chapter 11.)

852.10 Vagal nerve stimulation in rats increases parasympathetic tone and reduces anxiety-related behaviors.

852.15 Patients diagnosed with borderline personality disorder who have a history of childhood trauma, including loss, parental separation, and verbal, sexual, and physical abuse are thought to have a dysfunction of limbic structures and a lower threshold for autonomic reactivity. Kindling has been implicated in the pathophysiology, as measured by galvanic skin response (GSR) to viewing affectively laden pictures. Even a neuroscientific Carl Lewis would be hard-pressed to make the inductive leap from GSR to kindling.

854.3 The discriminative stimulus properties of amphetamine, as well as its locomotor and behavioral effects, can be enhanced by the beta-receptor antagonist propranolol.

854.18 MK-801, a noncompetitive NMDA antagonist, produces increased locomotor activity through the NAc in a DA-independent manner. Blocking the motor nuclei of the thalamus, ventroposterior ventromedial thalamus (VMT), and ventrolateral VMT inhibits this response.

854.19 Wasps, bees, and yellow jackets are Hymenoptera. Wasp venom blocks nicotinic receptors. Perhaps honey bee venom has this effect also.

855.2 The effect of amantadine and IV guaifenesin on IBS, for which there is no published effective treatment, is outstanding in my fairly wide experience and the limited experience of others. The hypervigilance shown by my IBS patients is usually generalized and does not include only visceral pain and other enteroceptive stimuli.

857.1 Activation of mGlu3R enhances de novo synthesis of TGF-beta$_1$ through the activation of the MAP kinase pathway and is neuroprotective against NMDA toxicity via a novel form of glial-neuronal interaction. Activation of mGluR2, 7, 8 may provide slight neuroprotection by other mechanisms.

857.12 Besides being cholesterol-lowering agents and immunosuppressants (Kwak B et al., 2000), the 3-hydroxy-3-methylglutaryl coenzyme A (HMGCoA) reductase inhibitor "statins" are protective against NMDA-mediated excitotoxicity. This effect occurs by reduction of NMDAR current. Simvastatin is the most potent of the statins in this regard. More will be published in the near future of serious immunosuppressive disorders linked to statin therapy. Statin variants may be used as ketamine-like drugs and may have neurocognitive effects.

857.14 Ginkgo biloba is a glycine-site antagonist at the NMDA receptor.

866.4 A group from McMaster University in Ontario, Canada found TGF-beta to be lowered in both bipolar patients and those with major depressive disorders, as compared to controls. They used a cDNA expression array that included up to 2,400 genes involved in signal transduction, receptors, and neurotransmitters to obtain their result. My grant proposal to test about 50 of these genes was rejected by the NIH because I was unqualified to diagnose fibromyalgia.

867.5   Forskolin, which may be obtained from the Life Extension Foundation in Florida as a nutritional supplement, inhibits adenyl cyclase and increases cAMP. It has been quite helpful to certain patients who respond to other agents that increase cAMP, such as stimulants, and has had no side effects thus far in a 10 to 20 mg a day dose. While autopsying the brains of suicide victims, $beta_2$-stimulated adenyl cyclase did not raise cAMP, suggesting the uncoupling of the G_S subunit of the postreceptor G protein of the $beta_2$ noradrenergic receptor. Because pure beta-agonists help almost none of my patients, depressed or not, I wonder whether this mechanism applies to them.

867.15 Chronic psychosocial stress in rats increases HPA activity and decreases neurogenesis in the dentate gyrus. These effects are reversed by repetitive transcranial magnetic stimulation.

867.18 A 24-hour period of maternal deprivation on postnatal day nine produced behavioral deficits in a cohort of adult rats, behavioral deficits similar to schizophrenia in humans. If an animal model for schizophrenia exists, I cannot think of it right now.

867.19 The thalamic posterior intralaminar nucleus (PIN) is a mediator of fear-potentiated emotional startle in rats in addition to the amygdala and PMd. A method of testing potential antidepressants in rats is reduction of immobility time in the Porsolt swim test. Right-sided PIN radiofrequency lesions reduced immobility time. There was loss of fibers projecting to the temporal cortex and the medial geniculate body after the PIN lesion. The geniculohypothalamic tract originates in the lateral geniculate.

868.4   Rolipram, a selective PDE4 inhibitor, increases cAMP. Depression causes atrophy of some brain structures, especially the hippocampus, and this atrophy can be reversed by some antidepressants. Rolipram, by a cascade of intracellular events, phosphorylates the immediate early gene (IEG) CREB, and its subsequent products induce neurogenesis.

868.18 Add Talwin (pentazocine) to the list of medications that block the binding of the glycine antagonist dichlorokynurenic acid to native NMDA receptors in rat forebrain neurons—or, at least, the brother of Talwin, igmesine, which has not been marketed yet. Igmesine requires no more than a single dose to block the binding of dichlorokynurenic acid.

869.17 MDMA (3,4-methylenedioxy-n-methylamphetamine, "ecstasy") produces selective degeneration of 5-HT terminals in the forebrain of the rat. This toxicity can be prevented or attenuated by citalopram, ascorbic acid, or baclofen.

871.7　Sigma$_1$ agonists (such as Talwin) and 5-HT$_{1A}$ agonists (such as buspirone) synergize in their antidepressant effects. They probably have antipsychotic effects as well.

871.11　A$_1$-receptor agonists reverse the PCP-induced decrement in PPI (prepulse inhibition). PCP also disrupts attention, another effect that is prevented by an A$_1$-receptor agonist, which is being investigated for antipsychotic properties.

871.14　rTMS produces increases in CCK and BDNF mRNA, similar to those reported in antidepressant drug treatment and ECT, suggesting a common mode of antidepressant action. BDNF as monotherapy has antidepressant effects.

871.15　I had hoped that some constituents of St. John's wort, especially hypericin and hyperforin, would antagonize SP. Several studies show that they do, but a recent large double-blind study in *JAMA*, February 23, 2001, showed no benefit of St. John's wort over placebo. I have also given up on kava kava. Too many different adverse reactions have been reported in the past 18 months.

Part III:
Pathophysiology and Treatment

Chapter 10

Treatment of Neurosomatic Disorders

[William Harvey] had long hesitated to publish his conclusions, knowing the conservatism of the medical profession of his time. He predicted that no one over forty years of age would accept his theory. "I have heard him say," reported Aubrey, "that after his book of the *Circulation of the Blood* came out, he fell mightily in his practice, and 'twas believed by the vulgar that he was crack-brained."

Will Durant and Ariel Durant (1961)
The Age of Reason Begins

Aspects of attention-related processes include arousal (the general level of responsivity), orientation (the realignment of sensory organs), selective attention (the preference for some stimuli over others), sustained attention (vigilance), and divided attention (the simultaneous heeding of several events). Attention can be distributed globally or focally. It can act upon stimuli in parallel or serially. And it can be attracted exogenously by external events or directed endogenously by mental phenomena related to motivation and volition.

M.-Marsel Mesulam (2000)
Principles of Behavioral and Cognitive Neurology

ABECARNIL AND ACAMPROSATE

Abecarnil is a partial agonist at the benzodiazepine receptor. It is one of a group of agents called beta-carbolines and has been studied for some time. A partial agonist is on the anxiolytic end of the spectrum between a full agonist and a neutral antagonist, such as flumazenil. Abecarnil has a high affinity for benzodiazepine receptors, and it has side effects typical of benzodiazepine-like anxiolytics, i.e., dizziness, fatigue, and unsteady gait, appearing in a dose-related fashion. Abecarnil, like buspirone, does not work immediately but takes a week or so to have its effect. It does not work quite as well as alprazolam but is superior to placebo in the treatment of anxiety disorders, particularly by week two and certainly after week four, when it is almost equal in efficacy to alprazolam. Little or no physical dependence is found with abecarnil, which has minimal withdrawal symptoms after a rapid taper and exhibits continued residual therapeutic effects after discontinuation. Not all studies have found abecarnil equal in efficacy to alprazolam, but it does appear to be better than placebo. The use of abecarnil in the treatment of anxiety was reviewed in the *Journal of Clinical Psychiatry Monograph* 1997, Volume 58, Supplement 11. More recent studies suggest that abecarnil may ameliorate benzodiazepine withdrawal.

Acamprosate is an experimental agent that reduces craving for alcohol and is one of a number of similar agents that are in development. Acamprosate binds to the polyamine site of the NMDA receptor where it acts as an antagonist. Acamprosate is a derivative of the amino acid homotaurine. It modulates NMDA receptor function by an allosteric action at the polyamine site. Its modulation "seems to be altered by previous exposure to ethanol which enhances inhibitory effects of acamprosate on NMDA receptor function." It may also be an antagonist at taurine receptors causing an increase in intracellular calcium $[Ca^{2+}]_i$, which could be neurotoxic. Thus, acamprosate would be more effective in alcoholics than in alcohol-naive subjects.

A current review of acamprosate pharmacology is available (Cole JC et al., 2000). Acamprosate, however, is an experimental drug and is not available for clinical use at this time. Neither is a similarly acting drug, ifenprodil. Ifenprodil has the additional action of being a preferential noncompetitive NR1/NR2B receptor antagonist that markedly diminishes NMDA-receptor activation in rat mesencephalic neurons (Allgaier C et al., 1999). An agent with this particular type of receptor antagonism could be extremely valuable for the treatment of neurosomatic disorders. Its efficacy has been described anecdotally in a report from Japan (Masuda Y, 1999). Acamprosate is available in Europe, where it is used to reduce relapse in weaned alcoholics. Medications are available in the United States that have a similar mode of action, i.e., antagonists at the polyamine site of the NMDA receptor. These agents are nylidrin, 6 to 12 mg t.i.d. p.o. or compounded as a 1.2 percent concentration in PLO, and isoxsuprine. Both medications have beta-agonist properties as well as being polyamine-receptor antagonists. They are very effective agents, nylidrin a bit more so than isoxsuprine (Whittemore ER et al., 1997).

STIMULANTS

Adderall is a mixture of several types of amphetamines. It is marketed for use in ADHD. Adderall is the stimulant of choice for most neurosomatic patients. It has a fairly gradual onset of action, does not usually make patients jittery, and has a fairly slow drop-off in its activity so that patients do not "crash" when it wears off. Adderall was initially developed as an anorectic agent, and some authorities in ADHD still believe no difference exists between Adderall and other amphetamines, particularly dextroamphetamine, but my experience has been that Adderall is superior. Although ADHD is not a condition I usually list under neurosomatic disorders, a double-blind placebo-controlled study has shown Adderall to be better than methylphenidate (Ritalin) in the treatment of ADHD (Pliszka S et al., 2000).

Amphetamines may produce long-lasting behavioral and neurochemical changes in the CNS after even a single dose. Rats, when electrically stimulated in the nucleus accumbens, have an increased release of [^{3}H] dopamine from the NAc, caudate-putamen, and medial PFC, as well as increased [^{14}C] acetylcholine from accumbens and caudate. The HPA response to stimuli is permanently altered. Behavioral changes ("conceptual") are noted when the rats are placed in the environment in which the amphetamine is administered and there is cross-sensitization to cocaine (Louk JMJ et al., 1998).

Adderall works both by inhibition of dopamine reuptake and by increasing secretion of norepinephrine and dopamine. Inhibition of dopamine reuptake by blocking the plasma membrane dopamine transporter is the primary mechanism of action of methylphenidate (MPH, Ritalin) and cocaine. Inhibition of dopamine reuptake increases the extracellular and synaptic concentrations as well as the life span of dopamine which leads to prolonged stimulation of dopamine receptors. The dopamine transporter (DAT) is the defining molecule of the dopamine neuron. The action of the stimulants may be prolonged and sometimes enhanced by concomitantly prescribing niacinamide.

A vesicular monoamine transporter (VMAT2) is also responsible for reuptake of 5-HT, norepinephrine, epinephrine, and histamine in their respective neurons, which suggests that the selectivity of monoaminergic neurotransmission is determined by the plasma membrane transporters (Miller, GW et al., 1997). Both the DAT and the VMAT have clear roles in specific neuronal injury, but they may also be involved in more general pathological conditions. Research has been done to determine whether inhibiting VMAT2 might cause depression, but the results of this work are inconclusive thus far. Patients who chronically abuse methamphetamine and cocaine have a down-regulation of the dopamine transporter that is not necessarily correlated with neurotoxicity. Patients with ADHD react to amphetamines and similar drugs with a paradoxical calming activity. This effect also occurs in dopamine transporter knock-out mice.

The increase in synaptic dopamine caused by amphetamine is derived from the cytosol, while elevated DA is a result of enhanced vesicular release. Cocaine has a much higher affinity for the serotonin transporter, and increases 5-HT levels manyfold, while amphetamine raises 5-HT levels only slightly. Both D_1 and D_2 receptors are stimulatory. The D_1 component is G-protein-coupled to adenylate cyclase and PKA. Forskolin, a stimulator of adenylate cyclase, may augment the effect of amphetamines.

Chronic use of amphetamines causes reverse transport through the vesicular dopamine transporter. If the dopamine transporter is deficient, and perhaps to an extent under normal circumstances, DA levels are amplified by inhibition of the norepinephrine transporter (Spanagel R, Weiss F, 1999). DA increase is activated through alpha$_1$ receptors, which stimulate release of DA, as is also seen with the NE-reuptake inhibitor reboxetine. Amphetamines and reboxetine often synergize nicely. By increasing DA release, stimulants activate feedback mechanisms that inhibit DA cell firing. D-amphetamine has a stimulatory effect on these cells even when both D_1 and D_2 receptors are blocked, suggesting the stimulatory effect of D-amphetamine is not mediated by DA receptors. NE-reuptake blockers, such as reboxetine or nisoxetine, mimic the effect of D-amphetamine in vivo. Thus, D-amphetamine has two effects on DA cells, a DA-mediated inhibition and a non-DA-mediated excitation. The latter is mediated in part through alpha$_1$ adrenergic receptors (Shi WX et al., 2000). Despite this experimental finding in rats, the alpha$_1$ agonist midodrine does not substitute for psychostimulants in my patients.

Self-administration of stimulant compounds such as cocaine and amphetamine enhances monoaminergic neurotransmission (Figure 2). It appears that activated dopaminergic neurotransmission in the mesocorticolimbic system mediates the reinforcing effect of stimulants. The effect of serotonin is less clear in this regard. Norepinephrine neurotransmission does not appear to significantly modulate stimulant self-administration, even though stimulants enhance NE neurotransmission. However, cocaine self-administration increases dopamine and serotonin levels in the nucleus accumbens. Lidocaine enhances the stimulant effects of cocaine, although it is not a stimulant when used as monotherapy. Local anesthetics with vasoconstrictive properties, such as procaine, are more apt to have stimulant effects. Other areas of the brain that might be involved in the acute reinforcing effects of stimulants include the ventral pallidum, the amygdala, and the bed nucleus of the stria terminalis. Chronic cocaine use enhances CRH release in the amygdala, compared to saline-treated rats. Dopamine dependence produces a decrease in CRH receptors in mesolimbocortical brain structures, indicating that cocaine administration enhances CRH neurotransmission, which may lead to a compensatory down-regulation of CRH receptors. The effect of neuropeptide Y may oppose that of cocaine-stimulated CRH.

CRH antagonists, when injected into the amygdala, can attenuate some of the symptoms of morphine withdrawal (Heinrichs SC et al., 1995).

Only about 25 percent of neurosomatic patients will have a good reaction to stimulants. Otherwise, they will have no reaction at all, even to very high doses, or stimulants will not only surprisingly calm them but will paradoxically make them sleepy or exacerbate their symptoms in general. This response indicates an abnormality of the dopamine transporter or autoreceptor hypersensitivity and also suggests the use of an agent that will inhibit the secretion of catecholamines, such as guanfacine (Taylor FB, Russo J, 2001). Alpha$_1$ adrenergic-receptor antagonists have not been particularly useful in my patient population, but beta-receptor antagonists are occasionally helpful. Alpha$_1$ antagonists combined with antagonists of ATP (such as suramin), which is cosecreted from noradrenergic terminals, may be more effective (Park SK et al., 2000). My few trials of reserpine have had no effect.

Returning to use of stimulants, it appears that increasing DA is a major effect of both modafinil and D-amphetamine in wakefulness promotion and is independent of the Hcrt-2 receptor. The orexin, or Hcrt, receptor does increase DA-mediated behavior, however. Orexin-A induces an increase in $[Ca^{2+}]_i$ in isolated A10 (VTA) dopamine neurons in a dose-dependent manner. The VTA effects are blocked by D$_1$- or D$_2$-receptor antagonists (Nakamura T et al., 2000). DA transporter knock-out mice were unresponsive to modafinil or amphetamine (Wisor JP et al., 2001). It appears that modafinil stimulates the tuberomammillary nucleus (histamine) and the perifornical area (orexin, Hcrt). These are regions involved in wakefulness (Scammell TE et al., 2001). Modafinil also may have anti-Parkinsonian effects (Jenner P et al., 2000) and amplifies the electro-neurosecretory coupling mechanism not involving the reuptake process (Ferraro L et al., 2000). Modafinil increases NE and DA in the PFC by spectral EEG criteria (Sebban C et al., 1999) and increases cortical activation on fMRI (Ellis CM et al., 1999). Modafinil does not ameliorate ADHD, which is characterized by hypertrophic A10 dopamine neurons. More direct dopamine agonists must be administered to decrease the firing of these A10 neurons, which give rise to the mesocorticolimbic system (MCL). The MCL, not to be confused with the medial collateral ligament, innervates the frontal cortex, NAc, BST, and the amygdala complex (Viggiano D, Sadele AG, 2000).

Because modafinil is a new type of drug, a Hcrt/orexin agonist and possibly an H_3 antagonist, we should consider it in more detail. The SCN projects to orexin neurons in the posterior hypothalamus. Hcrt-1 can cause hyperactivity by binding to the hcrt-B receptor. Hcrt is involved in feeding, sleep, and other homeostatic behaviors. Hcrt, when administered centrally, activates the HPA axis and is involved in the stress response in rats (Ida T et al., 2000). Hcrt modulates the RVLM and has histochemical relationships to TRH, NPY, MCH, and CART (Broberger C, 1999).

MCH, like Hcrt, is expressed in the neurons of the lateral hypothalamus. It is thought to stimulate food intake and modulate cardiovascular and immune function, learning, memory and pigmentation. There are five MCH subtypes. The crucial receptor for energy balance is MCHR4, working in part by modulation of the leptin receptor. The precursor for MCH is POMC, which may be decreased in neurosomatic disorders. CART is found in many regions of the brain and acts like a very pale version of cocaine. It limits food intake. Even though orexin may increase food intake, it has no effect on body weight. Modafinil modulates TRH secretion, and it may have effects on other related neuropeptides.

Phentermine is a stimulant, the still legal half of Fen-Phen. It is becoming increasingly clear that phentermine should not be prescribed either. Fen-Phen may cause satiety by producing a supraadditive effect on Ach levels in the NAc. Phentermine is a monoamine oxidase A inhibitor and increases serotonin levels. When mixed with ephedrine and estradiol, both of which are also MAOI(A)s, the effect on serotonin is additive (Ulus IH et al., 2000). These agents are being added to SRIs as an anorectic "cocktail." No resultant cases of serotonin syndrome have been reported, and I do not know why.

Little is new about methylphenidate (Ritalin) since *Betrayal*. It is primarily a DAT blocker, which makes only some individuals "high" with excessive use. It increases metabolism in people who have up-regulation of D_2 receptors in the superior cingulate, right thalamus, and cerebellum, as measured by PET. Those who crave MPH have increased metabolism in the right OFC and right striatum, and those who find MPH to elevate mood have increased PFC metabolism (Volkow NP et al., 1999). The regions involved with craving are abnormal in OCD as well. These results suggest laterality of reinforcing responses. Because MPH is used widely in ADHD, it is of interest that this disorder has been suggested to be one of right-hemisphere DA hypofunction, or atypical frontal-striatal function. MPH increased striatal activation in ADHD children in a task requiring response inhibition (Vaidya CJ et al., 1998). The most effective medications for ADHD increase the transmission of both NE and DA (Zametkin AJ, Liutta W, 1998).

Methylphenidate improves working-memory performance in normal subjects by task-related reductions in regional cerebral blood flow in the DLPFC and the posterior parietal cortex. It has the greatest effect on subjects with lower baseline working-memory capacity (Mehta MA et al., 2000).

ADHD, characterized by impulsivity and hyperactivity, is not often encountered in a neurosomatic practice. Inattentive ADD is seen frequently, however. Children with ADHD have a defect in response inhibition, which results in difficulty in self-regulating response to stimuli (Barkley RA, 1997). They have a hyperresponsiveness to stimuli because they are impaired in delaying responses. The inattentiveness is thought to be a result of this dysregulation. Effective treatment of ADHD would then activate the motor inhibitory system of the OFC-limbic axis, thus increasing delayed responding.

Using this paradigm, CFS might consist of hypersensitivity to stimuli, inattentiveness, and overactivity of the sensory inhibitory system. Sensory distractibility refers to this inability to screen out irrelevant stimuli and focus on or attend to relevant input. Sensory distractibility occurs following lesions to the pulvinar, which is not implicated in neurosomatic functional brain imaging. Sensorimotor distractibility has been noted following lesions of the PFC, which is almost always hypoperfused in CFS and FMS. Thus, attention to the background is enhanced and SNR is lowered. This dysfunction is related to a NE deficit in *tuning*. With normal NE function, information of high salience is preferentially processed and the SNR is high. NE can enhance responses of neural networks to excitatory or inhibitory stimuli, perhaps by enhancement of GABA-mediated inhibition. NE, particularly via $alpha_{2A}$ receptors, is important in cognitive tasks that require working memory. DA is also important in working memory, the ability to keep something in mind for a brief period of time. DA increases the firing of the PFC and striatum and increases SNR in this manner.

The CSTC systems are extremely complicated, much more so than I have indicated in this book so far. DA is a primary component of this complexity, along with glutamate and GABA as major transmitters and VIP, SP, NPY, TRH, and dynorphin as minor ones. DA helps to determine salience, the stimuli associated with reward or aversion. Aversion mechanisms are still controversial, but as of now it seems that DA transiently rises and then falls. The controllability of the aversive stimulus is important. DA falls considerably when the aversive stimulus is perceived as random, or uncontrollable. This is why coping skills have been so emphasized in CBT of neurosomatic disorders.

When I began to treat patients with CFS, I was amazed to see many of them fall asleep after taking dextroamphetamine (Dexedrine) and similar agents such as methylphenidate (Ritalin), phentermine (Ionamin), and pemoline (Cylert). Later, when amphetamine salts (Adderall) were introduced, the same paradoxical response often occurred. The cause of this sedation is central to the etiology of *neurosomatic disorders* (my term for inappropriate handling of sensory and cognitive input by the brain).

The nucleus accumbens is a part of the brain involved with reward, particularly expectation of reward. It has both a core and a shell, and the shell is germane to the present discussion. Its primary neurotransmitter is dopamine, although others, particularly norepinephrine and glutamate are also involved. For reasons too complicated to explain here, either not enough DA is available in the NAc or the receptors for it are not sensitive enough ("down-regulated").

Decreased DA in the NAc has profound effects on how an individual feels and thinks and how the parts of the brain with which it communicates function. Many, perhaps most, CFS and FMS symptoms are related to DA and NE. Fatigue, pain, and attentional problems are common consequences.

Somnolence after taking stimulants is analogous to relapse after ejaculation. Both are due to absolute or functional DA and NE deficiency and could not be easily explained by receptor down-regulation. Stimulants enhance secretion of these neurotransmitters. If the levels of the these substances are too low in the secreting ("presynaptic") neuron to begin with, squeezing out a little bit more may result in marked worsening of symptoms subsequently.

It pains me to write this, but the situation is more complicated than I have just described. Presynaptic DA may be totally depleted or the mechanism by which stored DA moves to the edge of the presynaptic membrane where it is secreted (the "ready-releasable pool") may be dysfunctional.

Neither of these explanations can account for the rapid symptom fluctuations commonly seen in neurosomatic disorders and certainly could not demonstrate why increasing DA transmitters can cause a relapse. These phenomena can be interpreted, however, as stemming from hypersensitivity of the DA autoreceptor.

What is an autoreceptor? The presynaptic neuron, which secretes most transmitters, must have a mechanism to sense how much transmitter it has secreted (i.e., how much is in the synapse). How autoreceptors themselves are regulated is imperfectly understood, but calcium ions are thought to be involved. Calcium is perhaps the most important intracellular regulating element.

If the DA autoreceptor is hypersensitive, small amounts of secreted DA will result in a marked decrease of further DA secretion. Such a scenario may be applicable to patients with neurosomatic disorders. An ideal drug, therefore, would block the DA autoreceptor and "fool" the neuron so that a low DA concentration is sensed in the surrounding environment. Researchers have been trying to develop a drug that blocks the DA autoreceptors without affecting similar receptors postsynaptically since the 1970s. It has recently been reported that Arvid Carlsson, who shared the Nobel Prize in Physiology or Medicine in 2000, has developed such an agent, currently named (-)-OSU6162, and is testing it on human patients. Its most obvious use would be in Parkinson's disease, which is similar to neurosomatic disorders in certain ways. Increasing DA in the NAc shell, which is difficult to do without using drugs of possible abuse, should be facilitated by a DA autoreceptor antagonist.

THE CORTICOSTRIATAL-
THALAMOCORTICAL (CSTC) CIRCUIT IN REVERSE

The corticothalamic projection is 90 percent afferent, i.e., from the cortex to the thalamus. The thalamic relay nuclei that carry basal ganglia output to the cortex, the ventral anterior (VA), ventral lateral (VL), and mediodorsal (MD) nuclei, project back to the basal ganglia directly (Haber S, McFarland NR, 2001). I have been hesitant to discuss the further complexity of the CSTC circuit but have concluded that I would be doing readers a disservice if I did not.

The flow of information from the cortex through basal ganglia structures to the thalamus and back to the cortex is topographically organized. I have earlier reviewed the direct and indirect pathways. To summarize, the direct pathway consists of two gabergic synapses, striatum/globus pallidis internal (GPi)/substania nigra pars reticulata (SNr) and GPi/SNr/ thalamus. Activation of the direct pathway results in disinhibition of the thalamic output to the cortex. The indirect pathway, globus pallidus external (Gpe)/subthalamic nucleus (STN)/Gpi/thalamus results in inhibition of thalamic output to the cortex because the output of the STN is glutamatergic. The two pathways have opposite effects on thalamic output to the cortex. The direct pathway provides reinforcement of cortically driven behavior and is modulated by the indirect pathway, which acts as a filter for irrelevant behavior, and participates with (primarily) the DLPFC in changing context when appropriate.

Primary, supplementary, premotor, cingulate, lateral prefrontal cortex (LPFC), OFC, and mPFC project to the striatum in a functionally topographic manner. I shall discuss the reticular nucleus of the thalamus here because I believe it to be a key structure in neurosomatic medicine (see *Betrayal,* pp. 81-84). A current review of the RTN has been published by R. W. Guillery and colleagues (1998). Guillery is perhaps the world's leading expert on the RTN, and his work has greatly influenced my understanding of its function. Others are studying the RTN. I have discussed the work of J. W. Crabtree and colleagues (1998) on thalamic nuclear intercommunication via the RTN. A major function of the RTN is to reduce the sizes of the receptive fields of its target neurons. If excitatory inputs to the RTN are reduced (corticothalamic and collaterals from the ascending reticular activating system [ARAS]), the result will be large increases in receptive fields of thalamic neurons, a state that would worsen neurosomatic symptoms and increase central sensitization. Flexibility in the activity of the RTN causes the size of receptive fields in the cortex to appropriately vary with stimulus contingencies (Kaas J, Ebner F, 1998). The situation is further complicated by mGluRs on the RTN. Activation of group II receptors inhibits the RTN, while stimulation of group I receptors activates it. Both actions result from a linear modification of K^+ conductance (Cox CL, Sherman SM, 1999).

GABA receptors in the RTN have a limited number of subunit mRNAs. The $beta_1$ subunit is highly expressed and is absent in relay nuclei. One of its primary functions is facilitating inhibition of neurons within the RTN GABA neurons in the RTN inhibit one another. $Beta_3$ knock-out mice have a decreased duration of thalamic inhibition (via inhibitory postsynaptic potentials [IPSPs]), promoting abnormal synchronization and predisposing to seizure activity (Huntsman MM et al., 1999).

All fibers going either way between the thalamus and the cortex must pass through the RTN, which acts as a sieve. It thereby functions as a regulator of what stimuli should be attended to. Several anatomically distinct thalamocortical and corticothalamic pathways interact in each functional section of the RTN (two or more).

> The important point is that each sector provides a nexus for the interaction of several thalamocortical and corticothalamic circuits, and will prove to be a key site where many cortical areas concerned with one modality can interact. The nature of interactions in this nexus is likely to prove crucial for the cortical and reticular control of relay properties of thalamic cells as they switch from one mode of firing to another, possibly changing as attentional foci shift across cortical areas and within cortical areas. (Guillery RW et al., 1998, p. 32)

Motor areas of the cortex project to the putamen and dorsolateral caudate. The DLPFC projects to the head and body of the caudate and the rostral putamen. This area has been hypoperfused in the brain SPECTs of fibromyalgia patients from Laurence Bradley and colleagues at the University of Alabama-Birmingham. Lesions of this region of the caudate produce impairments in working memory. The OFC and mPFC are referred to here as the OMPFC and project to the ventral and rostral striatum, including the

NAc and ventromedial caudate. Other terminations are less relevant to neurosomatic illness. Each functional region of the cortex projects topographically to the striatum. The topography is maintained in the projections from the striatum to the globus pallidus (GP)/SNr, and from the GP/SNr to the thalamus.

The MD and midline thalamic nuclei innervate distinct cortical areas of concern here: the DLPFC, OMPFC, and ACC. Thalamic nuclei may alter their oscillation patterns of frequency and synchrony, thereby altering the dynamics of cortical processing. Mircea Steriade and colleagues at the University of Laval in Quebec, Canada, have been instrumental in my understanding of these processes. Both the direct and the indirect pathways and, to a lesser extent, differential discharge rates of GP neurons, *gate* information to the cortex in relation to the task at hand (Contreras-Vidal JL, 1999). This gating function has been related to movement disorders but should apply to neurosomatic medicine as well.

Most neural pathways are reciprocal, and thalamocortical projections are no exception. The oscillatory firing pattern of the thalamus is controlled by the corticothalamic pathway (Steriade M, 1999). The cortex projects back to its innervating thalamic nucleus but also to a region of the thalamus that does not send an input. Corticothalamic terminal fields are wider than the reciprocal thalamocortical fields. The nonreciprocal component fires rapidly and derives from large cells in layer V, the reciprocal regions from small cells in layer VI. Thus, larger V cells can produce moment-to-moment change in thalamic oscillatory patterns which would, in turn, affect a different part of the cortex. Corticothalamic interactions can, by this mechanism, affect general global cortical activity. By the same route, primary sensory (unimodal) cortical areas can transmit information to heteromodal and "supramodal" (DLPFC) association areas.

Pertinent to neurosomatic pathophysiology is that the OMPFC, which is involved in neural-based learning, has a nonreciprocal connection to thalamic areas associated with the executive function of the DLPFC. This pattern of information transfer applies to the other cortical areas and their thalamic relay nuclei listed at the beginning of this section. The thalamic inputs and outputs to the basal ganglia are influenced by nonreciprocal corticothalamic innervation. The process is further complicated by basal ganglia loops and their transfer of information to the cortex. The information flow is ordered, from limbic to cognitive to motor output (Haber SN et al., 2000). The GP/substantia nigra (SN) may influence the effect of corticothalamic feedback on oscillatory thalamocortical patterns.

If the foregoing is not sufficiently explanatory, consider the role of thalamostriatal projections. After the cortex, the thalamus provides the largest source of excitatory input to the striatum. The midline and intralaminar nuclei, which I highlighted in *Betrayal* as part of the "nonspecific" thalamic nuclei, provide the majority of the thalamostriatal excitation. They are probably dysfunctional in neurosomatic disorders, being terminals of the ascending reticular activating system and producing cortical desynchronization and arousal when stimulated. They may "alert" the striatum for receipt of subsequent cortical input. There are also direct projections to the striatum from VA, VL, and MD, allowing the basal ganglia to influence the function of specific cortical areas. Thalamostriatal projections are, again, organized in a functionally topographic manner. The projections relevant to neurosomatic disorders were discussed in *Betrayal*. The thalamostriatal projections from relay nuclei *converge* with corticostriatal afferents. The same regions of the thalamus that convey basal ganglia output to the cortex also project back to the striatum. Thus, the CSTC circuit simultaneously operates in reverse, adding an immense degree of sophistication to allocation of salience and attention to exteroceptive and enteroceptive stimuli and their subsequent processing. This degree of complexity in functional neuroanatomy alone, disregarding other regions of the brain, all other transmitter substances, postreceptor cascades, and other possible etiologies is intricate enough to create errors that would result in neurosomatic symptomatology.

Spontaneous oscillation of $[Ca^{2+}]_i$ of glial cells surrounding developmental thalamocortical neurogenesis has recently been reported (Parri HR et al., 2001). These Ca^{2+} transients have been postulated to occur in adults. This experiment is the first to demonstrate that glial cells have activity *independent of neurons* in the "tripartite synapse," where one or more glial cells is associated spatially and functionally with a presynaptic and postsynaptic neuron. Glial Ca^{2+} activations occur every five minutes or so and can trigger glutamate-dependant activation of neurons, as well as propagating Ca^{2+} waves through neighboring astrocytes. This pathway can alter the strength of transmission at glutamatergic NMDA synapses, which is usually inhibitory (Rose CR, Konnerth A, 2001a).

Astrocytes appear to respond to the same medications as neurons. For example, the dihydropyridine L-type Ca^{2+}-channel blocker nifedipine dramatically reduces oscillations in astrocytic calcium levels. Spontaneous astrocytic Ca^{2+} oscillations correlate with Ca^{2+} transients in neurons and the neuronal currents are blocked with NMDA-receptor antagonists. Glutamate is released from astrocytes and neurons following stimuli that increase Ca^{2+}.

> [S]mall groups of astrocytes display correlated activity and lead to neuronal excitation. This suggests that a small and fairly specific cluster of neurons would be excited by an active astrocytic group at any one time. This property, and the potential for NMDA-induced depolarizations to elicit action potentials and therefore long-range sig-

naling, endow this form of astrocyte neuron signaling with properties required for a role in the topographic mapping of the thalamocortical loop. (Parri HP et al., 2001)

This loop is twisted into a Möbius strip, if not contorted into a tesseract, by Frank R. Sharp and colleagues (2001) as they seek to explain schizophrenia as a pathological alteration of limbic thalamocortical circuits similar to that produced by NMDA antagonists. They postulate that schizophrenia is a hypoglutamatergic, hyperdopaminergic state in a "psychosis circuit" activated by PCP and ketamine. The value of their strenuous efforts for our purposes is that the model they create is in some respects the opposite of neurosomatic and Parkinsonian pathophysiology. They note that blocking D_{1-4} receptors prevents the "neurotoxic" effects of NMDA antagonists in rats. They do admit that agents such as ketamine have never been shown to damage the brains of primates and humans, thereby doing their part to mute the tenor of opinion that created "reefer madness."

Production of heat shock protein (HSP) occurs when the neuron-glial unit is subjected to physical stress. MK-801, an NMDA antagonist, was injected into the thalamic VA and none of the relay nuclei, with the result that HSP 70 protein was produced in the retrosplenial cortex, an identical result to when MK-801 was administered systemically. Injecting it into the limbic cortex or the diagonal band of Broca did not induce HSP anywhere in the brain, but HSP 20 appeared in these regions when MK-801 was administered systemically. Injecting $GABA_A$ agonists into VA and MD bilaterally prevented expression of HSP 70 after MK-801 dosing.

Sharp and colleagues then leap a micron or so to posit that MK-801 blocks NMDA receptors on the RTN, which is composed entirely of gabergic neurons. Consequently, the RTN is less able to inhibit all thalamic nuclei, including the relay nuclei and the "nonspecific" nuclei. The relay nuclei would then secrete excessive glutamate onto AMPA/kainate receptors in the cortex, either damaging the neurons that expressed them or, at the least, overly exciting them. This process would eventuate in NMDA activation, since AMPA occupation is necessary before the Mg^{2+} block in the NMDA pore is removed. GABA in the cortex would decrease at the same time. These workers do not explain why thalamic hypersynchrony due to decreased RTN activity does not appear on schizophrenic EEGs on a routine basis.

The authors do not understand why only neurons in the limbic cortex are affected by MK-801 injection into the VA. They seem unaware that limbic neurons can be labeled by monoclonal antibodies, which serve as markers. These markers are thought to be directly involved in the pathophysiology of paraneoplastic limbic encephalitis, a long-recognized disorder. The fact that limbic neurons can be preferentially affected is perhaps the best case for retaining the concept of a limbic system. They are also selectively activated by "-caine" drugs.

NMDA antagonist effects can be blocked by DA antagonists. The action of DA on GABAergic neurons in the RTN is inhibitory as it is on GABAergic interneurons in the cortex. Whether DA itself could be neurotoxic and whether DA "neurotoxicity" occurs in humans is not considered by the authors (it can).

D_1-receptor antagonists are supposedly helpful in this situation. D_1 agonists are excitatory in the limbic cortex and could thus affect pyramidal neurons there. My recollection is that dopaminergic impairment of mitochondrial function often caused clinically by methamphetamine is not limited to cells that express the D_1 receptor.

NMDA antagonists block excitatory receptors on tonically inhibitory GABAergic neurons which project to the VTA and then to the NAc, in a manner analogous to the action of opioids as inhibitory heteroreceptors on the same neurons. The end result is increased mesocorticolimbic DA, bad for schizophrenics, good for neurosomatic patients.

The bottom line of the Sharp article is that dysfunctional thalamocortical responses could be involved with schizophrenia. They end the paper by qualifying many of their hypotheses. There is no excitotoxic cell death in the brains of schizophrenics. There is no impairment of the RTN or the retrosplenial cortex. They do cite recent evidence to support involvement of the "limbic" insular cortex, as well as the anterior nuclei of the thalamus in schizophrenia, i.e., atrophy of the VA and MD. They focus on GABA, glutamate, and DA almost exclusively but apologize for the necessary brevity of their article. To quote Albert Einstein: "Everything should be as simple as possible, but no simpler." Well, this article is simpler.

Attentional Processes in the CSTC System

Attentional processes are central to the CSTC circuit and its inputs, especially from the visual stream, the predominant sensory input. Attentional networks in this stream, the PFC and parietal cortices, project to the basal ganglia in topographically organized longitudinal stripes which then project to the thalamus in the same organizational manner. All these structures are involved in sensorimotor aspects of attentional behaviors through control of the frontal eye fields (FEF), responses to stimuli, and *gating* of incoming stimuli. Caudate lesions, which have been seen in brain SPECT of FMS patients, result in dysfunction of the attentional system.

Even though inattentive ADD is the only symptom, it is being conceptualized as *hypovigilance*. In a primary disorder of vigilance (PDV), there is a malfunction in the right inferior parietal lobule and a few associated structures. These patients will primarily be sleepy, inattentive, and fidgety. I have occasionally seen this type of patient in my practice.

In many areas in the CSTC circuit plus the extended amygdala, sensory projections are so wide, or diffuse, that focal or generalized malfunction of these projection areas can lead to pain, allodynia, dysesthesias, or hyperethesias in the entire body. The best example of such a disorder for me is the diffuse pain, which often unpredictably shifts, of fibromyalgia, which I have previously considered to be an example of dysfunction of the RTN (see *Betrayal*).

Although stimulants make some neurosomatic patients more alert, it is common that they decrease energy and increase other symptoms. Besides depleting dopamine, they may decrease energy as indicated by a lowered striatal ATP/ADP ratio, especially when taken with an NE reuptake inhibitor such as reboxetine or desipramine. Coadministration of nicotinamide prevents a decrease in ATP/ADP and elevates striatal nicotinic adenine dinucleotide (NAD) concentration. NAD is an electron carrier molecule (Wan FI et al., 1999).

NAD is converted to NADH (nicotine adenine dinucleotide, reduced form) via the citric acid cycle and participates in mitochondrial oxidative phosphorylation and ATP production. No evidence I am aware of suggests systemic administration of NADH has an effect on mitochondrial NADH levels. It has made a few of my patients feel "hyper," however. Amphetamine-induced bioenergetic deficits involve NMDA toxicity and resultant NO formation. NO can be a mitochondrial neurotoxin and can increase amphetamine-induced striatal DA depletion. Nicotinamide is converted to NAD, which is then energy repleting and protective against excitotoxic damage to the DA terminal. What I do now is give 500 mg of nicotinamide (niacinamide) per day to every patient who takes stimulants, with or without catecholaminergic antidepressants, and never prescribe nitroglycerin along with them. I advise most patients to take 500 mg of ascorbate and 10 to 20 mg of forskolin as well, even if they can't tell the difference. Patients who previously abused methamphetamine are among my most treatment refractory.

It is possible some individuals with neurosomatic disorders have a shortage of ATP, but then K_{ATP} openers such as gabapentin, morphine, and clonidine might make such patients more symptomatic by increasing energy demand. Although this response may aid in receptor profiling, it does not often occur.

The most effective stimulant is amphetamine. It is more effective than methylphenidate. Amphetamine salts (Adderall) are superior to dextroamphetamine and need only be administered twice a day. Pemoline (Cylert) may cause liver toxicity, and I do not use it. I have explained why I no longer prescribe phentermine and related agents. I still occasionally use diethylpropion (Tenuate), which is related to bupropion (Wellbutrin). Diethylpropion is also useful as an antidepressant. I hope it continues to be available. Mazindol (Sanorex) is not, an unfortunate situation, because it had D_1 and D_2 agonist activity. Some patients had their best response of any medication to mazindol, which was also an antidepressant and could occasionally alleviate all neurosomatic symptoms in an individual. Modafinil (Provigil), although a stimulant, or wakefulness-promoting agent, has a somewhat different spectrum of action since it is a central histamine agonist, and usually does not work as well as Adderall. If somewhat effective, however, modafinil may be combined with other stimulants. Adderall seems to be less anxiogenic and better tolerated than other stimulants.

There still is controversy about the mode of action of amphetamines. Glutamatergic neurons from the PFC innervate the VTA in an excitatory manner. Amphetamine decreases the excitation not by releasing dopamine but by releasing *serotonin* in the VTA (Jones S, Kaver JA, 1999). The substantia nigra has the highest concentration of 5-HT in the brain, more being in the pars reticulata than the pars compacta. Several types of 5-HT receptors have been detected in significant densities in the basal ganglia. As usual, 5-HT_1 is inhibitory and 5-HT_2 is excitatory. SSRIs, acting through the 5-HT_{2C} receptor, increase extracellular 5-HT which acts acutely on 5-HT_1 receptors of several types in the VTA to inhibit DA secretion. These fluctuations even out after chronic administration. VTA DA secretion is then no longer inhibited, and the 5-HT_{2C} receptors are down-regulated. This process may be a basic mode of action of SSRIs, which eventually enhance mesocorticolimbic DA function. 5-HT_{2C} receptors do not appear to have a relevant role in the nigrostriatal system. Specific 5-HT_{2C} receptor antagonists are being considered for antidepressants and for the treatment of the negative symptoms of schizophrenia (Di Matteo V et al., 2001).

When an NMDA receptor antagonist is administered simultaneously with an amphetamine in the mPFC-VTA circuit, behavioral sensitization, or hypersensitivity, to amphetamine is prevented, implicating both the mPFC glutamatergic projection and the dopaminergic cell bodies in the VTA in the process (Codor M et al., 1999). Hyperreactivity, or sensitization of the VTA DA neurons, can occur after even one exposure and persist for the remainder of an animal's life. Administration of amphetamine causes an increase in serum ascorbic acid, perhaps in exchange for glutamate in glial cells in the substantia nigra. Glutamate levels are decreased. Supplementing chronic amphetamine therapy with vitamin C might be warranted.

The NAc is a terminus of the mesolimbic DA system emanating from the VTA. The NAc has extensive and reciprocal connections with limbic and motor systems and is thought to be critical for generation of motor responses to emotionally relevant environmental and cognitive stimuli. These responses may be exploratory or goal directed and are motivated rather than random. When an amphetamine acts, a rise in NAc NE as well as DA occurs. From where does the NE come? Apparently not from the LC but from a dense projection of neurons in the NTS, surprisingly (Delfs JM et al., 1998).

Psychostimulant-induced DA amplification causes increased locomotion. This fact is well known and has been demonstrated repeatedly. Behavioral sensitization rapidly occurs. It has been found through experiment (Louk JMJ et al., 1999) that: (1) DA modulates NAc NE release through stimulatory D_1 and inhibitory D_2 receptors. (2) The effects of D_1 receptor stimulation on NAc NE release are not secondary to extracellular conversion of cAMP to adenosine. The D_1 receptor is coupled to cAMP, which is degraded after receptor occupation. Adenosine is one of the products and can alter neuronal activity through (at first) activation of A_1 receptors. Application of an A_1 agonist, however, has an entirely different effect (see the section on adenosine). (3) DA regulation of NE release does not occur in the mPFC and amygdala. (4) There is altered modulation of NAc NE release by DA in slices of amphetamine pretreated rats. Electric stimulation of this preparation evokes a 73 percent increase in DA and a 22 percent increase in NE. The increase in NE is almost abolished by a D_1-receptor antagonist.

These data were interpreted to show that NE release in the NAc is under opposing influences of stimulatory D_1 and inhibitory D_2 receptors located on the NE varicosities. A D_2 antagonist increases NAc NE release. Thus, released endogenous DA tonically inhibits NAc NE release via stimulation of D_2 receptors. Under normal in vivo conditions, the D_1 receptors are not activated. It seems that D_2 receptors are located in closer proximity to DA and NE nerve terminals, while D_1 receptors are farther away from the site of DA release. DA diffuses in a paracrine manner, a much more common form of neurotransmission than we used to think, up to 12 micrometers away from release sites. D_1 receptors would thus be activated at high rates of DA release or at later stages of the release of transmitter.

mPFC and amygdalar NE release is derived from the LC and is not modulated by DA. Furthermore, NAc NE release is additionally unique in that the NAc has no inhibitory alpha$_2$ autoreceptors. While in the NAc, DA, via D_1 receptors, inhibits both excitatory and facilitatory transmission. NE, via postsynaptic alpha receptors only, inhibits excitatory, but not inhibitory, transmission. Perhaps the balance of DA and NE within the NAc determines the balance of excitatory and inhibitory transmission. Of course, that is not all. Difference in tone of the NAc DA receptors regulates NE release also. To make some sense out of this information, imagine that moderate DA tone would inhibit NE release through local D_2 receptors. An increase in DA tone would allow enough DA to diffuse distally to the D_1 receptors. More DA at both D_1 and D_2 receptors preferentially increases D_1 receptor sensitivity, particularly in amphetamine pretreated rats resulting in a net increase in NAc NE release. If there is too great a predominance of D_1 activation over D_2 inhibition, behavioral changes could result and a person could go on a speed run, become addicted, or even develop an amphetamine psychosis. This puzzle is more complicated than I have described it, but as with much of neurobiology, each new piece seems to increase its intricacy while decreasing its comprehensibility. I have yet to consider the role of DA autoreceptors in this section. I can see nothing wrong with the methods of the experiment and can but hope there is an underlying simplicity ("What does this drug do, Dr. Goldstein? Explain it to me so I can understand it.").

CORTICOTROPIN-RELEASING HORMONE (CRH) AND HYPOCORTISOLISM

I have listed antalarmin, a CRH antagonist, as a near-future treatment option in neurosomatic disorders. It has not yet been established whether patients with neurosomatic disorders have deficits in their secretion of corticotropin-releasing hormone, also known as CRF (corticotropin-releasing factor). The pathophysiology of the illness suggests a deficiency in CRH, but ethanol withdrawal appears to be associated with enhanced CRH neurotransmission (Markou A et al., 1998). Patients with CFS and related disorders usually are hypersensitive to alcohol and usually have their symptomatology exacerbated not only by minimal alcohol administration but also by alcohol withdrawal. Thus, either there is a surfeit of CRH secretion with alcohol withdrawal, or CRH is not deficient to begin with. The topic of hypocortisolism in the pathophysiology of stress-related bodily disorders has recently been reviewed (Heim C et al., 2000). Increased CRH would raise cortisol levels by heightened ACTH stimulation of the adrenal cortex. Glucocorticoids antagonize the effects of NE to a considerable extent (Yehuda R, 2000), and the alcohol intolerance reported by at least two-thirds of CFS patients may be a result of a further decrease in already low NE levels.

Rachel Yehuda is the doyenne of post-traumatic stress disorder, which is similar in some respects to neurosomatic disorders. I have been reading her articles for at least a decade. She begins a discussion of PTSD, a chronic disorder, with comments about the neurobiology of fear, since she conceptualizes PTSD "as resulting from the cascade of biological and physiological responses following the activation of fear-related and other brain systems" (Yehuda R, 2000, p. 15). She cites the amygdala as assessing a stimulus and determining whether there should be a stress response. If so, in several milliseconds, it begins activating the neural network of fear. Amygdala projections activate the ANS, and pathways from the central amygdala to the bed nucleus of the stria terminalis initiate the hypothalamic-pituitary-adrenal response by stimulating the secretion of CRH from the hypothalamus.

Yehuda describes the synergy between the sympathetic nervous system and the HPA axis:

> Whereas catecholamines facilitate the availability of energy to the body's vital organs, cortisol's role in stress is to help contain or shut down sympathetic activation and other neuronal defensive actions that have been initiated by stress. In one sense, then, cortisol functions as the mediator of the termination of the stress response. (Yehuda R, 2000, p. 15)

Thus, by negative feedback, cortisol reduces levels of CRH and ACTH. NE and CRH stimulate each other in the first place. If alcohol or its withdrawal stimulates CRH secretion, one can discern how CRH secretion could result in noradrenergic synaptic fatigue. I shall return to Yehuda's work later. CRH administration to CFS patients results in a blunted ACTH response, as shall be seen.

CRH levels were measured in the cerebrospinal fluid in patients with CFS by Demitrack and colleagues in 1991 and were found to be normal. Cerebrospinal fluid CRH levels may not adequately reflect CRH activity in the hypothalamus or in brain areas involved in the regulation of arousal, and in fact, there may be CRH hypersecretion and down-regulation of pituitary CRH receptors. I tend to favor a CRH-depletion hypothesis, however. Endogenous CRH has been found to inhibit vagal activity when induced by conditioned fear (Nijsen MJ et al., 2000). In general, neurosomatic patients have a decreased level of vagal activity.

Several other CRH antagonists besides antalarmin are in clinical trials. One of these is astressin, which may be less sedating than antalarmin. It has no effect on CRH-induced locomotor activity but blocks other CRH effects. Thus, it would block CRH inhibition of gastric emptying and attenuate the increase of plasma interleukin-6 produced by one hour of immobilization stress in rats. Various other results suggest that "Astressin can antagonize CRF and CRF-like molecule action on physiology involved in the neuroendocrine and visceral responses to stress, but it may have less effect on those symptoms involved in behavioral response to stress, and very poor effect in the locomotor activation induced by CRF." This finding may be related to the fact that there are at least two types of CRH receptors (Spina MJ et al., 2000, p. 236).

Agents related to CRH have effects on pain when centrally administered. However, their therapeutic dose range is very narrow. Giving CRF intravenously also causes the release of beta-endorphin from the anterior pituitary gland, but CRH analgesia is not reversed by systemic administration of naloxone or the removal of the pituitary gland. CRH does not seem to be analgesic by its effect on the inflammatory process, nor does it directly affect peripheral nerve endings. There is reason to believe that peripherally administered CRH, a lipophilic agent, can cross the blood-brain barrier where it could then affect central mechanisms. When CRH has been given intravenously to human beings for postoperative dental pain, the patients report significant overall analgesia. The analgesia occurs on an affective scale but not on a sensory scale (Lariviere WR, Melzack R, 2000). Oral antalarmin attenuates the global response to stress in primates (Habib KE et al., 2000).

CRH has been found to produce analgesia in most experimental models. Increased CRH can cause hypercortisolism, which over time produces hippocampal atrophy, most noted in brain imaging of patients with major depressive disorder. Such atrophy is also found in those with PTSD. When PTSD is combat related, there is decreased benzodiazepine (BZD) binding in the prefrontal cortex (Bremner JD et al., 2000).

Hippocampal atrophy is not found in CFS patients. Unlike patients with post-traumatic stress disorder, in whom hypercortisolism is found, it is not present according to volumetric MRI hippocampal measurements on twelve CFS patients I studied about ten years ago. These results were published in *Limbic Hypothesis*. Certainly, stress early in life, as well as prenatal stress, may induce states of persistent hypocortisolism. It has been found that administration of ACTH or corticosteroids into pregnant rats results in decreased basal corticosteroid levels, reduced adrenocortical activity, and decreased adrenal volumes in the offspring. Female rats were more prone to develop adrenal dysfunction.

> Individual differences in behavioral and neuroendocrine responses to stress are, in part, derived from variations in maternal care. Such effects might serve as a mechanism by which selected traits could be transmitted from one generation to the next. . . . In humans, measures of parental bonding between a mother and daughter were highly correlated with the same measures of bonding between the daughter and her child. (Francis DD, Meaney MJ, 1999, p. 132)

A mother who is not stressed bonds well with her infant. She may have been genetically predisposed to bond well, but her neuroendocrine environment was also determined by her bonding experience with the infant's maternal grandmother. Poor bonding in rats produces increased CRH levels in response to stress, lower levels of glucocorticoid and GABA receptors, altered NE and 5-HT responses to stress, and fearful, timid adults. Rat pups from genetically fearful strains, when raised by mothers from less fearful strains, are considerably less fearful as adults than their home cage-raised litter mates. The less fearful mother rats licked their pups twice as often and had a decreased HPA axis response to stress than timid mother rats of another strain. Enhanced appreciation of intergenerational transmission of parental behavior has been for me one of the most significant shifts in my understanding of the developmental aspects of neurosomatic disorders in the past seven years.

Conceptualizing the role of hypocortisolism in neurosomatic disorders is advancing (Heim C et al., 2000). It is possible that some groups of patients with neurosomatic disorders may have hyposecretion of corticotropin-releasing hormone, and others may have hypersecretion of this polypeptide.

The relative hypocortisolism found in patients with neurosomatic disorders may reflect a lack of counter-regulation which enhances the adverse effect of hypercortisolism on immune function and thereby increases the risk of developing stress-related bodily disorders. It has been observed that patients with a genetically determined glucocorticoid resistance often present with symptoms of CFS and fibromyalgia (Stratakis CA et al., 1994).

Most experimental work evaluating immune up-regulation in neurosomatic disorders has focused on the HPA axis and not norepinephrine. However, as I have noted previously, the large majority of my neurosomatic patients also have allergic rhinitis or other disorders associated with immune-system up-regulation. Treatment of neurosomatic patients with corticosteroids does not usually benefit them. There have been two experiments in which CRH has been administered to patients with neurosomatic disorders. Such studies have implications both for pathophysiology and treatment. Both studies found a blunted ACTH response to CRH (Demitrack M et al., 1991; Scott LV et al., 1998). Sensitization of the HPA axis occurs in abdominal obesity which often accompanies CFS (Rosmond R et al., 1998). Brain insulin-receptor hyposensitivity may be involved (Bruning JC et al., 2000).

AGMATINE

Agmatine is decarboxylated L-arginine. The decarboxylating enzyme is appropriately termed arginine decarboxylase (ADC). Agmatine is hydrolyzed by the enzyme agmatinase. Most agmatine is found in the cerebral cortex and limbic system. Agmatine and glutamate are often released as cotransmitters. ADC is closely related to ornithine decarboxylase (ODC), an enzyme involved in polyamine biosynthesis. Nitric oxide synthase catalyzes the conversion of L-arginine to nitric oxide. Agmatine competitively inhibits NOS.

Verapamil, but not other Ca^{2+}-channel blockers, inhibits the uptake of agmatine. It may enter cells through the nicotinic and NMDA receptors. Agmatine releases LHRH, improves hyperalgesia, and dose-dependently enhances morphine analgesia. It prevents tolerance to mu- and delta-agonists, but not to kappa-agonists.

Agmatine binds to alpha$_2$ adrenoceptors as well as to imidazoline sites, although its binding is not comparable to any other agent. The I-2 binding site is located on the outer membrane of mitochondria where it is a constituent of the enzyme monoamine oxidase.

More significant to neurosomatic medicine is that agmatine can generate a voltage- and concentration-dependent block of the NMDA-receptor channel or pore. The location of the block is similar to that of ketamine and unlike that of the polyamine binding site. Agmatine is a cotransmitter with excitatory amino acids, especially glutamate, and antagonizes their postsynaptic actions. Agmatine may block several other catonic channels and inhibits all isoforms of NOS. Agmatine is analgesic and neuroprotective in ischemic models (Reis DJ, Dejunathan S, 2000). Many neuroprotective agents, as well as antiepileptic drugs, are effective agents in neurosomatic disorders. This widely distributed simple molecule is a good therapeutic candidate for neurosomatic disorders.

CHOLINESTERASE INHIBITORS

Aricept is also called donepezil. There is little more to say in neurosomatic medicine about the cholinesterase inhibitors since I wrote *Betrayal by the Brain*. Agents that inhibit acetylcholinesterase, the enzyme which metabolizes Ach, including pyridostigmine (Mestinon), may also be neurotoxic. I have not found these agents to be particularly useful in treating neurosomatic disorders. They are sometimes of benefit in individuals who appear to have a deficiency in glutamatergic secretion. Cholinergic agents may act as glutamate agonists, or they may stimulate the pedunculopontine nucleus to cholinergically activate afferents to the ventral tegmental area which secretes DA to the nucleus accumbens as well as to the mesolimbic and mesocortical dopaminergic tracts. It is usually the case that tacrine (Cognex) is more effective than donepezil, although the problems with t.i.d.

dosing as well as the requirements for frequent liver-function testing miti- gate against its utility.

Aricept may have some value in the treatment of the cognitive dysfunc- tion that occurs in up to 65 percent of patients with multiple sclerosis (MS) for which there had formerly been no accepted treatment. An open-label study was performed using Aricept for 12 weeks in patients with MS, and researchers found a significant difference in "several cognitive domains." The 10 mg dose seemed to be superior to the 5 mg dose. This is the most im- pressive study I have read to date on the use of a cholinesterase inhibitor in any sort of cognitive dysfunction (Greene YM et al., 2000). Galantamine (Reminyl), which also stimulates the nicotinic cholinergic receptor, should have greater benefit in selected neurosomatic patients. Rivastigmine (Exelon), which blocks two cholinesterases (dibutyryl cholinesterase is the other), may be preferred by an occasional patient.

Furthermore, the M_2 muscarinic receptor depresses GABAergic synaptic transmission in rat midbrain dopamine neurons, which would probably not be desirable in most neurosomatic patients (Grillner P et al., 2000). Overall, the cholinesterase inhibitors are not very useful in my practice. They benefit perhaps 5 percent of my patients. It is possible that some cholinesterases are not inhibited by available agents.

The present and future use of cholinesterase inhibitors in neuropsychiat- ric disorders has been recently reviewed (Cummings JL, 2000). They may be useful in the treatment of ADHD. They decrease opioid-induced sedation (Slatkin NE et al., 2001), and nicotinic agents may benefit the patient who has adverse drug reactions to ketamine and most antidepressants.

The ventral tegmental area secretes DA through terminals in the NAc and the MCL DA tracts. I had not realized until recently that the VTA has stimulatory muscarinic cholinergic receptors, perhaps part of the reason why a few neurosomatic patients have a good response to cholinesterase in- hibitors (Gronier B et al., 2000). When given under stressful situations, cholinesterase may disrupt the blood-brain barrier. Pyridostigmine, how- ever, has not been causally implicated in Gulf War syndrome.

The medication Artane (trihexyphenidyl) should, therefore, be more use- ful in neurosomatic disorders than it actually is. If cholinergic hyperactivity is present in some neurosomatic patients, the benefits of Artane, a mus- carinic cholinergic-receptor antagonist, should be more obvious than they have been in my patients. I have only an occasional patient who takes Artane on a regular basis, and even then it is part of a dopaminergic cocktail of various medications that have some utility in treating Parkinson's dis- ease. Patients often become tolerant to the effects of Artane.

What is more, central Ach systems are involved in sensory filtering, whereby irrelevant stimuli are excluded from sensory processing. This particular function of Ach does not appear applicable to neurosomatic patients, but hypothetically Artane could be anxiogenic (Smythe JW et al., 1996). It could also be sedating, since Ach is involved in the arousal network. Artane does not help or hinder cognition in my patients. If overlearning is a problem in neurosomatic disorders, Ach does not seem to be responsible.

ASCORBATE (VITAMIN C)

I have discussed the possible mechanisms of action of IV ascorbate in *Betrayal by the Brain* and have also updated this information in Chapter 8. Ascorbate appears to bind to a site on the NMDA receptor known as the redox site, which is characterized by having a disulfide bond. Redox is short for oxidation-reduction reaction, which refers to a reaction in which electrons are transferred from a donor to an acceptor molecule. Intravenous ascorbate remains a useful agent in the treatment of neurosomatic disorders, although it is still somewhat difficult to predict which patients will respond to it. Ascorbate may also act by lowering pH and by affecting the hydrogen ion site of the NMDA receptor.

The brain, spinal cord, and adrenal glands have the highest levels of ascorbate in the body. It enters the CNS by simple diffusion, carrier-mediated uptake, and active transport. Brain concentration of ascorbate is 20 times higher than plasma. The role of ascorbate in the brain has recently been reviewed (Rice MA, 2000). Amphetamine causes an increase in ascorbate levels in the striatum but not in other structures. The elevated brain ascorbate, [Asc]o, is linked to glutamate release and uptake in specific pathways. As glutamate is taken up, ascorbate is released in a molecular exchange process, which can be halted by glutamate-reuptake inhibitors but not by glutamate-receptor antagonists. This process occurs in a cortico-striatal-thalamocortical loop and is associated with the release of DA.

Ascorbate and glutathione (as GSH) form a "redox couple," in which they act synergistically. Increase in one substance can compensate for a deficiency in the other. Most research has focused on the role of ascorbate as a neuroprotectant against cell death, but increase in [Asc]o could decrease glutamate concentration. Ascorbate is also a neuromodulator for secretion of DA, NE, and Ach from synaptic vesicles. It is an essential cofactor for synthesis of neuropeptides and enhances their release at physiologic concentrations. Ascorbate is released by neurons as well as glia (Miele M et al., 2000). The redox modulatory site of the NMDA receptor acts as a gain control of receptor activity and is located on the NR1 subunit. Ascorbate would decrease calcium influx through the receptor pore.

AMANTADINE

Amantadine is a medication that has an antiviral activity against the influenza A virus, preventing its replication. It also is a weak NMDA-receptor antagonist with dopaminergic properties. Amantadine seems to work much better when it is placed in pluronic organogel. I have this substance made in a concentration of 400 milligrams per gram and usually apply two or three ml to one or both forearms. Onset of action occurs in two to three minutes. Although the gel and the 100 mg capsule are the same substance, the gel seems to be more effective, perhaps because it is directly absorbed into the systemic circulation and first-pass metabolism by the liver and vagal binding is avoided. It is not uncommon for other agents placed in PLO to work more effectively than when taken orally. Many patients report itching or burning at the application site when using amantadine gel. This contact irritation may be prevented by spraying a corticosteroid asthma inhaler on the site one minute prior to gel application.

Practitioners who use amantadine PLO should be aware that amantadine rapidly causes contact dermatitis in about 20 percent of the patients to whom it is applied. This process resolves after the medication is washed off and usually occurs 5 to 15 minutes after application. Most patients who develop contact dermatitis to amantadine will not have a therapeutic response to it.

The best review I have read of the preclinical studies of amantadine and related agents was written in 1997 (Danysz W et al., 1997). This review focused primarily on Memantine, which acts as an NMDA-receptor antagonist, and amantadine, for which there are about 12 different in vitro actions listed. As far as amantadine's enhancing dopamine release or inhibiting dopamine uptake, the authors find it unlikely that amantadine would have this property since the therapeutic concentrations in vivo are usually unobtainable (but see Eisenberg E, Pud D, 1998). Memantine also has a large number of actions in vitro, but the authors believe that its significant action is as an NMDA-receptor antagonist. Both are thought to be low-affinity, noncompetitive NMDA-receptor antagonists. Memantine has been used in countries outside the United States for postoperative analgesia, for which it seems to be very effective (Suzuki T et al., 1999). Most experts accept that NMDA-receptor antagonists manifest their anti-Parkinsonian effects by attenuating the imbalance between dopaminergic and glutamatergic pathways within the basal ganglia network. There are some differences between amantadine, which is currently available, and Memantine, which is not approved for use in the United States. Amantadine binds to the $sigma_1$ site at relevant concentrations, as does the medication pentazocine (Talwin). Amantadine has also been found to block neuronal nicotinic receptors and could be used if mecamylamine were not available. Amantadine, but not Memantine, increases norepinephrine release. It is thought that since both agents are NMDA-receptor antagonists, they might have neuroprotective effects. Intravenous amantadine, 200 mg in 500 ml of normal saline given over three hours, has been reported to *cure* some types of chronic pain, a word not often encountered in this context (Eisenberg E, Pud D, 1998). My use of IV amantadine in patients with fibromyalgia has helped some patients greatly but has not cured any, as of yet. I have seen it synergize with IV ascorbate to produce dissociation, when neither drug singly had that effect. Patients may become tolerant to the effects of IV amantadine and may even develop a schizophreniform disorder.

An interesting article by G. Northoff and colleagues (1999) reported amantadine was effective in acute akinetic crisis in Parkinson's disease, as well as in febrile catatonia. The authors thought that amantadine "may consequently be considered as a therapeutic alternative to lorazepam and amobarbital in akinetic catatonia." In addition, catatonic patients with fever, nonresponsive to lorazepam/amobarbital should be given a therapeutic trial of amantadine before undergoing ECT. Amantadine has been found to have good therapeutic efficacy with regard to catatonic symptoms in patients with schizoaffective psychosis. The authors relate catatonia to prefrontal/cingulate glutamatergic hypofunction (due to underlying psychosis) as well as to concomitant glutamatergic hyperfunction (due to therapeutic efficacy of an NMDA antagonist) in other cortical regions besides the cingulate. The authors hypothesize that glutamatergic hypofunction in the prefrontal cortex and anterior cingulate may lead to decreased excitation of inhibitory (i.e., GABAergic) projections from prefrontal cortex/anterior cingulate to premotor (i.e., supplementary motor area) and motor (i.e., motor cortex) cortical areas resulting in a paradoxical effect of frontostriatal glutamatergic hyperfunction. This frontostriatal glutamatergic hyperfunction may be antagonized by amantadine (Northoff G et al., 1999). One of my patients had a forme fruste of neuroleptic malignant syndrome two days after receiving her fourth amantadine infusion. It resolved spontaneously, but her creatine phosphokinase (CPK) was 5,000. She tolerated IV amantadine well subsequently.

MK-801, a noncompetitive NMDA receptor antagonist, inhibits amantadine-induced dopamine release in the rat striatum as demonstrated in an experiment by Takahashi and colleagues in 1996.

Perfusion of amantadine through a microdialysis probe in the rat striatum causes an increase in both extracellular dopamine and glutamate levels. This effect is not abolished by omega-conotoxin or by a P/Q calcium-channel blocker. Several studies have revealed amantadine inhibits dopamine uptake. One experiment suggested amantadine might facilitate dopamine release from striatal dopaminergic nerve endings in contrast to the view of

W. Danysz and colleagues (1997). The amantadine-induced dopamine release requires calcium influx, which is probably mediated by a calcium channel other than the N-type voltage-sensitive calcium channel since it is not inhibited by omega-conotoxin. In the rat striatum, dopamine agonists induce glutamate release, while glutamate induces dopamine release. These findings are the opposite of those reported more recently (Parkinson JP et al., 2000). Stimulation of the NMDA receptor on dopaminergic nerve terminals resulted in an increase of extracellular glutamate and aspartate in rat striatum. This NMDA-induced effect was abolished by prior perfusion with MK-801.

The stereotypical behavior that can be caused by amantadine is reduced by a low dose of haloperidol, a dopamine D_2-receptor antagonist. Thus, amantadine may be a D_2-receptor agonist. Hypothetically, an individual who responds to amantadine will also respond to lidocaine but not to ketamine. According to the experiment of T. Takahashi and colleagues (1996), lidocaine would act in a somewhat opposite manner, and its mild NMDA-receptor antagonism would not be significant. Other research does not support the view that amantadine is a D_2 agonist and attributes all its pharmacologic effects to NMDA antagonism. It may be worth mentioning in this context that nootropic agents such as piracetam, excepting levetiracetam, might have a stimulatory effect on AMPA receptors, another type of receptor for the EAA glutamate. When nootropic agents are combined with NMDA-receptor antagonists there is an additive response in state-dependent learning. Thus, it would be possible that nootropic agents might have their actions reversed by topiramate (Topamax), which has AMPA-receptor antagonism as one of its primary modes of action. It has been speculated that a balance between NMDA and AMPA receptors is required for successful learning. The action of topiramate is reversed in the office by piracetam 800 mg p.o. Piracetam is also an oxidant at the redox-modulatory site of the NMDA receptor (like ascorbate) and decreases receptor activity. Such oxidants may have antiepileptic activity (Laughlin SB, 2001). Levetiracetam has been used therapeutically as an antiepileptic drug.

ADENOSINE

Adenosine is a very useful agent in neurosomatic medicine. It is unique among nucleosides in its involvement in virtually every organ system through four receptors, A_1, A_{2A}, and A_{2B}, and A_3. The last two are involved only in pathological conditions. Adenosine-receptor activation influences the action of transmitters and modulators indirectly, in subtle ways. It has been termed the "modulator of modulators," and the interplay between its own receptors and receptors for other transmitters reminds me of interactions between G proteins (Figure 3). In this way it helps to "fine tune" synapses (Sebastiao AM, Ribeiro JA, 2000). Caffeine blocks the A_{2A} receptors and increases dopamine secretion. The A_{2A} receptors are hyperalgesic, and the A_1 receptors are hypoalgesic. The adenosine A_{2A} receptor is involved in sleep promotion (Satoh et al., 1998). The density of this receptor is especially high in the striatum, where it modulates the effects of DA. A_{2A} knockout mice are significantly less sensitive to the locomotor-stimulating effects of amphetamine than are wild-type mice (Chen JF et al., 2000).

Adenosine A_{2A} agonists have been suggested as a potential new type of atypical antipsychotic. They have an action somewhat like haloperidol and clozapine, antagonizing amphetamine-induced motor activity, and can "transactivate" Trk receptors for neurotrophins in the absence of neurotrophin ligands (Theonen H, Sendtner M, 2002). They also block the motor activity induced by phencyclidine. Thus, A_{2A}-receptor antagonists are thought to possibly act as "atypical" neuroleptics. Adenosine, in general, inhibits the release of neurotransmitters or increases potassium-channel conductance in the postsynaptic membrane. Activation of A_{2A}-adenosine receptors is reported to depress GABA release from the striatum. Adenosine A_{2A}-receptor activation decreases the ability of D_2-receptor agonists to reduce acetylcholine release. There are two main routes of adenosine disposition: deamination by adenosine deaminase to inosine or phosphorylation by adenosine kinase to 5'AMP. Adenosine formed from adenine nucleotides, e.g., ATP, preferentially acts on A_{2A} receptors, and adenine released as such acts on A_1.

Axons have numerous neurotransmitter receptors. Although their roles are unclear, axons are modulated by glutamate, acetylcholine, GABA, mu-opioid agonists, and the A_1 adenosine receptor. Adenosine A_3-receptor activation might be related to asthma but is otherwise unimportant in neurosomatic disorders except for skin diseases. A_3-receptor activation produces nociceptive behavior and edema by release of histamine and serotonin. The importance of adenosine as an analgesic agent or a hypoalgesic agent has been receiving increasing attention in the pain literature of late and has also been reported to have an effect on neuropathic pain. A report about this property was published recently (Karlsten R, Gordht T, 2000). The authors note that adenosine modulates spinal nociceptive transmission by inhibition of intrinsic neurons through an increase in potassium conductance and presynaptic inhibition of sensory nerve terminals to decrease the release of substance P, CGRP, and perhaps glutamate. They state that activation of the A_1 receptor mediates the antiallodynic effect of adenosine and that activation of the A_2 receptor mediates the adverse effect of motor dysfunction. An interesting slant is that CGRP receptors are positively coupled to adenylate cyclase with consequent activation of PKA and then ATP-sensitive K^+

(K_{ATP}) channels. A_{2A} receptors activate CGRP. K_{ATP} channels are opened by gabapentin, clonidine, morphine, minoxidil, and several other agents. They hyperpolarize the neuron when open and are thought to be an important aspect of the mode of action of gabapentin (Figure 4). Enhancement of several substances that increase transmitter release by stimulating adenylate cyclase is dependent on A_{2A}-receptor activation. VIP enhances ATP release from hippocampal synaptosomes, again with the requirement that the A_{2A} receptor be activated. In general A_1 and A_{2A} receptors have opposing effects.

Important for neurosomatic disorders, A_1-receptor activation inhibits NMDA-receptor-mediated currents in the hippocampus. On striatal medium spiny neurons, however, A_{2A}-receptor activation blocks the NMDA receptor via the phosphoinositide pathway (Wirkner K et al., 2000).

The A_{2A} receptor is a key player in transmitter and postreceptor interactions. The A_1 receptor fine tunes these events by acting as a brake on the A_{2A} receptor. Astrocytes possess A_{2B} receptors, which are being found to stimulate secretion of ever more substances, even interleukin-6 (IL-6). Using IV adenosine in patients with neuropathic pain decreases their allodynia.

Because adenosine is extremely expensive, has some side effects when it is administered intravenously, and also has a very short duration of action, other techniques to increase the action of adenosine must be employed.

Papaverine inhibits adenosine reuptake. Adenosine presynaptically inhibits catecholamine release. Injecting ATP produces increased levels of adenosine. Pentoxifylline, besides being a TNF-alpha antagonist, may block adenosine reuptake and may increase adenosine levels. Stimulating the adenosine-1 receptor plus the angiotensin II receptor may synergize to be antiepileptic. The effects of alcohol can be somewhat mimicked by stimulating the A_1 and A_2 receptors simultaneously. The A_{2A} receptors are fairly dense in the olfactory nerve, and this concentration is one reason why adenosine nasal spray is a good route of administration. Stimulating the olfactory nerve, which primarily projects to the piriform cortex, has different effects than stimulating the trigeminal nerve (Bereiter DA, Bereiter DF, 2000). Stimulating the A_{2A} receptor decreases dopamine D_2-receptor sensitivity. Such a decrease might not always be detrimental to neurosomatic disorders since the dopamine levels in the medial prefrontal cortex are inversely related to those in the nucleus accumbens. When one administers nasal adenosine or an adenosine-reuptake inhibitor such as pentoxifylline or dipyridamole, it is difficult to be certain what receptors are being preferentially stimulated, although one would expect that it would be those that are most up-regulated. Stimulating the A_{2A} receptor facilitates neurotransmission, and A_{2A} knock-out mice have increased anxiety. Adenosine has an effect somewhat similar to opioids and is analgesic, particularly when given intrathecally but also when given systemically, in models of windup and sensitization. The degree of the analgesia is very brief, however. Intravenous adenosine must be infused very rapidly, and the infusion process is unpleasant for the patient. I have tried adenosine infusions in the office on two or three occasions for patients with intractable fibromyalgia and have not found them to be effective. Stimulating the A_2 receptor may have an effect similar to indomethacin, haloperidol, or donepezil (Aricept). A_2 activation can decrease GABA levels while increasing glutamate levels.

Stimulating the A_1 receptor, on the other hand, has an NMDA and glutamate antagonist effect and inhibits the release of glutamate. It somewhat simulates the action of prostaglandin D2 and the atypical neuroleptics olanzapine (Zyprexa) and quetiapine (Seroquel). Agonists at the A_3 receptor inhibit the activity of adenyl cyclase. Calcium-channel blockers and indomethacin inhibit adenosine reuptake, and benzodiazepines increase the release of adenosine. A fairly successful way to perform benzodiazepine withdrawal in patients is to prescribe dipyridamole, an adenosine-reuptake inhibitor, and then much more rapidly taper the benzodiazepine than in a standard protocol.

Dipyridamole raises cAMP and cGMP levels as well as increasing adenosine by inhibiting its reuptake. Adenosine induces the synthesis of neurotrophins and pleiotrophins from glial cells and acts in concert with growth factors. It induces the release of growth factors and cytokines. Adenosine has been noted to be a mediator of interleukin-1 beta-induced hippocampal synaptic inhibition in an article from Harvey Moldofsky's group in Toronto, Canada. They found that brief application of subfemtomolar interleukin-1 beta causes a profound decrease of glutamate transmission but not GABAergic inhibition in hippocampal CA1 pyramidal neurons. This effect of interleukin-1 beta is prevented by pharmacologic blockade of adenosine A_1 receptors. Dipyridamole is thought to not cross the blood-brain barrier well but does so in a rat model of brain ischemia. It may also be more brain permeable in patients experiencing stressful conditions. Chronic adenosine therapy produces plasma adenosine elevations in normal human subjects. In the spinal dorsal horn, ATP is coreleased as a fast excitatory neurotransmitter at the P2X purinergic receptor concomitantly with the inhibitory neurotransmitter GABA, or with NE. ATP is metabolized into adenosine, which may fine tune GABA release in the dorsal horn and elsewhere.

"The co-release of an excitatory (ATP) and an inhibitory (GABA) neurotransmitter at the same synapse could have important functional implications, because it may allow a reversible switch between inhibitory and excitatory roles of a given synapse without any anatomical reorganization of the neuronal circuitry" (Jo Y-H, Schlichter R, 1999). This process would be an example of instantaneous neural-network reconfiguration. Manipulations that increase extracellular adenosine concentration enhance antinociception produced by opioids (Kyle GJ, DeLander GE, 1994).

I am not aware that dipyridamole has been tested in this manner. An adenosine A_1-receptor agonist has been shown to inhibit an NMDA-mediated windup in spinal neurons. It probably has this effect by decreasing the release of glutamate and may act as a neuroprotectant.

In the spinal cord, adenosine kinase is more important than adenosine deaminase in regulating adenosine levels. Adenosine-like gabapentin inhibits the release of the nociceptive mediators calcitonin gene-related peptide, and substance P. A_1- and A_3-receptor activation decreases intracellular cAMP, and A_2 activation increases it. A_1 agonists more than A_2 agonists have been found to block the effects of an NMDA-receptor antagonist and thus have been suggested as possible antipsychotics (Popoli P et al., 1997).

The functional neuroanatomy of adenosine-dopamine interactions has been discussed (Ferre S, 1997). Ferre suggests that A_2 and D_2, and A_1 and D_1 receptors oppose each other, i.e., adenosine and dopamine have essentially opposite effects. A_{2A} agonists could therefore be used as antipsychotics and/or administered concomitantly with D_2-receptor antagonists such as haloperidol to reduce extrapyramidal side effects. Dopaminergic D_2 innervation in the nucleus accumbens and other areas affects interpretation of which stimuli are salient and has arousing or alerting properties. The situation is complicated by the fact that the nucleus accumbens has a "core" and a "shell" with quite different functional properties. Its functional neuroanatomy is quite complex (Heimer L et al., 1997). A_2 agonists or antagonists could be used in this model to modulate salience, a critical determination in neurosomatic disorders.

Papaverine, which is also an inhibitor of adenosine uptake, may produce anxiolysis and may have antidepressant properties.

The fact that adenosine receptors are present on axons themselves and not just axon terminals is a complicating variable in the interpretation of adenosine administration by various routes such as eyedrops, nasal sprays, or oral swirls.

People who respond to benzodiazepines tend to respond to adenosine, although such is not always the case. Thyrotropin-releasing hormone when delivered in eyedrops or by intranasal application may modulate patients' symptomatology. One of the major effects of TRH is that of a benzodiazepine-receptor antagonist. It increases dopamine and serotonin and releases calcium from intracellular stores. It may also increase levels of nitric oxide. BZDs block adenosine uptake, decrease A_1-receptor binding, and downregulate A_2 receptors after chronic treatment.

Adenosine, therefore, would have a rationale for use in patients reacting negatively to topical TRH administered to modulate trigeminal nerve activity. There is not always concordance between the response to intranasal versus intravenous TRH. In this situation, I must consider that intranasal TRH does not affect the same receptor(s) as the fourth- or fifth-order neuron it ultimately influences. I am also stimulating trigeminal axonal receptors for TRH which have yet to be demonstrated. Usually, however, there is a similarity between the effects on trigeminal receptors (of whatever sort) and systemic administration.

Adenosine is unique among nucleotides in its involvement in virtually every organ system through four receptors, A_1, A_{2A}, A_{2B}, and A_3. Caffeine blocks A_{2A} receptors and increases dopamine secretion. A_{2A} receptors are hyperalgesic, A_1 receptors are hypoalgesic. Blocking A_{2A} receptors, which are inhibitory on some GABAergic neurons, can increase dopamine secretion in the striatum as well as the nucleus accumbens and olfactory tubercle. I use Adenocard (adenosine), which is prepared in a parenteral solution for treating supraventricular tachycardia, in 1:10 and 1:1 solutions for conjunctival and intranasal instillation. Those given by the conjunctival route work in about one second, since the speed of neural conduction is 250 miles per hour. Intranasal administration requires 15 seconds because the mucous barrier must be penetrated before the neurons in the second division of the trigeminal nerve are stimulated. I would like to stimulate the A_1 receptors so that I can reduce pain, although stimulating or blocking adenosine receptors have numerous other potential effects. Placing ligands in the eye or in the nose ultimately affects fourth- or fifth-order receptors. The sensitivity of peripheral targets may not represent the state of the adenosine receptor in target areas in the brain. For example, sometimes adenosine or haloperidol nasal sprays act as decongestants. Dipyridamole is an adenosine-reuptake inhibitor and a weak phosphodiesterase-5 (PDE5) inhibitor. The purported muscle relaxant Soma, or carisoprodol, is related to meprobamate. Both medications probably work by stimulating the adenosine A_1 receptor. In fact, many patients who respond to Soma can switch directly to dipyridamole without having any withdrawal symptoms. Adenosine A_{2A}-receptor antagonists may be new agents for the treatment of Parkinson's disease, and adenosine may have a neuroprotective effect. In many cases, adenosine is generated by extracellular metabolism of ATP and helps to finely tune GABAergic inhibitory postsynaptic currents. Viewed in this manner, adenosine would be a neuromodulator rather than a neurotransmitter since it is not secreted by a vesicular mechanism. The A_1 receptor is highly and widely expressed in the brain, particularly in the cortex, cerebellum, thalamus, and hippocampus. Adenosine-mediated effects that occur via the A_1 receptor include depression of neurotransmission, antinociception, A_{2A}-induced motor incoordination, autonomic control of cardiac function, bronchoconstriction, negative chronotropy, inotropy, and dromotropy, anti-beta-adrenoceptor action, and renal sodium retention. The functions of the adenosine receptors have been reviewed in many recent articles, particularly that of J. W. Nyce (1999).

There appears to be a site of action common to benzodiazepines, meprobamate, carisoprodol, and ideally buspirone which potentiates opioid antagonists. It has been well accepted for some time that removal of the opioidergic inhibition of GABAergic neurons with naloxone would reinforce the inhibitory effect of benzodiazepines on other neurons. Drugs such as meprobamate (propanediols) do not show this effect in response to naloxone, but one site involved in all of these potentially anxiolytic drugs is the adenosine receptor (Belzung C et al., 2000). Benzodiazepines, meprobamate, and carisoprodol may inhibit adenosine uptake. Because opioids inhibit adenyl cyclase, and activation of the A_2 receptor inhibits adenyl cyclase and has an anxiolytic effect, blockade of opioid receptors would, therefore, remove the opposing opioid action, which could potentiate activities at the A_1 receptor. Thus, anxiolytic medications may be potentiated by opioid antagonists, since opioids have multiple actions at the cellular level, including blocking calcium entry and activation of potassium channels. It is possible that clinically subeffective doses of anxiolytic drugs may be potentiated by substances such as naltrexone. Buspirone and fluoxetine can have an action on the 5-HT_{1A} receptor which can be augmented by the addition of naltrexone (Belzung C et al., 2000). Buspar acts as a P_2 antagonist and is metabolized into an alpha$_2$ adrenoceptor antagonist.

I have little to say about amoxapine except that it is an effective antidepressant as well as an effective antipsychotic. These properties make it somewhat useful in the treatment of schizoaffective disorder. Amoxapine may be used in the interval when switching from one antidepressant to another, particularly when using MAOIs. The problem of tardive dyskinesia is always an issue. Medications related to amoxapine, such as loxapine, are being marketed as atypical neuroleptics. Amoxapine is one of the antidepressants among many which have been found to decrease SP concentration in the striatum, substantia nigra, and amygdala. All antidepressants tested thus far have had this effect. Substance P antagonists, which do not have an analgesic effect, are being developed for use in treatment of mood disorders (Shirayama Y et al., 1996).

Amoxapine has been found to be a potent inhibitor of the glycine$_{2A}$ transporter (Nunez E et al., 2000) and may act as a unique type of NMDA/glycine antagonist. Glycine is excitatory as an NMDA-receptor coagonist and is a classical neurotransmitter at inhibitory ion-channel receptors. The majority of glycine receptors are found in the spinal cord and brainstem, but some are more rostral. GABA, glycine, and nicotine receptors belong to the same superfamily. GABA and glycine are the two major inhibitory neurotransmitters in the CNS. Receptors for both act by increasing chloride (Cl^-) conductance.

BACLOFEN

Baclofen remains one of the more useful agents in neurosomatic pharmacology. It is a $GABA_B$ agonist and could potentially be an abusable substance in that it may be biotransformed into gamma hydroxybutyrate (Bernasconi R et al., 1999). It is better known that gamma butyrolactone (GBL) can be hydrolyzed into GHB. GBL is more rapidly and more reproducibly absorbed than GHB. GHB has been reported to decrease pain and fatigue while enhancing slow-wave sleep in patients with fibromyalgia (Schorf MB et al., 1998).

(R)-baclofen is a structural analog of GABA and a specific agonist of $GABA_B$ receptors; it is inactive at $GABA_A$ and GHB binding sites. Baclofen inhibits the secretion of most neurotransmitters, except acetylcholine. GHB inhibits dopamine, and the actions of GHB can be indirectly antagonized by giving the nonspecific opioid-receptor antagonist naloxone. Numerous data suggest GHB interacts with $GABA_B$ receptors or with specific GHB receptors (Volpi R et al., 1997). As with GHB, baclofen protects against alcohol dependence and modifies cocaine self-administration in rats. People have gotten "high" from taking baclofen, although I have not observed this reaction in any of my patients. GHB and baclofen also modulate $GABA_A$ receptors. The benzodiazepine antagonist flumazenil, which acts at the $GABA_A$ receptor, attenuates the anxiolytic effect of GHB. There appears to be a functional interplay between receptors for GHB and $GABA_B$. It is thought that activation of both GHB and $GABA_B$ receptors might be required to produce the reinforcement of inhibitory post-synaptic potentials or the diminution of glutamate release, or both, which could explain misuse and abuse of GHB. GHB, however, differs from psychostimulants in that it appears to inhibit rather than activate dopamine release within the nucleus accumbens in rats. This property is shared by benzodiazepines and barbiturates. GHB may also have a cholinergic effect (Volpi R et al., 1997).

Baclofen is an interesting agent in other respects and is unique among medications available to the clinician. There is no direct baclofen antagonist at this time, although hydergine, forskolin, citalopram, triptans, oxytocin, valproate, ethosuximide, and reboxetine may serve that purpose.

The cellular basis of the antinociceptive action of baclofen seems to occur through a stimulation of presynaptic $GABA_B$ receptors, inhibiting release of glutamate and SP by blocking calcium channels in presynaptic nerve terminals. A postsynaptic $GABA_B$ receptor is also coupled to potassium channels. Activation of this receptor occurs at higher concentrations of baclofen, and its analgesic properties are uncertain. The anxiolytic action of baclofen may involve postsynaptic mechanisms. There may be subtypes of the $GABA_B$ receptor, but these have not been characterized yet. There do seem to be various $GABA_B$ receptor subunits, however (Ataka T et al., 2000). A $GABA_C$ receptor has been described (Zhang D et al., 2001).

All chronic antidepressant treatments upregulate $GABA_B$ receptors in the frontal cortex and hippocampus. It has been suggested that $GABA_B$ receptors do not appear to follow the "classical" rules of receptor regulation. Drugs that simulate the effect of GABA and are active at both the $GABA_A$ and $GABA_B$ receptors have been shown to be as effective as tricyclics in the treatment of depression. Such agents include progabide and the $GABA_A$-receptor agonist alprazolam (but not other benzodiazepines). A faster onset of therapeutic action occurs with alprazolam (Markou A et al., 1998).

GAMMA-AMINOBUTYRIC ACID (GABA)

Delineating GABAergic function succinctly is a daunting task, but some understanding is necessary to conceptualize the pathophysiology of neurosomatic disorders. When a postsynaptic glutamatergic neuron fires in response to a stimulus, GABAergic neurons that feed back to it are activated, and the response to a second stimulus will be smaller or inhibited. When an animal is in a learning mode, the feedback inhibition to the soma of the neuron is reduced and that to the dendrites is increased to maximize Hebbian function and to allow only strong signals to be processed ("filtering"). In order to permit the necessary sophistication of information processing, GABAergic cells, which are largely interneurons, are composed of distinct types that target different domains of the pyramidal cell membrane. It is not necessary to describe the various types (Paulsen O, Moser EI, 1998), but action potentials, begun at the initial segment of the axon, can back-propagate into the dendrites, possibly inducing LTP-like changes in concurrently active synapses. The GABAergic cells that target the dendrite could control the extent of the back-propagation and expression of (usually) NMDA activation in neighboring neurons, thereby regulating a type of synaptic plasticity. The activity of the pyramidal cell and GABAergic interneuron can oscillate, or resonate, producing phasing and synchronization. Such rhythmic activity occurs during encoding in the hippocampus.

In the hippocampus, pyramidal cells are termed "principal" cells. During the short-term learning (encoding) process just described, synaptic weights can be assigned to various stimuli by interneurons which specifically target dendrites, soma, or the axon initial segment. Synaptic weighting is dysfunctional in neurosomatic disorders. I discussed this problem in *Betrayal*. The GABAergic interneurons, which are modulated by other centers, determine the specificity of a synaptic network that is receiving input. The input neurons (NMDA) are probably modulated by the same centers that modulate the interneurons. In a typical situation, a generalized inhibition would be coupled with a disinhibition of relevant synapses. While the dendrites are receiving input, the axons would be inhibited until relevant input ceased. Back-propagation would be regulated, even rhythmically, by interneurons at the soma and dendrites so that only appropriately timed inputs will produce modification of the synaptic network (plasticity). If back-propagation is timed with input, the synapse is strengthened in a Hebbian manner.

GABAergic interneurons also help to determine *context,* or a stimulus environment changing much more slowly than the specific stimuli being learned. Context development in the hippocampus is thought to occur in the CA3 region. Rhythmic variance between afferent cells and different context-sensitive cells is switched by $GABA_B$-mediated conductance and thus can be disrupted by $GABA_B$ antagonists or, conversely, facilitated by baclofen. Stochastic resonance and Hebbian learning are also crucial to context formation (Wallenstein GB et al., 1998).

An example of decreased activity of GABAergic interneurons which inhibit pyramidal cell dendrites is seen in temporal lobe epilepsy. There is increased glutamatergic input for their targets, which include interneurons and the soma of principal cells. There is decreased function of the subset of GABAergic interneurons that innervate the dendrites, usually due to cell loss. Thus, excitatory input would be facilitated, as well as back-propagation of action potentials in neurons with NMDA receptors. The increase in somatic inhibition prevents status epilepticus. Increased excitatory input plus decreased dendritic inhibition would cause intermittent seizures (Cossart R et al., 2001).

GABA-mediated responses are quite heterogenous and occur rapidly. In addition to the domain-specific interneurons already discussed, we should examine GABAergic actions at the presynaptic, cleft, and postsynaptic levels. Besides presynaptic autoreceptors and heteroreceptors (often mu-opioid), GABA release can be modulated by astrocytes, which possess $GABA_B$ receptors. Binding of GABA to these receptors triggers glutamate release which activates glutamate receptors on interneurons, potentiating inhibitory synaptic transmission (Kang YS, Park JH, 2000).

In various proximities to the synapse are GABA transporters, or GATs (Figure 5). GAT-1 is localized in the vicinity of synapses and is inhibited by tiagabine, or Gabitril. GAT-2 and GAT-3 are more often found at a farther distance from the synapse and on astrocytes, where there is also an occasional GAT-1. The three GATs plus BGT-1 (not GAT-4) regulate the amount of GABA "spilled over" which could have a tonic GABA effect, desensitizing GABA receptors (GABARs) and autoreceptors (Cherubini E, Conti F, 2001).

The postsynaptic effects of GABA are determined in large part by GABARs, which consist of several of nineteen subunits, some of which have alternate splice variants. Different subunits are found in various areas of the brain. The alpha-6 subunit is found more in the cerebellum than elsewhere and confers sensitivity to blockade of the GABAR by furosemide, or Lasix, which is much less expensive than flumazenil to use in the office. An occasional patient, usually without fibromyalgia, will become more alert when given furosemide 20 mg. Its effect as a diuretic lasts two to three hours, but its effect as a GABAR antagonist may last 24 to 48 hours.

Zinc, which I have scarcely found useful at all, inhibits the GABAR to different degrees depending on subunit construction. Activation of the GABAR releases bicarbonate ion (HCO_3^-), raising pH. Increased pH can have increased, decreased, or no effect on the GABAR depending on its subunit composition, perhaps one reason why patient response to alkalinizing agents is so variable.

Neurosteroids also modulate the GABAR, again depending on its subunit composition. The subunit composition can change slightly in physiologic situations, decreasing inhibition produced by a substance such as allopregnanolone. Subunit alteration can trigger release of modulators that are usually tonically inhibited, such as oxytocin (Brussard AB, Herbison AE, 2000). Receptors containing certain subunits are insensitive to benzodiazepines (MacDonald RL, Olsen RW, 1994), perhaps explaining why certain patients have anxiety disorders that are benzodiazepine-insensitive.

The complexity of the GABAergic system is probably responsible for the GAT-1 inhibitor tiagabine being the most unpredictable medication I use. I certainly can't give a patient tiagabine who has responded to a BZD, AED, or any other agent and hope the response will be similar. Patients have become depressed, sedated, manic, or delirious, and I have little advance notion of the outcome. Mania and delirium have occurred when patients feel better after taking the first 4 mg and decided to take another rather than increasing the dose by 4 mg per week, as the manufacturers instruct. Adverse reactions to tiagabine are usually ameliorated by furosemide. Occasionally, I must administer flumazenil, which fortunately often works by nasal spray (1:10 is sufficient) rather than by the parenteral route, which is very expensive. Tiagabine is one of the least effective of the AEDs in treating neuro-somatic disorders, leading only levetiracetam, zonisamide, carbamazepine, oxcarbazepine, and ethosuximide in futility. At least Mysoline (primidone), which acts on the GABAR by metabolizing into phenobarbital, helps tremors and occasionally works as a hypnotic or a mood stabilizer.

In broader perspective, GABAergic agents are often indispensable in treating neurosomatic disorders, which are usually produced by NMDAR overactivity. Anxiety, or even hypervigilance, is not a necessary symptom for their effective use. Even ketamine, the single most useful medication in the neurosomatic pharmacopeia, has been shown to have $GABA_A$ agonist properties. Its anesthesia is potentiated by the $GABA_A$ antagonist bicuculline. Flumazenil, which is really a BZD antagonist, has no effect in this system (Irifune M et al., 2000).

The tuning of GABAergic interneurons and their intrinsic voltage-gated currents allows inhibitory neurons to generate and control rhythmic outputs of large populations of pyramidal/principal cells and often populations of inhibitory neurons. However, interneuronal populations are so diverse and are excited or inhibited by such a vast array of contributions of modulators that pharmacologic alteration of their function in any but the coarsest manner seems beyond the current state of the art and science. GABAergic neurons might be grouped, or "clustered," into anatomically defined populations that could lead to further functional understanding. Besides ionic channels and a multitude of receptors, interneurons also have "gap junctions," cellular appositions that allow for the passage of electric currents and small molecules through nonselective channels called "connexins," which are bidirectional. Rhythmic fluctuations of neuronal assembly membrane potentials can become salient for a neuronal coincidence detector of another assembly so that cross-modal communication can occur in the brain. Such "nesting of oscillations" has been suggested as a solution to the "binding problem"; i.e., how do different areas of the brain combine their information simultaneously (McBain CJ, Fisahn A, 2001)?

ADENOSINE TRIPHOSPHATE (ATP)

Because ATP is often cosecreted with NE, alpha$_1$-receptor antagonists might not be beneficial unless combined with an ATP blocker, such as a nontoxic version of suramin.

ATP receptors are also P_2 receptors. P_1 receptors are more sensitive to adenosine. "P" stands for purine. There are over ten P_2 receptors, subtyped as P2X and P2Y. ATP can be a cotransmitter with NE or Ach, or may be secreted alone from synaptic vesicles. It remains as ATP for about one second, before it is degraded into various compounds, notably adenosine mono-phosphate (AMP) and adenosine. ATP as a transmitter can have excitatory (via cAMP), biphasic, or inhibitory effects, based on its conversion to aden-osine, which inhibits cAMP (Figure 6).

P2X receptors are widespread in the brain, are excitatory, and are acted upon by ATP to open ligand-gated channels. P2X-receptor antagonists may have a role in glutamate release. P2Y receptors are G-protein coupled, acti-vate PLC, and increase $[Ca^{2+}]_i$ via IP_3 activation. P2Y receptors may medi-ate the ability of ATP to enhance the postsynaptic action of glutamate and may be involved in LTP.

A subject of recent investigation has been the role of ATP in extracellular signaling between neurons and glia (Fields DR, Stevens B, 2000). Astrocytes can detect the vesicular release of neurotransmitters. These glia can subse-quently regulate synaptic strength by releasing neurotransmitters, such as glutamate, into the synaptic cleft. ATP can be coreleased with mast cell se-cretory granules and stimulate an intracellular Ca^{2+} wave, in which levels of associated glial cells rapidly raise their Ca^{2+} and can affect the firing rate of neurons and release of neurotransmitters. This ATP-mediated wave is one possible method of communication within and between neural networks. The inhibitory effect of the adenosine derived from ATP may be reduced by inhibiting the ectonucleotidase that degrades ATP (Cotrina ML, Nedergaard M, 2000).

Synaptic transmission may propagate to neighboring glia and activate them by raising $[Ca^{2+}]_i$. The event stimulates gliotransmission to neurons or other glia. Stimulating glial AMPA receptors can result in enhanced pre-synaptic release of glutamate (Bergles DE et al., 2000). Gap junctions (electrotonic coupling) seem to be more common in neuron-glial or glial-glial communication.

GABAergic neurons also have electrical coupling through gap junctions. The proteins that form gap junctions are called connexins. Because electri-cal transmission is almost instantaneous, gap junctions are thought to partic-ipate in inducing or enhancing the synchronization of neighboring cells. Gap junctions are found between astrocytes and between astrocytes and neurons. Gap junctions between GABAergic interneurons have been found in the cerebellum, neocortex, hippocampus, neostriatum, and dorsal co-chlear nucleus. They are most commonly seen between two dendritic pro-cesses but also occur between dendrite and soma or two somata. The den-drites of GABAergic interneurons can extend to two hundred micrometers, and gap junctions can occur along the entire length of the process.

Networks of astrocytic or GABAergic cells joined by electrical synapses can facilitate precise synchronous spiking of a network of cells and also influ-ence oscillation frequency (Galarreta M, Hestrin S, 2001a) to coordinate such functions as sensory input, attention, and motor output. Synchronously firing neurons, even if widely separated, are responding to the same stimulus.

Astrocytes almost exclusively surround synapses with docked vesicles ("ready-release pool"). There are other pools of vesicles in neuron terminals, and the mechanism by which they enter the ready-release pool is not well understood. Dysregulated vesicular movement could be an aspect of synaptic fatigue. Perhaps astrocytes are involved in this process. Cytoskeletal protein function and BDNF play important roles. If physical exercise helps fibromyalgia, growth hormone secretion is increased. IGF-1 increases in the liver and is transported to the brain, where it stimulates BDNF secretion (Carro E et al., 2000).

One cause of synaptic fatigue could be inadequate synthesis of proteins involved in moving vesicles from storage pools into the ready-release pools. Synaptophysin and synaptobrevin are two proteins known to be involved in vesicle docking and fusion with the presynaptic membrane so that vesicle exocytosis occurs. Synthesis of these proteins is regulated by BDNF. If the neuron terminal is not exposed to sufficient BDNF, there is a significant reduction in docked vesicles. I have no reason yet to suspect that BDNF levels are low in patients with neurosomatic disorders. Such events occur in glial cells as well and are mediated by acetylcholine acting at muscarinic receptors. Paired-pulse depression, synaptic fatigue, and impairment of LTP can result from a decreased basal level of the activated Ca^{2+}/CaMKII. Dysregulation of other components of the kinase/phosphatase system might be implicated as well.

Small parts of the glia ("microdomains") can interact with neurons they ensheath and in which they elevate $[Ca^{2+}]_i$ an area of 100 square micrometers or less (Grosche J et al., 1999). Neuron-glia communication is much more complex than previously thought, as is everything else in neurobiology.

Glial activation in the perisynaptic area can occur with almost all classical neurotransmitters, as well as with adenosine, probably by overflow binding to glial receptors. $[Ca^{2+}]_i$ increases can start Ca^{2+} waves that can propagate for millimeters in a local neuron-glia network. Glutamate and ATP are involved in the propagation of the Ca^{2+} waves. Glia secrete ATP to bind to receptors on a neighboring glia cell, acting through the purinergic P2Y receptor, often at gap junctions. Prostaglandins are also involved in Ca^{2+} waves and release of gliotransmitters (Bezzi P, Volterra A, 2001). When glutamate receptors on an astrocyte are bound, NGF, PGE_2, and possibly NO are released to enhance calcium signaling. D-serine may be a similar neuromodulator, suggesting the use of cycloserine, NO-forming compounds, and essential fatty acids as pharmacotherapy for dysregulated glial neuromodulation. IP_3 molecules may pass through gap junctions. Heparin can block IP_3. Numerous agents which increase the activity of phospholipase C (as well as inositol) could stimulate IP_3 once it binds to the ER. IP_3 can be metabolized to other neuroactive compounds. Glial exocytosis, perhaps through vesicles, has been hypothesized. Immunoreactivity for D-serine is very high in glial cells. D-serine is released after AMPA binding to act as an agonist at the NMDA/glycine site. Proinflammatory cytokines may also be released after glial activation.

Astrocytes in the hippocampus have $GABA_B$ receptors. When occupied by GABA overflow, they increase $[Ca^{2+}]_i$, release glutamate, and potentiate inhibitory neurotransmission (Kang J et al., 1998).

Glial cells are involved in brain metabolic function, consuming most of the glucose that enters the glycolytic pathway. The astrocytes then export lactate to the neuron for oxidative metabolism. Astrocytic glycolysis is almost exclusively driven by glutamate uptake and cycling (Sibson NR et al., 1998).

ATP has been recognized as an important transmitter, often coreleased with glutamate, Ach, GABA, or glycine. The receptors for ATP are ligand-gated and ionic. They are designated $P2X_{1-7}$. $P2X_2$ receptors directly interact with nicotinic cholinergic receptors, and when they do, $P2X_2$ is the dominant partner (Kakh BS et al., 2000). The channel of P2X receptors is widened by ATP and by PKC-mediated phosphorylation of the P2X receptor (Robertson SJ et al., 2001).

Corelease of GABA and ATP may be common but seemingly counterproductive since GABA is a fast inhibitory neurotransmitter and ATP is a fast excitatory neurotransmitter. Depending on local conditions or firing rate, a synapse could switch from inhibitory to excitatory, perhaps involving GABA receptors modulated by Ca^{2+} influx and adenosine-receptor activation. P2X receptors can be blocked by several Ca^{2+}-channel antagonists. It is thought that the P2X receptor promotes Ca^{2+} influx. Presynaptically, P2X receptors modulate the release of GABA, glutamate, glycine, and vasopressin. This presynaptic modulation can be blocked by substance P. ATP release may be a double-edged sword. ATP can increase miniature glutamatergic excitatory postsynaptic potentials, but since ATP is rapidly metabolized to adenosine, activation and glutamate release can be inhibited by adenosine acting at the P1 receptor.

Realizing that the glial cells are complex and multipotential and probably have a role in nociception are important discoveries. It is not possible for me to determine at this time whether to target glia for my therapy. Even if I were to know, will the same medications I use now, ostensibly to modulate neuronal function, be effective in glial cells, or is their neurobiology so different they will require medications of their own? Probably the same drugs will affect both neurons and glia.

Numerous roles for ATP as a transmitter are not germane to this volume. The secretion of ATP, however, may be greatly attenuated by blocking sodium (Na^+) channels by tetrodotoxin (TTX) or by lidocaine and related substances. It is often difficult to understand the mechanism of action of these agents in a particular clinical situation. Decreasing ATP release and its binding to P2X and P2Y receptors might help clarify a particular situation, perhaps migraine headache, in which ATP may release inflammatory mediators.

Extracellular ATP may function as a phosphate donor acting as a cofactor for the phosphorylation of cell-surface proteins and extracellular ligands by ecto-protein kinases present in different cell types (Redgold FA et al., 1999). Ectophosphorylation is involved in regulation of neural cell adhesion, Ca^{2+} influx, and neurotransmitter and Mg^{2+} uptake. LTP is thought to be regulated by protein kinase activity present at the cell surface of hippocampal pyramidal neurons acting on protein kinase C. Ectophosphorylation stabilizes LTP. Ecto-protein kinases may be candidates for pharmacologic manipulation in neurosomatic disorders. Because behavior in these illnesses is overlearned, perhaps hippocampal function could be therapeutically inhibited.

LORAZEPAM NASAL SPRAY

I use Ativan (lorazepam) nasal spray 1:10. The primary benefit of this preparation is to abort panic attacks. It may also be used as an ophthalmic drop. The drops work in one or two seconds. The nasal spray works within 15 to 30 seconds. Ativan solution is helpful in receptor profiling and may reverse the effects of other medications. It is much appreciated by my patients with panic disorder.

ANTIBIOTICS

Almost all antibiotics appear to have psychotropic functions. These are mainly reported in the context of adverse reactions but can be used therapeutically. The neuropsychopharmacologic effect of most antibiotics is as GABA antagonists. They may have drug interactions with agents more commonly regarded as psychotropic. The prototypical antibiotic for inhibition of the synaptic activity of both the $GABA_A$ and the $GABA_B$ receptors is penicillin. I can recall during dog lab in my medical school physiology course inducing grand mal seizures by giving very high doses of intravenous penicillin, thereby inhibiting the main inhibitory neurotransmitter in the brain. Neurotoxic reactions with permanent behavioral and psychiatric features have been associated more with procaine penicillin than other penicillins. This phenomenon occurs because of inadvertent intravenous injection of procaine penicillin with liberation of free procaine, which has an epileptogenic effect of its own. All local anesthetics, when injected parenterally, may have an action somewhat like cocaine. Those with intrinsic vasoconstrictor properties, such as procaine, are more cocaine-like, although lidocaine can potentiate the action of cocaine. The cephalosporins and other beta-lactam agents antagonize GABA, as do the aminoglycosides.

The aminoglycosides activate the NMDA receptor at the polyamine site. This property is dissociable from their antibiotic activity and may be responsible for vestibular and cochlear toxicity (Harvey SC et al., 2000).

Oseltamivir phosphate (Tamiflu) is proving to be a useful agent in treating neurosomatic disorders. Its only known model of action is inhibiting viral neuraminidase, but many patients find that it makes them feel more alert.

Some antitubercular agents are MAOIs, e.g., isoniazid, or INH. INH can have an excitatory effect on the central nervous system causing apprehension, excitement, tremor, and seizures by lowering levels of GABA through inhibition of the enzyme responsible for GABA synthesis: L-glutamate decarboxylase. This enzyme requires the active form of vitamin B_6, or pyridoxine, as a coenzyme.

I have not had occasion to use rifampin therapeutically in neurosomatic patients since its main side effect is on liver drug-metabolizing enzymes. I prescribe cycloserine (Seromycin) frequently since it is a partial agonist at the glycine coagonist site of the NMDA receptor. I may use this agent or lamotrigine (Lamictal) when I treat patients with adverse reactions to NMDA-receptor antagonists. Lamictal blocks the action of ketamine by decreasing the secretion of glutamate (Anand A, Charney DS, et al., 2000). Pentazocine (Talwin) also may reverse the action of NMDA antagonists and decrease 5-HT and DA activity (Takahashi S et al., 1999). Chronic administration of a glycine partial agonist can alter the expression of NMDA receptor subunit mRNAs (Bovetto S et al., 1997). I know of no other therapeutic technique to alter subunit expression of any receptor. In the case of chronic cycloserine treatment, a decrease in NMDA-receptor sensitivity would be expected.

An interesting pharmacologic dissection can be made by giving an individual ketamine nasal spray, observing an adverse reaction, then giving glutamate nasal spray, a preparation which will stimulate receptors on the trigeminal nerve. Sometimes the adverse reactions are not entirely eliminated. Glutamate would theoretically overcome an NMDA-receptor block.

However, if the problem is hypersensitivity of the AMPA/kainate receptors produced by blocking the NMDA receptor, more glutamate would be made available for binding to the AMPA/kainate receptors. In this situation, it would be appropriate to administer an agent that blocks AMPA receptors, such as topiramate (Topamax), which I have yet to use as a nasal spray. Cycloserine has been administered to treat negative symptoms of schizophrenia with mixed results and is probably not a good agent for this purpose. Better results have been obtained when using this drug to improve general alertness in normal young and middle-aged patients. I primarily use cycloserine 250 mg when an individual has an adverse reaction to an NMDA-receptor antagonist such as ketamine. It may sometimes act as a narcotic antagonist, since ketamine potentiates opioids. Cycloserine is most effective in antagonizing adverse reactions to probenecid, which slows CSF excretion of kynurenate, an endogenous glycine-site antagonist. $5-HT_3$ receptor antagonists, such as ondansetron and tropisetron, are glycine-site antagonists, as is atropine; the latter drug has rarely helped any of my patients except those with seasickness. Intravenous tropisetron has been reported effective in treating fibromyalgia. Some Ca^{2+}-channel blockers (I think diltiazem is the best) are glycine-site antagonists, as is (I think) guaifenesin. $5-HT_3$-receptor antagonists, probenecid, and ketamine do not synergize. I shall discuss this subject further on the section on the many ways to antagonize the NMDA receptor.

A biologically active form of the amino acid glycine called Bioglycin acts like cycloserine. It seems to work as a cognitive enhancer, but in experimental groups "Bioglycin significantly improved retrieval from episodic memory in both the young and the middle-aged groups, but it did not affect focused or undivided attention . . . it primarily improved memory rather than attention" (File SE et al., 1999, p. 506). The macrolides include clarithromycin, erythromycin, troleandomycin, and azithromycin. Biaxin (clarithromycin) is the one that I have chosen to put on my treatment list since it is well tolerated. It appears to have a GABA antagonist effect and has the potential to stimulate the brain motilin receptor.

Another group of antibiotic agents are the quinolones. Nalidixic acid is the prototypical quinolone, and more recently, norfloxacin, ciprofloxacin, and others have been added to the therapeutic armamentarium. Quinolones have had many adverse neuropsychiatric reactions reported in association with their administration, and it has been suggested that the CNS excitation seen with quinolones is a result of displacement of GABA from its receptors. When investigating the kynurenic pathway of tryptophan metabolism, one sees that quinolones are a major end product of the kynurenic acid shunt which begins with tryptophan. Some of the quinolones have properties of an NMDA-receptor agonist. This propensity may be another mechanism of action for the neurotoxicity of quinolones. Pro-drugs, agents which are metabolized into active drugs, for kynurenine or inhibitors of enzymes that manufacture quinolones from tryptophan are in development (Stone TW, 2000).

Metronidazole (Flagyl) may cause temporary activation of psychosis in some patients and could increase their responsiveness to subsequent psychotropic drug treatment. Metronidazole may have a dose window in which excitation can occur. Agitated depression and atypical postpartum psychosis as well as panic attacks have been reported with the use of metronidazole. The combination of disulfiram (Antabuse) with metronidazole has been reported to cause paranoid delusions with auditory and visual hallucinations in six of 29 men treated with it for chronic alcohol dependence. One must wonder whether the use of metronidazole to treat alleged intestinal infections with *Giardia* may be having a neuropsychopharmacologic effect to improve the patient's well-being rather than by eliminating putative chronic giardiasis. It should be noted that chronic giardiasis can produce an immunologic cytokine response which can have an effect on neurobehavioral function.

The primary exception to most antibiotics (and acyclovir) being GABA antagonists is found with tetracycline and minocycline but not with doxycycline and others of the group. The tetracyclines may have an effect similar to lithium. Antiemetic and antidepressant effects appear to be associated with tetracyclines (Sternbach H, State R, 1997). Tetracylines, particularly minocycline, are NMDA-receptor antagonists and often have that effect 30 minutes after administration. Both minocycline and tetracycline, but not doxycycline, can block NMDA-induced excitotoxicity by inhibiting NMDA-induced increases in $[Ca^{2+}]_i$, most likely via a direct action with the NMDA receptor itself.

ENDOTHELIN (ET)

I have included bosentan in my medication list because I believe endothelin to be significantly involved in neurosomatic disorders. I have demonstrated a possible hypersecretion of this substance in the spinal fluid of patients with fibromyalgia which I published in *Betrayal by the Brain* in association with I. Jon Russell. The vasoconstriction that we see in almost all functional brain imaging of patients with neurosomatic disorders may be due to excess endothelin production rather than decreased metabolic activity, and bosentan is an endothelin-receptor antagonist. The physiology of brain endothelin has been recently reviewed, and the substance is "thought to be deeply involved in the central autonomic control and consequent cardiorespiratory homeostasis" (Kuwaki T et al., 1997, p. 545). I have believed for several years that blood flow as visualized in functional brain imaging is not always coupled to metabolism and is often an epiphenomenon of release of vasoactive substances with numerous other effects on neuronglial function. This view diverges from mainstream research findings (Heeger DJ, Ress D, 2002).

Endothelin is strategically located in a region of the brain to regulate autonomic activity and is present in the cerebrospinal fluid at concentrations higher than in the plasma. Endothelin is released by primary cultures of hypothalamic neurons, and when endothelin binds to its receptors, intracellular calcium mobilization occurs in neurons and glia via PLC activation and/or by opening the calcium channels. In this manner, it acts similarly to TRH and honey bee venom and could be opposed by heparin.

Endothelin, the Autonomic Nervous System, and Neurosomatic Disorders

As if I didn't know already that researchers were reinventing the wheel, I read an astonishing editorial that fibromyalgia symptoms may be caused by autonomic nervous system dysfunction (Martinez-Levin M, Hermosillo AG, 2000). I tremble to read that the earth revolves around the sun.

It has been proposed that we dispense with the term and concept of the autonomic nervous system (Blessing WW, 1997). The term ANS implies a separation from the brain, with a greater degree of independence than actually exists. The programs that code for the physiologic and behavioral patterning we associate with the ANS are set in the brain, not in the autonomic ganglia. Blessing suggests that we use terms "visceral afferents and efferents" so that these neurons can be viewed as representing one mechanism whereby the brain communicates with the bodily organs to maintain homeostasis (or allostasis).

I shall also mourn the passing of the term "limbic system." It is certainly, as Broca noted, "limbic," but unfortunately it is not a system. Its parts do not work in a unified manner, and, in an attempt to make it a system in my book *Chronic Fatigue Syndromes: The Limbic Hypothesis* (1993), I eventually included so many areas of the brain that the concept became unwieldy. Yet I cannot ignore paraneoplastic limbic encephalitis. This disorder must occur because limbic neurons have distinctive antigens. Why is it so? The concepts of the ANS and the limbic system still require integration.

So, too, for the brainstem neuronal groups still called the ascending reticular activating system, once conceived as a chain of neurons with short dendrites. The activating fields of these neurons eventually, with further study, became so overlapping that they ceased to have a place in functional neuroanatomy.

Blessing suggests what seems like a good working model: There should be three classes of CNS neurons: (1) those that receive direct input from visceral afferents, (2) those that innervate visceral motoneurons in peripheral ganglia, and (3) interneurons that are monosynaptically connected to central input and output neurons. Using these reference points, loops, circuits, and networks may be described that operate as part of a unified whole. I shall defer such changes in nomenclature to my next book, if then.

RESPIRATORY RHYTHM REGULATION IN FIBROMYALGIA SYNDROME

Knock-out mice for endothelin-1 exhibit cardiorespiratory abnormalities including elevation of arterial pressure, sympathetic overactivity, and impairment of the respiratory reflex. One of the most reproducible findings in my patients with fibromyalgia came from the exercise physiology laboratory. I reported it in *Betrayal* but did not understand enough about respiratory rhythm generation to integrate this unusual abnormality into neurosomatic pathophysiology. I'm not sure that I do even now, but at least I can give it a try.

Patients rode a bicycle and had various functions monitored, receiving a brain SPECT before and after exercise. A marked variability in tidal volume (the amount of air inhaled and exhaled) was noted at maximal tolerated exertion, a strange result not previously noted in any patient population. An individual should inhale and exhale as much as possible when maximally exercising, but tidal volumes were almost random. This abnormality was much more common in patients with diffuse pain and tender points than in neurosomatic patients without diffuse pain. In fact, it was the only objective way that I could differentiate FMS patients from non-FMS patients ten years ago. Since then, considerable research in the neurophysiology of breathing has been summarized (Richter DW et al., 2000; Richter DW, Spyer KM, 2001).

Although the respiratory arrhythmia found in my FMS patients was not discussed, the oscillatory network of early inspiratory and postinspiratory neurons was described in this article. Respiratory rhythm is generated in and around the pre-Botzinger complex, a morphologically defined region in the lower brainstem. The network is regulated by various neuromodulators, all of which are important in neurosomatic disorders (Figure 7), especially SP acting at the neurokinin-1R. Because patients with fibromyalgia have elevated CSF SP and NGF, these substances may be responsible for the tidal volume irregularity we saw.

Such disturbances most often originate from an unbalanced activation of excitatory processes in the network while inhibitory processes are weakened (Richter DW et al., 2000). This sentence refers to breath holding, which can be caused by brainstem lesions and can be treated with the 5-HT_{1A} agonist buspirone (Figure 8). It does not appear that variable tidal volume is related to inspiring or expiring too much.

Adenosine A_1 agonists depress respiration when given systemically, and A_1 antagonists stimulate it. A_1-receptor agonists hyperpolarize respiratory neurons via cAMP-mediated activation of various potassium currents, including opening the K_{ATP} channel. The K_{ATP} channel is opened depending on the availability of intracellular ATP to which it is coupled. Both adenosine and gabapentin decrease pain in many patients with FMS by decreasing hyperactive neuronal activity. Gabapentin selectively opens K_{ATP} channels. K^+ channels open after each inspiration to inhibit "burst-firing" neurons that stimulate inspiration. The opening and closing of the K_{ATP} channel is regulated by transmitters and receptors, prime candidates being metabotropic glutamate receptors. mGluR1 and mGluR5 inhibit K_{ATP} channels, while mGluR2 and mGluR3 activate them.

Richter and colleagues (2000) further state: "Enhanced synaptic interactions within the respiratory network lead to spillover of glutamate out of the synaptic cleft, which results in a long-lasting stimulation of para- or extrasynaptic mGluRs" (p. 192). This situation would apply in a patient with NMDA-receptor hyperactivity. If the neurons of the pre-Botzinger complex have both inhibitory and facilitatory mGluRs, than glutamate spillover could affect them randomly, which is just what seems to happen with the tidal volume fluctuations of the exercising fibromyalgia patients. Ligands for mGluRs should therefore be important agents in neurosomatic medicine when they become available.

When we published our results of brain SPECT in CFS patients with and without fibromyalgia (Goldstein JA et al., 1995), we found the same regional hypoperfusion in both groups, but the degree of hypoperfusion was greater in FMS patients. I could hypothesize that FMS patients have a greater NMDA hyperactivity and more spillover, while CFS patients without diffuse pain may have a greater relative deficit in DA/NE modulation of the NMDA-receptor complex. This model would account for the greater propensity of CFS patients to respond to agents that primarily increase DA and NE neurotransmission. All neurosomatic patients who respond to treatment reduce their global cerebral blood flow. DA and NE are vasoconstrictors. Central DA has been associated with cerebral cortical microcirculation. DA terminals are closely apposed to microvessels within the cortex, and exogenous DA causes microvessels in the brain to contract (Krimer LS et al., 1998). DA terminals are found in apposition to NE terminals on microvessels on a much more frequent basis, particularly in the frontal cortex. They can thus adjust microcirculation and neuronal activity in a discrete cortical location simultaneously. I speculated about the role of DA in cortical circulation but did not have enough information to draw a conclusion. The action of NO as a vasodilator might be important. If NMDA-receptor blockade is a final common pathway of therapeutic improvement in neurosomatic disorders, then NO secretion would be decreased, since NMDA postreceptor events are important in the regulation of NO synthesis.

There are three different kinds of endothelin, 1, 2 and 3, and two endothelin receptors for them, A and B. I have discussed endothelin fairly extensively in *Betrayal by the Brain* and see no reason to alter the opinions expressed in that volume. Many, if not most, of the symptoms related to neurosomatic disorders are caused by autonomic dysfunction which may be a result of inappropriate endothelin secretion. Blocking endothelin receptors may be an important way to treat neurosomatic disorders in the future, and numerous agents are in development to affect endothelin function. I use bosentan only as an example because it was one of the first endothelin antagonists to be synthesized. Endothelin seems to preferentially affect those parts of the sensorimotor system that are related to the stress response. Endothelin also regulates oxytocin and vasopressin secretion as well as supraspinal brainstem neurons that control sympathetic activity. The ET(B) receptor is present in dopaminergic neurons in the ventral striatum, and endothelin causes DA release by ET(B) activation.

Patients with CFS are usually hypotensive, although they may have rapid and marked perturbations in blood pressure that seem to be indicative of impaired central cardiovascular regulation. Endothelin-1 is a constitutive substance involved in normal central neural control of cardiorespiratory and sympathetic function. Endothelin-1 is the most potent vasoconstrictor of the three, but it also acts at ET(B) receptors on vascular endothelial cells to produce vasodilators such as nitric oxide and prostaglandin E2 which partly offset the increase in the vascular tone. If endothelin-1 is applied iontophoretically to single vasomotor and respiratory-related neurons in the rostral ventrolateral medulla, a presumed site of the cardiorespiratory center, a vast majority of these neurons respond to it.

Endothelin-1 may be involved in pain, particularly inflammatory pain, and this nociception is mediated largely via ET(A) receptors. Endothelin-1-induced nociception can be effectively prevented by prior IV treatment with the mixed ET(A)/ET(B)-receptor antagonist bosentan or a selective ET(A)-receptor antagonist. A selective ET(B)-receptor antagonist will not prevent endothelin-1-induced nociception.

Most sympathetic ganglionic neurons can express considerable quantities of both endothelin-3 and endothelin-1 and have been suggested to rapidly release the former into the circulation during exercise. The reversibility of interactions of endothelins with their receptors can be remarkably slow, and thus it is possible that postexertional relapse of neurosomatic disorders, especially pain, may be caused in part by a dysfunctional reaction to endothelin secretion (De-Melo JD et al., 1998). We saw the same reduction in global cerebral blood flow 24 to 48 hours after exercise as we did immediately afterward (Goldstein JA, 1996).

Endothelin stimulates phospholipase-D in striatal astrocytes. In glial cells endothelin can act as a growth factor, stimulating both the synthesis and secretion of NGF. Nerve growth factor has been found to be elevated in the spinal fluid of patients with fibromyalgia, one of the few distinguishing differences between fibromyalgia and CFS (Giovengo et al., 1999). Endothelin receptors are members of the G-protein-coupled receptor family, and endothelin causes an IP_3- evoked mobilization of calcium from intracellular stores. Endothelin also activates PLA_2 and inhibits adenylate cyclase activity while increasing tyrosine phosphorylation of several proteins including MAP kinase (Desagher S et al., 1997).

Endothelin-induced nociception appears to be a unique kind of pain. It is not alleviated by cyclooxygenase inhibitors but is reduced by certain benzodiazepines. Such patients might respond well to benzodiazepines in the treatment of their fibromyalgia. BZDs appear to antagonize the effect of endothelin-1, but the site of the antagonism is presumably not at the endothelin receptors. BZDs might be involved with the mechanism of ischemic pain in general (Raffa RB et al., 1996).

When endothelin agonists are administered centrally in the rat, blood pressure is lowered and sympathetic nerve activity is decreased by 61 percent (Gulati A et al., 1997). This finding is even more suggestive of the dysautonomia that is seen in patients with neurosomatic disorders. Endothelin has also been implicated in migraine headaches, a very common entity in patients with neurosomatic disorders. In migraine, endothelin, acting through ET(B) receptors, may play an important role in mediating neurogenic inflammation in the meninges of rats. It was noted that the profile of activity of bosentan was similar to that of the $5\text{-HT}_{1B/D}$ agonists sumatriptan and ergot alkaloids: "One may speculate that ET receptor antagonists might be potentially effective in the treatment of acute migraine attacks" (Brändli P et al., 1995).

These authors believe that since bosentan does not inhibit SP extravasation, then it antagonizes prejunctional ET(B) receptors, thereby preventing the release of inflammatory neuropeptides such as calcium gene-related peptide by perivascular nerve fibers. Brändli and colleagues present an impressive case for their hypothesis and implicate endothelin-3 as a trigger for endothelin action in neurogenic inflammation via prejunctional ET(B) receptors. They note that "Endothelin promotes tachykinin release from nociceptive neurons, whereas plasma protein extravasation is mainly caused by binding of the released tachykinins to the post-junctional receptors on endothelial cells of blood vessels in the dura matter."

PH AND PANIC DISORDER

The pH dependency of the integrity of neuronal activity is not highly emphasized in neuropsychopharmacology. It has been my observation, though, that some agents which increase pH, i.e., make the plasma more alkaline, are often effective treatments for neurosomatic disorders. With decreasing pH, cerebral metabolic rate decreases. Common processes such as incomplete oxidation and production of lactate or keto acids all decrease local pH. Substances that inhibit carbonic anhydrase, thereby raising pH, are often helpful. These include Diamox and some of the newer antiepileptic drugs. Many of my patients remark they feel better for a few days when they take a trip to the mountains. This improvement may occur because they hyperventilate, raising their plasma pH. They also increase their oxygen-carrying capacity by increasing red cell mass via erythropoietin, an agent which often improves neurosomatic symptoms when prescribed for treatment-refractory anemia.

The activation of the NMDA receptor can be allosterically inhibited by pH. As the environment around the NMDA-receptor channel becomes more acidic, receptor activation is suppressed, so at a pH of 6.0, receptor activation is suppressed nearly completely. Ascorbic acid could have a role in this process as well as acting at the redox site of the NMDA receptor to produce NMDA-receptor blockade. Citrates, in the form of sodium citrate or potassium citrate, are alkalinizing agents primarily used in patients with renal tubular acidosis. Sodium bicarbonate can also be prescribed to increase pH, but higher volumes of bicarbonate than citrate are required to have the same effect. Potassium citrate in the form of Polycitra-K does not impose a sodium load on the individual yet is an effective alkalinizing agent. Some of my patients have their best responses to agents that either acidify in very high doses, such as ascorbic acid, or that alkalinize, such as the citrates or sodium bicarbonate. This treatment option is simple and not particularly expensive or hazardous. It should be tried in most treatment-refractory patients. It is still difficult for me to tell by symptoms or by how patients respond to other agents whether they would respond to an acidifying or an alkalinizing agent.

Inhalation of carbon dioxide, which combines with water when catalyzed by the enzyme carbonic anhydrase to form carbonic acid, can cause a panic attack in a susceptible individual, as can intravenous infusion of sodium lactate. Both of these agents can lower pH. Thus, alkalinizing agents that would raise pH could conceivably have an antipanic effect, although how a panic attack is caused by pH change is not well understood. It may be related to activity of the NMDA receptor. NMDA-receptor activity is reduced as pH is lowered, but $GABA_A$-receptor occupancy increases pH. Carbonic anhydrase is said to function as an attentional gate by raising HCO_3^- flux through synaptic $GABA_A$-receptor channels, altering postsynaptic neural responses to GABA (Sun M-K, Alkon DL, 2002).

The transmitter ATP, usually coreleased with NE, is extremely nociceptive and has been implicated in the pathophysiology of reflex sympathetic dystrophy, also known as complex regional pain syndrome. It is released from microvascular endothelial cells during migraine headache and angina. ATP release is associated with distension of the tubular viscera (Burnstock G, 2001). There are two classes of purine receptors, P1 (adenosine) and P2X (mostly for ATP). The $P2X_2$ and $P2X_3$ receptors can be coexpressed to produce a channel with a slowly desensitizing response. $P2X_3$ receptors are not affected by pH, but recombinant $P2X_2$ receptors are strongly pH sensitive. The combination of the two is still pH sensitive but to a lesser extent (Stoop R et al., 1997). Acid pH augments the excitatory actions of ATP on dissociated mammalian sensory neurons. Because prescribing suramin, a general antagonist of all PX receptors, is not feasible, and receptor-specific antagonists are not yet available, consideration should be given to mild alkalinization of patients with painful neurosomatic disorders. The response is prompt, and the alkalinizing agent may be titrated by tolerance and effectiveness.

It should be noted that other panicogens such as cholecystokinin-B (CCK_B), as well as flumazenil and yohimbine, do not alter pH. Conceivably, DHEA and pregnenolone could be panicogens, and pregnenolone has been reported to cause epileptic seizures. Thus, there is no well understood unitary mechanism for causing panic disorder, although low levels of progesterone, GABA, and serotonin (and dysregulation of certain serotonin receptors) may predispose an individual to panic attacks. Low GABA causes GABAR up-regulation, a fairly constant finding in panic disorder. Neuroactive steroids such as allopregnenolone may be protective against panic attacks. It has been suggested that the anatomic locus of panic behavior resides within a neural substrate in the dorsolateral and lateral sectors of the midbrain periaqueductal gray area. Nitric oxide may also be involved in this system, particularly when GABA levels are reduced. The mechanism appears to be a hyperexcitability state due to malfunction of the neuronal gate control system in the dorsal PAG. Changes in $GABA_A$ subunit expression within the midbrain PAG could also predispose to the development of the neuronal malfunction that underlies panic disorder (Lovick TA, 2000).

The $gamma_2$ subunit of the $GABA_A$ receptor is involved in panic anxiety and is required for formation of the benzodiazepine site of the $GABA_A$ receptors. The $gamma_2$-subunit is necessary for synaptic clustering of $GABA_A$ receptors but not for synaptic function (Rudolph U et al., 2001). The sedative and anticonvulsant properties of the $GABA_A$ receptor primarily reside in the $alpha_1$ subunit. Eighteen $GABA_A$ subunits have been identified at the time of this writing, and considerable effort is being expended for subtype-specific agents. For example, zolpidem (Ambien) and zaleplon (Sonata), marketed as sleeping pills, are fairly $alpha_1$ specific. Anxiolytic drugs, in general, should be targeted for neuronal receptors containing the $alpha_2$ subunit. $Alpha_2$-containing $GABA_A$ receptors are very dense in the amygdala, the principal cells of the cerebral cortex, and the hippocampus, all areas associated with emotional stmulus processing (Fritschy JM et al., 1998). Ligands that targeted only GABARs containing $alpha_2$ subunits (constituting only 15 percent of all GABA receptors) would be expected to have a much reduced side-effect profile.

BUSPIRONE/BUSPAR

BuSpar is notable for its ineffectiveness in most patients, perhaps because its mode of action is not understood sufficiently so that it can be appropriately targeted. A comment, perhaps apocryphal, was attributed to Jerrold Rosenbaum, a psychopharmacologist at Harvard, who was purported to say that buspirone is the ideal anxiolytic in every way except for effectiveness. That has certainly been my experience with the medication until the last three years or so. It works best in patients with psychomotor retardation who have an anxiety component to their disorder but do not have fibromyalgia pain or many other neurosomatic symptoms. It is sometimes effective in ketamine responders, those who do well with atypical neuroleptics (especially ziprasidone), and those who respond adversely to pindolol, a $5\text{-}HT_{1A}$ antagonist which BuSpar often can reverse but is more effectively antagonized by ziprasidone.

The mechanism of action of buspirone has been debated for some time. For many years it was thought to be a $5\text{-}HT_{1A}$-receptor agonist with the $5\text{-}HT_{1A}$ receptor being primarily but not entirely a presynaptic autoreceptor. Thus, buspirone would decrease the secretion of serotonin. The ultimate action of the serotonin-reuptake inhibitors was thought to involve subsensitivity of the 5-HT_{1A} receptor which could be augmented by concomitant administration of buspirone. This is probably untrue.

A recent article reviews the neuropharmacology of buspirone (Gobert A et al., 1999). To make a long story short, it seems that buspirone has its main effect as an alpha$_2$-receptor antagonist, like yohimbine or oxytocin. It is metabolized into "1-PP," a potent alpha$_2$-adrenergic-receptor antagonist which elicits a pronounced increase in levels of DA in the frontal cortex. Among the numerous possible pathways for the action of antidepressants, the alteration of dopamine in the prefrontal cortex is one of the major contenders. Gobert and colleagues decided that all other effects of buspirone are secondary to the antagonist properties of 1-PP via alpha$_2$-adrenergic receptors which increase DA and NE in the frontal cortex.

The fact that buspirone is so ineffective in most, but not all, patients may relate to its alpha$_2$-adrenergic-receptor antagonistic properties, which usually are anxiogenic in populations in whom it has been tested, e.g., patients with panic disorder, generalized anxiety disorder, and PTSD. Buspirone augmentation of serotonin-reuptake inhibitors has a weak antidepressant effect, but buspirone remains more effective than placebo in treating GAD. Buspirone is not as effective as imipramine in treating depression in the elderly and has been tried in ADHD, brain injury, and headaches with inconclusive results. Buspirone may be useful for treating symptoms of anxiety and irritability in children with progressive developmental disorder.

One experiment related buspirone to fatigue (Marvin G et al., 1997). Subjects were given an exercise task after administration of either placebo or 45 mg of buspirone. Buspirone actually made the patients in the study feel fatigued earlier than those who received placebo. Another experiment compared buspirone and abecarnil in the treatment of GAD (Pollack MH et al., 1997). Abecarnil had a more rapid onset of action, but some withdrawal symptoms were noted with abecarnil which were not seen with buspirone.

One of buspirone's main advantages is that it is not habit forming and patients do not become dependent on it. It is thus perhaps a treatment of choice for the practitioner inexperienced in using psychotropic agents. Buspirone has not proven to be effective in obsessive-compulsive disorder or alcoholism. Body dysmorphic disorder may respond to buspirone, but this problem responds so well to serotonin-reuptake inhibitors and Neurontin that there is little need for buspirone in this situation. For me, buspirone has a niche as a better tolerated alternative to yohimbine.

Buspirone is still on the laundry list of substances that may be used in augmentation of antidepressant response since some experiments find a weak effect and some find a more robust effect. One study even combined buspirone and pindolol, an interesting combination, because buspirone is supposedly a 5-HT$_{1A}$ autoreceptor agonist and pindolol is a 5-HT$_{1A}$ autoreceptor antagonist. The experiment was done because pindolol had been reported in some cases to decrease the time of onset of response to serotonin-reuptake inhibitors. Buspirone was used to selectively activate postsynaptic weak 5-HT$_{1A}$ receptors. The authors found this combination produced greater than 50 percent symptom reduction in the first week in eight of ten patients and the response was sustained for the remainder of the trial. They also noted that the buspirone plus pindolol combination acted more rapidly than the combination of the SSRI fluvoxamine with pindolol. I must say that every serotonergic agent I have tried to augment with pindolol to increase its onset of action has had neither a rapid nor a robust response in the patient population I treat. I have tried pindolol with buspirone a number of times without benefit and have tried pindolol plus SSRIs at least fifty times without one success. It may be that my patient population is different from that of the experimenters (Blier P et al., 1997), or that a higher dose of pindolol than 5 mg p.o. b.i.d. should be prescribed before the receptors are saturated.

It appears pindolol, the weak 5-HT$_{1A}$ antagonist, may accelerate the response to electroconvulsive therapy in patients with major depression. A recent trial is the first double-blind, placebo-controlled study to demonstrate that result. I have never used pindolol to augment the action of ECT, but treatment responses allegedly occur more rapidly with the addition of pindolol. However, the total number of ECT treatments within a course or the overall efficacy of ECT treatment was not altered by the addition of pindolol (Schiah I-S et al., 2000). Pindolol also may enhance the action of tramadol (Ultram). Pindolol blocks the 5-HT$_{1A}$ presynaptic autoreceptor but not the postsynaptic receptor, which is present in the raphe nuclei (Beique JC et al., 2000).

The situation, of course, is complicated by the fact that 5-HT$_{1B/1D}$ agonists also have their own autoreceptors in the DRN which reduce 5-HT secretion and that propanolol is a 5-HT$_{1B}$>5-HT$_{1D}$ antagonist. The triptans, as 5-HT$_{1B/1D}$ agonists, act in the DRN primarily on the 5-HT$_{1B}$ receptor, because their effect is not changed by ketanserin, a selective 5-HT$_{1D}$ antagonist. Furthermore, the median raphe nucleus (MRN), which projects to the PFC, is less affected than the DRN by 5-HT$_{1A}$ agonists and not affected at all by 5-HT$_{1B/1D}$ agonists.

Administering the direct alpha$_2$-receptor antagonist yohimbine to patients who respond to BuSpar, however, does not augment the beneficial response. Rather, it usually makes the individual somewhat jittery, a reaction fairly predictably reversed by administering the alpha$_2$-receptor agonist clonidine. Buspirone might be more effective when combined with high-dose venlafaxine or with reboxetine, both of which are NE-reuptake inhibitors. There must be more to the action of buspirone than meets the eye, but it remains of somewhat limited utility in treating neurosomatic disorders. Buspirone may be augmented by naloxone which may also increase the effect of propanediols such as meprobamate and Soma (Belzung C et al., 2000) or even BZDs.

The dopaminergic system is in part an extrathalamic component of the ascending reticular activating system, which is involved in bottom-up modulation of attentional tone. The ARAS contains two major axes: One facilitates transmission through the thalamus to the cerebral cortex and is regulated predominantly by acetylcholine and excitatory amino acids. The other acts via extrathalamic pathways regulated by dopamine, serotonin, norepinephrine, acetylcholine, and GABA. The ARAS influences not only the maintenance of wakefulness but also the fine tuning of attentional tone during wakefulness. Many collaterals of the ARAS such as those to the intralaminar nuclei of the thalamus modulate signal-to-noise ratio during attentional focusing and sensory discrimination.

THALAMIC RETICULAR NUCLEUS

I have discussed the reticular nucleus of the thalamus extensively in the *Betrayal by the Brain.* I would like to remind the reader that the reticular nucleus may act as an attentional valve for regulating thalamocortical transmission, according to the integrated influence of the cortex and the brainstem reticular core. The thalamic reticular nucleus receives projections from the brainstem and the cerebral cortex. It does not project back to the cerebral cortex but inhibits the activity of the other thalamic nuclei. Top-down modulation of attention occurs in a network involving the parietal, temporal, and prefrontal cortices and is complementary to that of the ARAS. Feedback projections in the feed-forward connections between the two are very numerous. There appears to be specialization of the right hemisphere in the regulation of the attentional matrix. If the right hemisphere is involved in attention, it must also be specialized in representing salience. The right hemisphere attentional mechanisms distribute salience and attentional shifts more equally between both hemispheres and in both directions, although there is a slight leftward predominance. In the case of the left hemisphere, attentional mechanisms are more likely to endow the right side of events with salience and tend to coordinate the distribution of attention almost exclusively within the right hemispace (Figure 9).

Some recent discoveries about the thalamic reticular nucleus have enhanced my understanding of corticothalamic communication. The TRN is composed of GABAergic neurons which have subtypes of mGluRs. Glutamatergic projections from the cortex to the TRN are usually excitatory and increase GABAergic intrathalamic and TRN-cortical neurotransmission. Group II mGluRs exist on the TRN which can inhibit it, thus disinhibiting intrathalamic and thalamocortical transmission. Such disinhibition seems to have chaotic effects, turning its assumed functional role upside down.

It has been dogma that intrathalamic nuclei were functionally separate and could not communicate with one another. However, they do communicate in closed loops via the TRN. Previously, the TRN had been viewed as projecting in a highly topographic manner in that axons from each restricted region of the thalamus terminate on the same TRN neurons that project back to that region of the thalamus. Thus, the TRN neurons would inhibit the same thalamic nuclei that project to them. However, it has been found that neurons from one thalamic nucleus can excite an area of the TRN which could then inhibit another thalamic nucleus. Thalamic nuclei with wide receptive fields can project to the sensory cortex (SII, e.g.), which can then decrease its excitatory projection to the GABAergic TRN, one of the main functions of which is to decrease the size of receptive fields. During peak periods of arousal action of the TRN is suppressed because receptive fields should be as wide as possible to evaluate potential danger (Crabtree JW et al., 1998). This scenario has obvious relevance to neurosomatic disorders. I have lectured and written for years that the TRN could be malfunctioning as a result of inappropriate cortical input and that such malfunction could be a cause of neurosomatic disorders (Figure 10).

THE ATTENTIONAL NETWORK

The setting of visual-spatial salience involves the parietoccipital cortices. Exploratory behaviors, selection, sequencing, and execution of attentional shifts are more associated with the frontal lobe. Mesulam has described a large-scale distributed network for spatial attention which involves the posterior parietal cortex, frontal eye fields, cingulate gyrus, thalamus, striatum, superior colliculus, and ARAS (Mesulam M-M, 2000) (Figure 11).

Because shifting attention based on motivational salience is related significantly to dopaminergic function, one can understand how dysregulation of the network can lead to the cognitive and perceptual disorders prominently seen in patients with neurosomatic illnesses. Neurons in this network do not respond as actively if perceived events do not have motivational significance. However, if too many events are perceived as being cognitively and behaviorally salient, then almost every cognitive sensorimotor operation could be dysregulated. The frontal eye fields, which are at the junction of the precentral and superior frontal sulci, are activated during covert attentional shifts, even when controlling for other potentially confounding factors involved in attention. The function of the frontal eye fields is to regulate eye movements from left to right; hence the visual system dominates other sensory input systems and significance of sensory input.

It appears that any task relating to attention activates the frontal eye field. Mesulam considers it to be "the frontal core of the attentional network" (Mesulam M-M, 2000, p. 227). It is involved with tasks of spatial and auditory attention, as well as tasks of visual attention. It may influence visual information at a relatively early stage of analysis, because the limbic innervation of the FEF from the cingulate gyrus provides information about motivationally relevant segments of the extrapersonal space. Thus, the FEF and the superior colliculus are much more than command neurons for eye movements but are involved in an extensive neural network. The FEF "may thus encode the type of sensorimotor working memory which is essential for the systemic exploration of a visual scene under the guidance of mental representations" (p. 228). I emphasize the FEF because despite conflicting current research, a psychotherapeutic technique termed *eye movement desensitization and reprocessing* (EMDR) which must affect the function of the FEF. EMDR and other attentional reprogramming may be incorporated with cognitive-behavioral therapy. All attentional processes involve the FEF.

I have been impressed with the results of EMDR in some of my patients with fibromyalgia and look for a refinement of the technique to be much more valuable in future treatment of these disorders. I suspect a more sophisticated form of an extracranial technique such as transcranial magnetic stimulation or altering resonance of nodal neurons could be integrated into the procedure.

The cingulate cortex of the brain has a complex organization, and numerous behavioral affiliations are dependent upon the area of the cingulate gyrus involved. The ventral cingulate is predominantly limbic, the posterodorsal cingulate is visuospatial, and the anterodorsal cingulate is predominantly somatomotor. The neurons in the dorsal part of the anterior cingulate fire in response to behaviorally relevant cues and during the planning and execution of reaching movements. The activity of the posterior cingulate neurons increases immediately following back and forth (saccadic) eye movements. These neurons encode how far the eyes should move, but since their activity occurs after the eye movements, they are thought to be monitoring rather than controlling overt shifts in the direction of visual attention. There are numerous other nexi in Mesulan's attentional network which I will not be discussing since I do not want to be overly focused on mechanisms to the exclusion of treatments.

I have continually emphasized function of the PFC in my writing about CFS and other neurosomatic disorders. The prefrontal cortex is one of the possible "bottlenecks" in the attentional network where lesions may have the most severe impact on the integrity of directed attention. All three cortical components of the attentional network, that is, the posterior parietal cortex, the frontal eye fields including the prefrontal cortex, and the cingulate gyrus are engaged simultaneously in attentional behaviors. No matter what attentional task is performed, it seems that shifts of spatial attention automatically engage oculomotor mechanisms even when the attentional shifts do not involve eye movements. Much of this recent work involving distributed networks and parallel processing for attention has been done with the aid of functional brain imaging. Because the key to allocating attention is salience and the most important neurotransmitter involved with motivation is dopamine (Horvitz JC, 2000), it behooves us to consider this neurotransmitter and its receptors in a subsequent section.

CLONIDINE

Clonidine is an $alpha_1/alpha_{2ABC}$ receptor agonist, having more affinity for the $alpha_2$ receptor than the $alpha_1$ receptor. It induces Ach secretion. The $alpha_2$ receptor is primarily located presynaptically on noradrenergic neurons, where it functions as an autoreceptor serving to decrease the secretion of norepinephrine, but postsynaptic $alpha_2$ receptors of the A, B, and C types also mediate various functions. $Alpha_2$ receptors may be heteroreceptors on other neurons. The drug clonidine may be an agonist at the imidazoline receptor, of which there are three types, $I_{1,2,3}$. Clonidine is thought to be an agonist at the I_1 receptor where it could regulate blood pressure, but it probably has no other function at that receptor. Cimetidine is also a putative imidazoline receptor ligand. Because we have no specific imidazoline receptor ligands for use in clinical medicine at this time, it is probably not necessary to discuss this aspect of the neuropharmacology of clonidine at length.

There are several $alpha_2$ adrenoceptor antagonists, of which yohimbine would be the most familiar to practicing physicians. One used experimentally is idazoxan. Yohimbine and idazoxan are antagonistic at the I_1 receptor for blood pressure regulation, but they are less potent antagonists at somatodentric $alpha_2$ adrenoceptors in the locus coeruleus. Administration of clonidine often leads to improved performance on certain cognitive tasks. This effect of clonidine is not antagonized by idazoxan (Middleton HC et al., 1999). Oxytocin appears to be an $alpha_2$-adrenoceptor antagonist, at least in regard to the facilitatory effect of clonidine on food intake (Diaz-Cabale Z, Navarez JA, et al., 2000).

The alpha$_{2C}$ adrenoceptors are located on rat striatal GABAergic projection neurons. These receptors are thought to decrease the secretion of dopamine, which would be one of the considerations in giving clonidine rather than the more specific alpha$_{2A}$ agonist guanfacine. The alpha$_{2C}$ adrenoceptors are somewhat involved in the regulation of brain serotonin turnover but not in the release of norepinephrine or other monoamines (Holmberg M et al., 1999).

It has been known for some time that clonidine has antinociceptive properties. The pharmacology of this antinociception is somewhat complex. Clonidine appears to open K$_{ATP}$ channels. Agents that block the opening of these channels prevent alpha$_2$-adrenoceptor agonist-induced analgesia (Galeotti N et al., 1999). Gabapentin is also a K$_{ATP}$ channel opener, thereby hyperpolarizing the neuron and decreasing release of neurotransmitters (Lohman AB, Welch SP, 1999).

Clonidine has an analgesic effect when given intrathecally, but this mode of administration is not particularly germane to my current practice of neurosomatic medicine. Patients with chronic back and leg pain may be treated with long-term intrathecal infusions of drug combinations for up to 3.5 years. The drugs are infused by an intrathecal programmable pump-controlled method (Rainov NG et al., 2001) to which patient control may easily be added. Ultra-low-dose naloxone may prevent morphine tolerance in this system. This type of pain is fairly easily controlled by less invasive techniques. In the past ten years, only one of my patients has required long-term intrathecal analgesia. Clonidine may also bind to mu-opioid receptors directly and thus have an opioidergic mechanism as an aspect of its analgesia. A selective imidazoline/A$_2$ adrenergic-receptor agonist, moxonidine, may synergize with morphine and also deltorphin II to inhibit SP-induced behavior in mice (Fairbanks CA et al., 2000).

Work with moxonidine demonstrated that the analgesia it produces is independent of the alpha$_{2A}$ adrenoceptor, which is in contrast to antinociception mediated by clonidine. Clonidine acts primarily on the alpha$_{2A}$ adrenoceptor to relieve pain but appears to me to be more analgesic than guanfacine. Clonidine is a delta-opioid receptor agonist by virtue of its alpha$_{2BC}$ agonism. Moxonidine is selective for the I$_1$ imidazoline receptor. Coadministration of diverse alpha$_2$-adrenoceptor and diverse opioid-receptor agonists can produce a multiplicative spinal analgesic effect, often defined as "synergy." Moxonidine, which is not yet clinically available, acts primarily at an alpha$_2$- adrenoreceptor subtype different from that activated by clonidine, and this alpha$_2$-adrenoceptor subtype synergizes with the delta-opioid receptor but not the mu-opioid receptor. Thus, at this time, moxonidine would seem to be a rather unique substance. It may act at delta-opioid-receptor subtypes other than those affected by clonidine. Alpha$_2$-adrenoceptor subtypes have also been found to regulate the secretion of ACTH and beta endorphin during stress in the rat (Zelena D et al., 1999). The inhibitory effect of clonidine in the locus coeruleus is potentiated by 5-HT$_{1A}$ receptors. This result is an experimental finding primarily. I have not seen any clinical benefit from combining buspirone with clonidine, perhaps because buspirone is metabolized into an alpha$_2$ antagonist. However, both the 5-HT$_{1A}$ and the alpha$_2$ adrenoceptors inhibit the activity of locus coeruleus neurons. Clonidine not only reduces dopamine in the corpus striatum, including the nucleus accumbens, but also increases GABA$_A$ binding sites. The increase in GABA$_A$ binding sites in the nucleus accumbens diminishes striatal dopamine release. Clonidine administration increases NPY activity in the rat cerebral cortex. As we develop more specific NPY agonists, the importance of this effect should be further appreciated. Recall that NPY in many situations has an opposite effect to that of CRH (Smilaowska M et al., 1997).

Clonidine can potentiate the neuropathic pain-relieving action of NMDA-receptor antagonists such as MK-801 while attenuating their neurotoxic and hyperactivity side effects. It may in some situations potentiate the activity of MK-801 to the extent the dosage requirement for this antagonist may be cut in half "thereby achieving prolonged neuropathic pain relief while doubling the margin of safety against any type of side effect that may be mediated by blockade of NMDA receptors" (Jevtovic-Todorovic V et al., 1998).

I have used clonidine in this manner when treating patients with ketamine and find the dosage of ketamine required to become analgesic is lowered, although not by half. The mechanism of action of clonidine in this system has not been satisfactorily explained. An endogenous substance which has not been well characterized is clonidine-displacing substance (CDS), a putative endogenous ligand. CDS is thought to act at the imidazoline binding sites. As far as neurosomatic disorders are concerned, the most important imidazoline binding site would be the I$_2$ site, also an agmatine binding site, which possibly exerts a modulatory function on the enzyme monoamine oxidase. Whether the I$_2$ site would inhibit or facilitate the action of monoamine oxidase has not yet been determined to my knowledge.

The medication tizanidine (Zanaflex) is marketed fairly aggressively as a muscle relaxant/analgesic. Tizanidine is purportedly an alpha$_2$ agonist. Because I can use such agents much more effectively if I know their subtype specificity, I once asked the Zanaflex representative who visited my office at which receptor subtypes it was an agonist. She became quite flustered and said she did not know. Furthermore, no one had ever asked her that question. The information was not available in the promotional material in her briefcase. She gave me the number of the Zanaflex research department at her company headquarters. I called immediately, and after only three transfers, spoke to one of the head honchos. "Why would you want to know that?" he asked, incredulously. "So that I can prescribe the medication more precisely," I replied. In our subsequent conversation, I felt unsure he even knew what a receptor subtype was. Although I thought I had lost my capacity for amazement at scientific ignorance, I became quite nonplussed as it dawned upon me that the drug company had probably spent $400 million to launch Zanaflex but had only the foggiest notion of its basic pharmacology. I would almost certainly prescribe Zanaflex more frequently if I knew its mechanism of action. My receptor profiling process requires some knowledge of a drug's pharmacology. As a result, I prescribe Zanaflex only as option number 11 for sleeping pills.

Alpha$_2$-receptor agonists might be useful in the treatment of premenstrual dysphoric disorder. It has been found that during the luteal phase, i.e., after ovulation, alpha$_2$-adrenergic receptor density correlates positively with symptom severity in patients. High follicular alpha$_2$-adrenoreceptor density (prior to ovulation) predicts more severe luteal symptoms in patients with PMDD. Thus, it appears that alpha$_2$-adrenergic receptor agonists such as clonidine, guanfacine, and even Zanaflex may be of value in treating neurosomatic patients who have a premenstrual exacerbation of their symptomatology. Clonidine may work the best, since it is superior to the other two agents as an analgesic.

CATECHOLAMINES

One of the best articles I have read in the past several years is by Amy Arnsten (1998). Arnsten discusses the fact that the PFC is very sensitive to changes in the neuromodulatory input it receives from NE and DA systems. This sensitivity can lead to marked changes in its working memory functions. She notes, "While NMDA has important beneficial influences on processing in this area, very high levels of catecholamine release, for example, during exposure to uncontrollable stress, disrupt the cognitive functions of the PFC" (Amsten A, 1998, p. 46).

People with neurosomatic disorders often have a problem with "working memory," a form of short-term memory distinct from longer-term episodic (for events) or semantic (actual) memory. The information held within working memory is active for only a short period of time and, therefore, is continually updated. The PFC is thought to hold ideas "on-line" to guide behavior effectively in the absence of environmental cues. It is able to carry salient signals linking sensation to action and allow inhibition of inappropriate responses or distracting stimuli, thereby facilitating planning and execution of effective organized behavior (Constantinidis C et al., 2001). Working memory in the PFC permits assessment of similar stimuli while forming decisions that guide actions. Neural correlates of experiential modulation of percepts in working memory based on probable reward or punishment can be detected by measurement of single neuron activity in the PFC (Gold JI, Shadlen MN, 2001).

Catecholamines are essential to the organization of function in the PFC. They help to regulate attention, organization, hyperactivity, and impulsivity. In an acutely dangerous situation it might be adaptive to shut down "sensitive" PFC functions in order to respond to threat. Many of the cognitive abilities associated with the PFC are impaired by exposure to stress, particularly when the subjects feel they are not in control of the stressful situation. Catecholamines such as DA and NE have powerful actions that can switch the PFC on- or off-line. Both catecholamines must be depleted to substantially affect PFC function, but certain operations within the same region of the PFC may have differing neurochemical requirements. DA dysregulation may cause one sort of dysfunction, while NE dysregulation might cause another.

Significant working memory impairment, however, is probably related to depletion of both NE and DA. NE works predominantly at the $alpha_{2A}$-adrenergic receptor as far as working memory is concerned, and DA works predominantly at the D_1 receptor. DA release is sensitive to cues or to the anticipation of reward. DA has a longer-lasting effect on PFC cells than does NE, presumably by actions at postreceptor mechanisms. At least five DA receptors can be divided into two major families: the D_1 receptors (D_1 and D_5) and the D_2 receptors (D_2, D_3, and D_4). Because of the spatial synaptic organization of the PFC, DA is in the position to modulate excitatory inputs to pyramidal cell spines through D_1/D_5 receptor stimulation. The D_5 receptor can bind directly to a type of GABAR ($alpha_1$- $beta_2$-$gamma_2$) and reduce its inhibitory function. Conversely, $GABA_AR$ activation reduces D_5-mediated cAMP accumulation (Liu F et al., 2000).

Such stimulation can have a powerful modulatory input on neural activity, decreasing the calcium currents that convey signal from dendrite to soma. This mechanism may serve to focus signal transmission in PFC pyramidal cells. The D_5 receptor may be more important than the D_1 receptor in this focusing, particularly if it functions as an autoreceptor. I consider the role of the NE receptor families $alpha_1$, $alpha_2$, and $beta_{123}$ adrenergic next.

The catecholamines may have paracrine effects, i.e., they may diffuse from their presynaptic terminals to affect receptors at a distance. As has been mentioned previously, $alpha_2$ agonists can improve working memory deficits. These agents are more effective in elderly monkeys than young monkeys because there is an alpha$_2$ denervation hypersensitivity postsynaptically due to decreased NE secretion in elderly monkeys. The alpha$_{2A}$-selective agonist guanfacine is the most effective noradrenergic compound for enhancing working memory without producing side effects such as sedation. Guanfacine does not inhibit firing of the locus coeruleus nearly as well as does clonidine, but it is much more potent in improving working memory in aged monkeys. I have found guanfacine to be of some value in the treatment of Alzheimer's disease. Alpha$_2$ agonists are particularly effective in enhancing working memory during distracting conditions, a finding consistent with studies showing PFC NE depletion increases distractibility. Clonidine may be a suboptimal drug for many neurosomatic patients because it too greatly inhibits LC firing and is less potent at the alpha$_{2A}$ receptor than is guanfacine.

If catecholamines are secreted in excess, working memory can be impaired. This impairment has been observed with application of D$_1$ or alpha$_1$-adrenergic agonists. D$_1$ agonists have an inverted U-shaped dose-response curve, meaning either too little or too much D$_1$-receptor stimulation can impair working memory, whereas in contrast, NE appears to have opposing actions at alpha$_2$ versus alpha$_1$ receptors. Therefore, it would in theory be ideal to prescribe an alpha$_{2A}$ agonist such as guanfacine along with an alpha$_1$ antagonist such as prazosin. Prazosin and related compounds are not specific for the alpha$_1$ receptor (of which there are three types, alpha$_{1A, 1B, 1D}$), but other selective alpha$_1$-receptor antagonists besides the "-azosins," and tamsulosin (Flomax for prostatism) are not available for clinical use. In actual practice, combining alpha$_{2A}$ agonists with alpha$_1$ antagonists has not been very helpful for most patients, although excessive alpha$_1$-receptor stimulation may underlie PFC deficits in mania. Alpha$_1$-receptor agonists such as midodrine are more effectively combined with guanfacine in many patients. They may be used, as may stimulants, in the bipolar patient whose symptoms are first controlled with mood stabilizers. Lithium, a drug commonly used for mania, blocks the PFC cognitive deficits caused by alpha$_1$ agonists such as midodrine. Lithium has almost no other value in neurosomatic medicine, however, except as an antagonist to lidocaine. It has not been an effective augmentation strategy for my depressed patients who are treatment refractory. It is still effective for preventing hypomanic episodes in bipolar II patients. Perhaps these individuals have "atypical" depression for which lithium is less valuable. Midodrine's primary indication is to raise blood pressure. When a patient has excessive alpha$_1$-adrenoceptor stimulation, he or she will feel as if "my hair is standing on end," because the muscles that contract to raise the hairs, called the erector pilae, have alpha$_1$ adrenergic innervation. Flomax, which does not enter the brain, can be useful in this instance.

In rats, the degree of working memory impairment during stress is corre-lated with the amount of DA turnover in the PFC. Stress-induced cognitive deficits can be blocked by pretreatment with a selective D_1- or D_4-receptor antagonist but cannot be reversed by serotonergic-reuptake blockers such as Prozac. Selective D_1 and D_4 agents are not available yet for clinical practice, although olanzapine may be a D_4 antagonist.

Stress-induced working memory deficits may be attenuated by infusion of an alpha$_1$-receptor antagonist, suggesting that DA and NE synergize to take the PFC "off -line" during stress. Because a high SNR is desirable in patients with neurosomatic disorders, optimal levels of D_1-receptor stimula-tion appear to focus signal transmission, conveying only large or temporally coincident signals to the cell body. Alpha$_1$-receptor stimulation can increase excitatory postsynaptic current in apical dendrites, resulting in an increase in background noise. This process could interfere with signal transfer from dendrite to soma. Thus, the mechanism of stress-induced working memory deficit in neurosomatic disorders could be an impairment in the signal trans-fer mechanism.

NOREPINEPHRINE, DOPAMINE, SALIENCE, AND ATTENTION

A current popular view holds that the input from dopaminergic neurons to the striatum provides the reinforcement signal required to adjust the prob-abilities of subsequent action selection. A short-latency and short-duration response of dopaminergic cells is observed after the unexpected presenta-tion of a behaviorally significant stimulus (Redgrave P et al., 1999). These sensorimotor integrations have also been termed "flexible approach re-sponses," as contrasted to fixed instrumental approach responses, or habits (Ikemoto S, Panksepp J, 1999). Habits are more likely to involve nigro-striatal DA than mesocorticolimbic DA gateways involving the NAc. NAc DA is involved in both appetitive and aversive contexts. NAc DA would be instrumental in avoiding aversive situations and would be secreted when an organism felt "safe," as well as in similar environmental contexts in the fu-ture. Neurosomatic patients who have not learned to feel safe will be less likely to secrete DA into the NAc and mesocorticolimbic pathways.

Attentional resources are allocated in favor of unexpected salient events. The term "switching" is used to denote reallocation processes, and "salient" is used to refer to stimuli with special biological significance. Dopamin-ergic output is also involved in "behavioral orienting," the allocation of at-tention to a particular stimulus. This response in normal individuals extin-guishes rapidly. Unexpected rewards or punishments lead to the acquisition of new conditioned responses. Dopaminergic neuron activity is associated with unexpected rewards or with stimuli previously associated with reward. Dopaminergic activity is suppressed when expected rewards fail to materialize, and short dopaminergic responses may be quite suppressed, or in some situations, activated, if aversive consequences are associated with perceiving too many stimuli as novel and, therefore, salient. Redgrave and colleagues (1999) have proposed that the vertebrate basal ganglia have evolved as a centralized selection drive specialized to resolve conflicts between multiple subsystems competing for access to limited motor or cognitive resources. Thus, the neurons involved in attending to the most salient stimuli will receive most of the dopaminergic input, while those involved in perceiving decreased reward salience will receive much less. This process has been termed "winner take all" and has been described most extensively in the visual cortex. Thus, one of the core functions of the basal ganglia is considered to be selection. Dopaminergic secretion has been proposed to promote behavioral switching as part of its general modulatory role. Unexpected incongruous or intense stimuli always elicit a robust short-latency dopamine response.

As will be discussed further, there is sustained activation of several areas of the brain during learning tasks. DA is involved in firing delay-active neurons in working memory in the PFC. Extracellular DA in the amygdala nuclei closely related to the OFC and DLPFC is elevated during working memory and associative tasks but also during the reading of simple words. In some subjects the amplitude of increase is greater than 100 percent above baseline. Fewer DA neurons respond when a task is learned and expected, but DA neurons respond robustly to novel situations, leading to the view that DA is particularly important during learning, when behavior is adapted to new situations and attention is paid to salient stimuli in the environment. The amygdala, along with the medial OFC, is involved with "incentive salience." Dopamine is usually fired in very short bursts. For sustained DA secretion to occur in cognitive tasks, presynaptic regulation of DA release must be altered. Like NE before it, DA is increasingly being conceptualized as a mechanism for stabilizing active neural representations by providing protection from distractors and facilitating sustained information processing in the human brain (Fried I et al., 2001).

The frontal eye fields bring visual stimuli into the most active perceptual area of the retina (the fovea), so its potential reward significance may be determined. The computations of the possibility of reward occur before a behavioral switch occurs, and a signal is often lost before the identity of the stimulus is fully known. Thus, dopaminergic cells must extract the specific reinforcement value of a stimulus. A transient decrease in the dopaminergic activity follows reward omission as well as perception of aversive stimuli.

The exact role of dopamine in aversive and stressful events is somewhat unclear at this time. Extensive literature shows both aversive and stressful events can increase the release of dopamine, and also that behavior motivated by these stimuli is impaired by dopamine depletion. The tuning of these dopaminergic cells by the attentional network seems to be a very important aspect of neurosomatic disorders. Reductions in dopamine-mediated neurotransmission can impair attentional switching and may be involved in the unpleasant symptoms that occur when neurosomatic patients are in conditions of stimulus overload. Both dopaminergic neurons and noradrenergic neurons from the locus coeruleus show strikingly similar responses to salient events, having a slow spontaneous rate of discharge interrupted by a short-latency, short-duration burst of pulses in response to unexpected novel stimuli in all modalities. DA and NE are the two primary reinforcing neurotransmitters. These neurons are maximally activated by unexpected stimuli made salient by virtue of their novelty, their status as primary reinforcers, or their association with primary reinforcers. This response is, as Mesulam discusses, involved in the regulation of attention to the external environment and the readiness to respond to unexpected events. The neurosomatic patient has inappropriate activity of this system. Dopamine D_1-receptor activation can be suppressed by an L-type calcium antagonist such as nimodipine, and this D_1 response is facilitated by an AMPA-mediated neuronal transmission when glutamatergic GABA heteroreceptors are blocked. Selective dopamine depletion within the medial PFC produces anxiogenic effects in rats (Espejo EF, 1997).

The PFC and NE systems are both important for attentional regulation. PFC lesions impair the ability to sustain attention to relevant information and to inhibit processing of irrelevant stimuli. As has been noted several times in this book, this problem is perhaps the core deficit in neurosomatic pathophysiology. Attentional mechanisms are intertwined with working memory, and NE has important effects on several types of attentional processes. The cell bodies of many neurons in the LC fire in relation to the attentional state of the animal. The PFC is one of the few high-order inputs to the LC and is an important regulator of LC activity. This circular relationship, as I outlined in *Betrayal by the Brain,* may have powerful effects on attentional regulation.

There is poor attentional regulation, therefore, under conditions of very low or very high NE release. NE is known to enhance signal-to-noise ratio in sensory cortices. Therefore, with insufficient NE stimulation, small signals may be obscured (targets) while potent stimuli may be processed (distractors). Once again, this is one of the core deficits in patients with neurosomatic disorders. If NE were hypersecreted, it would take the PFC "off-line" because of high levels of alpha$_1$-receptor stimulation, and since the PFC was off-line it would no longer be in the position to inhibit processing of irrelevant stimuli. Alteration of NE release in the PFC may also shift control to subcortical regulation of behavior. Alpha$_1$-receptor stimulation in the PFC augments DA-mediated responses in the nucleus accumbens, e.g., amphetamine-induced locomotor activation. This finding suggests patients who are developing tolerance to stimulant medications may have alpha$_1$ agonists such as midodrine added to their therapeutic regimen to enhance stimulant efficacy. Supplemental ascorbate may also be beneficial.

It has been noted that pretreatment with the alpha$_1$/alpha$_{2BC}$ antagonist prazosin prevented the increase in ACTH and beta endorphin in rats who inhaled ether, but an alpha$_1$/alpha$_{2A}$ antagonist was unable to counteract the inhibitory effect of clonidine. Prazosin alone had no effect on ether-induced plasma ACTH and beta endorphin elevation, suggesting NE in the CNS may inhibit stress-induced HPA axis activation. NE also decreases pituitary beta endorphin activation via alpha$_{2BC}$ adrenoceptor subtypes; thus prazosin and suramin may antagonize NE effect on alpha$_{2BC}$ receptors. It would theoretically be desirable to increase the secretion of ACTH and beta endorphin in neurosomatic disorders, but unfortunately, prazosin and related agents alone have not significantly improved the clinical status of the large majority of neurosomatic patients to whom I have administered them. Giving an alpha$_1$ adrenergic agonist can stimulate the secretion of ACTH and beta endorphin but does not influence the effect of ether on either of these hormones, confirming that alpha$_1$ adrenoreceptors are not involved in the action of clonidine on ether-induced ACTH and beta endorphin release. The inhibitory effect of clonidine on the ether stress-induced ACTH level appears to be localized presynaptically via an alpha$_2$ heteroreceptor on ACTH-secreting neurons. Thus, chronic clonidine administration may alter endocrine responsiveness, and the effects of chronic administration of an alpha$_2$ agonist may be enhanced by giving an alpha$_1$ antagonist such as prazosin with suramin. Clonidine or prazosin alone does not produce the same result.

DOPAMINE AND REWARD

Prefrontal dopamine activation appears to be necessary for coping with an anxiogenic challenge, at least in rats, so the animal may display adaptive exploratory responses in a fear-inducing environment. Prefrontocortical dopamine levels increase during anxiety and stress fairly routinely. There is a complex regulation of prefrontal dopamine and limbic dopamine, and reduction of prefrontocortical dopamine input is known to disinhibit the excitatory projection to the mesolimbic dopamine system, perhaps by activation of mGluR2 heteroreceptors on dopaminergic neurons.

Midbrain dopaminergic neurons respond to natural rewards such as food and liquid, but the activity of these neurons depends on the predictability of the reward presentation. This conceptual shift that dopamine itself is not rewarding has influenced my thinking in the last seven years. Thus, the response of midbrain dopaminergic neurons represents a learning signal for the codes of the reward. Another interpretation is that the allocation of limited DA resources induces targeting of any unexpected event of behavioral significance and that associative learning is linked to enhanced DA release in the NAc. This response involves associative learning in general, not just reward. The novelty of the reward, or the deprivation of it (such as food and water), has been termed "incentive salience."

Much of this work on secretion of midbrain dopamine into various areas such as the NAc, mesocorticolimbic tracts, or the lateral and medial OFC has been done studying drug abuse, which is not a major problem in neurosomatic medicine. Some interesting findings have emerged, however: DA-induced euphoria is not blocked by the DA antagonist pimozide, and cocaine and amphetamine act primarily in the PFC by increasing NE, which then increases DA via the $alpha_1$ receptor. Mu-opioids can be stimulating in part by activation inhibiting mu-opioid heteroreceptors on GABAergic neurons which tonically inhibit DA secretion from the A20 dopaminergic nucleus in the VTA (Figure 12). This mechanism was published in 1992 and subsequently at least twice a year (or so it seems). The general medical and psychiatric community is largely unaware of it, as far as I can tell (Spanagel R, Weiss F, 1999), just as they are of the antidepressant effects of opioids.

One of the common actions of antidepressants is to increase dopamine in the PFC. However, fluoxetine (Prozac), when used chronically, is associated with normal presynaptic dopamine transmission in the prefrontal cortex, since tolerance develops to acute fluoxetine-induced dopamine increase. Desipramine, however, a noradrenergic reuptake inhibitor, chronically increases prefrontal dopamine. Release of dopamine by SSRIs may occur by activating $5\text{-}HT_3$ receptors on dopaminergic neurons. Desipramine can increase PFC dopamine levels by blocking DA uptake by the NE terminal, a process termed "heterologous uptake" (Tanda G et al., 1996).

Most types of antidepressants increase PFC dopamine. However, dopamine increase does not appear to be required for their antidepressant effect. More attention has been paid in recent years to the D_4 receptor. It is of interest that both epinephrine and norepinephrine bind to the D_4 receptor.

Glutamatergic efferents from the DLPFC have been shown to regulate caudate dopamine release in the monkey. Hypoperfusion of the dorsoventral caudate nucleus has been found fairly consistently in brain SPECTs of patients with CFS and fibromyalgia done by the group at the University of Alabama, Birmingham, but not by other investigators.

Quite germane to neurosomatic disorders is that chronic stress can induce in rats a decreased reactivity toward noxious stimuli, termed an "escape deficit." This deficit can be reversed by antidepressants. The behavioral deficit is accompanied by a decreased level of extracellular dopamine in the nucleus accumbens shell, the region of the ventral striatum that is the most behaviorally important.

The increases in dopamine output after cocaine administration observed in stressed animals are significantly lower than those in control rats, (Gambarana C et al., 1999), in which it is quite elevated. Synaptic fatigue may play a role in the stressed rats.

A similar condition may apply to patients with neurosomatic disorders no matter what the etiology of their dopaminergic dysfunction. Rats with chemical lesions in the medial PFC which reduce dopamine levels in this area demonstrate a delayed extinction of a conditioned fear response without an overall increase in the initial conditioned response. It has been known for some time that mesoprefrontal dopamine neurons are involved in maintaining the animals' response adaptability with regard to stress-related changes in the external environment, but this finding, again, implicates dopamine deficiency in the etiology of misperception of salience of events in patients with neurosomatic disorders (Morrow BA et al., 1999).

The lateral area of the orbitofrontal cortex is activated following a punishing outcome, and the medial OFC is activated following a reward outcome. The degree of the activations reflects the magnitude of the reward or punishment delivered. The medial and lateral OFCs are two separate networks. There is no difference in the region or extent of OFC activation between the two hemispheres. Information used from rewarding or punishing choices is processed primarily in the OFC (other brain areas are less involved) and is used to guide behavioral choice (O'Doherty JO et al., 2001).

Neurosomatic disorders are encountered more often in women than men. Can this discrepancy be accounted for by gender differences in D_2-receptor levels? As assessed on a high sensitivity three-dimensional PET which used a new, highly specific D_2 ligand, [^{11}C]FLB 457, women had increased D_2-receptor density in the frontal and temporal cortices and the thalamus. Although these studies were performed on healthy subjects, the results suggest gender differences in susceptibility to certain neuropsychiatric disorders (Kaasinen V et al., 2001).

A similar depletion of dopamine in the prefrontal cortex has been found to decrease the basal activity of mesolimbic dopamine neurons. There are at least two pathways by which mesocortical dopamine neurons may ultimately regulate the activity of mesolimbic dopamine neurons. DA projections in the medial PFC decrease the spontaneous activity of pyramidal cells in this region. These pyramidal cells give rise to glutamatergic efferents that project directly to the nucleus accumbens where they frequently terminate on the same spine as tyrosine hydroxylase in immunoreactive terminals. Tyrosine hydroxylase is the enzyme that converts tyrosine to L-dopa. The supply of phenylalanine and tyrosine is almost always adequate, and although TH is rate limiting, it is extremely difficult to overwhelm its capacity for the biosynthesis of DA. The corticoaccumbens pathway influences mesolimbic DA neurons either by a direct action on the terminal or via polysynaptic pathways originating in the NAc and terminating on DA cell bodies in the ventral tegmental area. The second pathway involves a direct projection from the medial PFC to the VTA, which then projects to the NAc and enhances dopamine secretion via a VTA-NAc route. Recent experiments, however, have shown these subcortical DA neurons do not normally inhibit the activity of cortical pyramidal cells. It has been demonstrated that the glutamatergic efferents from the medial PFC are selective. Certain PFC terminals synapse on VTA DA/TH neurons and others specifically on GABAergic neurons, some of which may play a role in inhibiting the electrophysiological activity of VTA-DA neurons. Thus, a chemical lesion that induces disinhibition of pyramidal cell activity may increase the activity of GABAergic interneurons within the VTA and, thereby, increase tonic GABA-mediated inhibition of DA cell activity. Feedback regulation from the NAc to the VTA may also decrease activity of the DA cells in the VTA. Thus, DA depletion of the mPFC disinhibits glutamatergic input to the VTA, causing inhibition or facilitation of VTA DA neurons, depending on the predominant type of neuron to receive mPFC glutamate axonal synapses (Corr DB, Sesack SR, 2000).

After a period of time, a compensatory process takes place in order to restore basal extracellular DA in the NAc to control levels despite diminished electrophysiological activity of VTA-DA neurons which occurs if GABAergic neurons are preferentially activated and DA autoreceptors are stimulated. The DA concentration may be maintained by a decrease in the sensitivity of release-modulating autoreceptors on DA or GABA terminals. If these compensatory changes take place, a stimulus that activates DA cell firing, such as stress, would be expected to produce an augmented response. This pathway may be dysregulated in the neurosomatic patient (Harden DG et al., 1998). This work indicates that a specific D_1-receptor antagonist could be quite beneficial. I attempted to create a D_1 agonist by combining the D_1/D_2 agonist mazindol with the primarily D_2 antagonist haloperidol, but this combination did not improve the symptomatology of a single patient. Next I should try apomorphine/haloperidol. Apomorphine (APO) is also a D_1/D_2 agonist. A more specific D_2 antagonist, such as raclopride, could supplant haloperidol. Chronic stress produces an increase in D_1-receptor density in the PFC and a decrease in working memory. Memory impairment is reversed by a specific D_1-receptor antagonist, indicating that up-regulation of the PFC D_1 receptor is a result/cause of a *hypo*dopaminergic state (Mizoguchi K et al., 2000). Specific DA_2/DA_3 autoreceptor antagonists are in the pipeline. Human trials have begun on OSU6162 from Arvid Carlsson's group in Gothenborg, Sweden (Carlsson A, 2001). Such an agent could be of great benefit in neurosomatic disorders and Parkinson's disease.

The brain of a neurosomatic patient is not analogous to an automobile gasoline tank that just needs to be filled with dopamine. There might be abnormalities in dopamine transporter density or autoreceptor sensitivity, as well as in postreceptor events (Dougherty DD et al., 1999).

Atypical neuroleptics, which are of only moderate utility in neurosomatic disorders, increase PFC dopamine output. This enhancement is significantly potentiated by the alpha$_2$-adrenoceptor antagonist idazoxan (Hirtel P et al., 1999).

I have not found the combination of olanzapine and yohimbine, one of the few alpha$_2$-adrenoceptor antagonists available to me in clinical practice, to be an effective therapeutic intervention. Oxytocin, which has many other actions, is also an alpha$_2$ antagonist (Diaz-Cabale Z, Petersson M, et al., 2000). Remeron (mirtazapine), which inhibits alpha$_2$-autoreceptors, is occasionally strikingly effective in 30 minutes. Alpha$_2$ adrenoceptor antagonists facilitate norepinephrine efflux. It has been found that the norepinephrine transporter contributes to the clearance of dopamine from the extracellular compartment within the cortex, and so the concentrations of extracellular norepinephrine may affect cortical dopamine levels by competing for the same transporter. Another treatment combination that might hypothetically work by this mechanism would be methylphenidate (Ritalin) and yohimbine, although it is clinically ineffective. Olanzapine is known to have an alpha$_2$-adrenoceptor blocking action and could conceivably synergize with yohimbine. Using both drugs might enable lower doses of either drug to be administered. Yohimbine and reboxetine may be a beneficial combination. Alpha$_2$ antagonists also enhance the release of serotonin, but this effect of yohimbine does not appear to be clinically important. In fact, yohimbine has been a relatively useless drug in the treatment of neurosomatic disorders except when one seeks to reverse alpha$_2$-agonist ADRs. A rare patient with marked hypofunction of the monoaminergic system contributing to fatigue may benefit from yohimbine, but the drug invariably exacerbates PTSD and panic disorder, illnesses similar to neurosomatic disorders in many respects. Furthermore, although NMDA-receptor antagonists may increase dopamine in some areas of the brain, they seem to reduce dopamine utilization in the prefrontal cortex of monkeys who have been treated chronically with the NMDA-receptor antagonist PCP (Kretschmer BO, 1999).

The way that I access the dopaminergic system is by using dopamine eyedrops, nasal sprays, or oral swirls in either a 1:10 or 1:1 concentration. The eyedrops usually work within one second, and I do not use greater than a 1:10 concentration because most patients remark that the drops initially sting when instilled. The onset of action of the nasal drops and the oral swirl is about 15 seconds. There appears to be no similar use of dopaminergic agonists or any other agonist or antagonist in the pharmacologic literature. One article described intranasal administration of dopaminergic agonists, but this experiment was designed to illustrate that serum levels of these agonists could be raised after intranasal administration to treat Parkinson's disease. The onset of action was measured in several minutes rather than seconds, and, other than by describing a different route of drug delivery, the article casts no light on the use of dopaminergic agonists to alter sensory gating (De Souza F et al., 1997). Nasal instillation of 25 mg of ketamine (the highest dose I use is 1 to 2 mg and is an excellent treatment for headache) has been reported to be effective in familial hemiplegic migraine. I have found that gabapentin 240 mg/gm in PLO applied to the posterior neck rapidly eliminates migraine aura and subsequent headaches in many patients.

Dopamine appears to activate the descending pathways from the rostral agranular insular cortex (RAIC), a cortical area that receives a dense dopaminergic projection and is involved in descending antinociception. Injection of a dopamine-reuptake inhibitor into the RAIC can increase antinociception. Tianeptine, an antidepressant which is also a dopamine-reuptake inhibitor, may have some utility in pain management, if it is ever marketed (Burkey AR et al., 1999).

The complexity of the dopaminergic regulatory system is such that it is often difficult to know what receptor one should stimulate or block because of receptor interactions. For example, up-regulation of the cortical dopamine D_2 receptors is accompanied by a down-regulation of the D_1 sites. This change routinely occurs when using D_2 antagonists but makes almost every neurosomatic patient feel groggy and not improved in any way. The cerebral cortex expresses much higher levels of D_1 than D_2 receptors, but there is no D_1-specific agonist or antagonist with which one might take advantage of this circumstance. I am able to give dopamine by the peripheral trigeminal route and then try to block its effect at the D_2 receptors by using haloperidol, either peripherally or centrally. Until recently, the drug mazindol (Sanorex) was available, which is a psychostimulant selective for D_1 and D_2 receptors only. Combining mazindol and haloperidol, however, which would hypothetically preferentially stimulate D_1 receptors, was not ever a successful strategy while the medication was still on the market. Similarly, I have noted that the D_2 receptor appears to be preferentially involved in neurosomatic patients. If there is an adverse reaction to topical dopaminergic agents at the level of the distal trigeminal nerve, it can almost always be completely reversed by using haloperidol solution. Haloperidol is a fairly specific D_2-receptor antagonist. There has not been any benefit to stimulating D_1 receptors by using dopamine nasal spray while concomitantly blocking D_2 receptors in an attempt to achieve some receptor selectivity in the treatment approach. Haloperidol spray usually completely reverses the effect of dopamine nasal spray. When D_2 receptors are up-regulated, both D_1 receptors and D_5 receptors are down-regulated. When D_2 receptors are blocked, it takes a significant amount of time, at least one month, to see D_1-receptor up-regulation. Enhancement of normal cognitive performance, as noted previously, occurs only within a limited range of dopamine D_1-receptor activation, and overstimulation of these receptors attenuates memory fields of neurons in the primate PFC (Lidow MS et al., 1998). Radioactive ligands to label the density of these receptors by functional brain imaging have existed for many years. They would be of great help to me and others, but the FDA has not approved them.

Low levels of a D_1-receptor agonist can potentiate glutamate-evoked activity, whereas higher levels always suppress activity. It has been suggested that D_1-receptor modulation of neuronal activity includes both facilitation, possibly by increasing high-threshold calcium influx and potentiating an NMDA-evoked activity, and inhibition, possibly mediated by the attenuation of a slow inward sodium conductance or, indirectly, via action on GABA-containing interneurons. Thus, we once again encounter the inverted U-shaped function in which there is an optimal range of dopamine concentration and cortical D_1-receptor activation for normal cognitive performance. "Too little or too much D_1 receptor activation leads to deficient operation of the neural mechanisms required for working memory (due to lack of facilitation or extensive inhibition, respectively), thus resulting in diminished cognitive performance" (Lidow MS et al., 1998).

It is not yet known how D_2 antagonists reduce the levels of cortical D_1 and D_5 receptors. It is thought that there might be a compensatory reaction of these receptors to an overflow in cortical dopamine release resulting from the block of D_2 pre- and postsynaptic sites. Neostriatal D_1 and D_5 receptors, however, quickly develop tolerance to chronic D_2-antagonist treatment, and so this down-regulation would not occur in the basal ganglia. There is also a strong interaction between D_1 and D_2 second messenger systems, as previously noted. Therefore, increase in the sensitivity of D_2-associated adenylate cyclase could conceivably be accompanied by an increase in the sensitivity of D_1-coupled postreceptor enzymes which, in turn, could constitute a signal for down-regulation of the D_1-receptor class. The D_1 and D_2 receptors have an opposing role in modulation of rat nucleus accumbens norepinephrine release (Van der Schuren LJ et al., 1999).

There is no dopaminergic modulation of norepinephrine release in rat medial PFC or amygdala, and, although under a moderate dopaminergic tone, accumbens norepinephrine release is primarily regulated by inhibitory D_2 receptors. This finding is important because the nucleus accumbens shell receives a dense NE-containing projection originating in the nucleus tractus solitarii. The NTS contains vagal fibers, as well as other types, in a thalamo-cortical projection with numerous collaterals. Thus, NE release in the rat NAc is under the opposing influence of stimulatory D_1 and inhibitory D_2 receptors. These NE release-modulatory DA heteroreceptors are presumably localized on nerve terminals of NE neurons originating in the NTS. The D_1 and D_2 receptors are probably differentially located on or near NE nerve terminals, and secreted dopamine may diffuse up to twelve micrometers away from release sites to contact extrasynaptic D_1 receptors. In the case of DA modulation of NAc NE release, this paracrine action would imply that DA released from mesolimbic neurons preferentially interacts with D_2 receptors located in the vicinity of the site of release (Figure 13). D_1 receptors located further away might be stimulated in case of higher rates of release and/or during later phases of neurotransmission by DA that diffused away from the synapse. The noradrenergic projections to the medial PFC and amygdala originate in the locus coeruleus, which is regulated differently than the NTS. It appears NAc NE release may be modulated in a unique manner. For example, NAc NE release is not under the inhibitory influence of alpha$_2$ autoreceptors (Schoffelmeer NAM et al., 1998).

The interaction in the nucleus accumbens of NE and DA release suggests the existence of a catecholaminergic fine-tuning mechanism modulating the generation of adaptive behavioral responses. The balance of DA and NE neurotransmission in the NAc might determine whether excitatory or inhibitory input into NAc neurons will prevail. Thus, under circumstances of moderate DA tone, stimulating D_2 receptors tonically suppresses NAc NE release, whereas extrasynaptically located D_1 receptors play a less prominent role in the regulation of NE release. When DA tone is increased, such as in amphetamine pretreated rats, enhanced DA release from the mesolimbic terminal increases the tonic D_2-receptor-mediated suppression of NE release. In addition, augmented DA release will stimulate extrasynaptic D_1 receptors, resulting in a net increase of NAc NE release. Intrauterine influences, neonatal trauma, or early childhood stress may alter the structure and function of the ventral hippocampus. If such a lesion occurs, there is a blunted DA stress response in the right PFC, consistent with the idea that a

DA-sensitive mechanism in the PFC exerts an inhibitory influence on NAc DA transmission. Mesocorticolimbic DA function is mediated by the ventral hippocampus in rats and can permanently alter the DA stress response. This lesion is more likely to occur in early development than in an adult but may explain some of the dopaminergic abnormalities seen in patients with neurosomatic disorders (Brake WG et al., 1999). Fortunately for these patients, ketamine increases both striatal DA and NE (Kubota T, Hirota K, Yoshida H, et al., 1999).

Looking at neurosomatic disorders from a different perspective, memory and learning related to emotions occur in a hippocampal-amygdala circuit. The salience of these memories and their contextual importance is always being updated by a circuit involving the prefrontal cortex. I have discussed this circuit in regard to memory in *Betrayal by the Brain*. There is hypofunction of the prefrontal cortex commonly noted in patients with neurosomatic disorders and perhaps in the caudate nucleus. These regions are related to memory and continually update the learned associations in the amygdala and make them more flexible.

> Thus, in the face of frontal hypoactivity, limbic structures may be relatively disconnected from normal cortical modulatory influences and may promote more rigid stimulus-response linkages. Emotional biases driven by more primitive amygdaloid and hypothalamic processes may thus escape the modulatory cognitive influences mediated by the frontal lobe. In the absence of effective frontal modulation, early experiences of real or threatened loss or lack of social support may become embedded in the limbic system and generate fixed negative biases toward the self, the world, and the future without the possibility of modulation by a more realistic and adaptive cognitive assessment. (Post RM, 2000)

Thus, in patients with neurosomatic disorders which include mood and anxiety disorders, there is inappropriate modulation of this hippocampal-amygdala circuit, as well as of the hedonic (nucleus accumbens) system. Most neurotransmission from the PFC to other structures is glutamatergic, but, as I have previously noted in *Betrayal by the Brain,* the PFC also regulates secretion of classical neurotransmitters moment to moment, according to the stimulus environment. It also regulates neurotransmitter input to the NAc and hippocampal-amygdala circuits.

Other recent work has elaborated Post's disconnection hypothesis between the prefrontal cortex and the amygdala-hippocampal circuit. In my previous writing, I had emphasized the role of Brodmann's area 46 of the dorsolateral prefrontal cortex and the hippocampus. It appears that the

DLPFC is important in modulating salience since activation of area 46 is associated with selection of an item from memory to guide a response (Row EJB et al., 2000).

In this model, area 46 would be involved in selection of memories to associate with a stimulus by top-down attentional mechanisms. This process has also been termed "attentional selection." Although I heartily endorse the attentional network described by Mesulam, I still believe that area 46 of the DLPFC has a special role to play in determining salience. Knowledge or experiences are voluntarily recalled out of awareness from memory by reactivation of their neural representations in the association cortex. "Associative codes" are created by neurons that have the ability to link the representations of temporally associated stimuli. The frontal eye field, for example, represents locations of relevant objects based on visual salience and knowledge (Miyashita Y, Hayashi T, 2000).

Ketamine-induced NE release from the mPFC can be antagonized by the cholinesterase inhibitor physostigmine. Such inhibitors tend to increase glutamatergic function (Kubota T, Hirota K, Anzawa N, et al., 1999).

Finally, it is worthy of mention that I often notice impaired wound healing in my patients. I was unsure how this phenomenon related to neurosomatic disorders until I read a recent article relating norepinephrine to the rate of wound healing (Kim LR, Pomeranz B, 1999).

The sympathetic nervous system has recently been shown to contribute to neurogenic inflammation, and 6-hydroxydopamine, a sympathetic agonist in low concentrations, was found to accelerate the rate of cutaneous wound healing at both the epidermal and dermal levels. This process is thought to occur by the release of proinflammatory peptides and purines from the sympathetic terminals such as NPY, adenosine (acting at the A_2 receptor), ATP, and the biosynthesis of prostaglandin E2, a potent proinflammatory mediator, as well as a stimulator of collagen synthesis and epidermal keratinization. The increased incidence of Ehlers-Danlos syndrome seen in patients with fibromyalgia may be reflective of a cutaneous noradrenergic hypoactivity.

EFFEXOR (VENLAFAXINE)

I shall discuss in general the use of antidepressants in this section about Effexor, which is probably the most useful single antidepressant one can prescribe in neurosomatic disorders. It is a serotonin/norepinephrine-reuptake inhibitor with a mild inhibition of dopamine reuptake. Its structure is quite similar to tramadol (Ultram), and its analgesic effect is even naloxone reversible. Tramadol has been used as monotherapy in treatment-refractory depression (Shapiro NA et al., 2001).

The primary reason for using nontricyclic antidepressants in neurosomatic disorders is to treat depression. They are not particularly effective in treating somatic symptoms. They are somewhat effective in treating anxiety, although not as effective as they would be in an individual with generalized anxiety disorder or panic disorder. For example, I have not had much luck with them in treating PTSD or OCD. When seen comorbidly with neurosomatic disorders and for severe cases of mixed anxiety and depression, I often find the atypical neuroleptics to be a better choice for monotherapy or as add-on therapy to antidepressants than a serotonin- and/or norepinephrine-reuptake inhibitor.

Effexor has been shown to be superior to most serotonin-reuptake inhibitors in the treatment of depression in several double-blind placebo-controlled experiments. Although it can cause hypertension, most of my patients are hypotensive anyway, so this adverse reaction has not been a problem in my practice. The extended-release form of Effexor is far superior to the immediate-acting form which I had discontinued using because of the high incidence of nausea and vertigo. If I am starting an antidepressant now in a fatigued patient, I will usually begin with Effexor, which has the added benefit of an analgesic effect which is naloxone reversible (Pernia A et al., 2000). If I am using an antidepressant in an individual who appears to have a dopamine deficiency disorder, I might prescribe Wellbutrin (bupropion) as initial therapy, screening for this agent by a positive response to a nicotine patch, although all second-generation antidepressants antagonize the nicotinic cholinergic receptor to some extent. Particularly in patients with sleep disorders, Remeron (mirtazapine), in a dose of 45 to 60 mg at bedtime, is an effective antidepressant as monotherapy, and it can be added on to any of the other antidepressants because it has a unique mode of action. It should be remembered the sedative effect of Remeron is inversely proportional to the dose, which is counterintuitive to most physicians and patients. Therefore, if Remeron is being used as a sleeping pill, it should be prescribed in a low dose, such as 7.5 mg at bedtime. Because it has an effect on the alpha$_2$ autoreceptor, the higher the dose of Remeron that is ingested, the more norepinephrine is released. NE tends to counteract the sedating effects of Remeron, which are caused by its H$_1$ receptor antagonism.

Remeron and Zyprexa (olanzapine) are probably about tied for the medications that cause the most weight gain. Zyprexa does so by increasing hunger, while Remeron acts by delaying satiety. Remeron has proven to be occasionally effective in patients with diffuse pain. In this setting, it has an immediate onset of action. It should be mentioned that the alpha$_{2A}$ agonist guanfacine, although usually conceptualized as a sedative and as possibly causing depression, may act as an antidepressant. It has been reported to induce mania in children, proving "Bunney's rule" that any medication which can cause mania may be used as an antidepressant (Horrigan JP, Barnhill LJ, 1999; Garcia-Sevilla JA et al., 1999).

I find guanfacine to be one of the most useful medications in the neurosomatic pharmacologic armamentarium. Fairly high doses of guanfacine are well tolerated, particularly if the medication is increased gradually and given b.i.d. It should be remembered by both physicians and patients that treating depression in a neurosomatic disorder such as CFS is unlikely to diminish reporting of pain in medically unexplained symptoms but may improve social function (Morris RK et al., 1999).

Numerous medicines I use to treat neurosomatic disorders have an antidepressant effect either immediately, which would probably be nongenomic, or delayed for two to four weeks, which would indicate a possible genomic mechanism such as many antidepressants are presumed to have. These medications may be used as monotherapy for depression or may be used to augment existing antidepressant medications. They include Adderall, Adenocard spray, amantadine, Amerge, intravenous ascorbate, most opioids, particularly methadone, which is a serotonin-reuptake inhibitor, an NMDA-receptor antagonist, and mu-opioid-receptor agonist. Also effective are Dexedrine, DHEA, dipyridamole, dopamine sprays, Gabitril, gamma globulin, guaifenesin, guanfacine, honey bee venom, hydergine, inositol, isoxsuprine, ketamine, Kutapressin, Lamictal, lidocaine, Marinol, modafinil, NADH, naltrexone (usually as augmentation only), Neurontin, nicotine patch, nimodipine (which acts as a $5-HT_2$-receptor antagonist with chronic use), nylidrin, omega-3 and -6 fatty acids, oxytocin, papaverine, pindolol, Ponstel, Requip, Rilutek, Ritalin, Talwin, Tasmar, Topamax, TRH, Ultram (which should not be used with serotonin-reuptake inhibitors or triptans), enalapril or other ACE inhibitors, and Zantac.

Thyroid or lithium augmentation of antidepressants has not been a successful strategy in the neurosomatic population, and, as of this writing, I have induced iatrogenic hyperthyroidism in about ten patients with treatment-resistant depression, and none of them has responded to this intervention. Depression could be considered a neurosomatic disorder having to do with inappropriate cognitions about oneself, just as could anxiety or delusional disorder.

IVIG is very effective in treatment-refractory OCD which, perhaps, has an autoimmune basis. Even more effective in this regard is plasma exchange. Antineuronal antibodies are usually present in those who respond, and the disorder is poststreptococcal in such cases (Perlmutter SJ et al., 1999). Both opioid agonists and antagonists are effective in OCD. An ideal strategy would be to give opioids with ultra-low-dose naltrexone to retard the development of tolerance.

Guanfacine has been found to be as effective as dextroamphetamine in the treatment of ADHD in adults (Taylor FB, Russo JR, 2001). It is a specific agonist at the $alpha_{2A}R$, which is particularly abundant in the PFC and LC. Guanfacine is also a fairly good anxiolytic and may increase cognition in the elderly. By modulating LC NE discharge rates, DA secretion may be indirectly tuned so that attention may be better focused. By increasing NE, such as with the specific reuptake inhibitor reboxetine, DA may also be increased via the effect of alpha-1 receptors on dopaminergic nuclei.

Monoamine oxidase inhibitors are greatly underused in neurosomatic medicine. Some younger psychiatrists have never prescribed them in their careers. They are very effective. Tranylcypromine (Parnate) is better for the patient in whom fatigue is the primary complaint, and phenelzine (Nardil) is preferable in others. MAOIs are safe if used appropriately. Despite warnings in the *PDR,* they can be augmented with stimulants, bupropion, and reboxetine. Nardil is an excellent treatment for headaches resistant to other medications. Selegiline may be used transdermally in a 2 percent PLO and works in about a week. It will be available in a transdermal patch shortly. There are no dietary restrictions with transdermal selegiline, as far as I know.

Executive function is often impaired in patients with neurosomatic disorders. Executive processes are implicated in complex cognition, such as novel problem solving, which entails identifying and coordinating the steps to a new goal, evaluating the intermediate outcome, and modifying the plan as needed. Executive processes are also associated with task-set control, modifying behavior as appropriate in light of changes in the environment, such as in inhibiting prepotent or previous responses. Working memory has been operationalized primarily as the processes and structures that keep information available over a relatively short time. In this standard perspective, executive processes manipulate the contents of the working memory buffers (Carpenter PA et al., 2000).

There is a question about whether executive processes are localized in the prefrontal regions and control lower-level processes in more posterior regions. This notion of singularity, or modality specificity, in the heteromodal cortex is increasingly outdated. The emerging view is that each associated cortical region has more than one function and that the functions of distinct areas might overlap. This idea may not extend to only executive function or working memory but may be a general principle of cortical organization. Thus, neural networks can be viewed as overlapping rather than dissociated, although different regions of the brain may make differential contributions to a specific cognitive function. The extent of activation of a particular region, such as area 46, would depend on the degree of specificity of the involved task for the particular functions of that area.

For example, it has been suggested that available evidence does not support a modality-based system of organization with the DLPFC. The DLPFC may contribute to the manipulation of information within memory, while the ventral PFC may be more involved in salience selection (Rushworth MFS, Owen AM, 1998).

Although there is still considerable debate in the literature about whether there is functional specificity in the PFC, I am most swayed by functional brain imaging that reveals roughtly the same patterns of activation in the frontal lobe associated with a broad range of different cognitive demands, including aspects of perception, response selection, executive control, working memory, episodic memory, and problem solving. For all these demands, there is a striking recruitment of middorsolateral, midventrolateral, and dorsoanterior cingulate cortex. It seems there is a specific network of prefrontal neurons recruited to solve various cognitive problems (Duncan J, Owen AM, 2000). Unfortunately, Duncan and Owen do not discuss the "deactivations" (decreases in neural activity associated with increased demand) commonly seen in functional brain imaging of neurosomatic patients (Gusnard DA, Raichk NE, 2001; Leslie RA, 2001; Logothetis NK et al., 2001).

To further discuss how the effective intensity of a stimulus is regulated or "attentional weighting" is given to a stimulus, I shall review the habituation of the orienting response (OR) to visual stimuli. "The OR is modulated by associative learning and this modulation is abnormal in rats with selective damage to the dorsal hippocampus" (Honey RC, Good M, 2000).

A novel stimulus often provokes a response that habituates during repeated encounters with that stimulus. If, indeed, one stimulus is attended to in the first place, many novel stimuli are not attended to. The initial response to a novel stimulus may be triggered by the fact that an animal does not possess a memory of that stimulus. This response is inhibited when the stimulus present in the environment has a matching stored memory and is, again, triggered by a novel stimulus for which no memory exists. Thus, patients with neurosomatic disorders who have an inappropriate perception of the salience or novelty of a repeated stimulus may have a dysfunction in habituation and dishabituation in the neural mechanisms that underlie recognition memory. The hippocampus, the anterior cingulate, and the DLPFC are important components of a system that detects or acts on mismatches between the current stream of sensory input and stored memories of previous sensory streams. Hippocampal dysfunction in neurosomatic disorders may give too much weight to the presentation of a stimulus because of inappropriate storage of memories. Normally, these memories should be relatively inactive.

Disruption of the associative modulation of an OR in an organism with hippocampal dysfunction may contribute to hypervigilance.

In neurosomatic disorders, an accentuation of the attentional weighting is given to elements of a stimulus that, in actuality, have a very tenuous relationship to the state of activation of the long-term memory store. Unlike the individual with a normally functioning neural network for associative learning, the activated memory store to which the stimulus is associated does not rapidly decay but continues to be highly weighted, even if this weighting occurs outside of the individual's attention. This mechanism is somewhat related to that of PTSD (Newport DJ, Nemeroff CV, 2000).

One of the differences, however, is that there does not appear to be global neurosomatic noradrenergic hyperactivity in neurosomatic disorders, although there may be enhancement of whatever noradrenergic tone there is by glutamate. There is no hippocampal atrophy in patients with CFS. This atrophy has been related to glutamatergic excitotoxicity. Patients with neurosomatic disorders seem to respond better than those with PTSD to NMDA-receptor antagonists. The notion of overactivity of the amygdala, a rapid subcortical information processing unit involved in aversive classical conditioning, has survival advantages for an organism. Amygdala processing speed of behaviorally relevant and possibly dangerous stimuli is rapid, but a fast nonspecific subcortical system with a deliberately high false alarm rate is constantly "under supervision of the more specific cortical system" (Buchel C, Dolan RJ, 2000).

Certain subnuclei of the amygdala may be continuously activated without temporal decay by an overly broad range of conditioned stimuli. Evidence from functional MRI studies shows such activation of the amygdala with no decreases over time during classical fear conditioning (Figures 14 and 15). The hippocampal response, however, to the conditioned stimulus is more likely to be attenuated (Buchel C, Dolan RJ, 2000).

Classical fear conditioning has been recently reviewed (Schafe GE et al., 2001). The results are what I would expect. Conditioned stimulus (CS) and unconditional stimulus (US) inputs converge onto individual cells in the lateral amygdala (LA). When fear is expressed in behavior, the LA engages the central nucleus of the amygdala (CE), which as the principal output nucleus of the fear system projects to areas of the hypothalamus and brainstem that control behavioral, endocrine, and autonomic conditional responses (CRs) associated with fear learning. Input neurons of the LA demonstrate Hebbian learning and LTP in association with fear learning.

LTP has early and late phases, which overlap. They both involve the kinase cascade, but late LTP is maintained genomically by synthesis of new proteins, in contrast to early LTP, in which changes in protein activity and activation are sufficient. Early LTP can persist because of *autophosphory-*

lation, or the capacity of kinases to be activated for much longer than usual in the absence of Ca^{2+} for a period of time following LTP induction (Figure 16). PKA and CAMKII are the kinases most likely to be initially auto-phosphorylated, and they, in turn, can phosphorylate a large number of target proteins. NMDA blockade in the LA disrupts fear acquisition but not fear expression, as well as short- and long-term memory of the fear-provoking event.

LTP-inducing stimulation of the hippocampus or LA by the cAMP agonist forskolin leads to increases in the phosphorylation of CREB and subsequent activation of ERK/MAPK (Figure 17). Thus, CS:US → LA → principal cells → Ca^{2+} influx through NMDA receptor. Increased $[Ca^{2+}]_i$ → activation of alpha CaMKII, PKC, PKA, ERK/MAPK → cell nucleus → activation of transcription factors such as CREB → further gene transcription and the synthesis of new proteins. Variations of this pathway can be applied to numerous other situations.

A postulate to which I shall continually refer in this book is that patients with neurosomatic disorders have overly learned and overly generalized associative responses and that the primary molecular basis of this memory dysfunction involves the NMDA receptor. In the subsequent discussion, I shall be referring considerably to a recent article by Joe Z. Tsien (2000).

SYNAPTIC PLASTICITY AND LONG-TERM POTENTIATION IN NEUROSOMATIC DISORDERS

The pharmacologic manipulation of neurosomatic neurocognitive dysfunction will be addressed in my discussion about the NMDA-receptor antagonist ketamine. One aspect of the pharmacology of ketamine relevant to the subsequent sections is that ketamine decreases one's ability to attend to stimuli, and neurosomatic disorders may be conceptualized as overattending to nonsalient stimuli. In 1949, Donald Hebb postulated learning and memory occurred by strengthening the synaptic connection between a presynaptic and postsynaptic neuron by activating both simultaneously (Hebb DO, 1949).

A continuum of associative synaptic changes is determined by the relationship between the specific level of postsynaptic depolarization paired with presynaptic activity. Strong depolarization leads to potentiation. A widely used model for studying learning in mammals experimentally is that of long-term potentiation, particularly in the CA1 region of the hippocampus (Malenka RC, Nicoll RA, 1999).

Patients with neurosomatic disorders may have genetically and/or developmentally induced enhancement of long-term potentiation. LTP in the

CA1 region requires the activation of the NMDA receptors and numerous protein kinases, phosphatases, transcription factors, and immediate early genes.

Various types of glutamate-receptor knock-out mice have been bred. These mice have deficits in LTP which can be overcome by pretreating or environmental enrichment. Patients with neurosomatic disorders may have overexpression of NMDA receptors or of certain NMDA-receptor subunits. NMDA-receptor activation is directly associated with release of intracellular calcium stores and subsequent engagement of intracellular calcium-related mechanisms.

Enhanced LTP is related to reduced GABAergic inhibition, an alteration which appears to occur in many individuals with neurosomatic disorders. There are two major types of intracellular calcium-release mechanisms. These have been discussed previously and will be discussed further in the section on heparin, but one is IP_3-induced calcium release, and the other is calcium-induced calcium release (CICR) occurring via a ryanodine-sensitive receptor. There are three types of ryanodine receptors. RyR_3 is present in the brain where it may be activated by calcium, ATP, and caffeine. The RyR_2 receptor is also highly prevalent in the brain. It can be activated by calcium in calcium channels, calmodulin kinase, and protein kinase A. It can be augmented pharmacologically by caffeine and suramin. Mice lacking RyR_3 may have LTP facilitated by electrical stimulation. This type of LTP is independent of the NMDA receptor and is partially dependent on L-type voltage-dependent calcium channels and metabotropic glutamate receptors. This fact illustrates the utility of pharmacologic agents that can block L-type calcium channels at the present time in the treatment of neurosomatic disorders and in the future by subtype selective agonists or antagonists of metabotropic glutamate receptors. Transgenic mice overexpressing the gene encoding tissue plasminogen activator (tPA) have increased hippocampal LTP evoked by theta burst stimulation, a type of electrical stimulation (Medani R et al., 1999). tPA enhances NMDA receptor-mediated signaling (Nicole O et al., 2001).

tPA is an immediate early gene known to be induced by LTP and kindling. Several years ago, I investigated tPA levels in patients with CFS, and sometimes found them to be elevated (Goldstein J, 1990).

Thus, an overexpression of tPA, interacting with the NR1 subunit of the NMDA receptor, might lead to overly enhanced associative learning which could be characteristic of patients with neurosomatic disorders. tPA is best known in general medical practice for its use in acute arterial occlusion, particularly occurring in the myocardium. tPA in the presence of thrombin, which forms clots, becomes greatly activated and induces the formation of plasmin, which is a thrombolytic substance. tPA is also an immediate early gene found in increased concentrations in the granule cells of the dentate gyrus in the hippocampus after an epileptic seizure.

It is significant that the majority of patients with neurosomatic disorders are quite sensitive to caffeine. If certain subunits of the CA1 NMDA receptors are deleted in knock-out mice, some forms of learning and memory are significantly impaired. Important for understanding neurosomatic disorders, the conditional knock-out of the gene encoding the NR1 subunit results in a complete loss of NMDA currents, short-term potentiation, LTP, and long-term depression (LTD) in the CA1 region. NR1 knock-out mice are also impaired in three hippocampal dependent, nonspatial memory tasks, namely novel object recognition tasks, social transfer of food preference, and contextual fear conditioning. Novel object recognition and contextual fear conditioning are overly enhanced in many patients with neurosomatic disorders. All of these learning deficits can be "rescued" by daily exposure to an enriched environment that induces an increase in the synapse density of the CA1 region in knock-outs, as well as in control littermates (Rampon C et al., 2000).

The opposite side of the coin is that NMDA-receptor overexpression or overactivity, which may be present at birth, may be enhanced by an early childhood environment that places a premium on learning to detect potentially threatening (novel) events, or not (Raphael KG et al., 2001). Such a case would occur in a child raised in an unsafe environment. Tsien, when discussing learning and allostasis, writes,

> How can we get around these uncertainties and roadblocks? A simple way appears to focus on the upstream master switches that are essential for controlling major classes of synaptic plasticity. The best example of this kind of master switch is the NMDA receptor, which has been consistently shown to be required for the induction of many forms of plasticity, such as LTP . . . The reason that the NMDA receptor is unique is because the activation of NMDA receptors requires both the release of glutamate from pre-synaptic cells and the depolarization of the post-synaptic cells. It serves as a molecular coincidence detector for detecting the two simultaneous events, thus implementing Hebb's rule at the synapse . . . (Tsien JZ, 2000, p. 269)

NMDA receptors are known to be heteromeric complexes consisting of a core NR1 subunit and various modulatory NR2 subunits. NMDA-receptor complexes consist of more than 80 different proteins, many of which might have their functions pharmacologically modulated to create novel neurosomatic treatments (Kind PC, Neumann PE, 2001; Kemp JA, McKernan RM, 2002).

The NR2A and NR2B subunits, unlike NR2C and NR2D, are strongly blocked by extracellular magnesium. This reason is one among several that explain why the NR2A and NR2B subunits are better suited for the coincidence detection of presynaptic and postsynaptic activities. Thus, one might hypothesize that administering parenteral doses of magnesium sulfate would function as an NMDA-receptor antagonist. Perhaps this antagonism occurs in vitro or in certain areas of the brain not relevant to neurosomatic disorders, but after numerous trials, I abandoned the use of intravenous magnesium sulfate as monotherapy when I was doing therapeutic trials of various NMDA-receptor antagonists. On the other hand, it would be useful to have a selective antagonist at the glycine site of the NMDA receptor, since glycine is an essential coagonist for glutamatergic activation of the NMDA receptor. Until quite recently, it was possible to specifically stimulate only the glycine coagonist site, but now there is a potent and selective antagonist, gavestinel. In a randomized controlled trial of this agent in patients with acute stroke, hoping it would be a neuroprotective agent, administration of gavestinel within six hours of acute ischemic stroke did not improve outcome (Lees KR et al., 2000). Other glycine-site antagonists used for other indications are in development and could be used concurrently with probenecid (Stone TW, 2000), which decreases the excretion of the endogenous NMDA/ glycine antagonist kynurenate.

Numerous antagonists at various sites of the NMDA receptor, such as lubeluzole, selfotel, aptiganel, eliprodil, and many others, have not been effective neuroprotective agents in acute stroke when used as monotherapy. However, all of these agents could be useful modulations of the NMDA receptor in the treatment of neurosomatic disorders (DeKeyser J et al., 1999).

"Furthermore, during the transition from juvenile to adult, there is a developmental switch from NR2B to NR2A, as the preferred partner for NR1 in the forebrain. Therefore, the increase in the ratio of NR2A over NR2B may explain the age-dependent decline in the slow component of NMDA currents during the transition period" (Tsien JZ, 2000, p. 220). Mice have been bred that overexpress the NR2B receptor (Tang Y, 1999).

Overexpression of the NR2B subunit leads to enhanced NMDA function and facilitated performance in certain behavioral tasks including a recognition test, contextual and cued fear conditioning, and contextual and cued fear extinction. The NR2B overexpressing mice have much longer memory retention and significantly enhanced learning ability in two types of fear extinction tests. Thus, NR2B transgenic mice are able to associate paired events two to three times faster than controls. This finding may explain why the NR2A subunit might be the preferred partner for NR1 in the forebrain, but NR1 is associated with NR2B instead. This combination could possibly impair learning to dissociate previously paired events and may lead to enhanced NMDA-receptor-mediated coincidence detection and stimulus generalization. Partly because of the NR1/NR2B subunit predominance, a different type of learning occurs in preadolescence. Tsien writes that "[t]he NMDA receptor, indeed, acts as a common molecular master switch for various forms of associative learning and memory" (2000, p. 220). Tsien describes the

> NMDA receptor-gated terrain model, [in which] learned information or memory trace is registered by the patterns of a specific group of neurons in the entire memory circuit which are tightly coordinated by common sensory information. In addition, in a given local network, the neurons that are most effectively connected weight heavily on the network properties. As a result, firing patterns of these neurons dominate the network output . . . (Tsien JZ, 2000, p. 221)

The NMDA receptors and such "nodal neurons" can often be pharmacologically modulated without altering their subunits. This sort of modulation can occur so rapidly it has been termed "instantaneous neural network reconfiguration" and is commonly seen in the rapid symptomatic amelioration that occurs on a daily basis in my office practice of neurosomatic medicine. I shall discuss instantaneous neural network reconfiguration in a subsequent section.

THE POSTRECEPTOR PHOSPHORYLATION CASCADE

Postreceptor events can be increasingly targeted at the present time, and knowledge of these processes greatly enhances one's options in neuropsychopharmacology. Such mechanisms would include various G-protein-coupled receptors related to second messengers and ion channels. Thus, if a patient seems to respond to a certain type of neurotransmitter, one can select agents that target the postreceptor changes occurring after the ligand binds to the receptor. For example, there are numerous receptor subtypes for acetylcholine, serotonin, norepinephrine, dopamine, GABA, tachykinins, NPY, VIP, opioids, and glutamate. These are G-protein-coupled receptors, and the types of G-protein receptors to which they are coupled differ. By knowing what the G proteins are, it is possible to predict elevations or depressions in second messengers such as IP_3, diacylglycerol, and cAMP. Levels of these second messengers may rise or fall depending on the G-protein receptor.

Ion channels, particularly potassium and calcium ion channels, also may be opened or closed, producing excitation, inhibition, or a variable physiologic response. This subject is vast. Whizzing through the literature, we find neurotransmitter-gated ion channels, protein-tyrosine-kinase receptors which bind to growth factors, and Src-homology domains (SH_2 and SRH_3) which bind to various intracellular peptide sequences. Other channels include the JAK- and STAT-coupled receptors for polypeptide messengers such as cytokines, interferons, growth hormone, prolactin, leptin, and others related to a cytoplasmic tyrosine kinase belonging to the Janustyrosine kinase (JAK) subfamily. Activation of this class of receptor can regulate gene expression via a single family of intermediary proteins called STAT (signal transducer and activator of transcription). There are also receptors for steroid hormones, which are both nongenomic and occur on the neuronal membrane, and genomic, which bind to a hormone and then diffuse into the nucleus where the complex attaches to specific DNA promoter sequences.

Among the various G proteins are small G proteins, simple molecular switches such as Rab which inhibits exocytosis of the vesicles in proximity to one which is expelling its contents. These activate the exchange of guanosine diphosphate (GDP) for guanosine triphosphate (GTP). There are also larger G proteins composed of three subunits. The alpha subunit binds to GTP, and the beta/gamma subunit can activate or inhibit adenyl cyclase, K^+ channels, the MAP kinase pathway, and recruit G-protein-coupled receptor kinases (Figures 18 and 19). The Ras MAP- kinase pathway (Figure 20) is activated after stimulation of growth factor receptors and numerous other receptors (Chang L, Karin M, 2001), and on and on and on.

Cyclic AMP is an important compound formed from ATP by a class of transmembrane enzymes termed adenyl cyclases, which are usually activated by subtypes of G proteins. Cyclic AMP has numerous intracellular functions, the most prominent of which involves binding to cAMP-dependent protein kinase, which is present in all cells. Various protein kinases can then become activated by associating their catalytic subunits. There are phospholipid metabolites catalyzed by phospholipases; phospholipase A_2 will be discussed in some detail in the section on honey bee venom. Other phospholipases include stimulated phospholipase C, an important enzyme to consider in neurosomatic disorders.

Inositol triphosphate has been discussed previously and will be discussed further in the section on heparin. Calcium is an important divalent cation. Calcium concentrations in the extracellular space are much higher than in the cytoplasm. Some intracellular organelles, particularly mitochondria and the endoplasmic reticulum, contain high concentrations of calcium which can be released by various pharmacologic substances. Nitric oxide is a highly diffusible gas which acts intracellularly and also extracellularly on a different region of the neuron from which it was secreted. NO is also an intercellular retrograde neurotransmitter. I discussed nitric oxide extensively in *Betrayal by the Brain* and shall discuss it further in this book. Recall that nitroglycerin exerts its effect by being transformed into nitric oxide. Protein phosphorylation is an important intracellular process carried out by protein kinases in the presence of magnesium which transfer phosphate groups to various amino acids. Protein kinases form a very large group of related enzymes, each of which has its own localization, regulation, and substrate specificity. Some protein kinases are either receptors for extracellular signals or are associated with such receptors. More of them are activated directly by postreceptor messengers. There are neuronal phosphoprotein phosphatases best known for their relationship to DARPP-32.

In general, protein phosphatases and protein kinases have opposite effects. Many immediate early genes are encoded very rapidly by various signal transduction pathways, often within minutes, following a host of extracellular signals or membrane depolarization. Phosphorylation of transcription factors activates IEGs. One example of an IEG activated by the cAMP pathway is CREB. There are numerous other IEGs. Obviously, these topics are too complex for me to discuss at great length, but I shall allude to them in subsequent pharmacologic discussions.

THE TREATMENT OF ATTENTIONAL DISORDERS

The neuropharmacology of attention is in such a primitive state that it can best be described as pitiful (Robbins TW, 1998).

The level of sophistication in treating attentional disorders primarily relates to attention deficit hyperactivity disorder, and has focused primarily on manipulation of acetylcholine, dopamine, and norepinephrine. Almost all medications I use to treat neurosomatic disorders can ameliorate attentional difficulties in selected individuals. For example, for "inattentive ADD," that is, ADD without hyperactivity, the best single treatment is gabapentin. Inattentive ADD is almost impossible for me to differentiate from CFS unless the only deficit the patient presents with is an attentional problem, in which case inattentive ADD would be the proper diagnosis. However, treating inattentive ADD with stimulants is largely unsatisfactory, and stimulants may, indeed, make this disorder worse. Alpha$_{2A}$-receptor agonists such as guanfacine would be preferable if the choice is made to treat this disorder within a framework of catecholaminergic modulation (Seahill L et al., 2001). In the very near future, it should be common practice to use cholinergic agonists to treat ADHD, but it may be many years before attentional disorders in general will be treated as they should within the neurosomatic paradigm. In contrast to the paucity of work in attentional clinical pharmacology, research in the pharmacologic alterations of the mechanisms of memory formation in brain slices or in living animals is fairly advanced (McGaugh JL, Izquierdo I, 2000).

The cognitive deficits characteristically found in neurosomatic disorders can simplistically be viewed as problems with overallocation of attentional resources. Because recognizing the salience of information and giving it appropriate synaptic weight is required both for attention and encoding (making of new memories), pharmacologic manipulation of memory formation should benefit attentional disorders of the sort found in neurosomatic patients. Thus, agents that inhibit the making of new memories in normal individuals would facilitate the making of new memories in patients with neurosomatic disorders. McGaugh and Izquierdo list several types of medications which can induce irreversible amnesia for single-trial inhibitory avoidance in major tasks.

> One, specific antagonists of AMPA, and NMDA or mGlu receptors, CaMKII (calmodulin kinase II) inhibitors or inhibitors of guanylate cyclase or PKG infused into CA1 immediately after treating; two, PKC inhibitors infused within the first 32-120 minutes after treating; three, inhibitors of either PKA or MAPK [MAP kinase] infused either immediately or three to six hours after treating; or, four, anisomycin infused shortly before or after treating or three hours after treating. (McGaugh JL, Izquierdo I, 2000)

For example, a protein synthesis inhibitor could be combined with CBT and EMDR in treating PTSD in patients receiving cancer chemotherapy (Nader K et al., 2000). These drugs may be used in the treatment of patients with neurosomatic disorders when they present to the physician. Agents that improve encoding, as listed by McGaugh and Izquierdo, include

> glutamate receptor agonists or some of the above mentioned enzymes (e.g., PKG, and PKA), infused into CA1 at the appropriate times [to] enhance memory. The activity of PKG, PKC or CaMKII, and the phosphorylation of GAP42 and GluR1 increase in the CA1 shortly after treating whereas the activity of PKA and MAPK increases in two peaks that are concomitant with increases in the concentration of nuclear CREB phosphorylated at the serine 133 residue. (McGaugh JL, Izquierdo I, 2000; Figures 21 and 22)

Virtually every extracellular signal produces its physiological effects by regulating phosphorylation of neuronal phosphoproteins. Protein phosphorylation is by far the most prominent mechanism of neural plasticity. Kinases phosphorylate proteins. Thus, medications that would enhance memory in a normal individual should result in a memory decrement in patients with neurosomatic disorders, although this postulate would apply only to those with hyperactivity of the NMDA receptor complex. As I have mentioned previously, a group of generally hypoactive patients, usually identified by an almost completely normal score on the Beck Anxiety Inventory and a paucity of symptoms on my CFS checklist, often respond in the opposite manner. Some of these patients, if sleep apnea has been ruled out, may have a primary disorder of vigilance. It has also been observed that mitochondria have a role in memory consolidation (Bevilaqua LR et al., 1999), which results in the inclusion of mitochondrial encephalomyopathy and subtler mitochondrial dysfunctions in the differential diagnosis. Narcoleptic variant should be considered in difficult case presentation, as well as idiopathic recurring stupor, dissociative disorder, complex migraine (e.g., basilar), other sleep disorders, simple deteriorative disorder, and atypical depression.

I shall be discussing mitochondrial function further when I discuss the pathophysiology of fatigue. McGaugh and Izquierdo make a distinction between "core" and modulatory mechanisms of memory. They state:

> Amnesia that is produced by mechanisms that involve the core mechanism (e.g., CaMKII or PKA inhibitors microinfused into CA1) is not reversed by the subsequent infusion of PKA stimulant into CA1 or by systemic adrenocorticotropin (ACTH) or vasopressin administered at the time of retrieval. (McGaugh JL, Izquierdo I, 2000)

These findings would support my own observations that neither DDAVP, a form of vasopressin, nor ACTH improve symptoms in patients with neurosomatic disorders. Specific CaMKII or PKA inhibitors are not available to me for clinical use. However, memory impairment in neurosomatic disorders can be reversed by numerous other agents. Medications that might inhibit casein Kinase II (CKII), another calcium-dependent kinase, include nylidrin and isoxsuprine, which block the spermine activation site of the NMDA receptor. They also activate $D_{2,3,4}$ receptors, $beta_2$ receptors, and sigma receptors. They block alpha receptors and voltage-gated Na^+, K^+, and Ca^{2+} channels.

Spermine is a nociceptive substance. Its algogenic effect may possibly be antagonized by Ca^{2+}-channel blockers, SAMe, morphine, and various NMDA antagonists, especially those acting at the polyamine site. Blockers of the NK-1 receptor for SP are ineffective in eliminating spermine-induced nociception. SP is a cotransmitter with glutamate in the spinal cord dorsal horn (Tan-No K et al., 2000).

CKII, one of many serine-threonine kinases, is constitutively active in controlling the basal function of NMDA-receptor channels. Spermine stimulates CKII and up-regulates NMDA-channel activity, probably through coupling to the spermine modulatory site on the receptor. Several agents block the spermine site. They include acamprosate (which may reduce alcohol craving), ifenprodil (which may decrease symptoms of somatoform disorder; Masuda Y, 1999), eliprodil, and haloperidol (Figure 23). Nylidrin and isoxsuprine were developed in the 1960s as beta-adrenoceptor agonists (Whittemore ER et al., 1997) and do not cross-react with other site-specific NMDA-receptor antagonists or, indeed, with each other. Nylidrin and isoxsuprine are useful agents in the practice of neurosomatic medicine.

DRB (5,6-dichloro-1-β-D-ribofuranosyl benzimidazole) is a cell-permeable CKII inhibitor. Its effect on NMDA-channel openings is reproduced by heparin, which reduces NMDA-channel open durations (Lieberman DN, Mody I, 1999). I include heparin (and warfarin) among the NMDA antagonists. Heparin also blocks the intracellular IP_3 receptor, which regulates release of calcium from cytoplasmic stores. The dose of heparin required for a therapeutic effect in neurosomatic disorders is ten- to fiftyfold less than the anticoagulant dose. McGaugh and Izquierdo go on to state:

> Therefore, memory impairment that is induced by drug treatments that block core memory mechanisms seems to be irreversible. By contrast, memory impairment induced by treatments that act upon modulatory systems, such as electroconvulsive shock, systemic beta endorphin, or intra-amygdala CaMKII inhibitors can be attenuated by the subsequent injection or infusion of several drugs and hormones. (McGaugh JL, Izquierdo I, 2000)

Certainly, all my patients who have received ECT have developed the characteristic anterograde and retrograde amnesia which usually attenuates with time. The lone exception to this phenomenon has been patients with depressive or subcortical pseudodementia who, after they recover from the amnesic effects of the ECT, have enhanced memory function. Most of these patients, however, develop Alzheimer's disease in five years or so.

Attention is a process to which I shall repeatedly return, since neurosomatic disorders are attentional disorders. Stephen Grossberg (Grossberg S, 2000) discusses that the brain is organized into parallel processing streams with complementary properties. Grossberg's work is too complex to summarize in this book. He reviews the complementary processes of resonance and reset which are related to properties of attention and memory search, respectively. His work has recently been summarized and updated, emphasizing synchronous oscillations (Engel AK et al., 2001).

Resonance is an easily measurable property that describes the ability of neurons to respond selectively to inputs at preferred frequencies. Neuronal resonance is an important mechanism in tuning the brain. Because all events in the brain act in frequencies and rhythms, the brain has found a set of mechanisms capable of tuning neurons to specific frequencies. There are circumstances in which strongly amplified resonances are used to coordinate the emergent pattern of network activity around a preferred frequency. Such is the case in thalamic participation in delta and spindle wave generation, which I discussed in *Betrayal by the Brain*. There are functions for subthreshold oscillations in many areas of the brain. The widespread disposition of a resonance of whatever strength aids neurons in the integration of their input. "In effect the establishment of even a weak resonance makes a neuron a good listener for activity within a specialized frequency band. This phenomenon has been termed stochastic resonance. A host of good listeners, mutually connected, should tune networks to operate in frequency ranges in special biological meaning" (Hutcheon B, Yarom Y, 2000). A type of resonance termed "neural synchrony" has been related to arousal, attentional selection, and working memory. Neural synchrony involves fast oscillations in the gamma range and has been invoked to explain the "binding" occurring in fast parallel processing (if not due to glial calcium waves), as well as consciousness itself (Engel AK, Singer W, 2001).

Resonance and synchronization may be accomplished by pacemaker cells synaptically driving follower cells as a network oscillator, i.e., the neural network itself may oscillate. One way in which this phenomenon may occur has been described in a culture network through synapses that release glutamate, activating a heteromultimeric AMPA-type receptor containing a GluR2 subunit associated with a high-conduction channel for sodium and potassium. Rhythmic activity is controlled by synapses that release GABA to activate $GABA_A$ receptors. The presumed function of the two receptor types is facilitated by their respective location, $GABA_A$ receptors predominating on the soma and AMPA receptors being abundant in dendrites. It may be that neural network oscillators are more important than the activity of pacemaker or nodal neurons (Misgeld U et al., 1998). Amplified resonances can coordinate neural activity at the outset around a preferred frequency. I have discussed this phenomenon in the section on the work of Mircea Steriade. Weaker resonances may aid neurons in the integration of their inputs, or "tuning."

The other world "maven" in thalamocortical synchrony is Edward G. Jones, now at UC-Davis. Jones describes a matrix of calbindin-immunoreactive neurons, explaining that "their superficial terminations can synchronize specific and nonspecific elements of the thalamocortical network in coherent activity that underlies cognitive events" (Jones EG, 2001). Jones deals with the "binding problem," as well as the mind itself, via the calbindin synchronous thalamocortical neuron.

Attention and memory search enable the brain to discover and stably learn new representations for novel events in an efficient way. Grossberg highlights the relationship between matching top-down expectations with bottom-up data, a process which focuses attention on those feature clusters in the bottom-up input that are expected. The interaction of attention-learning and orienting-search subsystems and how they interact has been developed into adaptive resonance theory, or ART. ART reaffirms the processes of the attentional network of Mesulam and uses the word "pattern" to refer to the hypothesis that the brain's functional units of short-term representation of information and of long-term learning about this information are distributed patterns of activation and of synaptic weight, respectively, across a neuronal network. "Energy" refers to the mechanisms by which pattern processing is turned on and off by activity-dependent modulatory processes. The neurosomatic pattern processing network in the cerebral cortex, particularly in the DLPFC, could be viewed as dysfunctional in ART theory, because decreased signal-to-noise ratio inappropriately gives synaptic weight to irrelevant stimuli. If thalamocortical representations of recently presented sensory events viewed either in a classical or instrumental conditioning paradigm do not constitute a proper pattern because too many events have become conditioned stimuli, then too many sensory events will amplify their own activity via learned motivational feedback signals which have the role of "energy" in this example. Usually, if there is not inappropriate stimulus generalization, then amplified representations can, in turn, attentionally block or inhibit the representations of irrelevant sensory events. Grossberg states, "Attentional blocking is one of the key mechanisms whereby animals learn which consequences are causally predicted by their antecedent sensory cues and actions, and which consequences are merely accidental" (Grossberg S, 2000, p. 242). Conditioned stimuli activate sensory categories which compete among themselves for limited-capacity short-term memory activation and storage. With appropriate allocation of salience, attention, and synaptic weighting, sensory representations that win the competition in response to the balance of external inputs and internal motivational signals are able to activate neural networks and provide cognitive and sensory motor regulation. The ART theory is quite compatible with my own conceptions of the pathophysiology of neurosomatic disorders. Many other attentional theories could also be cited to explain essentially the same process.

Recently, an event-related brain potential, error-related negativity (ERN), has been developed to monitor medial frontal cortex activity. ERN has been proposed to reflect anterior cingulate action monitoring. "In demanding task situations, it is important to detect when actions are (or are likely to be) erroneous—and to correct for the problem" (Gehring WJ, Knight RT, 2000).

Activation of the lateral PFC and the anterior cingulate cortex show a co-occurrence of activity related to error processing observed in single neuron recordings from nonhuman primates. One view of this interaction is that the anterior cingulate monitors for response, conflict, or errors, and other systems further downstream actually implement the compensatory behavior. One such candidate system is the basal ganglia. Several models postulate that the prefrontal cortex maintains representations which define the contextually appropriate perceptual-response mappings used for decision making. Such a map would be analogous to the "pattern" in ART. Without such representations, the ACC would not be able to determine what was correct and what was not. Therefore, if the representations maintained by the PFC are weak or inappropriate, multiple competing responses might become active, causing response conflict subsequently detected by the anterior cingulate. In either case, the alerting signal produced by the anterior cingulate would be less reliable. This system matches up well with the models previously discussed, even though dysfunction of the ACC has not been demonstrated in neurosomatic disorders without concurrent mood disorders. Compensatory systems may have been unable to act on such an unreliable alerting signal, or they may have made strategic adjustments to weaken the coupling between the less reliable alerting signal and the compensatory action, thus producing a deleterious effect of PFC dysfunction on compensatory behavior. The ACC, when detecting a mismatch, may mobilize affective systems, perhaps the cingulate connections with the amygdala and brainstem autonomic nuclei. Findings from various ERN experiments support this view. Thus, PFC dysfunction may disinhibit an ACC response that normally occurs only in response to errors. Gehring and Knight's study has been somewhat refined by adding in an error-modulatory system, the locus coeruleus, that increases responsivity of processing units globally, perhaps by a change in gain. Alteration in gain would modulate selective attention by its influence on representation of specific task demands in the PFC, as well as motor preparation by its influence on response units. Thus, the primary function of such control is to favor the processing of past relevant information and allow it to competitively suppress processing of distracting information. A disturbance in this mechanism assigns decreased synaptic weight to relevant information and increased power to distractors, one of the major aspects of neurosomatic disorders (Cohen JD et al., 2000). Other work also supports the point of view of Gehring and Knight (McDonald AW et al., 2000).

INSTANTANEOUS NEURAL NETWORK
RECONFIGURATION

For many years, I have viewed brain function as a coruscation of electro-chemical impulses continually flashing through the brain. These neural networks often can be modulated fairly simply by tuning them. Sometimes one may tune "nodal neurons" in the neural networks in order to achieve this result. One of the problems I have had over the years when addressing groups of learned clinicians and researchers has been either the disbelief or total nonacceptance of my everyday observations that patients with brain function disorders may be successfully treated in an extremely short time, sometimes as short as one second. This transformation is termed instantaneous neural network reconfiguration (Nicolelis M, 1997) or immediate plastic remapping. The modification involves changes in the dynamic balance of excitation and inhibition throughout the neural axis, primarily due to the reduction of afferent-driven tonic inhibition. Converse remodeling may occur in certain individuals. The fact that the somatosensory system is capable of undergoing considerable and almost instantaneous plastic reorganization (Marder E, 1997) has profound implications about how the somatosensory system actually operates.

Functional brain imaging in recent years has highlighted this process. As recently as six years ago, however, I described functional remapping to a group of CFS researchers only to have no one in the audience understand the concept and only one individual ask a question about neural networks that had to do with lesions of the brain, i.e., permanent changes such as those in stroke. One good description of the coruscating aspect of brain function states "Nevertheless, recent evidence suggests that these maps cannot be viewed any longer as static spatial representations. Instead they seem to be better defined as spatiotemporal representations in which the coupling of spatial and temporal domains results from a dynamic equilibrium between asynchronously convergent excitatory and inhibitory afferents. One can argue, therefore, that the dynamic and distributed nature of these somatosensory representations offers the perfect functional medium for the occurrence of very fast sensory reorganization following changes in the pattern of ascending sensory information" (Nicolelis M, 1997, p. 28).

There are time-dependent variations in receptive fields, particularly in the thalamus but also in the cortex, and as Nicolelis states, "receptive fields cannot be seen as hardwired properties of single neurons; instead they more closely resemble spatiotemporal probabilistic distributions, a configuration that can be easily altered by minimal changes in synaptic strength which would modify the delicate balance of excitation and inhibition that defines a central neuron sensory response" (1997, p. 28). Every day in my office, I witness patients' symptoms dramatically altered in seconds by using eye-drops, nasal sprays, or oral swirls that modulate the gating of the peripheral axons of the trigeminal nerve and result in second- to fifth-order changes in neuronal function. Such a global response has been demonstrated repeatedly in pre- and posttreatment brain SPECT, which I stopped doing long ago, since the point had been proven completely to my satisfaction that global changes in cerebral blood flow occur immediately upon symptomatic change. As Nicolelis goes on to say:

> Moreover, since these perturbations would affect cortical and subcortical structures alike, one should not be surprised by the observation that this reorganization occurs at all levels of the somatosensory system. If anything, the appearance of isolated immediate cortical reorganization would be rather unexpected. Instead, most of the effects associated with an immediate cortical reorganization likely reflect modifications at subcortical levels, which are superimposed on alterations in intrinsic cortico-cortical interactions. Such a change could occur, for example, by an alteration in the firing of the locus ceruleus, either by a reduction or an increase in the amount of afferent induced inhibition and an aggravation of the imbalance of excitation and inhibition. Once a threshold is crossed this imbalance triggers a series of mechanisms which are responsible for the establishment of long-lasting functional and anatomical reorganization of cortical and subcortical circuits. This involves alterations in synaptic efficacy needed by the activation [*or inhibition*] of NMDA receptors and sprouting of new connections induced by the activity-dependent release of neurotrophins. (Nicolelis, 1997, p. 29)

Since *Betrayal by the Brain* was published in 1996, immediate reconfiguration of neural networks has been demonstrated numerous times by functional brain imaging in cluster headaches, migraine headaches, seizures, changes in multiple personality, and the like. Normal people change their neural networks all the time by switching from one task to another or one cognitive process to another. The point I have been trying to make for many years is that this process may be pharmacologically regulated extremely rapidly in a manner which does not yet seem to be recognized by the medical profession. Pharmacologic induction of immediate remapping does not seem to have been mentioned in the literature as yet, although the use of transcranial magnetic stimulation and vagal nerve stimulation, both of which alter neural network function, have received a good deal of attention. Transcranial magnetic stimulation has not worked very well in my patients with neurosomatic disorders; in fact, it has only worked in one of them. No one has had vagal nerve stimulation yet. I have referred eight patients to a center performing an experiment in vagal nerve stimulation for depression. All have been excluded because their histories were too complex and/or they were too treatment refractory. As I write this part of the book, others are hoping to try it. In general, their case histories show so much treatment refractoriness that they are excluded from the sample lest they bias it toward failure. Vagal nerve stimulation may stop epilepsy and may treat depression with psychomotor retardation. It also may improve patients with pervasive developmental disorder (PDD) or those in that spectrum (personal unpublished observation). Patients with neurosomatic disorders who would respond to glutamatergic agonists (the minority) would also benefit by this electric stimulation, since glutamate is the primary neurotransmitter in the vagus nerve with acetylcholine probably being second. However, low-intensity stimulation of the vagus nerve has been reported to increase pain (Ness TJ et al., 2000). Because the core deficit of neurosomatic disorders appears to be an NMDA-receptor hypersensitivity, increasing glutamate might be expected to make symptoms worse. It may be possible, however, to vary the frequency and amplitude of the pulse so that optimum stimulation of the vagus could be achieved for an individual neurosomatic patient.

I have not discussed AMPA receptors thus far, since techniques to manipulate them are limited. The NMDA and AMPA receptors, however, must often be viewed as a unit, and the AMPA receptor is certainly glutamatergic. In the normal individual, synaptic plasticity in the form of NMDAR stimulation, mGluR activation, Ca^{2+} influx, and second messenger signaling occurs within the first hour after the train of stimuli. Subsequently, it is maintained by AMPA receptors and is resistant to NMDA antagonists. It might be destabilized by topiramate (Topamax), an AMPA-receptor antagonist. It could be augmented by piracetam, an AMPA agonist (Husi H et al., 2000). Agents named *ampakines* were the first allosteric modulators of AMPA function to augment excitatory transmission in the brain. They modify desensitization and deactivation and are being used experimentally for memory enhancement and the treatment of schizophrenia and ADHD (Lynch G, 2002).

I shall further discuss the AMPA receptor when I describe the action of topiramate. The idea of instantaneous reconfiguration of neural networks and the role of attention in this process has been known for some time.

> It is well known, however, that any brain area can be anatomically connected to any other one by either direct or indirect routes. In higher cognition, the act of attending organizes the circuitry between brain areas. . . . the last five years has seen a tremendous increase in our understanding of these networks, each of which carries out a function

important to selective attention, such as orienting, detecting events, or maintaining the alert state. (Posner MI, Raichle ME, 1995)

Work on neural networks and attention has been enhanced in recent years by finding the corticolimbic-striatal-pallidal circuitry involved in the reward process, particularly involving the dopamine-dependent functioning of the nucleus accumbens (Robbins TW, Everitt BJ, 1996; Sherman SM, 2001). One of the usual goals of my treatment is to increase dopaminergic activity in the nucleus accumbens. Neural networks have temporal irregularities in their function that are responsible for neurosecretion. The NAc is involved in numerous responses and has been most studied for its role in drug addiction (Nestler ER, 2001). Interestingly, dynorphin, a leading candidate in the pathophysiology of neurosomatic disorders, is excessively secreted during withdrawal (Human SE, Malenke RC, 2001).

Relative to human behavior and also to pharmacologic intervention in neurosomatic disorders, particularly when giving high doses of intravenous medications slowly, is the fact that neural networks may respond with long-lasting periods of activity to brief input signals. Such an input response can occur if the activity of ion channels that are bound to G proteins alters after hyperpolarization. In this case, K^+ channels will especially be modified, thereby altering the action potential frequency in single cells.

Changing the properties of network neurons will in turn produce specific changes in the network output pattern. For example, serotonin reduces the availability of K_{Ca} channels and thereby the amplification of the afterhyperpolarization period. In the network, this will result in longer bursts of locomotor activity and the coordination between body segments will become modified. Activation of each modulator system in the spinal cord (serotonin, dopamine, tachykinins, somatostatin, and neurotensin) will affect single or groups of ion channels in certain cell types; this in turn will produce specific, predictable changes at the network level and in motor behavior. (Grillner S, 1997)

A discussion of neural networks may become very complex and will lead in part to computational neuroscience, a discipline relatively inaccessible to many readers of this book. A review of this subject has recently been published (Jennings C, Aamodt S, 2000), and I shall attempt to summarize it, at the risk of oversimplifying for the sake of brevity. Mathematical biophysical models, often computer generated, are used to make testable predictions about behavior. These models range from the single neuron to large regions such as the cerebellum or complex processes such as attention. Models are developed to discover the laws governing the brain's information-processing functions. I must understand these rules as well as possible in order to practice neurosomatic medicine: remediating dysfunctional information input. The hackneyed phrase "Garbage in, garbage out" is the simplest way to describe neurosomatic pathophysiology.

At the level of the single neuron, activation mechanisms occurring through the NMDA receptor result in simultaneous depolarization, or "clustering," of other neurons which respond to the same stimulus. The neurons thus far studied have been spatially related, but clustering may involve distant functionally-related neurons as well (binding). An example would be a cortical pyramidal neuron that responds to a specific orientation of a line or bar placed in its receptive field. This neuron could be "tuned" to its optimal orientation by NMDA receptors on its dendrites. These receptors could regulate Na^+, K^+, and Ca^{2+} fluxes on an instantaneous basis, which the neuron could compute in the process of gain control.

OTHER ASPECTS OF SYNAPTIC PLASTICITY

Synaptic plasticity, the basis for learning and memory, is the process by which activity modifies synapses and the response properties of neurons. Neuronal circuits must be modified efficiently, safely, and reliably. Network modification must occur at varying strengths across its constituent synapses. Synaptic strengths are determined by receptor sensitivity, amount of transmitter release and the timing of the firing of pre- and postsynaptic neurons. Synaptic depression may occur when there are insufficient synaptic vesicles in a ready-release pool. It is characteristic of rapid "burst-firing" neurons, which secrete most of their neurotransmitter in the ready-releasable pool, with one neuronal spike. Neurons can be entrained to a burst-firing mode in a process termed "synaptic redistribution." The efficiency of all synapses is decreased in direct proportion to the postsynaptic firing rate. For example, NMDA receptors could decrease and AMPA receptors could increase in response to glutamate secretion. This principle is called "synaptic scaling" and is more sophisticated than the concepts of receptor up- or down-regulation. I shall elaborate on synaptic depression, an aspect of synaptic fatigue, shortly.

The PFC is the brain structure most linked to working memory, the ability to hold and manipulate information to guide forthcoming actions. Working memory is impaired in most patients with neurosomatic disorders. There must be elevated firing rates in subpopulations of PFC neurons for working memory to occur. This elevation is termed "delay activity," which is task driven and more prominent in the PFC than in other brain areas. Most researchers believe delay activity is sustained through strong recurrent excitation in a "cell assembly," related to the notion of "clustering." An assembly is a spatially distributed set of cells activated in a coherent fashion and part of the same representations causing the generation of actions optimally adapted to particular situations. There are numerous variations on this theme. Neurons in an assembly are "wired" to respond to what they perceive as salient and may maintain their activation for a period of time after the stimulus is withdrawn. A problem with this mode is that overlearned stimulus-response associations (as may occur in neurosomatic disorders) evoke decreased PFC activity, perhaps via the "disconnection" model of Post.

The PFC has the highest NMDA-receptor density of all cortical areas. In the normal brain, a nearly constant synaptic drive of NMDA-receptor currents, which last eighty milliseconds, can account for delay activity resistant to noise. AMPA receptor currents have the opposite effect. Dopaminergic activity increases during working memory tasks. It enhances delay period SNR by strengthening currently active neuronal assemblies. Overactivity of PFC neuronal assemblies may lead to response perseveration: the inability to appropriately shift to a new response type. Dopamine is also necessary to stimulate PFC $GABA_A$ receptors to suppress task-irrelevant representations. The effect of PFC dopamine is particularly dependent on the balance between D_1- and D_2-type receptors. These and other aspects of PFC function are amenable to modeling.

The medial prefrontal cortex is highly activated by stress and modulates neuroendocrine and autonomic function. Dopaminergic inputs to the mPFC facilitate coping ability and demonstrate considerable hemispheric functional lateralization. In acutely restrained rats, only right, not left, mPFC lesions decrease prestress corticosterone levels and stress ulcer development. Thus, mPFC dopaminergic neurons demonstrate an intrinsic right-brain specialization in both neuroendocrine and autonomic activation (Sullivan RM, Gratton A, 1999).

Selective attention, inferred from classical conditioning studies, concerns what items should be attended to and how responsibility for making predictions, a type of learning, should be competitively allocated. Cholinergic activity is related to the attentional state via the hippocampus and parietal cortex, and prediction is mediated by dopaminergic projections to the NAc. A distinction is made between which stimuli are *appropriate* for a given task and the assessment of *relevant* inputs in different tasks. In regard to neurosomatic medicine, overlearned behavior produces decreased dopaminergic activity in the NAc, part of the ventral striatum. The hypothesis is put forth that in normal information processing the ventral striatum and its associated basal ganglia structures are involved in attentional competition.

Modification of various adhesion molecules, such as the neural cell adhesion molecule (NCAM) helps to regulate synaptic plasticity. Even one domain of the NCAM molecule may be altered (the polysialic acid residue) causing dysfunction in important aspects of behavior such as circadian rhythmicity and long-term potentiation. Various other molecules, such as proteases, may inhibit plasminogen activators expressed in brain areas involved in memory processing and storage, thereby regulating structural modifications that result in neuronal plasticity (Brosamlee C, 1998). I know of no proteases that might affect tPA. Proteases are ubiquitous enzymes which degrade proteins and are specific for a simple peptide bond, e.g., trypsin. They may exert their effects indirectly via warfarin, and somewhat more directly by genestein, a tyrosine kinase inhibitor, and Gleevec (imatinib), an antineoplastic Trk blocker used for thrombocytosis (Gingrich MB, Traynelis SF, 2000).

For several years researchers have known that rapid functional changes are accompanied by structural changes, particularly in the dendritic spines. Remodeling of spine patterns and density has been demonstrated after chronic epileptic activity and through phases in the menstrual cycle. Chronic neuropathic pain observed after peripheral injuries causes release of nerve growth factor from lesioned C nerve fibers which causes A fibers to sprout and ectopically innervate surrounding regions. Inappropriate response to NGF is related to pain in neurosomatic disorders by a variety of mechanisms.

Thinly myelinated A fibers and unmyelinated C fibers are nociceptors. About half of them express neuropeptides such as SP and CGRP. All small-diameter sensory fibers express TrkA, the high-affinity receptor for NGF, at some time during their lives, especially during the prenatal period. Postnatally TrkA is expressed by a smaller population, but the non-peptidergic population has a domain sensitive to brain-derived neurotrophic factor. The latter population is also sensitive to purine nociceptors such as ATP and $P2X_{2/3}$.

NGF tonically regulates the sensitivity of peripheral, cranial, and some central nerves to nociception. It is directly involved in thermal and inflammatory hyperalgesia and, particularly relevant to neurosomatic pain, evokes mediator release from mast cells (Figure 24). It regulates receptor proteins for bradykinin and is involved in the increase and clustering of sodium channels at nociceptive sites providing a rationale for use of kutapressin, a BK antagonist, and lidocaine, a Na^+-channel blocker. Secretion of SP and CGRP is strongly regulated by NGF. These peptides are involved in numerous neurosomatic processes, especially migraine headache. Some NGF-sensitive nociceptors also express BDNF.

The high-affinity receptor for BDNF is TrkB. Through TrkB, BDNF regulates the gain of nociceptive information processing. TrkB phosphorylates intracellular targets such as the NMDA receptor, increasing its sensitivity. NGF and BDNF antagonists will be important therapeutic agents in the future (Bennett DLH, 2001). BDNF agonists may be used as antidepressants and as broad-spectrum agents to increase synaptic transmission.

The neurobiology and neurochemistry of the brain can be explained in symbolic concepts. I would recommend reading "The Brain As a Symbol Processing Machine" by A. F. Rocha (1997), and any of the prolific works of Konstantin Baev. I will discuss a recent paper of his: "Highest Level Automatisms in the Nervous System, a Theory of Functional Principles Underlying the Highest Form of Brain Function" (1997). This sophisticated work refers to topics I discuss in this volume and in previous works. Baev describes changes in state as being regulated by higher centers:

> When moving from lower to higher levels, generalization or abstraction of the parameters within the hierarchy occurs. The parameters of higher levels change less frequently than the parameters of lower levels. In general, the hierarchy present within a control system has to be considered as a consequence of the object state hierarchy. (Baev C, 1997)

Rather than speaking of nodal neurons or oscillatory networks, he describes "command areas" that occur in the brainstem and spinal cord which activate fully organized neural systems or inborn behaviors. These command areas respond to a higher level of command neurons, regulated in part by expectations and in part by input from lower centers. When the input is viewed as novel or a "mismatch" it ascends in the hierarchal structure of the brain until it reaches a command level that can detect it. "It is noteworthy that higher sensory levels can send initiating and informational signals to lower detectors and consequently *tune them* to concentrate on any desirable feature because new minimization criteria become available to the lower levels" (Baev C, 1997). As I speculated in *Betrayal by the Brain*, cortico-cerebellar circuits have been recognized as being more and more important in learning and detection of novelty. Baev (1997) considers that "[t]he circuitry of the cerebellum can be considered to be an optimal filter that is also capable of computing mismatched signals that help to separate any novel stimuli that do not coincide with the expected afferent flow."

HORMONAL MODULATION IN NEUROSOMATIC MEDICINE

It is very difficult to use hormonal modulation in the treatment of neurosomatic disorders. The results of giving a substance such as estradiol are extremely variable. In general, estrogen has effects opposite to those of progesterone, but this fact is complicated by estrogen's increasing the levels of progesterone receptors. Estrogen can also have an immediate receptor-mediated effect which is nongenomic and can modulate the response of neurons to various transmitter substances. It appears to rapidly up- or down-regulate excitability of neurons in a wide variety of brain regions, which suggests estrogen may act broadly through G-protein-dependent mechanisms when it acts within seconds or minutes (Figure 25). The phase of the menstrual cycle alters response to exogenous estrogens. Different investigators have found that pain threshold is elevated when estrogen levels are high (Giamberardino MA et al., 1997) or that estrogen can decrease pain threshold (Kayser V et al., 1996). Menopausal women with fibromyalgia develop increased pain when treated with estrogen replacement. It has also been suggested that estrogen deficit is a promoting factor in patients with fibromyalgia syndrome (Waxman J, Zatzkis SM, 1999).

The classical mechanism of estrogen action is through nuclear receptors that act as transcription factors by binding as dimers to specific response elements in DNA and regulating the expression of target genes. Two estrogen receptors have been cloned, alpha and beta, which are differently up- or down-regulated by estradiol in different brain regions. Some neurons co-express estrogen receptor alpha protein and estrogen receptor beta mRNA. There are multiple variants of estrogen receptor beta (Woolley CS, 1999).

Estrogen appears to be an agonist at NMDA and non-NMDA glutamate receptors, a response which involves a G protein and a protein kinase A-dependent increase in cAMP. Because the ovary makes three estrogenic hormones, estradiol, estriol, and estrone, I prefer to use a topical tri-estrogen preparation 5 mg/gram. It also can be prepared in an oral form. Estradiol causes an increase in dendritic spines which is probably NMDA-related. There is an interaction between estradiol, GABAergic interneurons, and brain-derived neurotrophic factor in the induction of new dendritic spines. The decrease in hippocampal BDNF may be caused by its retrograde transport to the septum (Gibbs RB, 1999).

Estradiol treatment causes an immediate decrease in GABA levels and subsequently an increase (Murphy DD, Cole NB, Greenberger V, Segal M, 1998) resulting in increased excitatory drive in dendritic spines causing an increase in spine density. Estradiol treatment of hippocampal cultures decreases levels of BDNF which again causes disinhibition, allowing an activity-dependent increase in dendritic spine density (Murphy DD, Cole NB, Segal M, 1998). Estrogen also increases spinal cord enkephalin gene expression (Amandusson A et al., 1999).

The pain threshold of female rats is elevated when their levels of sex hormones are high as occurs during pregnancy. This elevation is abolished by the opioid antagonist naltrexone (Gintzler AR, Bohan MC, 1990). Some believe that the hormone relaxin, elevated in pregnancy, is an effective treatment for FMS. It is being extracted from pigs and used as a nutraceutical. My results with relaxin have been mixed, as with all other agents. Sedation is the most common adverse reaction. It usually relaxes patients, sometimes is analgesic, and occasionally elevates mood and energy.

Estrogen and progesterone modulate delta- and kappa-opioid receptors in the spinal cord as well as the spinal content of the endogenous opioid dynorphin. This molecule is an antagonist at the other opioid receptors and an agonist at the NMDA receptor.

Estrogen may increase cognitive function in females by a general activating effect and also potentiates norepinephrine secretion and sensitivity of noradrenergic receptors. Estrogen acts to stimulate dopamine receptors as well (Simonian SX et al., 1998; Pasqualini C et al., 1996; Hogervorst E et al., 1999).

Estradiol has an effect on benzodiazepine function. It prevents the potentiation of benzodiazepine binding in nonstressed and stressed animals. Progesterone produces the opposite outcome, and a combination of estradiol and progesterone has an intermediate action (Bitran D, Dowd JA, 1996).

Estradiol has an effect somewhat the opposite of the $GABA_B$ agonist baclofen in hypothalamic neurons. $GABA_B$ and mu-opioid receptor agonists clonidine, minoxidil, L-lysine, diazoxide, and gabapentin open the same K_{ATP} channels. The response to $GABA_B$ agonists and mu-opioid agonists is rapidly attenuated by 17-beta-estradiol. Some hypothalamic neurons are very sensitive to baclofen, and others are only mildly sensitive. Thus, a discrete subpopulation of hypothalamic neurons is sensitive to the role of estrogen to decrease inhibitory transmission (Lagrange AH et al., 1996).

This situation is complicated by the fact that GABA receptors can inhibit mu-opioid neurons and vice versa. Activation of mu-opioid receptors on beta-endorphin neurons represents autoinhibition, thereby reducing subsequent beta-endorphin release. Thus, 17-beta-estradiol may rapidly release beta-endorphin neurons from inhibition by $GABA_B$ and mu-opioid receptor activation. Nearly every hypothalamic cell responds to GABAergic drugs, but the $GABA_A$ and $GABA_B$ responses vary among cells. $GABA_B$ receptors are coupled to calcium channels. The uncoupling of $GABA_B$ and mu-opioid receptors in the arcuate nucleus of the hypothalamus occurs within only a few minutes and is, therefore, nongenomic.

Estrogen has been known for some time to be a monoamine oxidase inhibitor (Chakravoty SG, Halbriech U, 1997). There are two types of monoamine oxidase, A and B. The isoenzyme MAOA is found mainly in the brain and is thought to be involved in the pathogenesis of mood and thought disorders. The isoenzyme MAOB, which is found in the substantia nigra, is thought to play a role in neurodegenerative disorders by indirect production of toxic free radicals. The activity of MAOB is increased by acute and chronic estrogen treatment, whereas MAOA is decreased in the locus coeruleus and the cerebellum, indicating a region-specific and reversible activity of estrogen on monoamine oxidase. Monoamine oxidase A primarily metabolizes norepinephrine and serotonin, and monoamine oxidase B is involved with dopamine metabolism. Other bioactive amines may be affected by monoamine oxidase as well.

The sudden postpartum withdrawal of supraphysiologic levels of gonadal steroids can precipitate depression in women with a differential sensitivity to changing levels of estradiol and progesterone (Bloch M et al., 2000). The same differential sensitivity to fluctuating hormone levels is probably responsible for LLPDD, as I have mentioned in previous works and has been discussed recently by others. Estrogen also modulates the activity of the HPA axis to stress and creates a considerable gender dimorphism (as does progesterone to a lesser extent) to the effects of central serotonin. In short, women are more sensitive to serotonin than men.

Estrogen has been reported to increase numbers of adrenergic receptors in humans and may act as an antidepressant, particularly in postpartum depression (Hakoas A et al., 1999). Estrogen may have an augmenting effect when administered adjunctively with antidepressants (Stahl SM, 1998).

Estrogen increases the number of serotonin transporters and tends to normalize the blunted serotonin receptor responsiveness of postmenopausal women. It increases tyrosine hydroxylase activity, decreases norepinephrine reuptake, changes alpha$_2$ receptor binding sensitivity, beta$_2$ receptor binding activity, and the sensitivity of D$_2$ dopamine receptors. Although certain levels of estradiol may make a patient vigilant or more alert, higher levels may have an anxiogenic action. This effect is in contradistinction to the benzodiazepine-like effect of progesterone on GABA receptors. There it acts as a weak allosteric modulator of GABA activity and increases chloride conductance through the GABA$_A$ receptor complex. However, the administration of exogenous progesterone can have a mood destabilizing effect in certain women and mitigate some of the mood-stabilizing or even antidepressant-facilitating actions of estrogen. One of the profound actions of progesterone is its ability to dismantle synapses at the end of the menstrual cycle that were erected by estrogen at the beginning of the cycle. If unopposed estrogen were prescribed, this synapse dismantling would not occur. I am unsure of the effect of this alteration in normal physiology.

Estradiol modulates both presynaptic and postsynaptic 5-HT$_{1A}$ receptor function by reducing the action and/or activation of 5-HT$_{1A}$ receptors within the ventral medial nucleus of the hypothalamus (Jackson A, Uphouse

L, 1998). Thus, it would act somewhat like pindolol, the only 5-HT$_{1A}$ antagonist currently available. SSRIs (Prozac) are indicated for LLPDD probably because they increase the neurosteroid allpregnanolone (Guidotti A, Costa E, 1998).

Estrogen stimulates a significant increase in the density of 5-HT$_{2A}$ binding sites in the anterior cingulate, primary olfactory cortex, and nucleus accumbens, areas of the brain concerned with the control of mood, mental state, cognition, emotion, and behavior. Thus, estrogen therapy and/or serotonin-reuptake inhibitors may treat the depressive symptoms of premenstrual syndrome, which may be conceptualized as an estrogen deficiency syndrome. Patients intolerant of estrogen usually become tolerant to this hormone after their neurosomatic disorder is pharmacologically alleviated. In view of the possible up-regulation of the 5-HT$_{2A}$ receptors in these women, consideration might be given to utilizing 5-HT$_2$ antagonists such as risperidone, olanzapine, quetiapine, or mirtazapine. Nefazodone, although it is a 5-HT$_2$ receptor blocker also has some mild properties of a serotonin-reuptake inhibitor, and this combination seems, in my experience, to be poorly tolerated by estrogen-sensitive women with neurosomatic disorders (Wooley CS, 1999; Wickelgren I, 1997).

Estrogen augments the activity of several serotonergic systems. Increased plasma levels of estrogen are associated with up-regulated platelet imipramine receptor binding. Estrogen also augments the prolactin and cortisol responses to the serotonergic 5-HT$_{2C}$ agonist m-CPP. It enhances release of cortisol, thereby decreasing corticotropin-releasing hormone. Progesterone, perhaps acting in an opposite manner to the dopaminergic-enhancing function of estradiol, may restore the disruption of prepulse inhibition of the acoustic startle response caused by apomorphine, a characteristic finding in schizophrenia which can be reversed by traditional neuroleptics. In contrast, allopregnanolone, the neurosteroid I would most like to use in neurosomatic patients and one of the main CNS metabolites of progesterone, does not significantly antagonize the effect of apomorphine on prepulse inhibition. The behavioral profile of progesterone is compatible with the sedative properties of its metabolite allopregnanolone via the GABA$_A$ receptor. Progesterone itself shares some properties with atypical neuroleptics, which may be relevant for the development and treatment of psychotic disturbances (Rupprecht R et al., 1999).

Perhaps the most relevant aspect of the neuroregulatory aspects of gonadal steroids in neurosomatic disorers is that "estradiol enhances and testosterone attenuates novelty stress-stimulated increases in c-Fos mRNA in the hippocampus, with presumed consequent alterations in the transcription regulatory effects of c-Fos" (Roca CA et al., 1999). Until recently, I have been reluctant to use antiestrogen therapy in women, except in treatment-refractory bipolar disorder (Goldstein JA, 1986). I have used testosterone only in men who respond to nitroglycerin, since NO increases DA in the medial preoptic area of the brain. I may be liberalizing its use in transdermal treatment trials, however. When effective, it markedly increases alertness.

MODULATING THE N-METHYL-D-ASPARTATE (NMDA) RECEPTOR

It is better to die according to the rules than recover contrary to them.

Moliere (1665)
L'Amour Médicin

So-called "classical" neurotransmitters either excite or inhibit neural activity. Glutamate is the major excitatory neurotransmitter, and gamma-aminobutyric acid is the major inhibitory neurotransmitter. More neurons secrete glutamate and GABA in a 5:1 ratio than all the rest of the neurons put together. Glutamate acts at several receptors, which may be further subdivided by their subunit construction and so may GABA. There are two major types of glutamate receptor, ionotropic (NMDA, AMPA, kainate) and metabotropic (mGlu$_{1-8}$) (Figure 26). There are three types of GABA receptors, GABA$_A$, GABA$_B$, and GABA$_C$ (Figure 27). There are various classification systems for all receptors, including glutamate and GABA, which are constantly undergoing revision.

Neurosomatic disorders are disorders of attentional state and the "attentional template," or the schema used to determine salience of a stimulus and to focus attention on it. I have discussed this hypothesis frequently in my work of the last decade. Neurosomatic patients usually cannot focus attention well and are easily distracted. Their task performance dramatically decreases when confronted with multiple stimuli because their attentional template is too wide. As a corollary, it is likely that the *receptive field* is too wide.

The term *receptive field* was originally used to describe the area of the retina that must be excited to produce a response in a visual cortical neuron. The excitation is specific for the intensity of the stimulus, as well as for one or more attributes, such as direction of movement of the stimulus or its rate of change. The concept of receptive fields has subsequently been applied to all sensory systems, and I believe it should be applied to cognitive systems as well (Iversen SD, Muller RU, 1997).

Most sensory neurons are best adapted for detecting *change* in the internal or external environment. Change implies novelty, and novelty implies potential threat. Furthermore, it is more efficient to detect alterations in a usually static world than to attend to every possible aspect of it. A stimulus is processed in stages, from the point of initiation to its interpretation at the highest cortical level. Stimuli outside the receptive field are less attended to, are weaker, and lose in a competition to pass on the next stage of processing, a phenomenon which has been termed "winner take all." Thus, the receptive fields of higher-order neurons become large, since nonsalient stimuli should not get that far. Higher-order neurons, or neuronal assemblies which respond to the same stimulus attribute, are exquisitely sensitive to input the prefrontal cortex has selected via its attentional template. Because processing a stimulus is a multilevel task, the receptive fields enlarge at each stage. Competition between stimuli occurs at each level between input and output, whether exteroceptive, enteroceptive, or cognitive.

As the receptive fields increase in size, their inputs from various areas of the central nervous system increase. Filtering of the stimuli must occur or the system would be overwhelmed. The prefrontal attentional template regulates competition between stimuli so that an attended stimulus will achieve control over the output of a neuron or neuronal assembly and a nonattended stimulus will not. The prefrontal cortex is regarded as the most sophisticated section of the brain, or the "top." Everything else in the central nervous system is "below" it. Thus, the prefrontal attentional template can exert "top-down" control of other areas of the central nervous system. This "descending" influence can be modulated by "ascending" neuronal connections from "lower" areas of the CNS. The principle that attention regulates competition between stimuli ("objects" in the visual system) for access to neural receptive fields is discussed in virtually every recent neuroscience textbook, but the neurochemistry of the attentional process receives considerably less space. Structural disorders of the brain that produce attentional problems, e.g., parietal lobe "neglect," have been recognized for a century. The neurophysiology of neglect has been substantially described only in the last few years. The appreciation by physicians of the role that attention plays in the syndromes they encounter on a daily basis is sorrily lacking. Consequently, the feasibility of modifying the attentional template by pharmacologic and other means is quite misunderstood and underestimated, even in recent publications (Parasuraman R, 1998). A notable exception is the creative work of V. S. Ramachandran (Ramachandran VS, Blakeslee S, 1998).

Numerous models have been proposed to explain how attention is related to goal-directed behavior, or "executive attention." Because my purpose in writing this book is to explain "tuning" of the brain's attentional network in a clinical setting, I shall not exhaustively review each hypothetical construct but shall discuss my working syntheses of these views in relationship to treatment. A salient stimulus may be attended to because of one to several key attributes, such as finding your car in a parking lot, or as a reflection of one's attitude about the world, or weltanschauung. Many neurosomatic patients regard an inappropriately large number of stimuli as being salient. This propensity leads to overlearned responses in widened receptive fields with diffusion of attentional resources. Evidence for this assertion may be found in my previous book, *Betrayal by the Brain,* in the decreased amplitude and slope of the N-100 attentional wave on auditory evoked responses and the hypoperfusion of frontotemporal regions, suggesting overlearned attribution of salience and decreased requirement for activation. Neuropsychological testing shows a deficit in making new memories, perhaps because of overattribution of salience to too many stimuli, a decrement in performance with cues (additional input) which help a normal subject, and difficulty in planning and sequencing, which involves holding multiple stimulus representations (e.g., ideas) in working memory which is already filled to capacity. Salient stimuli are not appropriately enhanced, and competing stimuli are not appropriately muted. In focal attention, only one input modality may be used at a time. For example, it is difficult to appreciate the odor ("nose") of a wine and its taste simultaneously, even though these sensory modalities are quite interrelated. It would be much more difficult to enjoy its bouquet while contemplating the mode of distillation.

Based upon the foregoing, which many who follow my work already know, I have for years searched in vain for abnormalities in the activation of the anterior cingulate gyrus in neurosomatic disorders. This region of the cortex is involved in conflict resolution between competing stimuli in a novel situation. The only study to demonstrate any abnormality showed a slight increase in right anterior cingulate blood flow as measured by SPECT in anticipation of acute pain in women with fibromyalgia plus anxiety and depression (Alberts KR et al., 2000). The activity of the anterior cingulate is increased in antidepressant-responsive depressed patients anyway. The activation is reduced by antidepressant therapy. These results seem fairly trivial since the subjects were not controlled for depression. I might have expected to see some other area of the brain activated in an overlearned activity, but we have never seen any regions activated on CFS patients, with or without FMS, while performing various tasks. We most often see task-related decreased regional blood flow, e.g., in the left parietal region while doing calculations. The actual lack of cingulate activation, or even its decrease, in neurosomatic patients may reflect an absence of local amplification in neural activity that accompanies top-down selection of items. I would expect a decrease in ACC activity, which was not seen in the Alberts and colleagues study, since the rostral or ventral parts of the ACC play a role in assigning a positive or negative value to future outcomes, respectively, in the rat (Takenouchi K et al., 1999). Memory retention in mice is enhanced by Ach and

NMDA agonists, as well as $GABA_{A,B}$ antagonists and $5\text{-}HT_{1,2}$ antagonists. Because responses are overlearned in neurosomatic patients, medications that would impair memory in normal subjects often improve general symptoms, as well as memory specifically (Goldstein JA, 1996). The same neurochemistry is involved in the hippocampus, septum, amygdala, and mammilary bodies. Cingulate cortex lesions in monkeys decrease pain sensitivity, probably the component related to the affective response (Devinsky O et al., 1995), although not necessarily (Hutchison WD et al., 1999).

The pain and allodynia (a noxious response to an innocuous stimulus, such as rubbing the skin) is "central." It is generated by the brain itself. Central pain does not involve activation of any part of the cingulate gyrus, and peripheral nociceptive stimuli in patients with structural causes (e.g., stroke) for central pain activate regions other than the cingulate (Peyron R et al., 2000). The findings in the Alberts and colleagues study probably reflect the attentional aspect of pain sensation in the ACC, as shown by fMRI, which provides superior resolution to that of SPECT (Kwan CL et al., 2000).

Determining salience relates directly to the level of arousal, or alertness. If a subject is lethargic or jittery, perception of salience and allocation of attentional resources will be impaired (in different ways, of course). Transmitter substances other than glutamate or GABA serve to modulate neuronal activity triggered by glutamate and GABA and are thus involved in tuning the brain, or the gating of information. I have discussed this matter in much of my previous work and shall gloss over it here. Beta adrenoceptors augment GABA neuronal responses, and alpha-1 adrenoceptors increase glutamate reactivity and may contribute to stress-induced alterations in PFC cognitive function (Birnbaum S et al., 1999). Other findings show that alpha-1-adrenoceptor activation enhances memory for inhibitory avoidance training through an interaction with beta-adrenergic mechanisms in the basolateral nucleus of the amygdala (Ferry B et al., 1999). The locus coeruleus, the source of most NE neurons in the brain, is activated by salient stimuli, and perception of salience is usually conditioned.

When LC activity is low, a monkey is drowsy. When LC activity is consistently elevated, the monkey is distractible and makes more errors in classical conditioning tasks. The monkey is more apt to respond to nonsalient stimuli, i.e., those that do not produce a reward. Intermediate levels of LC activity produce stable, focused attention, and acute "phasic" elevations in NE secretion occur when learning to pair an unconditioned stimulus (e.g., banana) with a potential conditioned stimulus, such as a light. Dopamine secretion is associated with anticipation of reward and codes for the deviation of errors between the predicted and the actually experienced reward. All modulatory neurotransmitters project diffusely to a large number of postsynaptic neurons. Dopamine is frequently linked with NE secretion, and both of them increase signal-to-noise ratio. Phasic LC activity, superimposed on low continuous "tonic" NE release is the ideal situation (Aston-Jones G et al., 1999). In this condition, neurons would be appropriately able to scan the environment and respond to salient stimuli. If LC activity is tonically elevated, phasic activation is reduced. Applying this neurophysiology to clinical practice, patients who are hypersomnic will be more likely to benefit from "stimulant" medications than those who have a disorder of initiating and maintaining sleep; the latter group of patients will frequently have their symptoms exacerbated by stimulants. They are much more apt to have elevated scores on brief anxiety inventories, such as the Hamilton or the Beck. Please be advised that the relevant neuropharmacology is infinitely more complex than the preceding example.

The NMDA receptor has numerous modulatory sites. These include those for ketamine, polyamines, zinc, magnesium, pH, redox, glycosylation, glycine, heparin, dextromethorphan, and dynorphin. Dynorphin levels in the CSF of FM patients are normal (Russell IJ, 2001, personal communication). Ca^{2+}, Na^+, and Mg^{2+} flow in through the pore of the activated receptor, and K^+ flows out. A calcium-calmodulin site decreases open-channel probability, and the activity of the receptor can be rapidly modulated by phosphorylation. The NMDAR1 subunit is essential for receptor activity. There are at least eight types of NMDAR1 produced by RNA splicing, which confers functional diversity upon the receptor. There are also four NMDAR2 subunits, which can have splice variants as well. The NMDAR2 subunits can be rapidly exchanged, depending on changes in single neurons, neuronal assemblies, or neural networks. A physician has the capability, using existing medications, to modulate some of the NMDA binding sites and regulatory molecules, which perhaps number in the hundreds (Kemp JA, McKernan RM, 2002). It is not yet possible to alter subunit composition of the NMDA receptor through its pore so that ionic flow can be altered except by chronic cycloserine treatment, which should decrease Ca^{2+} flow by subunit switching. This tonic flow requires the binding of glutamate to the receptor and depolarization of the cell membrane. Depolarization is necessary because the pore is blocked by Mg^{2+} at resting potential. The receptor allows influx of Ca^{2+}, which activates numerous intracellular processes. The NMDA receptor has a glycine coagonist site, which makes it unique among receptors. The glycine site must also be bound (by glycine, alanine, or serine) in concert with NMDA-receptor agonists (NMDA, glutamate, or aspartate—glutamate is the most potent agonist). Kynurenic acid is an endogenous competitive antagonist at the glycine site. Kynurenate levels can be increased by administration of probenecid. Calcineurin is an endogenous phosphatase which inhibits Ca^{2+}/calmodulin NMDA-receptor activation but is not yet amenable to clinical modulation (Figure 28).

Ca^{2+}-activated enzymes include Ca^{2+}/calmodulin-dependent protein kinase II, calcineurin, PKC, phospholipase A_2, phospholipase C, nitric oxide synthase, and several endonucleases. Blocking the channel with high-dose intravenous ketamine administered over a three-hour period to avoid adverse reactions sometimes produces a therapeutic effect lasting a week or more. Apparently, blocking the NMDA receptor in this manner can produce long-lasting activity-dependent alterations in synaptic efficacy, perhaps related to changes in Ca^{2+}-dependent enzyme function and production of fos-related antigens (FRAs). Intravenous lidocaine and amantadine also have prolonged actions. This effect has been termed "wind-down" (Eisenberg E, Pud D, 1998).

The NMDA synapse is the unit of neural organization most involved in neurosomatic disorders. The dysfunction of this neurochemical connection is an example of Hebbian homosynaptic plasticity gone wrong.

In 1949, Donald Hebb proposed the theory, first suggested by Ramon Cajal in the 1890s, that information is stored in the brain as a result of anatomical changes between neurons. Memory, according to Hebb, occurred by strengthening the synapse(s) which were activated by the events being encoded. If the firing of the pre- and postsynaptic neurons is closely correlated in time ("temporally"), the connection between the two neurons will become stronger, and the synapse will be associated with increased neural activity in appropriate circumstances. Other synapses are unchanged by this single synaptic strengthening. If the synapse is modulated by a third neuron (heterosynaptic), it may strengthen or weaken the synapse in a different manner, particularly if the modulatory neuron fires in association with the presynaptic neuron (Figure 29).

Habituation occurs after frequent presentation of the same stimulus, due to a decrease in transmitter, e.g., glutamate, from the presynaptic neuron. *Sensitization*, the opposite of habituation, is found in most neurosomatic patients. Presynaptic glutamate secretion increases on a homosynaptic or heterosynaptic basis (via a third, modulatory neuron). Sensitization can also occur if the NMDA receptors for glutamate become up-regulated (increased in number or more easily activated). One way for this process to occur is by hypersensitization of mesocorticolimbic DA autoreceptors, resulting in less *regional* DA secretion. Neutral stimuli may become associated to a temporally distant noxious stimulus and result in inappropriate learned fear (Bailey CH et al., 2000). There are numerous genetic, developmental, and environmental influences on the propensity to develop learned fear or anxiety as a general response mode in a wide range of contexts. Sensitization can be a type of heterosynaptic facilitation. When I attempt to "tune" the brain, I am often trying to alter the function of the heterosynaptic modulatory neuron(s), which usually secretes one or more classical neurotransmitters, as well as a peptide cotransmitter. After multiple sensitizing stimuli, kinases are recruited which translocate to the nucleus and eventually result in morphologic enhancement of previously existing synapses or the development of new ones.

A widely studied form of homosynaptic Hebbian plasticity is termed long-term potentiation and is involved in making and storing new memories (Bailey CH et al., 2000; Eichenbaum H, 2000). It requires coincident pre- and postsynaptic firing and is specific to a certain type of input. LTP usually involves secretion of glutamate acting on AMPA and NMDA receptors (Figure 30). The NMDA receptor is more difficult to activate because the magnesium block of its pore must first be removed. In the usual circumstance, the AMPA receptor is activated first, depolarizing the postsynaptic cell which causes removal of the magnesium block and activation of the NMDA receptor channel, allowing influx of calcium ions into the postsynaptic cell. Ca^{2+} can activate numerous kinases, causing a cascade of events (Soderling TR, Derkach VA, 2000). This concatenation is why the NMDA receptor has been termed a "coincidence detector," because a synapse can be strengthened by coincident firing of pre- and postsynaptic neurons. Memory storage involves protein synthesis and is heterosynaptic. The modulatory neurotransmitters vary in different brain regions. More than one modulatory neuron can regulate a synapse simultaneously.

Classical conditioning involves the pairing of an unconditioned stimulus such as withdrawal of the finger when touching a hot surface, to a conditioned stimulus which is nonnoxious, such as hearing a tone. After repeated pairings of the US and CS the subject may withdraw his or her finger from a surface of normal temperature upon hearing the same tone. This response results from a strengthening of the synaptic connections between finger touch (sensory) and withdrawal (motor).

Classical conditioning is more potent than sensitization. The calcium influx produced by activation of the modulatory neuron greatly enhances the secretion of the homosynaptic transmitter, in this case, glutamate, by raising cAMP intracellularly. The increase in cAMP produced by classical conditioning is greater than the sum of the heterosynaptic and the homosynaptic processes alone. Furthermore, calcium flow through the pore of the NMDA channel causes secretion of a retrograde messenger (often nitric oxide) from the postsynaptic neuron to local firing presynaptic neurons, thereby increasing transmitter release.

ATYPICAL MESSENGERS

NO diffuses into monoamine neurons in an axosomatic or axodendritic manner and inhibits the function of monoamine transporters, thereby increasing the strength of their excitatory (presynaptic glutamatergic axon) or modulatory (NMDA synapses) activity. Because almost all of the neuronal nitric oxide synthase is associated with NMDA receptor activation, the nearby monoaminergic neurons can release transmitters without synaptic contact into the extracellular space (Figure 27). nNOS is directly connected to the NMDA receptor by a postsynaptic density protein (PSD-95) which allows nNOS to be exposed to a flood of Ca^{2+} when the NMDA channel opens. The monoamines diffuse in a paracrine manner into the extracellular space like NO does. Although the half-life of NO is only a few seconds, it is a gas and can diffuse a few hundred micrometers in that time and activate a large number of monoaminergic neurons and firing glutamatergic neurons in a sphere around the synapse (Kiss JP, Vizi ES, 2001). As we shall see, monoamines can inhibit the release of glutamate (Travagli RA, Williams JT, 1996), and the NO-mediated interaction can serve as a negative feedback loop. The monoaminergic cells do not require receptors for glutamate. They require only that glutamate can cross the neuronal membrane.

Atypical neural messengers such as NO have recently been reviewed (Baranano DE et al., 2001). The rather rigid criteria for proving that a substance was, indeed, a neurotransmitter which existed when I began to teach psychopharmacology are now quite elastic, and the recognition of the function of NO led the way for this reappraisal. I have discussed NO extensively in my previous work and will here only apprise the reader about the rapidly expanding discipline of studying atypical neural messengers. They are not called "retrograde messengers" any longer because they may affect the neuron from which they originate (Figure 31).

I have grown accustomed to thinking that NO diffuses into firing presynaptic neurons, catalyzes the conversion of GTP to cGMP by stimulating guanylyl cyclase (GC), and induces the secretion of more glutamate in a Hebbian manner. But NO can reversibly attach to cysteine in certain targeted proteins, a process called "S-nitrosylation," which tends to modulate the function of the protein. S-nitrosylation can even decrease NMDA-evoked processes in a voltage-dependent manner (Choi YB et al., 2000).

Numerous proteins are endogenously S-nitrosylated in the normal course of events, even the NR1 and NR2 NMDA-receptor subunits. Although neurons that manufacture NO are only about 1 percent of the cell bodies in the cerebral cortex, their axonal arborizations are so ramified that potentially every cell in the cortex is exposed to nNOS nerve terminals. NO affects the secretion of every classical neurotransmitter, and I can never predict who will respond to it. I do not administer it to patients with migraine or cluster headaches, which start in the rostral dorsal brainstem as seen on functional brain imaging. I have had an occasional patient who did not respond to nitroglycerin at all (it transforms into NO). One such patient took 22 0.3 mg tablets sublingually every three minutes. He did respond to hydralazine, however, which directly activates cGMP, so I assumed he had a congenital deficiency in conversion of guanylyl cyclase from its inactive to its active form. He was fatigued and had an extreme disorder of initiating and maintaining sleep, as did his sister. He was judged by an expert not to have familial fatal insomnia and to not be eligible for GHB. I unsuccessfully attempted to obtain for him a consultation with an MD researcher in NO. None of the physicians he contacted would see him. I tried pentazocine next, which catalyzes the conversion of inactive GC to active GC. It was quite effective as monotherapy and when coadministered with nitroglycerin.

When men have a good response to nitroglycerin, I try transdermal testosterone, which has an effect in 30 to 60 minutes or less. If it works, they feel much more energetic. Testosterone induces the secretion of NO, which in turn increases DA in the medial preoptic area (Du J, Hull EM, 1999), which is the area of the brain that determines an individual's response to sexual stimuli. I shall discuss the sexual response in neurosomatic disorders in the section on oxytocin. A much lower dose of transdermal testosterone can have a similar effect on women.

Carbon monoxide, or CO, has somewhat similar actions to NO and also activates soluble guanylate cylase. CO is formed by heme oxygenase which cleaves the porphyrin ring of heme, ultimately yielding a one carbon fragment as CO. CO may be a neurotransmitter of vas deferens innervation and is probably involved in ejaculation.

Hydrogen sulfide (H_2S) has been suggested as an atypical messenger (Kimura H, 2000). H_2S is a by-product of transmethylation and is an NMDA agonist. H_2S inhibits the stimulated release of CRH from rat hypothalamic explants (Navarra P et al., 2000). Zinc is an atypical messenger previously mentioned. It is a cotransmitter with glutamate and inhibits NMDA receptors somewhat like Mg^{2+}. It can modulate other currents as well, but treating my patients with various nontoxic doses of zinc has not had a significant effect (Paoletti P et al., 1997). If zinc can really help the common cold, perhaps it is an example of "psychoneuroimmunology in action"!

D-serine is released from astrocytes only and is thought to bind to the glycine site so that D-serine and glutamate can activate NMDA receptors together (Figure 32). D-serine, along with glycine, and the much more potent cycloserine bind to the glycine coagonist site of the NMDA receptor. D-serine is best antagonized by probenecid, which decreases the excretion of kynurenate, some of the metabolites of which specifically block the glycine site. 5-HT$_3$ antagonists also block the glycine site and include ondansetron and tropisetron, as well as diltiazem, other L-type Ca^{2+}-channel blockers, piracetam, felbamate, guaifenesin, and atropine. It is thought that the Ca^{2+}-channel antagonists either accelerate desensitization of the 5-HT$_3$ receptor or block its open channel. Dihydropyridine Ca^{2+}-channel blockers such as nimodipine (Nimotop) have been found to inhibit NMDA and nAch receptors (Taylor CW, Broad LM, 1998).

Probenecid and L-type Ca^{2+} blockers do not usually augment each other, however. Ondansetron may alleviate pain by being a glycine-site antagonist when given 4 mg by IV push over two to five minutes. NMDA antagonists of multiple types given intravenously and glycine-site antagonists may be combined in difficult cases. The procedure is usually safe if the rate of infusion is controlled, but I recently treated a young woman with 200 mg of IV amantadine and 2 mg of IV ondansetron over two hours without ill effects. She frequently received IV ascorbate, which, as discussed, has several effects on the NMDA synapse, with no adverse reactions. In this situation however, after she received about 100 ml of her usual dose of ascorbate, MgSO$_4$, and calcium gluconate, she began to dissociate and feel weird. The IV ascorbate was discontinued, and she decided her ADR was not severe enough to warrant pharmacologically reversing it, since I might reverse the benefit derived from the IV amantadine as well. The effects of IV amantadine are usually apparent by at least six hours after the infusion is completed. Infusions of two or three medications may have additive effects, e.g., lidocaine plus ketamine. Ondansetron and ketamine should not be combined—they are antagonistic. In particular, ondansetron will nullify the effects of ketamine.

Arousal and attention are optimized in emotionally charged LTP when the modulatory transmitters are NE and/or DA. NE and DA are secreted in anticipation of receiving a reward, so reward contingencies are attended to and learned. In areas of the brain involved with memory, NE and DA levels may also increase with an aversive or novel stimulus but decrease in areas that regulate motivation, e.g., the NAc. Secretion of modulatory neurotransmitters as well as the various atypical messengers and the resultant secretion of "classical" neurotransmitters from neuronal varicosities should be tonically low and then pulsatile when required, so that postsynaptic receptors will not desensitize. It has been suggested that modulatory neurons at NMDA synapses may be activated by a spillover or "paracrine" action of glutamate. In this scenario, the glutamate autoreceptor should be desensitized or one of the mGluRs stimulated. If the synapse is too strong, as may occur in neurosomatic patients, too much glutamate will activate modulatory neurons until they are unable to secrete additional NE or DA when appropriate. This tiring out is termed *synaptic fatigue* (Thomson AF, 2000).

Overly strengthened synapses produce overlearning, or a stereotyped response to stimuli. Synaptic fatigue would impair attention, motivation, and memory. Perception of the salience of stimuli would be impaired, and a low level of attention would be constantly allocated to weak stimuli. Directly or indirectly blocking the NMDA receptor would decrease calcium influx so that less retrograde transmitter would be secreted. Dantrolene has been touted as an NO inhibitor, but results are spotty. As a result, less glutamate would be available presynaptically, the spillover would be reduced, and modulatory neurons would respond appropriately to salience and need for selective attention. Overlearned behavior would decrease. Inhibiting the NMDA receptor, the presynaptic release of glutamate, and facilitating NE and DA secretion should be effective ways of treating neurosomatic disorders.

Most NMDA autoreceptors are "metabotropic" glutamate receptors. There are eight types of mGluRs, each with somewhat different properties. mGluRs in the neurosomatic patient might not decrease glutamate secretion appropriately; some increase it. Depolarization of the presynaptic neuron causes transmitter release via a voltage-dependent, as well as a Ca^{2+}-dependent, process. It may shift the autoreceptor from high to low affinity, thereby leading to dissociation of the transmitter from the autoreceptor. The free autoreceptor dissociates rapidly from the exocytic (synaptic vesicle-releasing) machinery, which interacts with Ca^{2+} in the presynaptic neuron, and glutamate secretion results (Feinstein N et al., 1998). Agonists and antagonists of the mGluRs have been developed, and some are in clinical trials. Autoreceptor mechanisms are incompletely understood.

SYNAPTIC FATIGUE

Synaptic fatigue is a term that used to make me think an axon terminal had been repetitively stimulated so frequently that its supply of transmitter-containing vesicles in the appropriate position at the membrane to be released ("docked") could not keep up with the demand. Such a process is termed "frequency-dependent depression." It occurs over minutes of repetitive firing and recovers slowly, eventually reaching an equilibrium with transmitter packaging into recycled vesicles. In the case of the catecholamines, using this scenario, there could also be

1. decreased precursor (phenylalanine and tyrosine—even L-dopa);
2. insufficient activity of tyrosine hydroxylase, the rate-limiting enzyme for catecholamine biosynthesis;

3. low levels of the various cofactors for the enzyme chain DA and NE;
4. impaired axonal transport to the terminal;
5. impaired manufacture, transport, and reuptake of DA and NE vesicles at the terminal;
6. problems with the Ca^{2+} channels (which open to initiate vesicle release); and
7. dysregulation of communication in the postsynaptic neuron.

I never really analyzed the process until now. It appears that factor number seven may be the most relevant for the pathophysiology of neurosomatic disorders. Autoreceptor hypersensitivity would affect most of these functions.

As I have with other mechanisms, I shall greatly simplify the process of synaptic neurotransmitter release, which is regulated by presynaptic Ca^{2+} channels. Of the various Ca^{2+} channels, the N-type is the most important for vesicle exocytosis. N-type Ca^{2+} channels can be modulated by various substances, including histamine, adenosine (A_1), NE (alpha$_2$), Ach (muscarinic), and FMRF (the peptide Phe-Met-Arg-Phe). The specific blocker of N^- channels is funnel spider web toxin, or omega-conotoxin. These various substances have individual postreceptor mechanisms by which they regulate the diameter of the channel and the time it is open or closed. Release of calcium from intracellular stores is also involved, including ryanodine-sensitive, IP_3-sensitive, and CICR (Fossier P et al., 1999).

The ryanodine receptor binding sites may be modulated by cyclic ADPribose (cADPR), which also releases Ca^{2+}, from intracellular stores to facilitate transmitter release. Ca^{2+} which enters through the N-channels may be sequestered by intracellular storage or by special synaptic vesicles. It can also activate CICR to increase $[Ca^{2+}]_i$. Which of these events predominates depends on the activity of the neuron. NO stimulates cGMP and PKG, activating ADPR. An enzyme synthesizes cADPR from NAD^+ (Figures 33a-c), which then releases Ca^{2+} from intracellular stores. Increasing $[Ca^{2+}]_i$ from intracellular stores does not supply as much $[Ca^{2+}]_i$ as voltage-gated channels but may have a large effect if $[Ca^{2+}]_i$ is subthreshold for vesicle (1) "docking" and "priming," (2) "unlocking," (3) membrane "zipping" (fusion of vesicle and plasma membranes) to form a "fusion-core complex," and (4) fusion, which occurs when a release-competent vesicle receives another little jolt of Ca^{2+} through adjoining channels and releases its contents into the synaptic cleft. Numerous molecular "brakes" retard this process, first by binding the vesicles to the cytoskeleton (synapsin) in the "reserve pool." Synapsin tethering is inhibited by activation of CAMKI and CAMKII. The vesicles then are "mobilized" and are available for the ready-releasable pool where brakes include the proteins and phospholipids synaptobrevin, synaptophysin, syntaxin, Munc-18 or -13, and cystine-string proteins. I suppose that "slamming on the brakes" could cause synaptic fatigue, but can think of no plausible excuse for inserting such a phenomenon into an integrated process. Small vesicular proteins called Rabs, associated with GTP, are also released when the vesicle is "liberated." They then diffuse and inhibit the exocytosis of neighboring docked vesicles by an unknown mechanism (Figure 34).

The Ca^{2+} sensor that initiates this release is thought to be the synaptic Ca^{2+}-binding protein synaptotagamin I. This protein is already present on docked vesicles and may bind syntaxin (Fernandez-Chacon R et al., 2001). BDNF (or other neurotrophins) is required for exocytosis, a surprisingly ubiquitous function for a neurotrophin. BDNF increases $[Ca^{2+}]_i$ and phosphorylates synaptic vesicle-associated proteins. Neurotrophins, which preferentially activate one of the tyrosine-binding kinases, may also cause membrane depolarization by Na^+-channel activation (Poo M, 2001). A deficiency of BDNF could be involved in a synaptic fatigue (Turrigiano GG, Nelson SB, 2000). BDNF, by activating TrKB receptors, enhances NMDA receptor opening and facilitates the induction of LTP in the postsynaptic cell (Manabe T, 2002).

Unc-13 drives syntaxin into an open conformation to promote core complex formation, after which a spritz of Ca^{2+} zippers it into vesicle fusion (Lloyd TE, Bellen HJ, 2001). RIM, or Rab-3-interacting molecule is specifically localized to the presynaptic active zone, and works with Munc-13 to "prime" vesicles. RIM may also be involved in stabilizing the vesicle pool of synapses. It is as yet unclear if spontaneous release frequency is due to a depressed pool of fusion-competent vesicles or RIM dysfunction.

In the hypothetical neurosomatic model of the hyperactive NMDA synapse, synaptic fatigue could occur at DA, NE, or even GABAergic modulatory neurons by frequency-dependent depression or by elevated levels of NO acting as an atypical messenger. NO from the postsynaptic NMDA neuron could diffuse into these modulatory neurons and increase cADPR-receptor release of $[Ca^{2+}]_i$. At some time, release of modulatory transmitters would be at maximal or near-maximal levels at relevant (perhaps even nodal) synapses on a chronic basis, and increased demand would exceed supply.

During learning or attention, hippocampal pyramidal cells fire at the negative phase of oscillatory waves. The cells that fire earliest in the cycle produce stronger inputs which are rapidly consolidated, so that a behaviorally relevant cue will be encoded. The context in which the cue occurs thereby alters synaptic plasticity, perhaps forever if early in development or very traumatic. Other neuronal firing is inhibited by interneurons, which open a temporal window when afferent impulses could have the most effect. The firing of the pyramidal cells stimulates and recruits interneurons that inhibit dendrites, blocking most inputs increasingly to a hypothetical maximal point when further glutamate secretion from firing neurons would be harmful. Glutamate release is thus maximally augmented by increasing $[Ca^{2+}]_i$ to a level past which intracellular damage would occur, and that intercellular excitoxicity from excessive glutamate secretion would destroy neuronalglial elements. I assume overlearning would occur in this situation and modulatory neurons, stimulated by NO to a state of chronic attentiveness, would be unable to further increase their transmitter output without "synaptic fatigue" causing an exacerbation of symptoms. Chronically restrained rats have a decrease in mesoaccumbens DA release. The reduction in DA secretion is not due to exhaustion of DA synthesis or depletion of DA pools since restrained rats are able to respond with a new increase of DA outflow to the release from the restraining apparatus (Cabib S, Puglisi-Allegra S, 1996).

The situation in which synaptic fatigue is most obvious is that of sexual arousal and ejaculation in the male with a neurosomatic disorder. Some males relapse after ejaculation. A few relapse, but in a different, milder way, after sexual arousal. Arousal seems to depend on activation of the medial preoptic area by testosterone, which facilitates NO synthase. NO increases the secretion of DA in the POA, which, as has been seen, is associated with anticipation of reward. Arousal can be augmented by dextroamphetamine, which also increases DA, particularly in the NAc. Lesions of the MPOA in animals decrease sexual behavior. Sexual arousal, causing increased DA secretion, can cause relapse.

Ejaculation is related to the actions of NE and oxytocin. All indicators of sympathetic function (heart rate, pupillary dilatation, blood pressure, plasma [NE]) rise during ejaculation. Furthermore, DA secretion must occur since the inability to sustain an erection or sexual desire after ejaculation is related to elevated levels of prolactin, the tonic secretion of which is inhibited by DA. Prolactin may act as a central and/or peripheral feedback signal in the control of sexual arousal following orgasm (Exton MS et al., 2001). There is a massive release of NE with ejaculation, which further explains relapse by a synaptic fatigue mechanism (Pfaus JG, 1999).

GLUTAMATE RECEPTORS, SUBUNITS, AND SYNAPTIC SCALING

Neurosomatic patients may genetically overexpress the NR2B subunit of the NMDA receptor (Wei F et al., 2001). An NMDA receptor composed of the NR1 and NR2B subunits in transgenic mice prolongs NMDA excitation (measured by EPSCs, or excitatory postsynaptic currents). Because activity of the NMDA receptor is associated with memory and learning, these mice are smarter than normal ("wild-type") mice but are also more sensitive to pain caused by tissue injury and inflammation. NR2B subunits are found primarily in the forebrain in mice, which would correspond to the ACC and PFC in humans. The NR2B subunit promotes the activity of CAMKII, which phosphorylates the NMDA receptor and prolongs its open time. These currents decay three to four times more slowly than those of the NR1-NR2A NMDA receptors. With more open time, more Ca^{2+} would enter the postsynaptic neuron and enhance its numerous calcium-dependent processes, including the secretion of retrograde (atypical) messengers to induce the presynaptic neuron to secrete more glutamate.

There are several potent and selective antagonists for the NR2B subunit. Protons inhibit the receptor by interacting with the extracellular protein sensor. Polyamines potentiate the NR2B-containing NMDA receptors by shielding the proton sensor and relieving tonic proton inhibition. Histamine has this property, as well. Antihistamines, which occasionally improve neurosomatic symptoms, may act here.

Ifenprodil and related compounds (isoxsuprine and nylidrin) selectively block sites at the NR1 and NR2B subunits, allosterically acting with the proton sensory and polyamine binding site. They provide analgesia by potentiating NMDA-receptor inhibition by endogenous protons, and because they are subtype selective, may have a better therapeutic index than many other NMDA antagonists (Chizh BA et al., 2001).

What might be the consequences of overly active NMDA receptors in the PFC and adjacent areas? The PFC is involved in numerous activities. Planning, sequencing, and working memory are only a few of its functions. The most pertinent to neurosomatic disorders is *salience,* i.e., which stimuli have been learned to be important to attend to other than those that are immediately novel or threatening? The PFC has overlapping connections with itself and most other parts of the brain. By using various types of learning, it exerts top-down cognitive control over a wide range of brain processes depending on the situation. The PFC can determine the context of a current situation from previous experiences and may thus guide a person to the appropriate thoughts and actions (Miller EK, 2000).

Most PFC neurons do not respond to a single stimulus. Rather, they are tuned to associate regularities among multiple stimuli in order to guide goal-directed behaviors. As neural assemblies in the PFC learn from experience, they are increasingly able to detect similarities in a current experience to previous learning, whether rewarding or aversive. Expectation of reward produces secretion of dopamine from the VTA into the mesocortical tract, which richly modulates the predominant glutamatergic neurons (Figure 35).

When there is no expectation of reward, or perhaps when sensory or cognitive context is predictive of no reward or an aversive consequence, DA secretion is turned off. Working memory is impaired under these conditions, and a fear-learning template may be imposed, so that attentional weighting is given to many stimuli. If DA is secreted, neurons firing at that time are likely to associate. As DA is secreted in rewarding situations, more and more neurons form associative connections so that they might be more prepared to recognize as many parameters of the stimulus configuration as possible. Recall that DA modulates a heterosynaptic connection and can block the NMDA pore. DA also may act as a gating signal to instruct a neural assembly to retain its pattern until secretion is interrupted, or a new goal-directed environment produces another pulse of DA from the VTA. NE from the locus coeruleus participates in these processes, helping the PFC to disregard distractors and maintain task behavior requiring a given activity state, regulating selective attention, working memories, and response selection (motor or autonomic nervous system output). Selective attention can prepare other areas of the brain to scan for a potentially rewarding stimulus. This property has been most studied in the visual cortex, where even the primary input area, V_1, may be tuned. Until quite recently, V_1 was regarded as impervious to PFC suasion (Kanwisher N, Wojciulik E, 2000). The PFC can also tune itself. It is the only area of the brain that can regulate its own modulatory classical transmitters according to task demands. PFC neurons (mostly glutamatergic) innervate secretory neurons in the LC (NE), VTA (DA), raphe nuclei (5-HT), and nucleus basalis (Ach) and is innervated by them.

LTP and LTD have been demonstrated to occur in the ventral striatum, which includes the NAc, especially in regard to motivationally significant behavior (Parkinson J et al., 2000). The ventral striatum receives converging glutamatergic afferents from various structures and contains the VTA, which secretes DA which may attenuate these afferents (Figure 36). A recent view is that the afferents may be attenuated selectively, according to their neuronal structure of origin (e.g., hippocampus versus amygdala), so gating of afferents to specific neuronal ensembles may occur (Figure 37).

Glutamate can also modulate DA secretion via mGluRs in the VTA. As learning occurs and reward or punishment becomes more predictable, as reflected by plasticity of glutamatergic afferents in the PFC, hippocampus, amygdala, and various thalamic nuclei, some VTA neurons may temporarily or permanently shift their firing activity. Such an outcome would be likely in the hyperglutamatergic state which I suggest underlies neurosomatic disorders (Figure 38).

The PFC continually selects other regions of the brain for task-related behavior. These regions eventually learn contextual cues also. Because the capacity of the PFC is finite, it eventually goes "off-line" when learning is completed. This eventual "automatic" performance is then regulated by other cortical areas. PFC "disconnection" can cause symptoms if behavior is prematurely overlearned, perhaps because of hyperfunction of PFC NMDA receptors composed of NR1/NR2B subunits. NMDA receptors help determine the "gain" allotted by attention. "Gain" multiplies the neural response. The PFC does not store memories. This function is performed by the hippocampus and perihippocampal areas, which transfer them to other areas of the brain by a protein-synthesis-requiring process that often occurs during sleep. The PFC detects regularities among different tasks so that it may appropriately organize responses. Conflict resolution between incompatible responses appears to be controlled, at least in part, by the ACC.

The subunit composition of both NMDA and AMPA receptors can be determined by the source of their input, e.g., from different locations in the auditory apparatus for AMPA receptors (GluR2 subunits versus GluR4). Different areas of the hippocampus have NR1 plus NR2A/B, or only NR1 plus NR2A. These have been termed "input-specific functional requirements" (Nusser Z, 2000), which should allow for "input-selective fine tuning of the postsynaptic responses within a single cell." Interestingly, AMPA receptors are never found postsynaptic to GABA terminals, although they are found on several intracellular organelles (Molnar E et al., 1993).

AMPA receptors are very common on GABAergic interneuron dendrites, where they await insertion into the cell membrane, a consideration if one wishes to alter interneuron function. The ratio of NMDA to AMPA receptors in the hippocampus is linearly related to synaptic diameter. They are co-localized in only 75 to 85 percent of hippocampal synapses, every one of which has an NMDA receptor.

Hippocampal CA1/CA3 glutamatergic synapses have a predominance of NR1/NR2B subunits composing the NMDA receptors, perhaps to maximize Hebbian coincidence detection. Such synapses may add AMPA receptors after repetitive firing, so-called "silent synapses." A "destructive mechanism" removes AMPA receptors during long-term depression. A "maintenance pathway" also replaces AMPA receptors on a one-for-one basis. GluR2/GluR3 receptors constantly cycle, and receptors of other subtypes, e.g., GluRx/GluRx enter the maintenance pathway after a special calcium signal. GluR1 subunits cannot be inserted until an LTP signal arrives. The availability of GluR1 is strictly controlled.

Silent synapses are postsynaptic responses mediated solely by activation of NMDA receptors (that do not produce a response when the cell is at resting potential). Thus, LTP results from the delivery of functional AMPA receptors to synapses from nonsynaptic sites, which may be intracellular. There may be different types of AMPA receptor complexes. Insertion of an

AMPA receptor seems to depend on its bonding to a specific element in the synaptic scaffolding in the postsynaptic density. The PSD is quite complex, and I shall consider it in passing from time to time as it relates to brain tuning. For example, expression of a peptide that interferes with the interaction of the PSD protein NSF, which interacts with the Glu2R, decreases synaptic transmission by 30 to 50 percent. AMPA receptor insertion and removal during LTP occurs through what has been termed the "constructive pathway" (Malmow R et al., 2000). After AMPA receptors are inserted, NR1/NR2B switches to NR1/NR2A. I suspect that neurosomatic patients have a lower than normal level of PFC AMPA receptors, because AMPA antagonists, such as topiramate (Topamax), are not particularly efficacious. One result of decreased AMPA-receptor levels would be a dysfunction of PFC LTP, which may be a contributing cause to the PFC being "off-line" in neurosomatic disorders. Because it blocks AMPA receptors in non-neurosomatic patients, Topamax may cause cognitive impairment and has been nicknamed "Dopamax" by some neurologists. This cognitive impairment does not usually occur when neurosomatic patients take Topamax, which acts somewhat like an NMDA antagonist. Hebbian plasticity resulting from correlation-based mechanisms induced by changes in pre- and postsynaptic elements, as well as activity of neurons modulating the synapse cannot be the whole story of higher brain function. I have learned over the years that when studying the brain, physiology and pathophysiology are always much, much, much more complicated than I originally appreciated. In the case of LTP, homeostatic mechanisms promote network stability (Turrigiano GG, Nelson SB, 2000).

Application of the Hebbian learning rule to in vivo neuronal systems occurs by correlation-based synaptic potentiation, which can be likened to a snowball rolling down a mountain. In LTP, the postsynaptic neuron will continually diffuse retrograde (atypical) messengers to firing presynaptic neurons, making input stronger and more broad-based. How is this mechanism regulated? I have mentioned the techniques previously.

"Synaptic scaling" adjusts levels of AMPA and all other receptors in a single neuron, up or down, to maintain a regulatory set point (Figure 39). This process might be impaired in patients with increased NR2B in the PFC, since expression of AMPA receptors in these synapses is little to none, the consequence being that LTP should be almost impossible, even with a hyperactive NMDA receptor (see Figure 30). LTP could conceivably occur if the presynaptic neuron becomes depolarized anyway and the Mg^{2+} block is removed.

LTP without prior activation of the AMPA receptor may not occur under normal circumstances, even given the remarkable flexibility for phosphorylation of NMDA receptors. Phosphorylation may be caused by tyrosine kin-

ases such as CAMKII, the action of which is prolonged by autophosphorylation, and inhibition of PP1 (a phosphatase) by PKA phosphorylation,
which prolongs the phosphorylation of CAMKII. To overcome dephosphorylation by protein phophatase 1 (PP1), the kinase reaction must proceed much faster than the dephosphorylation reaction (Glazewski S et al.,
2000). PKA can be activated by forskolin. Forskolin, which stimulates
adenyl cyclase, seems to work better when combined with an adenosine antagonist or an alpha-1 agonist. Cross talk between multiple kinases is involved with the activation of CAMKII (Soderling TR, Derkach VA, 2000).

Approaching this situation from the standpoint of mGluRs, Fagni and
colleagues (2000) suggest that an intense rise in $[Ca^{2+}]_i$ can cause glutamate
spillover and activate members of the mGluR1 (mGluR1 and mGluR5) family, which may inhibit $GABA_A$ receptors or potentiate NMDA receptors but
not AMPA receptors. The Mg^{2+} block in this scenario could be caused by
G-protein generation of phosphoinositides, a rise in cytosolic $[Ca^{2+}]_i$, and
binding of Ca^{2+} to calmodulin.

I cannot see at this point how the extremely complex process of dendritic
integration of excitatory synaptic input contributes to LTP except for the
possibility of activation (Magee JC, 2000). Filtering done by dendritic arbors attenuates AMPA-modulated EPSCs considerably more than NMDA
EPSCs. Distal synapses can increase their impact by increasing their ratio of
NMDA to AMPA receptors because of the kinetic features of the potential
change, a topic too arcane to discuss here (Rinzel J, Rall W, 1974), since I
am attempting to eschew electrophysiology and complex equations in this
volume. I must allude to the fact that in the pyramidal cells of the hippocampal CA1 region, excitatory synapses grow progressively stronger with
distance from the cell body. "The spatial distribution of synaptic efficacies
is a flexible design feature that the brain uses to accommodate its various information processing goals" (Mel BW, 2002, p. 1845).

Synaptic scaling does not depend on any particular receptor(s). It scales
up or down the activity of all synapses in a neuron equally, thus preserving
relative strengths of the preexisting synapses. Thus, excitatory and inhibitory synapses on an entire neuron may be separately "tuned." A similar process occurs at voltage-dependent conductances (Na^+, K^+, and possibly
Ca^{2+}). Synaptic scaling determines how fast a neuron fires for a given
amount of input drive. Neurons also have a property termed "intrinsic plasticity" and can adjust to fire less or more from a given amount of synaptic input. The scaling of the magnitude of currents generated by ion channels attempts to achieve homeostasis. If a neuronal receptor is blocked, Na^+
currents increase, and persistent K^+ currents decrease. The ability to selectively modify the balance of inward and outward ion channels can fine tune
neuronal outputs to match inputs and can regulate protrusion of dendritic

filopodia or formulation of new dendritic spines. The time needed for synaptic scaling is hours to days, which is about how long it takes a new dendritic spine to grow. If neural activity is blocked for much longer, the spines are retracted and lost after a failed attempt at compensation.

NEUROTROPHIC FACTORS

Neurotrophic factors bind to the high-affinity receptors TrkA, TrkB, TrkC, and low-affinity p75. They are a heterogenous group of proteins which have many functions and some unconventional modes of action. Some act as retrograde messengers in the manner of NO. Brain-derived neurotrophic factor perhaps has the most relevance to neurosomatic disorders. Neurotrophins function somewhat like neurotransmitters, and their synthesis, storage, and release are regulated by classical neurotransmitters. Neurotrophins regulate other neurons through Trk receptors, which act as tyrosine kinases intracellularly. Tyrosine kinases interact with other intracellular proteins to subsequently activate MAP kinases and the PLC gamma cascades. Tyrosine kinase inhibitors are marketed as nutritional supplements (e.g., the phytoestrogen genistein) as a component of "naturally occurring" soy protein precursors. Tyrosine kinases regulate a host of intracellular signal transduction mechanisms. BDNF regulates hippocampal LTP and does so in part by modulating synaptic vesicle exocytosis. Neurotrophins are permissive for LTP (Figure 40).

Acute exposure to BDNF enhances synaptic function in general and can greatly attenuate synaptic fatigue (Gotsschalk WA et al., 1999). Exogenous BDNF can alleviate depression and acts as an antidepressant when given chronically. Antidepressants increase the expression of BDNF and TrkB, potential targets of CREB, a common postreceptor target for antidepressants. Up-regulation of BDNF and TrkB influence the function of hippocampal 5-HT and NE neurons (Duman RS et al., 1997). BDNF alone has antidepressant effects, and reduction in BDNF can cause depression. This sort of depression is often associated with hippocampal atrophy, so it is by no means certain that neurosomatic patients have decreased BDNF activity.

Nerve growth factors enhance NMDA-mediated responses. NGF and SP (Evengard B et al., 1998) levels are increased in the spinal fluid of patients with fibromyalgia, one way to distinguish these individuals from patients with other neurosomatic disorders. NGF is nociceptive, and retrograde neuronal transport of NGF from sensory neuron terminals increases levels of BK, SP, CGRP, and BDNF (Bennett DLH, 2001). NGF has been studied extensively in relation to inflammatory pain. The pro-inflammatory cytokines IL-1 beta (IL-1ß) and tumor necrosis factor-alpha raise levels of NGF substantially. NGF has acute stimulatory effects on mast cell mediator release, sympathetic afferents, and activation of the 5-lipoxygenase pathway. Longer term effects include increases in vanilloid receptors, BK receptors, Na^+ channels, SP, CGRP, and BDNF present within TrkA-expressing neurons (which are NGF sensitive).

BDNF is chronically secreted at low levels. When activity falls and BDNF levels are reduced synaptic scaling occurs, excitation is increased, and inhibition is decreased in vitro. In neurons previously exposed to BDNF, however, repeated exposure causes excitation (Sherwood NT, Lo DC, 1999). Hours after a voltage-sensitive Ca^{2+}-channel opening, BDNF has been synthesized from its mRNA and has been secreted. The increase in BDNF can be eliminated by preadministration of a Ca^{2+}-channel blocker. Specific neurotrophins regulate long-term changes in functional activity and the connectivity of neurons within different neural networks or systems. The effect of chronic BDNF hypersecretion, as well as NGF hypersecretion in fibromyalgia patients, would be similar to that of hyperactivity of the NMDA receptor. Fibromyalgia patients have elevated CSF levels of NGF (probably) and SP. CFS patients allegedly do not (Evengard B et al., 1998). It is my belief that these elevations are state related, although genetic factors probably play a role. I have seen many patients who had diffuse pain characteristic of fibromyalgia at one time and did not have it at others. SP increases nociceptive, and no doubt other kinds, transmission, through the NMDA receptor. SP antagonists, although not particularly effective as experimental analgesics, are, at the time of this writing (Boyce S, Hill RG, 2000), in trials to reduce in the pain of fibromyalgia. SPR activation is G-protein coupled, activating PLC with subsequent formation of IP_3 and DAG. IP_3 increases intracellular Ca^{2+}, and DAG activates PKC, which phosphorylates the NMDA receptor and removes the Mg^{2+} block. If this process can occur without first activating the AMPA receptor, the concomitant increase in SP and NR2B could produce depolarization and NMDA receptor-mediated events, including central sensitization. SP antagonists should be effective antimigraine drugs (SP is secreted by V1 in the dura mater), antiemetics, and antidepressants, perhaps by virtue of their functional NMDA-receptor antagonism (Berman RM et al., 2000; Rupniak NMJ, Kramer MS, 1999). SP antagonists may also reduce c-fos (an immediate early gene) mRNA expression in the trigeminal nucleus caudalis of rats after trigeminal nerve stimulation (Shepheard SL et al., 1995). They may also be anxiolytic, since SP causes anxiety when injected into the lateral septal nucleus of rats, which receives a dense SP innervation (Gavioli EC et al., 1999). Neurokinins (NK-SP is NK_1) are often cotransmitters in Ach neurons and may have their own autoreceptors (Pattachini R et al., 2000). SP is involved with stress-induced activation of DA from the VTA and NE from the LC. SP can produce hypothalamic defensive rage in cats, an amygdala response blocked by antidepressants. SP content is high in areas of the brain known to mediate stress; antidepressants and anxiolytics decrease SP levels. SP increases DA and is *analgesic* when injected into the VTA (Altier N, Stewart J, 1997). There are large amounts of SP in the basal ganglia, where it is associated with modulating DA release from nigrostriatal neurons. Its highest basal ganglia concentration is in the caudate nucleus. Estrogen decreases SP levels in the anterior pituitary of the rat (Ma D et al., 1997). SP stimulates NO synthase but not by binding to a neurokinin receptor (Garcia-Villar R et al., 1996).

Angiotensin-converting enzyme is one of the two enzymes that degrade SP. ACE enzyme activity is genetically determined, and ACE is co-localized with SP in many areas where there is no angiotensin I, e.g., the caudate. ACE inhibitors decrease SP immunoreactivity (Arinami T et al., 1996). Angiotensin II causes an increase in SP. I have given ACE inhibitors and AII inhibitors to hundreds of neurosomatic patients. Not one continues to take them for noncardiovascular effects. Because ACE inhibitors increase BK levels (BK is a vasodilator), they can act as antidotes to kutapressin, a BK antagonist. Because BK increases SP and CGRP, kutapressin should have an antimigraine effect. Unfortunately, it does not.

NGF is an algesic substance. If NGF is administered on successive days to mouse pups, they will be hyperalgesic and hypervigilant as adults (Alleva E et al., 1996). In accordance with its putative role as an NMDA agonist, NGF improves LTP in elderly rats (Bergado JA et al., 1997). BDNF and NGF mRNA are increased by EAAs (Anderson H et al., 1997), especially glutamate. NGF appears to synergize with most other substances released by stress. Symptoms in fibromyalgia patients are apparently not directly caused by NGF, however, since administration of haloperidol, which dramatically reduces NGF levels, is usually of no benefit. NGF does not increase during pregnancy but does so during parturition and nursing, when it may synergize with oxytocin (Alleva E et al., 1997). One would thus expect oxytocin to be ineffective in fibromyalgia patients, or to possibly exacerbate their symptoms, but there have been few adverse reactions in my experience of administering oxytocin to at least 3,000 patients. Oxytocin causes an increase in hypothalamic NGF but is involved in stress reduction and improves hippocampal encoding during stress. The OXTRs are up-regulated by adrenal and gonadal steroids, but in different brain structures (Liberzon I, Young EA, 1997). Other stress hormones, including cytokines, regulate levels of neurotrophin mRNA. NGF appears to be another substance that alters "set point" and is doubtless involved in tuning the brain, perhaps by being cosecreted with NE in the modulation of the NMDA synapse. I view fibromyalgia pain as a manifestation of a dysfunctional corticostriatal-thalamocortical network with a slightly different locus of dysregulation than that existing in other neurosomatic disorders.

NGF regulates levels of SP in nociceptive sensory neurons (Levi-Montalcini R et al., 1996). It has a trophic effect on cholinergic neurons and sympathetic ganglia. NGF has been proposed to play a role in regulating corticothalamic structures, in particular the reticular nucleus of the thalamus. Cells of the reticular nucleus filter transmission from the thalamic relay nuclei to and from the PFC. The reticular nucleus contains the low-affinity neurotrophin receptor p75, which is greatly up-regulated by NGF. NGF stimulates the secretion of ACTH. Fibromyalgia patients have low CRH levels but no functional adrenal insufficiency.

Psychological stress produces elevations in NGF without changing levels of ACTH, cortisol, IL-1, or TNF-α. As noted previously, NGF is increasingly conceptualized as lowering the set point for neuroimmunoendocrine cells to fire by modulating their thresholds for triggering stimuli. It is involved in priming this system for noxious stimuli. Fibromyalgia patients may have sensitized intrathalamic mast cells (Silver R et al., 1996) which readily degranulate and hypersecrete preprotachykinin mRNA (SP precursor) when stimulated by cortical glutamatergic efferents, either directly or via the reticular nucleus. Because FMS patients may have a deficiency in their ability to increase the secretion of NE, central mast cell hyperplasia may occur (Bergerot A et al., 2000).

Anandamide, perhaps acting at mast cell CB_2 receptors, can suppress mast cell degranulation. Marinol, a synthetic de facto marijuana-like compound, has significant analgesic properties in many of my fibromyalgia patients, but certainly not all of them. It also ameliorates other neurosomatic symptoms, usually without significant adverse reactions. CB_2 receptors are not usually labelled in the brain, but perhaps an exception could be made for mast cells. CB_1- and CB_2- specific ligands should help sort out this problem. Rita Levi-Montalcini, who won the Nobel Prize for discovering NGF, has implicated it in chronic pain states.

The brain endogenous cannabinoid anandamide is dispatched by some neurons to fine-tune the signals they receive. One such process occurs in the hippocampus and is termed depolarization-induced suppression of inhibition (DSI). Cannabinoids block DSI and may enhance LTP. Marinol, however, is not secreted locally (it is taken orally), and when administered systemically, it could have a suppressive effect on the entire brain. Marinol is a useful agent in neurosomatic medicine, and I shall discuss it further in its own section.

When an animal is injected with subcutaneous formalin, it develops hyperalgesia over widespread parts of its body (widened receptive fields). Among the products secreted by neurons and glia in this process are EAAs,

NO, AA, IL-1beta, TNF, and NGF (Watkins LR et al., 1997). Antisera to IL-1 and NGF injected intrathecally reduce formalin hyperalgesia, a model of posttraumatic fibromyalgia. Thus, it is thought that central NGF facilitates pain and that its release from astrocytes is facilitated by IL-1 beta. NGF releases CGRP and SP from afferent neurons and might be inhibited by the triptans. Peripherally administered neurotrophins can gain access to the CNS (Pan W et al., 1998). Neurotrophins are but one more of the many influences that can hypersensitize the NMDA receptor and predispose to neurosomatic disorders. Neurotrophin interactions and signaling pathways are being identified at a rapid rate (Thoenen H, Sendtner M, 2002).

METABOTROPIC GLUTAMATE RECEPTORS

Although I have been loathe to add another layer of complexity to an already bewildering process, I would be derelict in my duty to the reader if I did not discuss metabotropic glutamate receptors to some extent. Although their mechanisms are not understood in great detail at the present time, I have no doubt that ligands for these receptors will be extensively prescribed as treatment in the neurosomatic medicine of the future. All of the glutamate receptors, including the mGluRs, are displayed in the illustrations.

mGluRs are linked by G proteins to cytoplasmic enzymes. They are divided into three classes, I (mGluR1 and 5), II (mGluR2 and 3), and III (mGluR4, 6, 7, 8). They are all activated by glutamate. Agonists and antagonists selective for a specific group or a specific mGluR have been, for the most part, synthesized. Group I receptors stimulate phosphoinositide-specific PLC (PI-PLC). When activated, they form IP_3 and release intracellular Ca^{2+}, which can be inhibited with heparin, and DAG, which activates PKC. Ca^{2+} is also released by activation of the ryanodine-sensitive receptor intracellularly. Activating most Group II and III receptors inhibits AC via an inhibitory G protein (G_1). To discuss every exception would needlessly complicate this brief section.

Agonism at any mGluR modulates L-type Ca^{2+} channels, and groups I and II inhibit N-type Ca^{2+} channels. Many ligand-gated channels are regulated in part by mGluRs, including AMPA, NMDA, DA, $GABA_A$, and NE receptors. Whether activation or inhibition occurs as a result of the mGluR modulation seems to depend on the cell type.

Some mGluRs are located presynaptically (II and III), in which case they inhibit release of neurotransmitter, probably by blocking presynaptic Ca^{2+} channels. When agonists or antagonists for the specific mGluR are not available, knock-out mice reveal the function of the receptor. Some of the mGluRs are (of course) subtyped, as in mGluR1$_A$, which has high immunostaining in the cerebellum and hippocampal CA1 interneurons (Fagni L et al., 2000). CA1 pyramidal cells stain for mGluR5. Both receptors are Type I, meaning they both release intracellular Ca^{2+}, either through IP_3Rs, RyRs, or both. There are three types of IP_3Rs and three types of RyRs, just one example of why I am not going to discuss mGluRs in detail. RyRs are activated by caffeine, among other substances, and blocked by dantrolene. Calcium-induced calcium release is also involved with RyR Ca^{2+} release. I have discussed this process previously. Recall that heparin is an IP_3R antagonist. Because dantrolene rarely relieves neurosomatic symptoms, the RyR must not contribute to their pathophysiology. I am surprised dantrolene is not more effective, because it also inhibits nitric oxide, a possible NMDA-receptor antagonist. Dantrolene is often effective when heparin is. It must be used with caution because of potential hepatotoxicity.

Group I mGluRs are more likely to be excitatory, either by inhibiting GABAergic receptors, potentiating NMDA receptors, or inhibiting K^+ channels. They have been studied more intensively than groups II and III. They can functionally couple RyRs and L-type Ca^{2+} channels, a process that can be blocked by nifedipine. Ca^{2+} influx through L-type Ca^{2+} channels can replenish intracellular Ca^{2+} stores (Ugolini A et al., 1997). It has been suggested that after accumulation of the glutamate in the synaptic cleft, spillover of glutamate molecules can reach the presynaptic receptors and trigger the mGluR-mediated response (Congar P et al., 1997). At present, my take on type I mGluRs is that they may be involved when a patient presents with symptoms suggestive of sympathetic overactivity. In such a case, dantrolene, an inhibitor of intracellular Ca^{2+} mobilization from RyRs only should be effective but hardly ever reduces symptoms, perhaps because I do not use it early in the therapeutic trials (it has some potential toxicity). Heparin is much more effective, acting somewhat like a downstream ketamine. Some other effects of dantrolene deserve mention. 3-hydroxykynurenine (3-HK) has toxic effects and has been implicated in certain neurodegenerative diseases. 3-HK produces neurotoxicity by generation of H_2O_2 (hydrogen peroxide) formed by 3-HK autoxidation in extracellular compartments. 3-HK can kill PC12 pheochromocytoma cells as well as GT1-7 hypothalamic secretory cells. 3-HK cells are protected from an untimely demise by dantrolene, which not only inhibits Ca^{2+} released from the endoplasmic reticulum but also increases the protein level of BC1-2, a prominent antiapoptotic gene product. Dantrolene's up-regulation of the BC1-2 gene product suppresses 3-HK toxicity (Wei H et al., 2000). In most cases, except when it is time for a cell to die, this result would be regarded as *good*. H_2O_2 can inhibit DA release, a property abolished when DA autoreceptors are blocked (Chen BT et al., 2001).

Although a nitric oxide antagonist would be quite useful in many clinical situations, one had not been known to exist, except for niacinamide, which had not been found to be very effective until a Chinese publication in 1999 (Wu CC et al., 1999). Dantrolene has clinically reversed a NO ADR, but one swallow does not make it to Goodman and Gilman.

Lipopolysaccharide, a bacterial endotoxin, increases production of NO and TNF and causes hypotension in the anesthetized rat. The hypotension is due in part to decreased response to NE. Dantrolene pre-treatment attenuates the overproduction of TNF-alpha and NO. Pretreatment with nifedipine prevents the decreased response to NE, perhaps by impeding refilling of Ca^{2+} in RyR-sensitive stores in the endoplasmic reticulum. If dantrolene acts to reduce NO in other circumstances (see previous sections on NO), it could be a very useful agent which could be used *right now.*

There are so many possible effects of mGluR agonism or antagonism that it almost seems the CNS could operate only with mGluRs. Here are some (brief) examples of mGluR functions:

1. Driving synchronized inhibition in the neocortex
2. Behavioral stimulation via the striatum and NAc (group II)
3. Involved in the action of amphetamine
4. Blocking kynurenine synthesis
5. Nociception or antinociception
6. Enhancing LC function
7. Modulation of K_{ATP} channels (site of action of gabapentin, morphine, minoxidil, diazoxide, clonidine and other alpha$_2$ agonists, sulfonylureas, and glucose)
8. LTP and LTD
9. Apoptosis
10. Vision
11. Anxiety

mGluR agonists and antagonists are in Phase II trials at the time of this writing. No results have appeared in the medical literature, but such agents will variously regulate NMDA transmission.

PKC-mediated desensitization regulates the physiological actions of mGluRs of all three groups. PKA is involved, as well, in modulating group II and III (Lariviere WR, Melzack R, 2000). Phosphorylation of mGluR1 changes the receptor when it is located presynaptically from an action of facilitation to one of inhibition of glutamate release, a condition which can be prolonged by inhibiting phosphatases. PKC may act on mGluRs selectively, depending on its type of G-protein coupling. One of the most important effects of mGluR1 is to potentiate ion flow through the NMDAR. There is a reciprocal relationship between NMDARs and group I mGluRs. Low concentrations of NMDA enhance the activity of group I mGluRs. In group I knock-out mice, LTP, spatial learning, and prepulse inhibition are impaired and EPSPs are reduced. The later finding suggests mGluRs are important in setting the tone of NMDA-mediated synaptic transmission. NMDARs and mGluRs may even physically interact, albeit indirectly, through scaffolding proteins at the postsynaptic density. NMDA may potentiate mGluR5 by dephosphorylating it via calcineurin.

Group II and III mGluRs inhibit synaptic transmission. This activity is reduced by PKC and PKA. Activation of adenosine A_3 receptors in the hippocampus inhibits these mGluRs by a PKC-dependent mechanism. PKA-mediated effects on presynaptic mGluR function can be elicited by beta-adrenoceptor activation in the hippocampus. This mechanism may be involved in encoding of brief important events (flashbulb memories). Much more is known about mGluRs than I am able to summarize here. For example, noncompetitive allosteric antagonists of mGluR5, as well as competitive antagonists, have been developed. These agents may be useful for inflammatory pain, anxiety, and depression. The mGluR7 receptor interacts with calmodulin, G-protein beta-gamma subunits, and PICK1, the protein that interacts with PKC. mGluR7 is involved with amygdala-dependent memory and behaviors. Its physiology is becoming increasingly well understood (Dev KK et al., 2001).

The ATP-sensitive K^+ channel (K_{ATP}) in glucose-responsive (GR) neurons is involved in the response to hypoglycemia. In addition to using glucose as fuel, GR neurons use it to regulate their firing rate by altering the activity of the K_{ATP} channel. It is composed of four pore-forming units for K^+ and four receptors for sulfonylureas (SUR1-4) (Figure 41).

Glucose uptake and metabolism increase the ATP/ADP ratio, which promotes ATP binding to the K_{ATP} receptor channel. This attachment closes the channel, increasing $[K^+_i]$, causing depolarization. When $[glucose_i]$ is decreased, ATP/ADP falls, the K_{ATP} channel opens and hyperpolarizes the neuron, decreasing firing. GR neurons are found in the hypothalamic ventromedial hypothalamus (VMH), arcuate nucleus, PVN, SN, LC, and NTS (Levin BE et al., 2001). K_{ATP} channels are found in other regions of the brain that do not have GR neurons. In these cases, the pore-forming unit is Kir6.2, which is joined to SUR1. If glucose or oxygen is limited and ATP/ADP falls, the K_{ATP} channel closes anyway to decrease neuronal activity and metabolic demand. Because neurosomatic patients rarely improve with sulfonylureas and often do with K_{ATP} openers, I assume there is excessive neurotransmission and no shortage of ATP in the usual case, although the brain and the liver have other glucosensing mechanisms.

Some K_{ATP} openers, perhaps all of them, enhance one another. This synergism is certainly seen with morphine and clonidine in treating pain, and I have observed it as well with minoxidil in PLO or taken orally. Hypotension is rarely a problem, nor are effects on behavior or motor coordination (Galeotti N, Ghelardini C, Vinci MC, Bartolini A, 1999).

Thus far, dantrolene has sometimes reversed the effects of nitroglycerin (NO) in my limited trials. Furthermore, if dantrolene acts by inhibition of phosphatidylinositol breakdown, it could have effects similar to lithium carbonate and valproic acid (Depakote). In general, I have noticed it sometimes sedates patients or reduces anxiety, but not often enough for me to try it frequently. I may not have been using it for the specific neurosomatic disorders that receptor profiling should have suggested.

Although I encounter it only about once every ten years, neuroleptic malignant syndrome, a disorder of autonomic hyperreactivity, fever, muscle breakdown, and apparent catatonia, is caused by standard neuroleptics and possibly by rapid cessation of IV amantadine infusion. CPK is almost always elevated. Dantrolene has been suggested as a treatment, but I have used neuroleptic discontinuation, dopamine agonists, and supportive measures with monitoring (Tsutsumi Y et al., 1998). I have restarted IV amantadine in one such patient for whom it was the only effective treatment and have encountered no problems so far.

CONCLUSION

When I was a psychiatry resident, one of the rotating assignments was to do "overdose rounds." For a county hospital, overdose rounds usually consisted of very rapid assessment of about fifty patients in a ward who were in various states of obtundation, delirium, or recovery. In the early 1970s, it was not unusual for me to discharge half the ward the same morning, because psychedelic drugs were frequently ingested at that time. I used intravenous niacin, or nicotinic acid, which can be synthesized from tryptophan quite easily. Because LSD and similar agents bound to the serotonin receptor (we didn't know about subtypes then), I would administer nicotinic acid in 200 mg boluses until the patient had a niacin flush, at which point he or she "came down." I assumed I was witnessing competitive inhibition for the 5-HT receptor. Hoffer and Osmond routinely terminated their LSD experiments of the late 1950s with niacin. As a probably predictable aside, I should mention no one evinced the slightest curiosity about how these results were accomplished, and this "antidote" remains little known thirty years later (Goldstein JA, 1983), much like my discovery in 1979 (Goldstein JA, 1983) that cimetidine made acute infectious mononucleosis in teenagers or adults (and varicella, too) resolve in one or two days. I am getting tired of whining about it, but hardly anyone is aware of this treatment, even now. Although I reported a 90 percent cure rate in over 100 patients (rather high for a placebo response), the results were "anecdotal." Naturally, I was unable to get a grant to perform a double-blind, placebo-controlled experiment. "But Tagamet [and later Zantac] is for ulcers," the reviewers would write. The fact that the chairman of the department of infectious diseases at the local medical school was my coinvestigator on the grant proposal did not grease the wheel at all.

Medications that increase dopamine and/or norepinephrine can have a stimulant effect, and some of these will also increase serotonin. Most of the agents that may act as stimulants are in the box [dopamine] in the receptor-profiling algorithm. Many more agents might be stimulatory, however, if they inhibit a neuron which is inhibiting a stimulating neurotransmitter. Mu-opioids are a prime example because there are inhibitory mu-opioid hetero-receptors on GABAergic neurons that inhibit dopaminergic tonic activation from the VTA/NAc. Almost any medication can be stimulatory in a certain person, and there are often inhibitory and excitatory subtypes of the same transmitter, such as adenosine (A_1 and A_{2A}), 5-HT($_{1A,B,D}$), NE (alpha$_{2ABC}$), and many more. Often a neurotransmitter or drug is stimulatory or inhibitory by a fourth- or fifth-order process. This phenomenon is seen with almost all of the eyedrops and nose drops. Every good reaction leads me a certain way, and so does every adverse reaction. Because the brain is so complicated, these observations might lead to a dead end, but along the way I should detect other good and bad responses which might give me more clues. After a while, in some patients, I will reach a point at which every medication but one has been eliminated on a certain pathway, and this intervention is almost always effective. I no longer seek to improve the patient's condition; I expect to make him or her feel virtually normal, and I often can, except for perhaps 2 to 3 percent of the cases. My job is usually not very difficult. Sometimes patients feel dramatically better in ten seconds. Other times it can take several days or longer. Some patients have tried 100 treatments until I found the right one. I am usually looking for a fairly immediate response, realizing it will be a receptor-mediated response and not genomic. Genomic responses take longer, as with antidepressants, but they may be longer lasting since an alteration in protein synthesis may be less perturbed by feed-forward and feedback influences than a change in protein conformation. When patients come to see me from thousands of miles away, I do not have the luxury, nor would I want it, of giving them Zoloft, for example, and telling them to come back in two months. In PTSD, which can take 24 weeks to resolve with SRIs, it is much better to make patients feel better on the first or second day of treatment and give antidepressants, or AEDs, as a backup.

Patients who are doing much better than before they first saw me are still encouraged to come in for a tune-up every six to 12 months. Because I already know (I think) the broad outlines of their neurochemical pathways, I can often replace a medication and raise their Karnofsky score from 80 to 90. The most important new idea is to tailor the treatment to the patient's neurochemistry. Many medications have powerful psychotropic properties but are used for entirely different indications in general medicine.

Currently, if I had to list the four medications that help the most patients the fastest, they would be (1) ketamine IV, p.o., gel, nose sprays, and eyedrops, (2) lidocaine IV or gel, (3) amantadine IV 200 to 400 mg, (4) and guaifenesin 250 mg slow IV infusion. Several patients take one spray of 1:1 ketamine three to four times a day. Each spray is about 0.5 mg. This dose is very low and very effective. Low doses of ketamine are nontoxic, and they are rarely abused. No physical dependence is associated with ketamine. Its primary effect is to enable patients to filter out less-relevant stimuli. I have discussed the neuropharmacology of ketamine and other NMDA antagonists frequently in this book. Patients can be premedicated with clonidine or benzodiazepines to eliminate most ADRs that may occur with intravenous administration, although this tactic is usually unnecessary. Despite its being a dissociative anesthetic, if administered at the proper rate, ketamine markedly improves dissociative disorders, as it does most symptoms related to panic, PTSD, hysteria, somatoform disorder, GAD, FMS, CFS, IBS, MDD, etc. Any disorder in which the patient attends to and magnifies irrelevant stimuli is a good candidate for ketamine. I would not give ketamine to most bipolar patients or to schizophrenics. Schizotypal patients are probably not good candidates either. Some borderline personality disorder patients seem to improve, but the severe borderlines remain almost untreatable (especially those with comorbid narcissistic and histrionic personality disorder).

Intolerance to lidocaine is uncommon. Some patients react to methylparaben used as the preservative. Procaine may be used in lidocaine allergy, but it has vasoconstrictive properties. I believe the way most physicians infuse IV lidocaine is wrong. They give the entire dose in 30 to 60 minutes, sometimes sedating the patient to avoid adverse reactions, which almost invariably occur. One patient who had been doing well with me for years, had been receiving IV lidocaine, 0.15 mg/kg every two to three weeks. She moved to another city. She went to a pain clinic, was put on a cardiac monitor, and was given the entire dose in 30 minutes. She felt anxious, confused, and disoriented while she was receiving it and relapsed after the infusion was completed. She never responded to lidocaine again. I infuse IV solutions at a rate at which patients have little or no adverse reactions. If they become a little jittery, they receive a low dose of clonidine or Xanax. This measure is rarely necessary since there are almost no adverse reactions. Lidocaine is particularly good for patients with allodynia but has the potential to help every symptom. It can be given subcutaneously in a dose of 5mg/kg, usually once or twice a day. Most people who respond to IV lidocaine have had some beneficial response to a transdermal gel.

I give lidocaine trigger-point injections now and then when patients have localized areas of pain. There are many solutions to use in the trigger-point injection, and I have used bupivicaine, Sarapin, triamcinolone, phentolamine, and ketamine. I am usually not impressed with the results. I do not often give trigger-point injections for fibromyalgia because frequently they do not work, sometimes they make a patient worse, and sometimes they last for only a few hours. Because many of my patients are indigent, I often do them for free. It is fairly easy to find 40 or more trigger points to inject at a time, and on some occasions, I must inject an entire constellation of them. If I miss one, the chance of recurrence is much greater. The patients are usually quite grateful, but I know they may feel worse the next day. The knowledge of trigger points, as is discussed in *The Trigger Point Manual* by Janet Travell and David Simons (Simons et al., 1999) is imperative to have for doctors in primary care, physical medicine, or rheumatology, but hardly anyone seems to. I sent a Boston patient who ran out of time while here to a pain clinic at Harvard for a pelvic muscle injection in the "piriform" muscle, a cause of pelvic pain and sciatica. "That's rare," said the clinician there. I have diagnosed piriformis myofascial pain on hundreds of occasions. He performed the injection incorrectly, her pain got worse, and she had to travel 3,000 miles back to California to have the injection done properly.

Both lidocaine and ketamine infusions typically are effective for about a week, and I usually do not order IV ketamine more frequently unless palliating a terminal patient. Many physicians insist on a cardiac monitor and continuous RN observation if giving IV lidocaine. When it is infused at a rate to avoid more than minor side effects, there is almost no risk at all. I have infused lidocaine thousands of times. Two patients developed urticaria, the most serious side effect yet, after which the lidocaine was no longer effective. I have discussed the possible mechanisms of lidocaine's action previously. IV lidocaine should be standard operating procedure in the emergency department and on the pain service as well as postoperatively.

There is considerable (unwarranted) concern over the possible neurotoxicity of ketamine (Sharp FR et al., 2001). I have administered intravenous ketamine by slow infusion less often than lidocaine, but still nearly 1,000 times and have never had a serious and/or permanent adverse reaction. Many physicians recoil at the idea of using ketamine for fear of precipitating a latter-day "reefer madness." I have had some very ill patients from middle-sized cities receive complete remission from IV lidocaine (which, after all, is routinely used in the coronary care unit) and not find one physician in their entire city who would administer it. Suicides have ensued after the patients reverted to crawling to the bathroom and being generally immobile otherwise. Nevertheless, some pharmacologists have suggested the NMDA receptor could be antagonized much more safely by doing so at the glycine coagonist site. Such a treatment approach is quite feasible and is often effective. Glycine-site antagonists have few adverse reactions, no effect on motor behavior, and no effect on nonnociceptive neurons. Their modulation of neuropathic pain, however, is quite significant (Bordi F, Quartaroli M, 2000).

D-cycloserine is an antituberculous drug no one uses any more. It is also a glycine-B partial agonist at the glycine-B binding site on the NMDA receptor/channel complex. It potentiates the action of most anticonvulsants except lamotrigine and phenytoin by an unknown mechanism (De Sarro G et al., 2000). Cycloserine also increases working memory and navigation (maze solving) in rats in a manner similar to an $alpha_1$ agonist. The two agents have no additive effect, however (Pussinen R, Sirvio J, 1999). This finding implies that cycloserine and alpha-1 agonists often impair the overlearned memories and responses of neurosomatic patients.

NMDA evokes release of NE in rat hippocampal slices. This effect is antagonized by several NMDA-receptor antagonists, including kynurenic acid, an endogenous glycine-site antagonist. The effect of kynurenine is blocked by nootropics such as aniracetam and oxiracetam, and also by D-cycloserine (Pittaluga A et al., 1999).

Kynurenine levels are raised by probenecid, which retards its excretion from the CSF as it does with penicillin. D-cycloserine is also antagonized by ondansetron (Zofran), diltiazem (which is also a $5\text{-}HT_3$ antagonist), and atropine, which I do not use at all, preferring trihexyphenidyl (Artane) as a centrally acting anticholinergic. I do not know how mirtazapine (Remeron) would work in this system, since it is also a $5\text{-}HT_3$ antagonist, but it has dramatically relieved pain on the first dose (in the office) in two individuals who had failed on many other medications.

When alosetron (Lotronex) was removed from the market by the FDA, to the dismay of many of my diarrhea-predominant IBS patients, I had little to offer them except

1. amelioration of their entire symptom complex, best done with lidocaine and/or ketamine, which also decreases intestinal motility;
2. smooth muscle relaxants which inhibit the NMDA receptor at the polyamine site (isoxsuprine) and the polyamine site plus the NR1/NR2B site (nylidrin);

3. opioids;
4. alpha$_2$ agonists;
5. cholestyramine;
6. low-dose oral naloxone;
7. ondansetron (Zofran); and
8. octreotide (Sandostatin).

Both ondansetron and alosetron are 5-HT$_3$-receptor antagonists. Patients who are wealthy or have good insurance can take two or three Zofran per day and often have much-reduced diarrhea. I wonder why this property is not better known? Zofran is also, to a degree, a blocker of NMDA-receptor antagonists (Suzuki T et al., 1999), and I try to control nausea in a patient receiving ketamine by other means. It is, nevertheless, a glycine-site antagonist and can be analgesic when combined, e.g., with probenecid. Zofran also potentiates the action of cocaine in the NAc.

Ondansetron, and probably other 5-HT$_3$ antagonists, may be an effective treatment for tardive dyskinesia (Sirota P et al., 2000). They can block motor hyperactivity induced by central administration of amphetamine and DA. The ability of DA to block the firing of mPFC neurons is inhibited by 5-HT$_3$ antagonists. Postsynaptic 5-HT$_3$ receptors are present on GABAergic interneurons and mediate fast synaptic transmission in the CNS. 5-HT$_3$ receptors may also be localized presynaptically (van Hooft JA, Vijverberg HP, 2000). The role of these receptors in mediating the release of various transmitters is ambiguous, even though they are Ca^{2+} permeable ion channels.

Guaifenesin is the best of the glycine-site antagonists. It synchronizes the EEG in anesthesized pigs as NMDA antagonists do in humans. It can relieve any and all symptom(s) in an individual patient. I use it initially in 10 percent PLO, usually 2 to 3 mL on both forearms. The response to the gel form correlates fairly well with the oral tablet. The usual dose is 1200 mg SR (sustained release) b.i.d. It is reliably reversed by cycloserine. There are other purported modes of action for guaifenesin in neurosomatic disorders, but they seem to have come from another space-time continuum. Guaifenesin is in my top ten oral medications. Except for a few unsuccessful trials in treatment-refractory patients about ten years ago, I did not use guaifenesin until I had discovered a mode of action that was rational and scientific. This process took several years, since the veterinarians who have been using it widely for decades ("You don't use it in human anesthesia! Why not?") have no clue about its neuropharmacology. I have tried IV guaifenesin on humans in extremis. Pigs are fairly similar immunologically. At *least* once a month a patient tells me that if I cannot help him, he is going to kill himself. No one has actually done so under my care, but I am widely regarded as "the end of the line." Three or four patients have almost exhausted their options, including ECT and multiple hospitalizations. Now that vagal nerve stimulation has been FDA-approved for epilepsy, perhaps I would try this modality first, but if vagal nerve stimulation is not possible (I can't find a neurosurgeon who will perform the procedure) or has adverse reactions, the risk/benefit ratio between IV guaifenesin versus ampligen versus skull-base surgery versus death looks pretty good. IV guaifenesin 250 mg in 500 mg normal saline appeared to be safe and is now in my top four medications.

Similar to reboxetine, the release of tegaserod, the 5-HT$_4$ partial agonist for constipation-predominant IBS, has been inexplicably delayed for over a year. Serotonin has a number of well-documented sensorimotor effects on the GI tract and can produce hyperalgesia in several models, especially at the 5-HT$_3$ and 5-HT$_4$ receptors, but also at the 5-HT$_{1B/1D}$ and 5-HT$_7$ receptors. I frequently use triptans (each one is a little different) for IBS pain and to decrease gut motility. Thus alosetron (Lotronex), a 5-HT$_3$ antagonist, can inhibit visceral sensitivity, increase compliance, and block excitatory receptors that increase peristalsis. Piboserod is a 5-HT$_4$ antagonist being developed for diarrhea-predominant IBS. Drug companies know that centrally acting IBS medications would be more effective, but since they may be labled "psychiatric," insurance companies might not pay for them.

We need a better prokinetic agent for those IBS patients with constipation. Metoclopramide has a very high incidence of extrapyramidal effects. Bethanechol is not too effective. Erythromycin in a dose of 50 to 100 mg is fairly good, but too few physicians know about it (binds to the motilin receptor in gut and brain). Domperidone (Motilium) is okay but is unavailable in the United States. Cisapride (Propulsid) had too many drug interactions for MDs to prescribe it appropriately, and it was withdrawn from the market because of prolongation of the QT interval. Now we are waiting for tegaserod and prucalopride, "second generation" agents, both like cisapride but devoid of effects on the QT interval. They may be more active than cisapride at the colonic level (DePonti F, Tonini M, 2000).

A list of effective neurosomatic medications would include ketamine, lidocaine, gabapentin (the best oral medication), lamotrigine, baclofen, IV amantadine, IV ascorbate, IV or subcutaneous TRH, and IV or p.o. guaifenesin. Then would come (in alphabetical order) Adderall, adenosine nasal spray, acetylcholinesterase inhibiters (for those who respond better to NMDA agonists), dipyridamole (not all those who respond to adenosine nasal spray respond to dipyridamole, but many do), methadone, modafinil, naphazoline eyedrops, nimodipine, oseltamivir oxytocin, ranitidine, reboxetine, relaxin, TRH (IV if it lasts a month or more, subcutaneous if it does not), Ultram, and ziprasidone (Geodon). I only recommend physicians trying them randomly like this if they have no idea what receptor profiling is and do not think they are capable of learning it. Doctors will still help the majority of their patients by making a list of these medications and throwing darts at it. I am at the point at which I expect new patients to become asymptomatic, or virtually so, and am surprised when they do not.

To finish my discussion of IBS, which is really quite easily treated, I would like to refer to the work of Emeran Mayer's group at UCLA. They study IBS well. Their work on pathophysiology is interesting and is ahead of anyone else. The following will summarize relevant points of a recent article (Mayer EA et al., 2001). As almost all others have found, those with chronic abdominal pain, or any chronic pain, have a greater history of traumatic events or losses during childhood than do healthy controls, or do they? IBS patients, like many neurosomatic patients in general, have differences in somatic threat appraisal, poor coping skills, and inadequate belief systems regarding management of life stresses and symptoms. Such findings, which have been confirmed many times in various settings, are a primary reason why cognitive-behavioral therapy is so widely recommended. Most researchers and clinicians do not seem to appreciate that inappropriate belief systems, consisting of cognitive information to which inappropriate attention is allocated, work on the same principle as does inappropriate perception of salience. Too many salient stimuli cause overloading of attentional resources and widening of receptive fields, thereby increasing the synaptic weight of these stimuli. The result is the processing of too much information in a dysfunctional manner. Ultimately, there are overlearned maladaptive cognitive and sensory networks—my deductions, not Mayer's. IBS patients are more likely to regard life events as threatening and more likely to seek out medical attention for their somatic symptoms.

Mayer discusses "CNS networks activated in response to perceived threat or fear and those activated in response to learned (or conditioned) fear" as causing anxiety and IBS symptoms, a duality he seems to perceive as being inextricably linked. He reifies an emotional motor system (EMS), parallel motor pathways used to manage allostatic load. He cites the rostral ACC, insula, and mPFC as representing the visceral motor cortex which projects to every central regulatory area of vigilance, arousal, and nociceptive functions.

He continues to follow the deeply trod academic path that CRH is the wellspring of the stress response, even (as in neurosomatic disorders) if CRH is low. Mayer fully describes the functional neuroanatomy of the amygdala, LC, and periaqueductal gray, which I outlined in both *Betrayal* and *Limbic Hypothesis*. "The findings are consistent with hyperactivity of ascending noradrenergic arousal systems in affective and functional visceral syndromes" (Mayer EA et al., 2001). His IBS patients are not sleepy? Their STR is good? They do not have comorbid CFS (two-thirds do)? To his credit, though, he does refer to NMDA and non-NMDA receptors, but unfortunately not in the context of treatment.

Mayer has been a leader in forming the hypothesis of visceral hypersensitivity. He finds that pure IBS patients have only gut hypersensitivity, not musculoskeletal hypersensitivity as is seen in FMS patients. IBS patients have "(1) hypervigilance toward expected aversive events arising from the viscera, and (2) hyperalgesia inducible in certain IBS patients, but not in healthy controls, by sustained noxious visceral stimulation" (Mayer EA et al., 2001). At the time he did the experiments to support these views, particularly in combination with PET and colonic balloon distension, they were pioneering, or even radical, in academic medicine. His latest work follows *Betrayal* as well as FMS researchers Daniel Clauw, whose work is very much like mine was in 1995, Robert Bennett, and I. Jon Russell: "The role of cognitive factors, such as selective attention and vigilance, in modulating the perception of visceral input to the brain is also supported by preliminary results from brain imaging studies" (Mayer EA et al., 2001).

He also has published work suggesting descending nociceptive inhibitory controls, particularly those involving endogenous opioids, may be hypofunctional in IBS. This research mirrors the same sort of findings in FMS. From my point of view, the locus of neurosomatic pain could extend from the amygdala through the pallidum, the basal ganglia, the thalamus (especially the reticular nucleus of the thalamus [RTN] and "nonspecific" nuclei), to the anterior insula and parietal operculum. The insula could be particularly important for visceral pain (Treede R-D et al., 2000). Thermal sensibility is exteroceptive—how hot or cold is it outside?—and enteroceptive, an aspect important for homeostasis, activity of the ANS, and thermoregulatory behavior. It may relate to other (often) exteroceptive sensations, such as pain. Temperature and pain sensation is integrated almost everywhere in the neuraxis. Cold usually inhibits pain, and this analgesia is lost in the post-stroke central pain syndrome (Craig AD, 1998). This pain is not diffuse but is aching, dysesthetic, and, in some locations, hyperesthetic. Brain lesions causing central pain and burning interrupt the ascending spinothalamic tract, leaving its ultimate termination, a parieto-insular region, deafferentiated, except for a dedicated region of the thalamus, the posterior part of the ventral medial nucleus, VM_{po}. Using cold stimuli with PET on human volunteers, the thermosensory cortex was located in the dorsal margin of the middle/posterior insula. Its degree of activation was directly correlated with stimulus intensity.

The VM_{po}, visible only in primates, is largest in humans. It projects to a cytoarchitectonically distinct field in the putative human thermosensory cortex, the terminus of the lamina 1 spinothalamocortical pathway. Thermal sensation, being integrated with homeostasis, influences behavior, affect, and the function of the ANS. Lamina 1 projects to many sites involved in sensory integration, including the hypothalamus, amygdala, vagus, and NTS, and to several brainstem nuclei, such as the parabrachial, PAG, raphe, and noradrenergic areas. The authors of the paper I am discussing, Craig and colleagues (2000), view the insula as limbic sensory cortex, the projections to which "seem to provide a highly resolved enteroceptive representation of the body's condition in humans, including the specific sensations of temperature, pain, and other 'feelings' from the body." Most of my patients are cold intolerant.

Aspects of primarily insular enteroceptive sensations include taste, hunger, thirst, hyperthermia, lactate- and CCK-induced panic, inspiration, isometric exercise, and various types of cutaneous and deep pain. Insular dysfunction could account for air hunger and the almost random tidal volume variability we see in (only) fibromyalgia patients performing submaximal exercise. The insula is also associated with internally generated emotions such as recall-generated sadness, anticipatory anxiety, panic, disgust, and visually evoked sexual arousal.

The right anterior insula is activated in anticipation of sensation of tonically evoked heat pain, and the right insula is considered to be part of the "somatic marker" hypothesis of consciousness (another topic I omitted in this book), or a "limbic sensory substrate that invests internal feelings with emotional significance" (Craig AD et al., 2000). When the thermal stimulus is unpleasant, the limbic motor cortex, i.e., ACC, is activated.

The human thermosensory cortex corresponds to that area of the cortex damaged in poststroke patients with central pain. Craig has proposed that disruption of thermal sensation may cause central pain (Craig AD, 1998). Post-stroke pain is not fibromyalgia pain, or IBS pain, or any of the other types of neurosomatic pain, but a stroke destroys nerves; neurosomatic illness produces a potentially reversible alteration of function.

The degree of dysfunction in the various regions could coruscate, analogous to Crick's "attentional spotlight." Symptoms could wax, wane, change, and shift in an apparently inexplicable manner probably regulated by cortico-cortical projections.

Mayer ends by comparing nonconstipated IBS to panic disorder. He states there is evidence for "aversive interoceptive conditioning" in both groups, a learned fear response to previously innocuous physical sensations. A hypervigilance for certain visceral stimuli develops, with associated catastrophizing, in or out of awareness (out, if there is pre-frontal-amygdalo-hippocampal disconnection). I admire Mayer's work.

I now segue into a discussion of stress and the mesolimbic dopamine system, which is, as it turns out, one of the central issues of this book. I have been thinking for a long time about what is the cause of fatigue in the patients I see. Doubtless there are several, but one stands out: mesolimbic dopamine.

Almost all my patients have a worsening of their symptoms by stress. It is not necessarily the stress (learned helplessness) that results in depression. Different strains of rats and neurochemically individual people respond to stress in various ways. Some victims of severe child abuse have no apparent sequelae at all. Primitive people living 20,000 years ago had the same brains as we do, yet life was hard and short, and I am sure most children did not feel safe—yet the species survived and prospered. I am certainly not advocating that we routinely beat our children because it will be good for them, a fairly common notion not too long ago, only that the rigors of a hunter-gatherer lifestyle may have selected for "hardiness." This quality may not be necessary in a civilized environment, in which natural selection has been rendered obsolete, because natural selection occurs too slowly to reflect the dizzily accelerating rate of change of our lifestyles.

The mesocortical, and probably the mesocorticolimbic, DA pathways respond to stressful stimuli. I had hoped to avoid venturing into the rapidly expanding universe of the stress response for fear I would never get out, but I must discuss stress to the degree it affects neurosomatic disorders. Stress can be defined operationally as a response of an organism to any stimulus that has the properties of novelty, threat, conflict, or homeostatic imbalance. It is related to the concept of "allostasis" (stability through change) I discussed in *Betrayal*. Dysfunction of allostasis could produce "allostatic load," producing adverse effects on the organism. Hypocortisolism is "type 4" allostasis and could produce CFS, FMS, and atopic dermatitis (McEwen BS, 1998). Stress usually increases but sometimes, if it is aversive, decreases DA. Dopamine-level alteration occurs to the greatest degree in the PFC, to a lesser but still large degree in the NAc, and mildly in the nigrostriatal tract, which is concerned more with execution of learned motor acts, or habits. The initial DA increase in an aversive situation may be related to defensive preparations.

If the stimulus is unavoidable or uncontrollable, mesoaccumbens DA is inhibited. If the organism is able to cope with the stress, even if it persists, DA does not fall. The degree to which the organism perceives that the stress can be handled is strain-specific in animals and individual in humans. Other influences, such as prenatal stress (Hayashi A et al., 1998) or early maternal care (Francis DD, Meaney MJ, 1999) seem to be just as important as genetic factors in the adult response, but I shall consider them in the briefest manner possible, since they do not lend themselves to amelioration in the office setting except for influencing the development of a patient's future children.

Stressed pregnant rats give birth to offspring with impaired behavioral indices later in life, in part due to decreased intrauterine 5-HT levels. Other maldevelopmental events may occur which are too numerous to list here. The role of early life events has been followed prospectively since Jerome Kagan began to do so in the 1960s. The best recent work has been done by Michael J. Meaney and colleagues, and I have referred to it in previous writings. A recent paper (Francis DD, Meaney MJ, 1999) discussed the role of CRH and glucocorticoids, *brief* handling and subsequent increased maternal attention producing decreases in CRH gene expression, increases in $GABA_A$ neuronal mRNA, and reductions in ascending 5-HT and NE neurotransmission. "Arched back nursing," making the nipples and milk more accessible to the neonate, produces a less stress-sensitive adult, despite any other modifiers. This type of nursing is exhibited when a rat pup is returned to its mother after a 10- to 15-minute absence.

Some strains of rats are bred for certain physiologic or behavioral characteristics, e.g., hypertension and fear. When rat pups of these strains are cross-fostered with mothers from strains that are relatively "mellow" and lick them a lot, the adult rat's behavior is midway between that of its siblings, who were not cross-fostered, and the strain of rat to which its adopted mother belongs. Nature combines with nurture to produce an adult best suited, within the limits of its genetic code, to adapt to its environment.

Any female pup that has been handled arches its back when nursing as an adult. Meaney cites this observation as one example of the *intergenerational transmission of parental behavior,* a rather Lamarckian viewpoint which is becoming increasingly appreciated. Daughters of rhesus monkeys who were nurtured became nurturing mothers themselves. Rhesus mothers who rejected their infants had, in all cases studied, been rejected by their mothers as well, independent of social rank in the tribe. Mothers who are not nurturing are more fearful than their nurturing counterparts in every behavior thus far studied. The neurobiological correlate to this phenomenon is that most mammalian mothers show an aversion to their offspring because they are novel, and adult rats, in particular, are neophobic. Oxytocin usually prevents this aversion. Lesions that decrease fearful responses, e.g., those made in the amygdala, which secretes CRH, increase maternal responsivity even in nulliparous females. The maternal behavior of rats can be easily manipulated; CRH is anxiogenic and reduces nurturance, while OXT has anxiolytic and bonding effects and promotes parental care (Uvnas-Moberg K, 1997). Adult children of nonnurturing mothers show increased levels of CSF CRH, indicative of altered catecholamine responses to stress. If environmental conditions remained stable, these characteristics would be transferred to the offspring. Lest I appear to be a neo-Freudian mother-blaming dogmatist, let me assure the reader that to a great extent, I regard the mother as a transducer of events in the external world (e.g., predators or lack thereof, feast or famine) to the pup, whose initial world in the burrow consists of its mother's body. Her type of maternal care is also determined by life circumstances. Many researchers seem to think CRH levels are destiny. I have been arguing against this simplistic attitude for many years to little avail. Knock-out rats with no CRH at all have intact behavioral responses to stress, even though they do not increase their cortisol after footshock. For such an important response as stress, the CNS must possess multiple redundant mechanisms (Dunn AJ, Swiergiel AH, 1999).

An enormous amount of money has been spent on investigating the HPA axis in neurosomatic disorders. The lack of consensus over the last 20 years has been recently summarized (Heim C et al., 2000) in 35 pages of what charitably may be termed (my opinion only) a yawn-provoking procession of meaningless facts casting pseudolight on nonproblems. Added to the five experiments already done giving low-dose corticosteroids to CFS patients is another by Stephen Straus and colleagues who concluded it is not worth doing. Perhaps they can found a cottage industry and do one every two or three years, or as long as it takes the public to forget the last one.

Several of us in CFS private practice had given corticosteroids to hundreds of patients prior to 1990, but our opinions were not elicited. Virtually every experiment done by the NIH about CFS/FMS/IBS has been done numerous times previously by one or more of us, although not in a rigorously controlled setting. British researchers have more of a propensity for hypothalamic stimulation tests. Probes of D-fenfluramine, ACTH, insulin, and buspirone, are the ones I recall. Lest the NIH miss out on the fun, vasopressin was infused and ACTH was measured as an indirect reflection of CRH sensitivity (Altemus M et al., 2001). All tests suggested that central CRH was either low or that its receptors were down-regulated.

Some time ago, a misguided researcher determined that CFS patients were alexithymic, meaning, more or less, that they have little emotion and do not enjoy anything. The term "alexithymia" is obsolete, and the condition is thought by many to not exist. Several experiments followed. I see CFS patients by the thousands, and if I encounter one alexithymic every five years, it is a lot.

As I mentioned before, the FMS researchers and the IBS researcher(s)— including G. F. Gebhardt—have done much better work than the CFS researchers. There is a lot less featherbedding in FMS research now than there was in the early 1990s.

Somehow, an interesting experiment got through the CFS/HPA ideological thought police. Hypocortisolism was viewed as a phenomenon linked to normal early developmental stress allowed an optimal response. The author (Dienstbier RA, 1989) was one of the developers of the concept of "physiological toughness," akin to the "hardiness" concepts of Sal Maddi (Kobasa

SC et al., 1985). Dienstbier thinks early childhood stress experiences combined with successful coping with stress in adulthood

> induced a certain neuroendocrine pattern, which is characterized by decreased basal adrenal activity, increased autonomic and blunted HPA axis responses to stress, and a fast termination of these stress responses. Physiologically, this pattern is thought to allow increased stress tolerance as well as better performance and optimal maintenance of physical health during stress conditions. Dienstbier suggests that hypocortisolism reflects an adaptive state of stress tolerance in functional individuals. (Heim C et al., 2000, p. 18)

And so would I, if I thought the HPA axis was preeminently important in the stress response—but I do not. Only one of my long list of treatments directly affects the HPA axis—prednisone. I use it to treat allergies and autoimmune diseases. Rarely (every two to three years) it helps a patient with a neurosomatic disorder, since it alters the secretion of so many neurotransmitters, as I discussed in *Limbic Hypothesis*.

Stressed rats with hypercortisolism are much more likely to self-administer cocaine, which releases DA as well as increasing levels of ACTH and corticosterone. Cocaine-naive rats who are adrenalectomized completely lose the ability to acquire cocaine self-administration behaviors. Ketoconazole (Nizoral), which blocks cortisol biosynthesis, results in patterns of cocaine administration virtually indistinguishable from saline placebo given to cocaine-dependent rats during a withdrawal period. These findings suggest corticosteroids may be necessary for cocaine reinforcement (Goeders NE, 1997).

The locus of initiation of cocaine self-administration may be the mPFC. It is the only region in which direct cocaine injection is reinforcing. The initiation (but not maintenance) of cocaine self-administration may be the D_2 receptor, since the process can be attenuated or blocked by a D_2 antagonist, and increased DA activity in the mPFC decreases DA activity in the VTA. Cocaine also increases transmission between glutamatergic nerve terminals and DA neurons in the VTA of the rat brain (Ungless MA et al., 2001). It enhances the postsynaptic effect of glutamate on VTA DA neurons similarly to those associated with LTP in the hippocampus and elsewhere. Cocaine could also alter the activity of target regions of the VTA, such as the PFC and amygdala. These regions reciprocally glutamatergically innervate the VTA. The NAc modulates emotional value, or strength, of memories encoded in the hippocampus. Animals will self-stimulate the amygdala, hippocampus, and NAc (ventral striatum). The striatal neurons direct habit memories and control compulsive behavior. Learning, memory, reward expectation, and addiction may form a neural network (Nestler ER, 2001).

The role of the HPA/catecholamine axis in regulating the stress response is too complex for me to discuss in detail, particularly since experimental results vary. The subject has been extensively reviewed in a special issue of *Psychoneuroendocrinology*, Volume 26, 2001.

I am being drawn ineluctably to the conclusion that fatigue is, at least in part, related to NAc DA release, or the insufficiency thereof. PFC, even mPFC, hypoactivity is common in neurosomatic disorders. Mesocortical mPFC lesions lead to mesolimbic (VTA, ventral pallidum) hyperfunction. Mechanisms include increased DA in the mPFC which leads to decreased activity of mPFC pyramidal neurons, which send direct EAA projections to the NAc. These frequently terminate on tyrosine hydroxylase-positive spines. Thus, the cortico-accumbens pathway is involved in the interaction between mPFC glutamatergic afferents and DA production in the NAc, either directly or via projections to the VTA. If mPFC DA is insufficient, there will be a hyperglutamatergic input to presynaptic D_2 autoreceptors on meso-accumbens DA neurons, which is the apparent situation in neurosomatic disorders. Glutamate projections may go from the mPFC to the TH-immunoreactive elements of the VTA. In this case, a hyperglutamatergic PFC would cause the VTA to be hyperdopaminergic. Thus, the PFC can increase or decrease mesoaccumbens DA depending on where it enhances glutamatergic input.

It appears, however, that mPFC neurons terminate primarily on GABA-ergic neurons within the VTA (Harden DG et al., 1998), which may inhibit VTA DA release. Furthermore, projections from the NAc to the VTA are largely inhibitory, and the NAc is stimulated by the medial PFC. Despite decreased VTA activity, the NAc can still increase its DA output in stressful situations because in its basal state there is a decreased sensitivity of the D_2 release-modifying autoreceptors. If stress is chronic, however, the autoreceptors will hypersensitize to the point that DA release could be markedly reduced. This scenario could depict an aspect of the neurosomatic neural network. Neither William of Ockham's razor nor Sir William Osler's rule would be worth wielding if fatigue could be simply explained by local deficiencies of NE and DA inhibition of the hyperactive neurosomatic NMDA synapse.

Chronic stress in rats produces a decreased reactivity to noxious stimuli. The behavioral deficit is accompanied by a decreased level of DA in the NAc shell (Gambarana C et al., 1999). The core is medial to the shell. The two regions have separate afferent and efferent neurons. The cytoarchitecture of the core is like that of the caudate nucleus. The shell is considered part of the extended amygdala since it has the highest expression of D_3 receptors in the brain. The dopaminergic deficits I have described thus far can usually be normalized by antidepressants, which is not the case in neurosomatic illness. I shall try to explain why this disorderly state of affairs exists, a challenging task since the mode of action of antidepressants is not well understood. Increasing DA in mesocorticolimbic tracts, blocking the NMDA receptor, and stimulating the immediate early gene CREB are the current leading contenders for antidepressant pharmacology.

Much of the pathophysiology of neurosomatic disorders involves the acquisition of conditioned fear at some time in the past, which is often out of awareness at the time of illness onset. Conditioned fear acquired before age four could not be retrieved in any event, because declarative memory accessible to retrieval does not exist before that age.

The mPFC DA neurons are sensitive to classical fear conditioning. When they are dysfunctional in rats and mPFC DA is significantly decreased, conditioned fear still increases NAc DA. NAc DA is important in behavior in several situations: (1) appetitive behavior arousal, (2) as a facilitator and inducer of neural processes, and (3) responses to aversive contexts. I have suggested that NAc DA increases in preparation for defense and then decreases if the animal cannot cope with the aversive stimulus. A broader viewpoint is expressed by Ikemoto and Panksepp (1999). They believe DA plays an important role in sensorimotor integration that facilitates flexible approach responses, not habits.

NAc DA is released when the organism is presented with a *salient* stimulus, both novel and incentive. In response to a US, NAc DA is released and enables stimulus representations to acquire incentive properties. Within a specific environmental context, NAc DA is not essential for cognitive perception of environmental stimuli. Another way to view increased NAc DA is in response to an aversive stimulus. An avoidance response, i.e., a movement toward "safety" is reinforcing, as it often is again when the animal encounters similar environmental contexts. In a rat with a mPFC dopamine deficit, *extinction* of the fear is markedly delayed. Rats do not live very long. Conditioned fears could last a human lifetime, and the original unconditioned stimulus could have been forgotten. Even the original conditioned stimulus might not be retrievable.

Delving further into DA, stimulants, and considering sensitization, we start once again at the VTA but then quickly branch out into the *motive circuit* (Figure 42). Behavioral sensitization to stimulants occurs in the rat VTA and begins at least several days after the last intermittent dose of stimulant. Chronic stimulant administration would lead to tolerance. The interconnected nuclei of the motive circuit work together to facilitate or prevent the expression of behavioral responses to environmental or pharmacologic stimuli. The motive circuit is viewed as a *gain-control* mechanism that determines both the threshold and response to a given behavioral stimulus. Sensitization increases the gain of the motive circuit to a given stimulus so that a greater response will be emitted. Neurosomatic patients may be said to have *behavioral desensitization* in this paradigm (Pierce RC, Kalivas PW, 1997) (Figure 43).

Altering transmission through the dopamine transporter is one of the primary actions of all psychostimulants. We have seen that much dopamine diffuses into surrounding areas, but it has its primary action at the axon terminal from which it was secreted. After 14 days of abstinence, behavioral sensitization occurs in almost every rat. Ca^{2+}-dependent protein kinases are critically involved in activity-dependent synaptic modifications. One of these changes is that the psychostimulant augmentation of DA release is blocked by systemic administration of L-type Ca^{2+} channel antagonists. Amphetamine-induced DA release is usually independent of L-type Ca^{2+} channels. The amphetamine-induced behavioral sensitization involves CaMKII phosphorylation of synapsin I (a protein that anchors synaptic vesicles to the cytoskeleton) which releases the "docking" vesicles for a Ca^{2+} signal and binding to synaptotagmin, which then triggers fusion and exocytosis.

In the NAc, however, vesicular exocytosis may not be a primary mode of transmitter release. Botulinum toxin, which blocks exocytotic release, has little effect on NAc DA secretion. The mere fact that CaMKII can undock a vesicle and amphetamine can widen the DAT pore may allow the vesicles to diffuse out of the axon terminal. CaMKII can also phosphorylate the DAT and increase the velocity of transport of undocked synaptic vesicles. Dopamine reuptake through the DAT is so enhanced by amphetamine that during early withdrawal some investigators are unable to measure extracellular DA after a simple psychostimulant challenge in this period. Changes in nigrostriatal excitability may persist for the life of the animal.

Amphetamine-induced behavioral sensitization has other consequences and may include decreased stimulation of NAc DA by glutamate and enduring sensitization of D_1 agonists. Pretreatment of the sensitized rat NAc with a D_1 antagonist prevents the stimulatory effects of amphetamine.

After one week, when behavioral sensitization should be well established, there are no increases in D_1 or D_3 number, but stimulation from amphetamine still occurs because of enhanced sensitivity of adenyl cyclase and PKA, which are G-protein coupled. During behavioral sensitization, the G_i inhibitory tone on AC decreases. There is a persistent elevation in Fos-related antigens which might be more meaningful and of longer duration than the elevations in CREB. Behavioral sensitization is less common in people than in animals and does not always occur in animals. A human version of behavioral sensitization may be paranoia and psychosis. Those in whom chronic intermittent use of stimulants had this effect would obviously not be prone to addiction. Neurosomatic patients are also not addiction prone, in the same way that chronic pain patients are not. I only deal with drug abuse in my practice two or three times a year, although I define drug abuse as craving higher doses and using amounts of medication that could cause acute harm to the patient. Some chronic-pain patients, although compliant, believe they require frequent dose escalation. It is these individuals in whom I am most apt to use augmentation or adjunctive strategies. Every two years or so, I must terminate my services to one of these individuals for noncompliance and related psychosocial issues, especially if he or she is not able or unwilling to obtain counseling.

Behavioral sensitization also encompasses the ability of stimulated NAc cells to secrete precursor peptides such as preprodynorphin and related substances. The increase in dynorphin by psychostimulants is D_1 mediated. In a direct feedback mechanism, however, "increased dynorphin transmission appears to inhibit, rather than support, the expression of behavioral sensitization" (Piece RC, Kalivas PW, 1997), perhaps by decreasing the release of DA. Dynorphin in this model, instead of being allostatic, may play a homeostatic role to inhibit behavioral sensitization.

There is considerable EAA input to the NAc from several cortical and allocortical areas, as well as from the periventricular thalamus. DA and EAA interact to determine information transfer from NAc to the VP and VTA/SN. DA and EAAs from the hippocampus and amygdala form synaptic contacts on the same NAc spiny neurons (Figure 44). As it does elsewhere, DA modulates EAA input to accumbal neurons. The NAc can thus be viewed as a node for information transfer from widely separated areas of a neural network. Projections from the DLPFC and mPFC (cortical projections are glutamatergic) to the NAc can be stimulated by cocaine to secrete more glutamate. This response can be blocked by tetrodotoxin, a Na^+-channel blocker with some of the same actions as lidocaine. Lesions in the PFC in amphetamine-treated rats do not impair the increase in glutamate. The reasons for the discrepancy involve transporter functions not relevant to this general discussion. The glutamate release from the PFC does not increase DA.

Amphetamines bind to 5-HT transporters, increasing 5-HT by blocking reuptake. Cocaine decreases 5-HT by 5-HT_{1A} agonism which reduces the firing of the dorsal raphe neurons. The sum of these effects is usually augmented 5-HT neurotransmission in the NAc, but the role of the enhancement is not yet clear. GABA and EAA afferents intermingle in the VTA and are both modulated by D_1 presynaptic heteroreceptors providing feedback regulation. D_1 receptors stimulate AC, producing cAMP, which dissociates into adenosine, thereby decreasing GABA transmission by binding to A_1 receptors on GABAergic terminals in the VTA. Repeated cocaine injections decrease PFC DA while amphetamine injections do not. Decreased PFC DA means PFC EAA projections to the NAC and VTA are enhanced and DA-dependent locomotor activity is increased. In amphetamine-treated rats, stress still has the same or an increased ability to increase PFC DA. An important principle is that *PFC DA is inversely related to VTA DA*. PFC DA directly inhibits EAA (usually glutamate) projections to the VTA, which actually manufactures some of the DA that travels in the mesocorticolimbic tract. This circuit is a direct example of how the PFC is the only brain area to regulate its own neurotransmitter input.

A corollary to this principle, important to neuropharmacology, is that antagonizing PFC DA receptors increases DA transmission in the NAc and the behavioral response to psychostimulants. These responses occur because EAA transmission from corticofugal neurons is disinhibited. Lest the reader think prematurely that this process is only mildly complex, I must mention that neurotrophins are involved, as well as most of the signal transduction pathways. Drugs which are possibly addicting induce TH, cause morphologic changes in VTA neurons, and up-regulate the cAMP pathway in the NAc. Administration of BDNF or related neurotrophins attenuates these changes, and it is thought that potentially addicting medications work in part by inhibiting the action of certain neurotrophins. This property may be relevant to the treatment of fibromyalgia. I recommend to the reader the work of Eric J. Nestler at University of Texas Southwestern Medical Center, whose work I have been following for the past decade. Originally working with Nobel Laureate Paul Greengard, he is one of the editors of *Neurobiology of Mental Illness*. His chapters on basic neurobiology and cellular mechanisms are outstanding, and I always try to make time to read any article that has his name on it. One of the points he makes is that all drugs of possible abuse increase levels of CREB. So do antidepressants. Heretical articles have begun to appear that perhaps opioids could be used as antidepressants. I wrote one myself in the mid-1980s about methadone. CREB, via a series of intermediates, produces Fos-related antigens which persist for several weeks after the drug is withdrawn. The reasons for the increase in synaptic dopamine after chronic administration of amphetamine but not cocaine is unclear but may involve increased inhibition of 5-HT on various potentially releasable pools of DA in the VTA neurons. I shall venture no farther into this labyrinth here except as it may apply to my nascent neurosomatic hypothesis: the excitatory glutamatergic projection from the PFC to the NAc is increased. The NAc sends GABA, dynorphin, NPY, and TRH projections to the VTA, which decrease its function. The PFC sends direct, potent glutamatergic projections to the VTA which are excitatory, but perhaps only at GABAergic interneurons.

What is the VTA to do? It does what is does best: projects DAergic neurons to the NAc, ventral pallidum, *and back to the PFC*. The NAc and the

VP inhibit each other, and the VP projects GABA to the beleaguered VTA and to the thalamus which has an excitatory dialogue with the PFC. Thus, the result of the hyperglutamatergic state of the PFC in this simplified motive circuit is, in general, to decrease VTA DA secretion, especially in the mesocortical tract. This dysfunction could produce fatigue, or "decreased locomotor activity," as well as deficits in short-term memory, working memory, and other cognitive operations. A DA deficit could inhibit, via GABA, the corticothalamic glutamatergic excitation causing the reticular nucleus of the thalamus to misfire in its role of coordinating interactions between the thalamic nuclei and their resultant projections, not the least of which is the now unpredictable RTN transmission back to the cortex. Hence, bizarre sensory information is filtered through the extended amygdala and PFC. Ultimately, the tone of numerous structures are preset by inappropriate cognitive classical conditioning of which the individual is unaware or "mis-aware" (see the section on false memory). Whole-body pain has been produced by lesions or stimulation of very wide dynamic range neurons in a circuit from the amygdala through the GPe (globus pallidus externa) to certain areas of the thalamus and cortex. Dysfunction of this circuit could cause fibromyalgia. The network can include the ACC, the thalamus, and the insula. Voila! IBS. It can primarily affect DA, NE, and GABA, as well as descending dysregulation of ascending Ach, NE, 5-HT, and DA arousal centers causing CFS and primary disorder of vigilance, which I actually do treat now and then. Doctors can try theophylline (and forskolin) on their next case to augment stimulants.

Neuropsychopharmacology is like psychoanalysis in the respect that it can explain *almost anything*. It is unlike psychoanalysis in that the explanation may be somewhat correct and can sometimes be scientifically tested. As a bonus, a neurosomatic doctor can help patients get better in an average of three days or so, in the office, testing very safe, very rapidly acting medications that are directed at their individual neurochemical dysfunction(s).

If neurosomatic disorders primarily consist of dysfunction of catecholamines, GABA receptors, and NMDA receptors in a hyperglutamatergic state causing a catecholaminergic deficit, how might the situation be remedied? There are hundreds of possible treatments, but they all cause vasoconstriction. I demonstrated this phenomenon with pre- and posttreatment brain SPECT in *Betrayal*. It has been shown to occur after successful ECT and antidepressant therapy (Nobler MS et al., 2001). My hypothesis then was the same as now: Baseline vasoconstriction is caused by endothelin, which releases PKC. Further vasoconstriction after exercise or other relapse-inducing activities is caused from more endothelin secretion. Successful pharmacotherapy, of whatever type, also causes vasoconstriction, probably via DA and NE. In all cases, the blood-vessel diameter is an epiphenomenon of the neurotransmitters that produce increased or decreased symptoms by effects on neuronal networks. I am not persuaded rCBF is always directly correlated to local metabolism.

In 1995, I thought the cerebral vasculature was noradrenergically innervated from the superior cervical ganglion. A more recent experiment shows there is extensive, perhaps predominant, dopaminergic regulation of cerebral cortical microcirculation even to the level of the capillaries (Krimer LS et al., 1998). NE innervates the network of *extraparenchymal* blood vessels. Cortical blood vessels are also innervated by 5-HT, Ach, several peptides, and other substances, as I discussed in *Betrayal,* but NE and DA are the only rational candidates for vasoconstrictive improvement of neurosomatic symptoms.

Ach is a vasodilator at muscarinic receptors and a vasoconstrictor at nicotinic receptors. Muscarinic agonists, however, can cause vasoconstriction by activation of muscarinic receptors in the VTA, which release DA and 5-HT but not NE (Gronier B et al., 2000). Muscarinic agents may have a more generalized activating effect by stimulating the pedunculopontine nucleus, an element of the ascending arousal system. The pedunculopontine nucleus also sends direct glutamatergic projections to the VTA. The subthalamic nucleus does so as well (Westerink BHC et al., 1997).

Other projections to the VTA come from the hippocampus. This structure is important in the learning of associations between environmental context and a US, such as cocaine. Stimulation of the ventral subiculum (VSUB) of the hippocampus induces long-lasting DA release in the NAc and enhances the firing of mesolimbic neurons that originate in the VTA (Vorel SR et al., 2001). NAc DA increase is blocked by intra-VTA kynurenate, a glycine/NMDA antagonist, which also inhibits reinstatement of cocaine craving in a manner similar to ketamine. Thus, projections from the hippocampus to the VTA reinstate cocaine seeking in rats by stimulating VTA glutamate activity, probably via the NMDA receptor. A control group receiving cerebellar stimulation did not evince reinstatement. The medial forebrain bundle (MFB) supports self-stimulation, which is dependent on NAc DA release. MFB stimulation did not elicit reinstatement, either. The VSUB stimulation may reflect the contextual association between the operant chamber and the previously available cocaine, since VTA DA release is predictive of reward. The MFB is much more successful at supporting self-stimulation in and of itself than is the hippocampus. MFB stimulation markedly increases VTA DA for less than five seconds, while VSUB stimulation increases it for 30 minutes. This experiment is one of the several reasons why NMDA antagonists are being used for cocaine addiction. The muscarinic agonists I administer in my office are usually cholinesterase inhibitors. They often help patients who respond to NMDA agonism or have their symptoms worsened by

NMDA antagonists. Muscarinic agonists may also stimulate a hyperactive pedunculopontine nucleus, and sometimes inhibit nicotinic agonists. The nAchRs can have a stimulatory or anxiogenic action, and ligands are increasingly being developed as analgesics which synergize with many other antinociceptive compounds such as clonidine. nAch agonists can release GABA, NE, DA, and 5-HT.

The first plausible explanation about the mode of action of amphetamine in ADHD is that inhibition of DA firing and activation of negative feedback mechanisms increases DA release by stimulating NE release. Alpha$_1$ heteroceptors on DA neurons stimulate DA release (Zametkin AJ, Liutta W, 1998). D$_1$ and D$_2$ antagonists do not affect amphetamine-induced stimulation, nor do alpha$_2$ antagonists or beta blockers (Shi WX et al., 2000). Alpha$_1$ antagonists block amphetamine-induced burst responses and diminish increase in firing rate. I should be able to administer the alpha$_1$ agonist midodrine to a patient and see the same response as I do with dextroamphetamine. My patients who have obtained the NE-reuptake inhibitor reboxetine should also have a similar effect, but they do not. The other effects of amphetamine I have discussed must play a role.

Reboxetine should be a useful agent in neurosomatic medicine when and if the FDA approves it. The drug is available in most countries. It increases burst firing in VTA DA neurons and in the mPFC but does not alter NAc DA. These localized effects suggest it may be particularly beneficial for drive and motivation (Linner L et al., 2001). Many neurosomatic patients (I hear) have no response to reboxetine or a worsening of symptoms. Some respond to it immediately and proclaim it to be the most effective medication they have tried. Neurosomatic patients with comorbid treatment-refractory depression occasionally respond to it as well. It may become part of my current "dopaminergic cocktail."

Reboxetine has some unique characteristics, the most notable of which is that it decreases binding of cAMP to the type II PKA regulatory subunit (Mori S et al., 2001). It also increases Ca^{2+}/calmodulin-dependent phosphorylation of presynaptic substrates. By day 14, it increases extracellular NE by 599 percent (Invernizzi RW et al., 2001). Reboxetine increases DA to a slightly lesser extent and has no greater effect on reducing cortical NE after 14 days than after two days. This finding has been attributed to desensitization of alpha$_2$ receptors with chronic treatment. Therefore, addition of an alpha$_2$ antagonist such as yohimbine for augmentation would be counterproductive, particularly since the alpha$_{2A}$ agonist guanfacine has been reported to induce mania in children taking it for ADHD. It also enhances working memory in monkeys by an action on the DLPFC (Avery RA et al., 2000).

Another way to pharmacologically enhance catecholamine levels is administering tolcapone (Tasmar). When tolcapone was released, I thought it would significantly enhance neurosomatic treatment. The report of hepatic failure in several elderly patients with Parkinson's disease taking tolcapone has put a damper on my willingness to prescribe tolcapone for an extended period of time. The FDA requires very frequent monitoring of liver function tests in tolcapone-treated patients. I typically use it only in single trials now, continuing it with informed consent if a very beneficial response ("magic bullet") is obtained. I would prefer to give tolcapone a six-week trial before assessing its efficacy but will not do so except in very special circumstances, e.g., a patient who has failed on over 150 treatments including ECT and is still suicidal. Perhaps I am being too cautious, but my practice is high risk (to me), although highly beneficial to my patients. If another centrally-acting catechol-orthomethyltransferase inhibitor is approved, I will use it much more freely. Perhaps I should use entacapone (Comtan), since there is some evidence that the COMT inhibition caused by tolcapone occurs in extracerebral tissue (Mercuri NB et al., 1999), as well as intracerebrally (Russ H et al., 1999). Tolcapone is very useful as adjunctive therapy for Parkinson's disease with levodopa/carbidopa but is not too effective at raising DA levels (it should rase NE levels also) when used as monotherapy. Because my goal is usually to increase NE as well, I use tolcapone in my current dopaminergic cocktail. One open experiment showed tolcapone to be effective in treating major depressive disorder, but 39 percent of the patients dropped out of the eight-week study (a fairly high rate) because of diarrhea, elevated liver function tests, increased anxiety, and noncompliance (Dingemanse J, 2000).

An agent I have been trying recently is forskolin. Many physicians may not be familiar with it. Forskolin has no adverse reactions in the recommended dose (10 to 20 mg per day), and its major known action is to stimulate adenyl cyclase. It also stimulates hypothalamic tyrosine hydroxylase, an effect attenuated by estradiol (Arbogast LA, Hyde JF, 2000). AC-cAMP-PKA form an intracellular signalling cascade which participates in most phosphorylation pathways, either directly or via cross talk. I typically use forskolin to augment drugs with stimulant properties, including adenosine blockers and PDE inhibitors. It enhances hippocampal LTP and impedes PFC LTP. Because there is usually overlearned information in most neurosomatic patients, agents that inhibit hippocampal LTP often make patients feel better in general and enhance their short-term memory in particular because working memory is full and selective attention is, therefore, impaired. The usual neurosomatic patient has symptoms of dysautonomia with or without anxiety or panic disorder. These patients generally have adverse reactions to stimulants and receive symptom relief from agents that decrease neural transmission. This rule is not absolute, of course, but stimulants are more likely to benefit those with decreased arousal than those who are hypervigilant. Most stimulants increase AC activity, which is blunted in those with MDD, a common comorbid disorder in neurosomatic patients. Antidepressants are often unsuccessful. They may reduce depression, perhaps through increasing neurotrophins such as BDNF and its receptor, TrkB, which may participate in increasing the activity of forskolin-stimulated $cAMP_G$ (Morbobos S et al., 1999) which then can increase CREB and FRAs. More germane to neurosomatic disorders is the finding that there are increases in alpha$_2$ receptor levels in antidepressant-free MDD suicide patients (Garcia-Sevilla JA et al., 1999). An alpha$_2$ receptor agonist, particularly alpha$_{2A}$ (guanfacine), can bind to postsynaptic alpha$_2$ receptors and act as an antidepressant while reducing (primarily) inappropriately elevated NE release by its presynaptic action. MDD patients, as well as those with neurosomatic disorders, probably have an abnormality in regional synaptic organization in the PFC. Indeed, that is one of the hypotheses of this book.

Although I have not observed any symptom exacerbation thus far, I use caution when administering forskolin to a patient with chronic pain. Forskolin sensitizes sensory neurons, creating hyperalgesia, which is mediated in part by the cAMP signal transduction cascade. Forskolin-induced hyperalgesia is prolonged by PDE inhibitors and attenuated by PKA antagonists. After forskolin, bradykinin-elicited action potentials increase, as does the release of SP and CGRP. Tolerance does not develop to the facilitation of evoked peptide release, but after forskolin is stopped, no matter how long it has been administered, "cells rapidly returned to their control state suggesting that chronic activation of the cAMP pathway does not result in maintained sensitization" (Bolyard LA et al., 2000). This response is quite unusual in a system characterized by plasticity and is more like an on-off switch. One patient of mine has had exacerbation of migraine headache from forskolin, which I might expect, given the increase in SP and CGRP and possible neurogenic inflammation when secreted by the first division of the trigeminal nerve. For most patients, forskolin augments the effect of stimulants. If it will be effective, the first dose will relieve symptoms. For a rare patient, forskolin is the magic bullet. A 43-year-old, single, white female attorney had graduated at the top of her class and was doing appellate work when she developed CFS. She became easily exhausted and was too cognitively impaired to work as a paralegal at a personal injury law firm. Adderall gave her enough energy to perform activities of daily living, but it was difficult for her to go to the supermarket. I had been treating her for seven years and she had tried over 100 medications. She settled with her disability insurer after the usual drawn-out, acrimonious harangue.

She came in for a routine office visit. I offered her 10 mg of forskolin, which, as do many of my long-term patients, she took without asking for, or wanting, any explanation of its mode of action. Most of them trust me, and some realize that they are too impaired to understand my simplified neuropharmacology. In 30 minutes, she burst out crying. When I asked her what was wrong, she said, "Nothing. Nothing! This is the first time I've felt normal in twelve years!" As in the cAMP sensitization experiment, the forskolin has continued to render her asymptomatic for the past year. Cases like hers are why I never stop trying new treatments, never give up on someone, and continue my lonely pursuit of learning about neurosomatic medicine.

In occasional patients, stimulants are barely effective and NMDA receptor antagonists worsen symptoms. After I try cholinesterase inhibitors, nasal dopamine, glutamate, TRH, oxytocin, aminophylline, hydergine, oral DA agonists (I favor pramipexole for its D_2/D_3 activity and pergolide for D_1/D_2), amantadine, isoxsuprine, nylidrin, opioids, propranolol, buspirone, yohimbine, midodrine (which should work as well as Dexedrine but does not), nicotine, pindolol, bupropion, venlafaxine, ranitidine, cycloserine, piracetam, NMDA/glycine antagonists (ondansetron, felbamate, diltiazem, probenecid, guaifenesin, verapamil, atropine), NADH, inositol, SAMe (methyl group donor for polyamine biosynthesis—good when nylidrin exacerbates symptoms), furosemide, flumazenil, sibutramine (which has just worked for my first patient), pentazocine, tramadol, Kutapressin and various other parenteral agents, naltrexone, tranylcypromine (Parnate)—which apparently is not metabolized into amphetamine in the brain, tolcapone, and all those I forgot to mention, I get to *honey bee venom*.

This agent has limited utility. The injection is painful, similar to a bee sting. Tolerance may develop to its effects, or it may seem to reverse its mode of action and exacerbate symptoms. It is somewhat expensive. The duration of action is highly variable, from a few hours to a few months. There is no apparent upper limit to the dosage, so if there is no response, I never know whether the amount injected was high enough. And, worst of all, patients can become allergic to bee venom even if they have a negative skin test and tolerate doses of 300 units (six bee stings) in the office. For some patients, generally those who fit the PDV spectrum (but not always—since bee venom has many active ingredients), it is the magic bullet. If they become allergic to it, they are quite distressed. In general, the actions of honey bee venom are just the opposite of what most neurosomatic patients need.

I tend to view honey bee venom as injectable arachidonic acid or as phospholipase A_2 in a bottle. As such, it can be metabolized into various eicosanoids or cannabinoids and can act as the most potent NMDA agonist I can give, although sometimes it acts as an NMDA antagonist. Some effects of PLA_2 are mimicked by endothelin (Rogalski SL et al., 1999).

Cytosolic PLA_2 ($cPLA_2$) is expressed in neurons and glial cells. It hydrolyzes the arachidonyl group from the SN-2 position of glycerophospholipids, generating arachidonic acid and lysophospholipids. These products are further metabolized into eicosanoids, platelet-activating factor (PAF), a retrograde messenger inhibited by doxepin, and lysphophosphatidic acid. The only areas of the forebrain that densely stain for $cPLA_2$ are the arcuate and mammilary nuclei. There is dense staining in various midbrain nuclei, as well as the dorsal horn.

$cPLA_2$ is stimulated by DA, NE, 5-HT, ATP, and glutamate and is synthesized routinely during receptor activation. Glutamate up-regulation of $cPLA_2$ is blocked by kynurenic acid. The Ca^{2+} influx that occurs after NMDA channels open translocates and activates $cPLA_2$. AA is one of the several identified diffusible retrograde ("atypical") messengers. DAG has also been shown to produce AA release. $cPLA_2$ is stimulated by various growth factors, cytokines, and interferons and increases glucose utilization by astrocytes. It diffuses presynaptically to activate PKC and participates in LTP.

AA has many intracellular functions. It modulates ion channels, PKA, PKC, nicotinamide adenine dinucleotide phosphate reduced form (NADPH) oxidase, and Na^+-K^+ ATPase. AA also inhibits glutamate uptake at the transporter level. Not only AA but all the eicosanoids are amphiphilic and can act as diffusible retrograde messengers. Eicosanoids may regulate the activity of IEGs expressed after NMDA receptor activation. High concentrations of AA, as seen in ischemia, can uncouple mitochondrial oxidative phosphorylation.

Lysphospholipids are precursors for PAF and affect a wide number of enzymes, increasing cellular adhesion molecules (CAMs), heparin-binding edothelial-derived growth factor (EDGF), platelet-derived growth factor (PDGFs), COX-2, NOS, NGF, and activator protein-1 (AP-1) (to name a few). They inhibit acyl-CoA, GC, and AC.

As with most biochemical substances, honey bee venom can be helpful or harmful in a certain patient, at a certain dose, and at a certain time. At present, I am unable to duplicate its action with a clinically available medication (I would only want to produce one effect at a time, anyway). High doses of inositol, to increase $[Ca^{2+}]_i$ would be the best alternative at present. Several compounds, such as resiniferatoxin, are in the works as fairly specific PKC activators.

Honey bee venom apparently acts on the vanilloid receptor (VR1) as well as the vanilloid-like receptor (VRL-2) as do capsaicin and anandamide. It activates many nociceptive receptors: NMDA, non-NMDA glutamate, ATP/P2X-purinoceptors, NK1/2 receptors, and it stimulates intracellular PKC, probably via its agonism at glutamate receptors. As with most venoms, it also has an anticoagulant effect and may also be a nicotinic agonist, as are some paralyzing wasp venoms. Other components of bee venom are serotonin (which is hyperalgesic), histamine, acetylcholine, and several kinins. There are also polypeptide toxins, such as melittin which damages cell membranes, mast cell degranulating protein, and apamin (a neurotoxin). Tertiapin blocks muscarinic K^+ channels. Enzymes include hyaluronidase, which helps the venom spread, and phospholipase A_2, which is the major allergen. Many of these substances are arousal inducing, and most cause central sensitization. If they widen receptive fields, the PDV patient may benefit, since his or her ascending arousal system is hyporesponsive in the basal state to exteroceptive or enteroceptive stimuli. PDV patients present very much like those with sleep apnea, although they do not have headaches upon arising. I am next going to discuss some miscellaneous treatments that are difficult to fit into any category.

Thioperamide, were it available, would be a novel agent. It is an H_3-receptor antagonist and increases neural transmission in histaminergic neurons. It inhibits forskolin-stimulated cAMP formation in response to the activating neurotransmitter histamine. Both thioperamide and cimetidine increase cortical Ach release (Cecchi M et al., 2001). This action is probably related to their purported memory-enhancing properties. The H_3 receptor is found only in the brain, where its primary function is as an autoreceptor. It increases the release and metabolism of neuronal histamine (Yates SL et al., 1999). Thioperamide increases DA synthesis in rat striatum by acting at H_3 receptors located on dopaminergic nerve terminals (Molina-Hernandez A et al., 2000). Most experimental work with thioperamide has been done with rodents. Usually the neuropharmacology of rats and primates is fairly similar. When thioperamide is administered to a monkey, however, it is much less potent than in a rat. Other H_3 antagonists have been more effective (West RE et al., 1999). H_3 antagonists might be a new type of stimulant, but the possibility remains that they might degranulate brain mast cells. I have written about these cells when discussing the neurobiology of fibromyalgia, but they also have the potential to cause migraine headaches. Thioperamide augments the release of 5-HT and histamine from brain mast cells (Rosniecki JJ et al., 1999). This action could be a sticking point for human trials. On the other hand, H_3 agonists could be antimigraine agents and might be useful in other neurosomatic disorders.

Pentazocine (Talwin) has been available for over 30 years and is more underused now than ever. I have written about it in previous books and will update my views on it here. First, a brief review: pentazocine is a $sigma_1$-receptor agonist. There are two sigma receptors. $Sigma_1$ receptors are expressed diffusely in the brain, and $sigma_1$ agonists attenuate the effect of NMDA-receptor antagonists. Pentazocine was thought to be an opioid for many years. That is why one of its formulations is with low-dose naloxone, to hopefully prevent abuse. I can remember the first patient I prescribed pentazocine for—he developed cartoon-like visual hallucinations. Fortunately, this adverse reaction is rare, and sigma$_1$ agonists are being developed as antipsychotics.

Haloperidol down-regulates sigma receptors and antagonzes pentazocine, even in the form of a nasal spray. Sigma receptors have been linked to cognition, neuroprotection, and locomotion in the central nervous system. Pentazocine inhibits potassium-stimulated [^{3}H] dopamine release and may activate guanylate cyclase, a stage in the nitric oxide/GMP pathway (Mamiya T et al., 2000). Usually, guanylate cyclase is changed from the inactive to the active configuration by nitric oxide. Sigma$_1$ agonists may be a treatment for the rare patient who has no response to any dose of nitroglycerin but vasodilates after hydralazine, a direct cGMP agonist.

Sigma$_2$ ligands may be potent anxiolytics without causing sedation or withdrawal anxiogenesis (Sanchez C et al., 1997). The sigma receptor modulates voltage-gated K$^+$ channels. No other K$^+$-channel modulator resembles the sigma receptor, and its mode of action appears to be a direct physical action on the K$^+$ channel, to which it is in very close proximity. Sigma receptors are located in peptidergic hypothalamic neurons, and their activation results in a very rapid release of peptide transmitter.

Sigma agonists initially increase and then decrease K$^+$-stimulated DA release in the striatum. NPY, a "proposed endogenous sigma receptor ligand," increases striatal DA release. NMDA antagonists attenuate the DA increase but not the DA decrease produced in the striatum by pentazocine (Gudelsky GA, 1999). Thus, NMDA agonists would possibly enhance the initial increase of extracellular DA caused by pentazocine. This suggestion is in accord with my clinical observations that pentazocine and ketamine antagonize each other.

Pentazocine and DHEA, another sigma agonist, potentiate the neuronal response to NMDA. Haloperidol and progesterone do the opposite and could be considered functional sigma antagonists. It is thought that the marked elevation of progesterone during pregnancy is responsible for reduction of brain sigma-receptor function and that perhaps some postpartum psychiatric disorders could be a result of removal of sigma-receptor antagonism by progesterone (Bergeron R et al., 1999). Despite its facilitation by NMDA, pentazocine still has neuroprotective effects. It also synergizes with DHEA and pregnenolone to ameliorate conditioned fear stress (Noda Y et al., 2000), and is an Ach agonist.

Pentazocine is often effective when lidocaine and lamotrigine are and sometimes when gabapentin is. It is given every four hours, can decrease any and all symptoms, and sometimes two tablets are required per dose. The drug is unique among available agents and, again, is a "magic bullet" for certain patients. Abuse of pentazocine has never been a problem in 20 years of neurosomatic practice. Of course, many physicians are still afraid to prescribe it. I would try it in most situations when an NMDA agonist seems indicated. It often has analgesic effects.

Omega-3 and omega-6 fatty acids were popularized over 20 years ago. They should inhibit PKC and function as NMDA antagonists, but they can also generate phosphatidylserine and be PKC agonists. They may promote release of neurotrophins, may help CFS, may be antidepressants, and may help bipolar disorder. They have done none of these things in my practice after fairly extensive trials following the work of David Horrobin 20 years ago or more. The party line is still that patients must use the right brand for enough of these essential fatty acids to be absorbed. I am not trying any more brands until some hard data comes through.

Another agent that should work but has not is the amino acid taurine, which works something like GABA and acamprosate. Lamotrigine increases rat hippocampal GABA shunt activity and elevates cerebral taurine levels (Hassel B et al., 2001). Taurine has no adverse reactions I know of and activates $GABA_A$ receptors in the rat CA1 hippocampal area (del Olmo S et al., 2000). I have begun to add taurine for patients on chronic lamotrigine therapy. It is too soon for me to know whether it will help. Acamprosate reduces NMDA-stimulated Ca^{2+} influx and motor cortex excitability from transcranial magnetic stimulation (TMS). TMS of frontal brain regions selectively modulates the release of biogenic amines, vasopressin, and amino acids in rat brain (Keck ME et al., 2000).

I have written most of what I know about TRH in previous chapters and books. It is again the "magic bullet" for some patients. Those who are fortunate have a duration of action of two to three months from 500 mcg IV over ten minutes. Most patients become nauseated during the initial stages, and all have urinary urgency. These feelings usually pass after 250 mcg have been injected. TRH is a BZD antagonist. I never use it in patients with panic disorder and use it in those with GAD only after those symptoms have been managed. It has an antidepressant effect on some patients, to which tolerance may develop. It is often stimulating, relaxing, analgesic, and cognition enhancing. ADRs can be managed acutely with BZDs, and if the benefits are great, BZD premedication is an option. William Philpott suggested a single dose regimen of subcutaneous TRH for CFS. In most patients this dose is too low, but occasional patients do respond to subcutaneous TRH which they can administer at home. It is very expensive.

About one-third of hypothalamic TRH goes into the brain rather than the pituitary gland. TRH receptors are expressed diffusely. In rats given ICV TRH, Fos-like immunoreactivity was observed in the inner layers of the medial PFC, the midline thalamus, the NTS, and the adjacent reticular formation. Fos-like immunoreactivity was reduced in most areas of the cerebral cortex, the NAc shell (part of the extended amygdala), the medial amygdalar nucleus, parts of the hypothalamus, and the PAG (Otake K, Nakamura Y, 2000). When TRH is effective, it is usually stimulating. mPFC DA is inversely related to NAc DA. The midline reuniens nucleus of the thalamus is also activated. This nucleus is alerting, regulates autonomic function, and projects to the mPFC layers V and VI. The pyramidal cells of these layers project to the thalamus and the brainstem reticular formation. TRH produces suppression of Fos-related immunoreactivity in columns of the PAG that regulate parasympathetic activity. This regulation would therefore be disinhibited, accounting in part for the mild tachycardia and blood pressure elevation sometimes seen after TRH. There is Fos-related immunoreactivity found in the RVLM in neurons that contain TH, which is the rate-limiting enzyme for catecholamine biosynthesis. These neurons project to special respiratory motoneurons and might be related to TRH-induced changes in respiratory activity and could dysregulate tidal volume in exercising fibromyalgia patients. The brain regions that show the most Fos-related immunoreactivity are those involved with behavior and emotional state: the mPFC, NAc, and amygdala, all of which have high densities of TRH receptors. A last note: A panic attack, or an ADR to TRH, can be terminated in ten seconds with Ativan 1:10 or 1:1 nasal spray.

I may not have discussed nylidrin and isoxsuprine extensively enough. They are in a class of other compounds unavailable in the United States used (successfully, it is claimed) to treat neurosomatic disorders. Ifenprodil is the best known, but there is also eliprodil and those known only by letters and numbers. They are highly selective for NMDA receptors composed of the NR1/NR2B subunit.

I mention nylidrin, which has an unsullied reputation, because it had little chance to be. Nylidrin was originally developed in the 1960s as a beta-adrenergic receptor agonist. It is a structural analog of the "-prodils" but has an open piperidine ring. The degree of inhibition of NR1A and NR2B is tighter than competitive binding usually is. The tight coupling is explained by a positive allosteric modulation between the nylidrin and protein regulatory sites. This alteration confers increased potency.

Nylidrin also binds to central alpha-adrenergic receptors. It may have an affinity for D_{123} and sigma 1 and 2, receptors and block K^+, Ca^{2+}, and Na^+ channels.

I have nylidrin 1.2 percent in PLO compounded in a 60 mL syringe, as I do with all my gels. I apply 2 mL to one ventral forearm and wait two minutes. If there is no effect, I apply it to the other arm and wait a little longer. If it is effective, the patient washes it off and takes 6 mg capsules 30 minutes apart while under observation. If these work, fine. If they cause an ADR, I try to reverse it with two 400 mg SAMe capsules. Sometimes this intervention works and sometimes it does not. The drug effects should resolve in about six hours. Nylidrin, and its cousin, isoxsuprine, are similar medications, with isoxsuprine having more of a $beta_2$ agonism. Both nylidrin and isoxsuprine bind to the inhibitory polyamine site. They can be displaced by polyamines that are synthesized from SAMe.

Nylidrin and isoxsuprine do not cross-react, however, and a lack of response to nylidrin does not guarantee the same result with isoxsuprine.

SAMe is also a precursor to hydrogen sulfide (H_2S), a gaseous transmitter which inhibits the release of CRH from rat hypothalamic explants. In vivo, it reduces the rise in corticosterone commonly seen in rats exposed to cold for one hour (Navarra P et al., 2000). S-adenosyl methionine is part of the transmethylation pathway, with which every neurosomatic physician should be familiar (Figure 45).

Chapter 11

Modulating Glutamatergic Neurotransmission

The number of methods by which glutamatergic neurotransmission may be hypothetically modulated is incalculable. Such control is maintained by the content of the genome and regulation of its expression at the DNA, RNA, and protein levels. It is affected by presynaptic glutamate release with one or more cotransmitters. The synaptic neurons are regulated by a multitude of extraneuronal factors, including the glial cells, gap junctions, stimulatory or inhibitory inputs and their rates, pH, and a vast network of other cells inside and outside the central nervous system that secrete transmitter substances. The intracellular machinery of synaptic cells may vary among individuals on a genetic, allelic, or proteonomic basis. Because we do not have the capability to regulate neural networks at present, I shall restrict subsequent observations to the single synapse. We are also limited in being able to alter transcription and translation, and so I shall discuss molecular genetics and pharmacogenomics fairly superficially.

KETAMINE

The most useful agent in neurosomatic medicine at the time of this writing is ketamine, which binds to the PCP site in the pore of the NMDA receptor (Figure 46). It may also bind to a membrane-associated site that does not require the channel to be open (Orser BA et al., 1997) but decreases the frequency of channel open time (Schmid RL et al., 1999). This pore, or channel, allows calcium and sodium to enter and potassium to exit. Certainly not every patient benefits from ketamine. Enough do, however, to warrant further discussion of its mode of action and of other techniques of altering glutamatergic function, especially at the NMDA receptor.

I came to use ketamine later than I should have because of the pervasive view that ketamine was addictive and neurotoxic (Olney JW, 1994) and that the therapeutic index (a risk benefit ratio) was low. Schizophrenia was thought to be mimicked by ketamine and similar NMDA-receptor antagonists, which caused an open-channel block. It had been a drug of abuse for many years, earning the sobriquet of "Special K." Ketamine, as well as other noncompetitive antagonists, such as PCP and MK-801, can cause severe memory impairment, dissociation, and schizophreniform reactions when given in too high a dose to a sensitive patient. Increases in the NR1 subunit of the NMDA receptor and decreases in GABAergic neurons have been found after chronic PCP or MK-801 use. Similar changes are seen in the frontal cortex of schizophrenics (Jentsch JD et al., 2000). These agents may also reduce cortical synaptic dopamine neurotransmission, as reflected by a relative decrease in D_1-receptor-mediated activity, which can be remedied by systemic administration of a D_1-receptor agonist. Prefrontal DA levels are inversely related to VTA and NAc DA levels (Goeders NE, 1997). Competitive NMDA antagonists, such as CPP-ene, may have similar effects. Neuronal vacuolization may be seen in the posterior cingulate cortex and retrosplenial areas, but such toxicity occurs at a dose of 40 mg/kg or greater (de Lima J et al., 2000). Benzodiazepines, pentazocine, cholinesterase inhibitors, barbiturates, haloperidol, and clonidine may be neuroprotective in an individual receiving ketamine. Other agents that inhibit NMDA-receptor function in a noncompetitive manner do not have a stigma associated with their use, e.g., amantadine, memantine, and dextromethorphan (which has its own NMDA binding site).

Nevertheless, ketamine is a fairly hot topic. A MEDLINE search for the past year turned up 93 articles with ketamine in the title (02/01/01). There is not yet agreement on the neurotransmitter changes that accompany ketamine administration in the normal subject or in the symptomatic patient or animal. Between 1967 and 1999 the MEDLINE identified 378 animal studies and 132 human studies on the NMDA receptor in relation to pain (Fisher K, Hagen NA, 1999). Its primary indication is as an anesthetic, although it is increasingly being used as an analgesic.

Striatal dopaminergic neurons are, of course, directly stimulated by glutamatergic fibers in the corticostriatal thalamocortical tract, which has many more connections than the name implies (Figure 47a-b). mPFC glutamatergic efferents, however, may be inhibited by DA neurons originating in the VTA, as well as by increased activity of GABAergic interneurons that are stimulated by DA neurons from the VTA (Beyer CE, Steketee JD, 1999).

Most believe that ketamine-like drugs acutely increase dopamine and decrease GABA, especially in the PFC, where NMDA receptors are distributed on the outer layers of the cortex and DA neurons terminate on the inner layers. $GABA_A$ interneurons are thought to inhibit these DA neurons and also pyramidal neurons in less than 1 ms. These fast-spiking (FS) cells can synchronize local neural networks by responding to other GABAergic FS cells both chemically and electrically (Galarreta M, Hestrin S, 2001b). The GABAergic interneurons may be topically excited by glutamatergic neurons acting at GABAergic NMDA heteroreceptors. GABAergic neurons may be suppressed by glutamate acting at kainate receptors, however (Frerking M, Nicoll RA, 2000). Kainate acts via $GABA_A$ and $GABA_B$ receptor modulation. Kainate has a "presynaptic metabotropic activity of an ionotropic receptor [which is] unique within the central nervous system" (Frerking M, Nicoll RA, 2000).

Ketamine would thus increase PFC dopamine by decreasing GABAergic inhibition of VTA dopaminergic neurons (Yonezawa Y et al., 1998), much as opioids have been speculated to do, via inhibitory mu-opioid heteroreceptors on GABAergic neurons that are tonically active (Figure 12). The situation is greatly complicated by how these three types of neurons are regulated in different regions of the brain. Ketamine may also increase the biosynthesis of dopamine from dopa by stimulating the activity of aromatic L-amino acid decarboxylase (Fisher A et al., 1998), which is usually unsaturated. NMDA receptors are quite dense in the thalamus, where they may mediate hyperalgesia.

Antagonists at the glycine coagonist site of the NMDA receptor are considered to be less toxic than ketamine, to have fewer adverse reactions, and to be more specific for treating chronic pain (Bordi F, Quartaroli M, 2000). Several of these agents are available for clinical use, but their existence is not widely known. Probenecid increases kynurenate levels (Veesei L et al., 1998). Kynurenate, a catabolite of 5-HT via the GABA shunt (Figure 48) antagonizes the glycine coagonist site. Kynurenine derivatives also inhibit binding of NGF to its low-affinity p75 receptor (Jaen JC et al., 1995). Cycloserine, a glycine-site agonist, reliably terminates adverse reactions to probenecid that involve exacerbation of existing symptoms. They antagonize each other in clinical practice.

I have had very few problems prescribing ketamine for patients. Although rats will self-administer ketamine, it does not appear to cause physical dependence in the rats. I have never seen a patient in ketamine withdrawal, and NMDA antagonists have been advocated as a possible treatment for addiction (Tzschenke TM, Schmidt WJ, 1998). They may prevent plastic changes that develop with repeated administration of drugs of abuse at the electrophysiological or receptor level. In the proper dose, mode, frequency, and rate of administration, ketamine has few adverse reactions in those whom it benefits. Ketamine abuse has been a rare problem in thousands of patient trials. I prescribe it in eyedrops, nose drops, oral swirls, transdermal gels (Crowley KL et al., 1998), oral capsules, and intravenous infusions. My experience coincides with the literature: Ketamine, when properly administered, does not cause hallucinations or impairment of cognitive functioning (Schmid RL et al., 1999). The intravenous dosage I use, less than 2.5 micrograms/kg per minute, does not produce plasma levels

greater than 50 mcg/ml. Although it has been widely published that ketamine synergizes with opioid analgesics, I have not observed this effect more
than occasionally. Thus, few of my chronic-pain patients take opioids and
ketamine concomitantly. I administer 25 to 100 mg of ketamine in 500 ml of
normal saline over three hours or so, adjusting the rate to the patient's side
effects, which should be minimal. If intravenous ketamine (or lidocaine) is
infused too rapidly (even with midazolam), the results will often be poor,
and sometimes the patient will no longer respond to the drug (Sorenson J
et al., 1997). In the typical patient, an infusion of ketamine has a beneficial
effect lasting up to a week. Unlike the results reported in the literature
(Shimoyama M et al., 1999; Fisher K, Hagen NA, 1999), I do not find oral
ketamine to be as effective as other routes of administration, and it is more
apt to cause sedation than the transdermal preparation, 240 mg/Gm in
pluronic organogel. I have noticed this tendency with other medications in
PLO, even with gabapentin, which is not metabolized, and wonder whether
the adverse p.o. effects may be caused by binding to the vagus. Other agents
that affect the NMDA receptor have this property as well. The frequency of
infusions should be titrated to the needs of the patient (Mitchell AC, 2001).
Amantadine as a transdermal gel (400 mg/Gm in PLO) often works better
than the oral route, although about 5 percent of patients experience contact
dermatitis (which can usually be prevented by spraying a nebulized corticosteroid from an asthma inhaler on the site first). It is much more effective
when given intraveously, a preparation that is available to me in a compounded form (Northoff G et al., 1997; Eisenberg E, Pud D, 1998). Intravenous amantadine for chronic pain may actually *cure* it, according to the authors, and has few adverse reactions. It has never cured any of my patients
but is effective for some. NMDA receptors are involved in normal visceral
neurotransmission to the brain and also transduce nociceptive stimuli. This
finding may account for poor oral tolerability of some medications, as well
as the effectiveness of using NMDA antagonists in the treatment of irritable
bowel syndrome. NMDA receptors in vagal afferents may function as
presynaptic autoreceptors (Aicher SA et al., 1999). I titrate the oral dose in
the office from 10 to 120 mg t.i.d. by giving 10 mg every 30 minutes
(Enarson MC et al., 1999).

PHARMACOLOGIC MODULATION OF SENSORY
INTEGRATION VIA THE TRIGEMINAL NERVE

Topical application of psychoactive agents to the three branches of the
trigeminal nerve does not seem to have been discovered by others (Goldstein JA, 1996). Ketamine 1:10 in artificial tears t.i.d., nasal spray 1:10 or

1:1, and oral swirl 1:1 work within seconds and last for several hours. The functional neuroanatomy of the trigeminal nerve involves the vagus and glossopharyngeal nerves and cervical nerves 1 and 2. The trigeminal nerve also regulates the autonomic nervous system and pain transmission in the thalamus (Bereiter DA, Bereiter DF, 2000), perhaps through a projection to the nucleus submedius, a medial thalamic nucleus associated with supraspinal control of pain pathways. I use ketamine by the conjunctival, intranasal, and intraoral route even more often than other topical agents, such as naphazoline 0.1 percent, a noradrenergic agonist, dopamine 1:10 eyedrops and nose drops, adenosine 1:10 and 1:1 nose drops, and TRH 1:10 eyedrops and nose drops. I also keep lorazepam 1:10 nasal spray around for necessary occasions. It relieves certain ADRs, particularly to TRH, which is a BZD antagonist, and it aborts panic attacks, working in about 10 seconds. Aminophylline 1:10 nasal spray and haloperidol 1:10 nasal spray are only occasionally helpful, but oxytocin 10 units/ml, one spray each nostril t.i.d. (each spray is about 1/60 ml), often obviates the need to give compounded oxytocin tablets 10 units p.o. or oxytocin 10 units intramuscularly (most effective) added to 0.5 ml of 0.5 percent lidocaine so it will sting less. Oxytocin benefits many patients. I discussed it at some length in *Betrayal* and shall have a few more words to say about it later in this chapter.

Sensory nerves that supply the temporomandibular joint (TMJ) region include branches of the trigeminal, upper cervical, and vagus nerves. Bereiter and Bereiter (2000), in an excellent paper, plotted neural pathways by detecting c-fos, an IEG, and FOS protein, a Fos product, in the neuraxis. Rats were given acute injuries in their TMJs by injection of mustard oil. Two hours later the rats were sacrificed, and Fos-positive neuronal nuclei were located after appropriate staining. These would be the nuclei activated after the injury. Microscopical sections were done into the cervical spinal cord and through the brainstem. The c-fos neurons present extended through the upper cervical cord (V1, V2, and solitary tract of the vagus nerve). The trigeminal spinal tract interdigitated with the solitary tract and the first and second cervical nerve roots (C1 and C2). These levels also had high immunoreactivity for morphine and NR1. If rats were pretreated with morphine, there were fewer Fos-positive neurons. MK-801 (a ketamine-like agent) did not have much of an effect in the lower brainstem but reduced Fos at the C2 level, where the subnucleus caudalis of the trigeminospinal tract is located. A combined dose of MK-801 and morphine produced a greater reduction in Fos than either alone and seemed to be synergistic, rather than additive, in the reduction. The synergy is probably not a result of generation of hydrogen cyanide after activation of the mu-opioid receptor. Cyanide does increase NMDAR-induced Ca^{2+} and appears to be a constitutive gaseous immunomodulator. Systemic administration of hydromorphone to rats increases brain cyanide levels by 61 percent in 15 minutes (Borowitz JL et al., 1997). Atypical transmitters, or "neural messengers," will be discussed a little later. Branches of the mandibular nerve terminate in the dorsal paratrigeminal area and the superior area of the trigeminal spinal tract and then project more rostrally by third-order neurons. There is convergent input from the vagus nerve at C1 and C2, where 80 percent of the vagus neurons are nociceptive.

Usually nociception and tissue injuries produce widespread and long-lasting expansion in the receptive field of dorsal horn neurons. The caudal spinal tract of the trigeminal nerve, which is organized in a manner similar to the spinal cord itself, has autonomic connections. More rostral levels of the trigeminal tract, such as dPa5, send projections to autonomic brainstem regulatory centers, such as the nucleus tractus solitarus, dorsal vagal complex, parabrachial nuclei, and hypothalamus (Figure 49).

Some branches act as an intertrigeminal relay for somatic-autonomic integration in trigeminal nociception. The connection of the trigeminal subnucleus interpolaris and the subnucleus caudatus is designated as V1/Vc-Vl. These are third-order neurons, synapsing with those from the gasserian ganglion. V1/Vc-Vl have a role in the trigeminal-evoked changes in autonomic function and are not much affected by morphine/MK-801. They may be better modulated by receptor-specific eyedrops, which have their onset of action in about a second, or nasal sprays, which are effective in ten seconds, presumably because they must cross a mucus barrier first. The V1/Vc-Vl transition projects to the nucleus submedius of the thalamus, which is involved in pain control. Top-down nociception and other pathways from cortical and subcortical regions may be recruited. I have seen remarkable changes, including total remission and even a manic switch, one to two seconds after instillation of an eyedrop suitable for an individual patient's neurochemical dysregulation.

ELECTROCONVULSIVE THERAPY (ECT)

ECT reduces NMDA-receptor function as well as facilitating an action between D_1 and D_2 receptors (Smith E et al., 1997). Repeated ECT is similar to injections of both D_1 and D_2 agonists into the NAc. Reduction in glutamatergic function is thought to enhance D_1-D_2 interactions in the NAc. When my patients have had ECT it usually helps their depression, but their pain and fatigue are reduced only for a week or two, if at all. A neurosomatic patient who comes to me after failed ECT is a therapeutic challenge. Similarly, antidepressants, particularly SRIs, often help depression but leave other symptoms unchanged. A successful course of ECT produces a global reduction in cerebral blood flow, as do rapidly acting treatments imaged by SPECT as described in *Betrayal*. A successful course of antidepressant therapy produces similar hemodynamic alterations. Such a reduction may be parsimoniously explained by NMDA-receptor antagonism with reduced stimulation of neuronal nitric oxide synthase.

KINASES AND PHOSPHATASES

It is generally agreed that stress increases NMDA activity. Reexposure to the stress reactivates the increase. The primary postreceptor event involved in this process, no matter what the stressful event, is influx of Ca^{2+}, translocation of protein kinase C to the membrane, and subsequent activation of a cascade of calcium/calmodulin kinases (CaM-kinases) that can extend into the cellular DNA to modulate protein synthesis.

In the brain, there are at least seven subtypes of PKC (Shors TJ et al., 1997). Stress-induced activation and translocation of PKC can be prevented by NMDA antagonists. Because stress causes an influx of Ca^{2+} through the NMDA open channel, as well as its release from intracellular stores, the PKCs activated by Ca^{2+} (at least four of them) would be most likely to be affected. One of these, PKC gamma, is expressed exclusively in the CNS. Phorbol esters, present in tung oil, activate PKC by directly stimulating diacylglycerol and have been possible triggers of neurosomatic disorders, a point I have been making for over a decade (Goldstein JA, 1990). The effect of phorbol esters can last for days, until they are eliminated from the cell. Symptoms could be caused by prolonged activation or by eventual degradation of the enzyme. A cell may be experimentally depleted of phorbol ester-binding isoforms of PKC in this manner. Not only can a stressor activate PKC, the *context* in which the stressor occurs also does.

In addition to the stressor itself, exposure to the context in which the stressful event occurred was sufficient to reactivate an increase in [phorbol-ester] binding in the amygdala and activate the thalamus and area of CA1 of the hippocampus [Figure 50 of hippocampus]. These results suggest that different anatomical substrates are activated in response to the learned vs. the unlearned response. It is perhaps not coincidental that the amygdala and hippocampus [and the PFC even more] have been specifically implicated in acquiring information about context. In addition, the stress-induced facilitation of learning can be similarly reactivated by re-exposure in the same context under the same conditions, with respect to PKC itself. The calcium-sensitive isoform, PKC gamma, is likewise sensitive to contextual conditioning.

Mutant mice deficient in the isoform are more impaired in their fear response to contextual cues vs. explicit cues associated with an aversive stimulus. (Shors TJ et al., 1997)

This description has obvious relevance to neurosomatic medicine. I shall discuss the neurobiology of the kinases next, and then relate kinases to LTP and LTD, the point being that neurosomatic disorders are produced by overlearned responses to an overly applied context. Irrelevant stimuli are attended to, producing a deficit in working memory (deFockert JW et al., 2001). Protein phosphorylation is, by far, the most prominent mechanism of neural plasticity. Regulation of protein phosphorylation involves a protein kinase, a protein phosphatase, and substrate protein. Protein kinases are molecules, which, when activated, transfer phosphate groups to other molecules, altering their conformation and activating them (usually) (Figure 51a-f). Phosphatases work in a manner opposite to kinases and deactivate molecules by removing phosphate moieties. There are two major types of kinase. The serine/threonine kinases have a phosphate group attached to either of the amino acids serine or threonine in their protein structure. They are the major kinases in the brain. Tyrosine kinases are about 1 percent of kinases but are important in neurotransmission, are a part of growth factor receptors, and phosphorylate the NR2A subunit of the NMDA receptor, increasing its activity. Tyrosine phosphorylation of the NR2B subunit in the dentate gyrus may be involved in LTP. Protein kinases are usually activated by Ca^{2+}. Autophosphorylated CaMKII can bind to the NR2B subunit.

Autophosphorylation refers to a process by which a protein kinase remains active after Ca^{2+} has returned to baseline. This mechanism can produce relatively long-lived alterations in neuronal function. Autophosphorylation blocks an inhibitory section of the kinase molecule and traps calmodulin in the molecule after Ca^{2+} levels decline to normal, thereby prolonging the active state of the kinase. Regulation of pre- and postsynaptic neuronal processes by phosphorylation can result in transient facilitation or inhibition of synaptic activity. Intracellular regulatory pathways function as complexes with interactions between them mediated by phosphorylation-dephosphorylation, for the most part. The function of the many kinases are so interrelated that it is difficult to determine their effects individually. For the most part, clinical pharmacologic agents do not exist to modulate them. Exceptions would include Gleevec (imatinib), an antineoplastic tyrosine kinase inhibitor, and genestein, a nonspecific tyrosine kinase inhibitor. There are fewer phosphatases, and enhancing the activity of one or more of them would be relevant to dephosphorylating the NMDAR and decreasing its activity.

For example, yotiao, an NMDAR-associated protein, binds both protein phosphatase 1 (PP1) and PKA. Yotiao is a "scaffold protein" to which postreceptor regulatory substances bind and attach to receptors (Figure 52). Anchored PP1 limits NMDA-channel activity by preventing phosphorylation of the receptor. The effect of PP1 can be overcome by cAMP, which activates PKA, releasing it from its anchored site to attach to the NMDA receptor (Westphal RS et al., 1999).

Some agents used to treat excitotoxicity in stroke may be adapted to neurosomatic medicine. One such agent is actually PP1, which reduces the ischemic penumbra in experimentally induced stroke in rats (Paul R et al., 2001). I shall be looking at phosphatases in more detail shortly. Erythropoietin is another neuroprotective substance. After binding to its receptor, it activates the MAPK and P13K pathways and inhibits nuclear factor kappa B (Dawson TM, 2002). PP1 has been found to be a suppressor of learning and memory and a potential mediator of cognitive decline during aging (Genoux D et al., 2002).

Glutamate overactivity is also one of the causes of epilepsy (several other EAAs may also be involved). Ketamine may be used to treat seizures in the emergency department, but if a patient is in status epilepticus, tolerance to its anticonvulsant effect may occur (Kofke WA et al., 1997). Despite the apparent glutamatergic hypersecretion in neurosomatic disorders, epilepsy is less common than in the general population, although antiepileptic drugs are often used in treatment. By the same token, cholinesterase inhibitors, used to improve memory (barely) in Alzheimer's disease, increase glutamatergic neurotransmission and antagonize ketamine, which increases DA and NE in the medial PFC (Kubota T, Hirota K, Anzawa N, et al., 1999). Ach is, however, presynaptic to sympathetic ganglia. NE, increased by the administration of desipramine, decreases the potency of the glycine co-agonist site of the NMDAR (Harkin A et al., 2000).

The ketamine-induced NE release can be blocked by clonidine. Although glutamate releases GABA by acting through the NMDA receptor, ketamine also has $GABA_A$ agonist properties, because muscimol, a $GABA_A$ agonist, can potentiate ketamine anesthesia (Irifune M et al., 2000). Nevertheless, I must still administer a benzodiazepine to an occasional patient who becomes jittery from ketamine, perhaps because too much NE and DA is released. Some physicians give clonidine or a benzodiazepine prophylactically to all patients receiving ketamine infusions.

THE NICOTINIC CHOLINERGIC RECEPTOR

Acetylcholine, acting at the ionotropic nicotinic acetylcholine receptor, has numerous functions related to neurosomatic disorders. nAchRs are expressed diffusely in the cortex, hippocampus, and reward centers. The nAchR is presynaptic to GABAergic neurons as well as to glutamatergic neurons and can increase the secretion of both neurotransmitters. The nAchR is composed of subunits. There are seven alpha subunits and four beta subunits, which can produce a wide variety of nAchRs. The $alpha_7$ subunit appears most involved with neurosomatic disorders. The $alpha_4$-$beta_4$ nAchR is highly expressed in the limbic system and is inhibited by ketamine, the only nonvolatile anesthetic that can block the nicotine receptor (Flood P, 1999). $Alpha_3$-$beta_4$ nAchRs mediate NE release, while $alpha_3$-$beta_2$-containing receptors mediate DA release (Luo S et al., 1998). The nAchRs containing the $beta_2$ subunit are therefore involved in mediating the reinforcing properties of nicotine. nAchRs are glutamate agonists, as are (usually) muscarinic acetylcholine receptors (mAchRs) (Jones S et al., 1999). Dopaminergic VTA neurons receive cholinergic presynaptic innervation from the pedunculopontine nucleus via nAchRs. Thus, Ach can cause release of DA and help neurosomatic patients who have ADRs to ketamine-like agents, one of which would be mecamylamine, a nicotinic receptor antagonist.

Nicotine use is related to the mechanism of opioid dependence and can be decreased by naltrexone (Almeida LE et al., 2000). Nicotine not only releases DA and prevents experimental Parkinsonism in rodents but also induces striatal increase of neurotrophic factors, in particular fibroblast growth factor 2 (FGF-2), which is also induced by MK-801 and BDNF (Maggio R et al., 1998).

Other compounds act at the nAchR in ways one might not expect. It is well known that bupropion blocks many of nicotine's behavioral effects. Preapplication of bupropion blocks Ach binding in the closed state of several types of AchRs (Slemmer JE et al., 1999). What is not well known is that other antidepressants (sertraline, paroxetine, fluoxetine, nefazodone, and venlafaxine) also have this property (Fryer JD, Lukas RJ, 1999). So does the diuretic amiloride, which blocks kidney sodium channels (Gupta T et al., 1996), and methadone, perhaps because it is also an SRI and an NMDA antagonist.

The nicotinic Ach receptor has many important functions. Its most important subunit in neurosomatic medicine is $alpha_7$, which regulates release of neurotransmitters and activates the MAPK pathway. It is regulated by NGF and interacts with the Src family of tyrosine kinases, which can phosphorylate the $alpha_7$ subunit and desensitize it. Forskolin, which activates adenyl cyclase and is available as a nutritional supplement, accelerates the desensitization of the $alpha_7$ subunit. Agents that stimulate PKC do not affect this process. There should be a higher incidence of symptom exacerbation by nicotine in FMS patients, who have elevated NGF, than in other patients. Alpha$_4$-beta$_2$ and alpha$_3$-beta$_4$ are the most common subunit assemblies for nicotine receptors. The alpha$_3$-beta$_4$ receptor is labeled by epibatidine, an effective analgesic too toxic for human use. The next few years will see a profusion of subtype-specific nicotinic agonists and antagonists. At present, all I have is the nicotine patch, the nonselective antagonist mecamylamine, and the second-generation antidepressants, the most potent of which is bupropion. Most second-generation antidepressants block the nAchR (Fryer JD, Lukas RJ, 1999). Mecamylamine has a mode of action analogous to ketamine. I prescribe it when a nicotine patch exacerbates pre-existing symptoms. Ketamine inhibits nicotinic receptors, particularly the alpha$_4$-beta$_4$ variety predominantly expressed in the limbic system (Flood P, 1999).

Epibatidine has analgesic potency two orders of magnitude greater than morphine. Thus far, nicotinic analgesics, known of since 1932, have had too poor a therapeutic index for clinical practice. Their mode of action is unclear, but they do activate multiple descending antinociceptive pathways. Another drawback is that nicotinic analgesia is very brief, peaking at 10 minutes and absent at 30 minutes (Gilbert SD et al., 2001).

The alpha$_7$ subtype, which can be homomeric, is predominantly presynaptic and is an excitatory heteroreceptor on many classical transmitter neurons, generally activating very fast calcium currents that cause neurotransmitter release (Stahl SM, 2000). Nicotinic agents also potentiate neuroleptic effects (Castellanos XF, 1999). Spinal nicotinic receptors may wind down central excitability-amplifying nociceptive processes and inhibit neurogenic and bradykinin-induced inflammation (Lawand NB et al., 1999).

In human studies, nicotine increases pain thresholds in male smokers and nonsmokers but has no effect on this parameter in females. Tolerance does not develop to the analgesic effects of nicotine (Flores CF, 2000).

nAchRs are involved in attention and performance in working and associative memory. nAchR activation excites GABAergic interneurons in the hippocampus. Fast-spiking GABAergic neurons can perhaps initiate the activity of large numbers of principal cells and play a large part in regulation of hippocampal output, apparently deranged in neurosomatic disorders (Galarreta M, Hestrin S, 2001b). They contribute to one or more types of synchronization of the principal cells, which underlies the theta component of the hippocampal rhythm (Jones S et al., 1999). FS cells are quite active in the PFC. Alpha$_7$ nAchR subtypes are also located postsynaptically in the CA1 area of the hippocampus and produce fast Ach transmission. Some hippocampal responses are blocked by mecamylamine, which affects alpha$_{2-5}$ and beta$_{2-4}$ containing AchRs, suggesting that not all hippocampal nicotinic responses are mediated by alpha$_7$ subtypes (Figure 53).

In the cortex, nAchR activation potentiates NMDA but not AMPA neurotransmission, perhaps participating in memory consolidation, as it does in LTP in the hippocampus. Alpha-7 subtypes may even contribute to synaptic strengthening.

Ach neurons project from the pedunculopontine tegmental nucleus (PPT) and the laterodorsal tegmental nucleus (LDT) to DA neurons in the VTA, which express nAchRs. Activation of neurons from these nuclei mediate tonic regulation of the DA VTA neurons and could physiologically activate the reward system. The SN and VTA project Ach neurons to nAchRs in the basal ganglia and NAc (Figure 54) (Cordero-Erausquin M et al., 2000). Nicotine could associate its use with reward and lead to addiction. Because the nAchRs rapidly desensitize, continued use of nicotine is necessary to maintain the reward state. Both mecamylamine and specific alpha$_7$ antagonists block different aspects of nAchR-mediated reward, indicating that distinct subpopulations of nAchRs exist in the VTA.

NMDA-receptor antagonists administered systemically prevent the effect of nicotine on behavior and on DA release. This finding suggests nAchR-elicited changes in DA neuron activity might also be due to the effects of presynaptic glutamate. Glutamate releases DA in the VTA and vice versa in the PFC. Beta$_2$ subunit knock-out mice do not release DA from the VTA in response to systemic nicotine. Both pre- and postsynaptic nAchRs can enhance neurotransmission.

Nimodipine (Nimotop) may be viewed as a nicotinic and NMDA antagonist (Taylor CW, Brood LM, 1998), as can heparin if it has bound to the IP$_3$ receptor prior to NMDAR activation. It could thereby decrease acute elevation of intracellular Ca^{2+}. Heparin also binds to a site on the NMDA receptor. Even warfarin (Coumadin), by decreasing the activity of thrombin, can be an NMDAR antagonist. Activation of the thrombin receptor PAR1 (protease-activated receptor) has been shown to potentiate NMDAR function (Gingrich MB et al., 2000). It may do so by cleaving the NR1 subunit, in a like manner to tissue plasminogen activator (Figures 55 and 56; Nicole O et al., 2001; Traynelis SF, Lipton SA, 2001). The brain contains some of the same proteases and protease-activated receptors that are involved in the coagulation cascade. Plasmin reduces GABAergic inhibition, and thrombin can generate seizures (Gingrich MB et al., 2000). It is thought that stress can or cannot cause increased permeability of the blood-brain barrier to various substances, including serine proteases. Pyridostigmine, a peripheral cholinesterase inhibitor, has been potentially implicated in Gulf War syndrome (GWS), a typical neurosomatic disorder (Eserink M, 2001), or not (Graver E et al., 2000).

One of the most effective treatments in neurosomatic medicine is gabapentin (Neurontin). It has complex effects on NMDAR function by virtue of its binding to the $alpha_2$-delta subunit of the L-type calcium channel. It inhibits glutamate release, but not in a simple manner, because it does not antagonize ketamine, as lamotrigine (Lamictal) does. Ketamine, by blocking the NMDA receptor, makes more glutamate available to bind to the other glutamate receptors (Shimoyama M et al., 2000). Gabapentin is compatible with ketamine and will be discussed in its own section. It may bind to the glycine/NMDA site because its action can often be reversed by cycloserine.

As might be expected, baclofen inhibits NMDA EPSPs by acting at pre- and postsynaptic $GABA_B$ receptors (Wu YN, Shen KZ, Johnson SW, 1999) and is one of the more effective treatments in neurosomatic medicine. It could be reversed by d-fenfluramine, but since this agent is no longer available, I use citalopram (Celexa) instead, which is a pure SRI, affecting no other transmitters. Forskolin, hydergine, oxytocin, mexiletine, and reboxetine may also antagonize baclofen, which surprisingly increases 5-HT release from the dorsal raphe nucleus.

In accordance with (virtually) all antimicrobials affecting neurotransmitters (Sternbach H, State R, 1997) so do aminoglycosides, which are excitotoxic via their activation of the polyamine site of the NMDA receptor. Their antibiotic action has no correlation with their excitotoxicity (Harvey SC et al., 2000), which can be reversed by vinpocetine, a Na^+-channel blocker and PDE 1 inhibitor. I would consider using a very low dose of an aminoglycoside, if all else failed, in a patient whose symptoms were greatly exacerbated by nylidrin or isoxsuprine and were not relieved by beta adrenergic receptor antagonists or SAMe. I know of no specific polyamine-site agonists except those made by viruses such as cytomegalovirus (CMV). *S*-adenosylmethionine, however, is the primary methyl group donor in polyamine biosynthesis, and a 400 mg dose is usually an effective antagonist.

To my surprise, buspirone (BuSpar), has been found to suppress NMDA activity in the rat visual cortex (Edagawa Y et al., 1998). I have found BuSpar to be somewhat useful to lower 5-HT concentration and as an $alpha_2$ antagonist that does not cause panic attacks. Its primary metabolite, 1-PP, is an $alpha_2$ adrenergic antagonist. It synergizes with cyproheptadine (Periactin), which blocks the $5\text{-}HT_2$ receptors, and ondansetron, a $5\text{-}HT_3$ antagonist. Periactin reverses SRIs and triptans. I particularly would not expect BuSpar to be an NMDA antagonist, since all of the atypical neuroleptics, especially ziprasidone, antagonize ketamine and are $5\text{-}HT_{1A}$ agonists. BuSpar reverses pindolol, a $5\text{-}HT_{1A}$ antagonist, fairly well, unless the pindolol ADRs are caused by beta blockade.

Glutamate release can be inhibited or increased by activation of one or more of the eight described metabotropic glutamate receptors. The result of activation of each of these receptors may also depend on where they are located in the brain. mGluRs 2, 4, and 7 inhibit voltage-dependent Ca^{2+} channels and decrease glutamate release at selected glutamatergic synapses. Their actions may depend on different types of G-protein coupling. Numerous drugs that act at mGluRs are in various stages of development. Some mGluR agonists might produce LTD by increasing $[Ca^{2+}]_i$, which could be beneficial in treatment of neurosomatic disorders (Fagni L et al., 2000). An interesting hypothesis involving cooperativity between D_1 and D_2 receptors and corticostriatal glutamate has been advanced. Dopamine-denervated mice do not generate LTD. Coactivation of D_1 and D_2 receptors may activate PLA_2, resulting in increased arachidonic acid that potentiates PKC (Calabresi P et al., 1996). This hypothesis does not distinguish between mGluRs, however, and would suggest that honey bee venom, which activates PLA_2, should be extremely effective in a wide range of patients (which it is not). AA can function as an NMDA antagonist in certain situations, however.

Adenosine A_1 and A_{2A} agonists block MK-801-induced EEG changes. This effect is thought to be a result of these agonists inhibiting D_1 and D_2 receptors, respectively. Thus, A_1 and A_{2A} agonists are being considered as novel antipsychotics (Popoli P et al., 1997; Ferre S, 1997). This finding is quite the opposite of my clinical experience. Adenosine 1:10 and 1:1 nasal spray is often quite anxiolytic, and dipyridamole, an adenosine-reuptake inhibitor, sometimes is effective in ketamine responders and is a weak PDE-5 inhibitor.

Before I go any further with this discussion, it occurs to me that I should define LTP and LTD.

LONG-TERM POTENTIATION AND DEPRESSION

LTP is the most widely studied activity-dependent form of synaptic plasticity in the CNS. It has been examined most extensively in the hippocampus because of the fairly simple architecture of this structure. For this reason, LTP has primarily been associated with memory but may occur anywhere there are NMDA synapses, which is almost everwhere in the CNS. LTP is greatly involved with chronic pain (Sandkuhler J, 2000).

If a one-second train of impulses at high frequency is transmitted from the presynaptic Schaeffer collateral pathway to area CA1 of the hippocampus, there will be a profound enhancement of long duration in subsequent responses of the CA1 neurons to low-frequency presynaptic signals. In the hippocampus, LTD occurs by depolarization of the NMDA synapses. LTP begins by activation of kinases, one of which, CaMKII, I shall discuss shortly. Protein synthesis is required for maintenance of LTP and for physical changes in the structure of the synapse to occur. The initiation of LTP can be blocked by decreasing the sensitivity of the NMDA receptor or by ketamine (Salami M et al., 2000). LTD, somewhat the opposite of LTP, occurs after lower-frequency synaptic transmission and probably involves phosphatases.

Because NMDA synapses operate electrically as well as chemically, postsynaptic changes are fairly specific. These alterations involve dendritic morphology and insertion of AMPA receptors. Dendritic spines have protrusions called filopodia, which can move by contraction or extension of a protein called actin. NMDA neurotransmission increases the activity and the number of filopodia, a process inhibited by NMDA antagonists. Filopodia sprouting can make new synapses, or NMDA transmission can maintain existing synapses (Smith SJ, 1999). This process may constitute Hebbian learning.

The dynamic modulation of dendritic spines in LTP has recently been discussed (Luscher C et al., 2000). Ca^{2+} release from intracellular stores is necessary for filopodia to move, perhaps because Ca^{2+} depolymerizes actin. As discussed earlier, AMPA receptors can be rapidly inserted into the synapse, as a result of an NMDA-mediated LTP induction protocol. The AMPA receptors that respond to synaptically released glutamate are found in an area of the dendrite called the postsynaptic density. As AMPA receptors are inserted into the PSD, its physical structure changes. First it widens, and then it splits in two. Subsequently, the presynaptic neuron, probably via a retrograde mechanism, forms two synaptic terminals (boutons) to contact the two PSDs (filopodia) (Figure 56). The intracellular processes involved in this structural modification are dependent largely upon Ca^{2+}-activated CaMKII. I shall consider this event next.

Ca^{2+} concentration intracellularly, denoted as $[Ca^{2+}]_i$, is tightly regulated by (1) ion channels (including the pore of the NMDAR) that let Ca^{2+} in; (2) pumps that expel it; and (3) release from two primary intracellular stores in the endoplasmic reticulum, the ryanodine-sensitive receptors (opened by caffeine and blocked by dantrolene) and the IP_3-sensitive receptors, blocked by heparin. Ca^{2+} is also concentrated in the mitochondria. Ca^{2+} can change locally, as within a dendrite or axon terminal, or through the entire cell, including the nucleus. Ca^{2+} waves, propagated by opening of the ryanodine receptor by Ca^{2+} itself (calcium-induced calcium release), can spread through the ER and into the nucleus, even activating the IEG CREB (Hardingham GE et al., 2001). Ca^{2+} alone can activate numerous molecules by varying amplitudes and frequencies of its waves. IP_3 is a product of phosphatidylinositol metabolism, triggered by neurotransmitters that act on G proteins, activating phospholipase C. PLC changes phosphotidylinositol-4-5-biphosphate into inositol triphosphate and diacyglycerol, which activates PKC (Figure 57a-c). I shall discuss these molecules in the context of drug therapy subsequently. Phosphoinositides are involved in many intracellular functions. These include generation of second messengers linked to Ca^{2+} homeostasis and protein phosphorylation. Inositol lipids also anchor certain cell-surface proteins and are involved in membrane trafficking, maintenance of the cytoskeleton, regulation of PKC activity (activation), and opposing apoptosis. Phosphoinositides must bind to synaptotagmin before catecholamine exocytosis can occur (Figure 58).

Ca^{2+} binds to intracellular buffering proteins and also to calmodulin, a protein which then undergoes a conformational change so that it can activate other proteins, particularly kinases, phosphatases, and enzymes. Blocking calmodulin, however, which may be accomplished by trifluoperazine (Stelazine), has no particular value in treating neurosomatic disorders.

Ca^{2+}/calmodulin kinases are a family of serine/threonine kinases, and CaM-KII constitutes 2 percent of the protein in the hippocampus (Soderling TR, 2000). CaMKII inhibits its own function at its catalytic domain until its protein structure is altered by calcium/calmodulin binding. I am indebted to the work of Thomas R. Soderling for my understanding of the CaMK cascade (Soderling TR, 2000). I paraphrase his work in the next section.

Just as PKC acts at the PSD, or TrKs for neurotrophins are protein kinases themselves (Kaplan DR, Miller FD, 2000), CaMKII translocates to the PSD (Figure 59) following calcium signaling, where it can act on other PSD proteins. The frequency of Ca^{2+} oscillations in the postsynaptic spine determines whether LTP or LTD is to occur. Various kinds of oscillations are integral to many neural, glial, or neural network activities (Ritz R, Sejnowski TJ, 1997; Perez-Velasquez JL, Carlea DJ, 2000).

CaMKII is autophosphorylated on the Thy286 amino acid, resulting in a prolonged physiological response triggered by a transient increase in duration, amplitude, and frequency of $[Ca^{2+}]_i$. "Two characteristics required for LTP are contained in the molecular properties of CaMKII: first, to decode the frequency of synaptic stimulation; and second, to give a prolonged response after a transient elevation in Ca^{2+}" (Ritz R, Sejnowski TJ, 1997).

When activated, CaMKII translocates to the PSD, where one of its binding partners is the activated NMDAR that is admitting Ca^{2+} through its pore (Shen K et al., 2000). It would be straightforward if CaMKII would phosphylate NR2. Brain mechanisms are never simple. There is usually a good reason for complexity (Brezina V, Weiss KR, 1997). Instead, the NMDAR admits Ca^{2+} that activates CaMKII which then phosphorylates (thereby inhibiting) synaptic Ras-GTPase activating protein (SynGAP), potentiating the mitogen-activated protein kinase pathway. MAP kinase is important in synaptic plasticity and will be considered in more detail in a later section. I will also look at DARPP-32 because (1) it modulates calcineurin, a protein phosphatase acting in the NMDAR; and (2) we have calcineurin inhibitors, albeit toxic ones (cyclosporin and tacrolimus).

SynGAP is a fast synaptic Ras-GTPase activating protein (Ras-GAP) that interacts with synaptic proteins PSD-95 and SNAP-102 and is found in a complex with NMDA receptors in the brain. Such proteins are termed "trafficking proteins" and affect the synaptic vesicle cycle (Figure 60). SynGAP also binds proteins with the assistance of phospholipids. Ca^{2+} entry after NMDA-receptor activation could regulate SynGAP function, as may activation of CaMKII, phosphorylating it and thereby inhibiting Ras-GAP activity and modulating Ras signaling, which is involved in many downstream pathways (Scannevin RH, Huganir RL, 2000). The complexity of pre- and postsynaptic organization precludes an extensive discussion. SynGAP is but one of a multitude of constituents. I shall refer to these proteins only when directly relevant, since we are currently unable to specifically regulate them in clinical practice (Figure 61).

Moreover, CaMKII can phosphorylate the NMDAR glutamate-gated ion channel and increase its conductance. We have seen how AMPARs activate "silent synapses." The GluR1 subunit of the AMPAR must be phosphorylated and then autophosphorylated for CA1 LTP to occur.

If LTP is to persist longer than two or three hours, gene transcription and protein synthesis must occur. Localized induction of LTP in dendrites takes place after manufacture of alpha-CaMKII protein, a process blocked by the protein synthesis inhibitor anisomycin (which also blocks reconsolidation of retrieved memories) (Nader K et al., 2000). Increased local protein synthesis of CaMKII can be promoted by "polyadenylation," a detail I shall not explain here. The IEG CREB can be activated by numerous methods, but the most relevant one for me is that activation of the NMDAR by L-type Ca^{2+} channels causes significant translocation of CaMKII into the cell nucleus. BDNF subsequently can combine with CaM-KII to modulate CREB-mediated transcription.

CaMKII is inactivated rapidly, within minutes, probably because it binds to PPA2, or calcineurin. Calcineurin blockers prevent the inactivation of PP1 and could therefore serve as NMDAR antagonists, if less-toxic compounds were available. This process could continue in the hippocampus if PPA2 could be turned off (Bito H et al., 1996).

Of esoteric interest is that new synapse formation is blocked by KN-93, a general inhibitor of CaMKII. Evidence is suggestive, however, that CaMKII is involved in remodeling or maintenance of PSDs. Mechanisms of producing LTD prolonged by low-frequency NMDAR stimulation have proven somewhat more elusive and may be effective only at normal resting potential or by activating phosphatases.

The NMDAR is not required to produce LTP. If a rat is spinalized and descending noxious inhibitory controls are removed, LTP can be produced just by adding NMDA or SP to C-fiber synapses in the spinal cord. This phenomenon suggests that synaptic transmission is not required for LTP induction. Diffusion of potentially algogenic transmitters may cause hyperalgesia and central sensitization in animals lacking (or perhaps with weakened) DNIC (Sandkuhler J, 2000).

Forming new spines may depend on the high calcium fluxes resulting from NMDAR activation. Maintaining them may involve AMPAR activation by CaMKII (Soderling TR, 2000), a type of which may be Ca^{2+} independent, with much less perturbation of Ca^{2+} dynamics (Fischer M et al., 2000). PKC and PKA can also phosphorylate Ser 831 in GluR1 of the AMPA receptor, perhaps contributing to spine formation.

Soderling also explains (Soderling TR, Der Kach VA, 2000) that NR1 and NR2 subunits are subject to tyrosine phosphorylation "and infusion of tyrosine kinases potentiates the current through NR1-NR2A or NR1-NR2B recombinant channels by phosphorylation of C-terminal tyrosine residues, thereby relieving a basal zinc inhibition of NMDA receptors." Zinc levels (Zn^{2+}) have been related to pain threshold in fibromyalgia, and Zn^{2+} has been found to be reduced in FM patients. My success with Zn^{2+} supplementation in FMS has been one patient, but months of this therapy might be necessary (Russell IJ, 2001, personal communication). Zinc is the second most abundant trace element in the brain, but it is usually associated with other molecules. Free Zn^{2+} is in the nanomolar range. Zinc is found in synaptic vesicles that contain glutamate and probably is a cotransmitter. It inhibits NMDA receptors in the manner of Mg^{2+} (Barañano DE et al., 2001).

Thus, four kinases are involved in phosphorylating the NMDA receptor: PKC, tyrosine kinases, casein kinase II, and CaMKII. The number of kinases involved in the kinase cascade is so high that I am not able to discern which is the most important. Indeed, kinase preeminence is probably a nonissue. I have briefly mentioned casein kinase II. This substance has been found to be constitutively active, unusual among protein kinases, and continuously controls the basal function of the NMDA-receptor channels (Lieberman DN, Mody I, 1999). CKII tonically controls the opening probability but not the duration. NR1, NR2A, and NR2B subunits have more phosphorylation sites for CKII than any other substance. One inhibitor of CKII, abbreviated DRB, somewhat mimics the action of calcineurin on CaMKII and is highly specific. CKII is stimulated by spermine, a polyamine, up-regulating channel activity, which can be down-regulated by calcineurin. The site on CKII that is stimulated by spermine might be inhibited by nylidrin and/or isoxsuprine. The "classical" inhibitor of CKII is heparin, which, in the presence of ATP, dramatically reduces NMDA-channel open duration. This effect is not related to heparin's action of blocking the IP_3 receptor. Heparin appears to bind to a site on the NMDA receptor, with a resultant decrease in receptor activity. It appears that the phosphorylation state of the NMDA-receptor channel complex is set by a balance between the tonic activity of the spermine-sensitive CKII and the calcium-mediated negative feedback provided by calcineurin.

In central neurons, CKII may modulate the activity of several key proteins but selectively controls the function of only the NMDA receptors. CKII participates in LTP, during which neurotrophins activate CKII through their effect on other PKs.

Protein phosphatase 1, PP2A, and PP2B (calcineurin) are effective in dephosphorylating serine/threonine kinases and CaMKII. Protein phosphatases can be inhibited, e.g., by inhibitor 11, which, when phosphorylated by PKA, inhibits PP1. For LTP induction to proceed, 11 must by phosphorylated and then inhibit PP1 (Figure 62). PP1 inhibition also prolongs the activity of CaMKII and that of the GluR1 subunit of the AMPA receptor.

Inhibiting the activity of PP2B (calcineurin) may increase the activity of PP1, because PP2B dephosphorylates DARPP-32 (dopamine cAMP-regulated phosphoprotein, molecular weight 32,000). Inhibiting PP2B might be desirable, since PP1 dephosphorylates NR1 glutamate receptors and calcium channels. The only PP2B inhibitors available are cyclosporin and tacrolimus, which are too toxic to be used in neurosomatic medicine without compelling evidence that such an intervention would be a "magic bullet." The dephosphorylating activity of PP1 and PP2A is quite nonspecific, however, and I would hesitate to increase their activity even if I could, because I would be unsure of the repercussions. Perhaps in a year or two additional predictive information will be available. In vivo, the phosphatases are tightly regulated by inhibitor proteins such as DARPP-32. Although other inhibitor proteins are widespread in mammalian tissues, DARPP-32 is primarily neuronal and is particularly found in neurons that express D_1 receptors. A specific pharmacologic intervention in the DARPP cascade might have less potential toxicity. Any measure to increase phosphatase activity should of necessity be very delicate. Forskolin, an available nutritional supplement, activates PKA via cAMP, and I use it for augmentation of PKA-dependent processes, recalling that forskolin (10 to 20 mg a day for about a month) can also desensitize the process. "These results are consistent with the hypothesis that stable synaptic potentiation is associated with prolonged CaMKII activation, which requires protein phosphatase inhibition, probably through phosphorylation of 11 by PKAs" (Soderling TR, 2000) (Figure 63).

In normal human learning, facilitating this operation could be helpful, and there are numerous ways by which it could be made faster and more efficient. Patients with neurosomatic disorders, however, have overlearned information that acts quickly, efficiently, and inappropriately in a dysfunctional PFC-limbic-hippocampal context, or template. Even though attention and short-term memory (STM) are markedly impaired in many neuro-somatic patients, who are often unable to organize and learn multitask new information, LTP must be weakened almost to the point of elimination to allow more appropriate attentional templates to synaptically weight stimuli for neural-network processing. In a manner of speaking, neurosomatic patients are more aware of stimuli and their associations as a result of a hyperfunctional information-gathering system. This hyperfunction makes patients more efficient, more aware, and, if you will, perhaps more intelligent, until it overheats the system and it breaks down (deFockert JW et al., 2001). Cross talk between multiple kinases and kinases with other signaling mechanisms produce prolonged activation of some of these kinases. The example that has been best described is that of CaMKII. What we must do in the treatment of neurosomatic disorders is to produce a slowdown (LTD) rather than a complete stop (apoptosis).

This goal can be accomplished by reducing $[Ca^{2+}]_i$, modulating release of many transmitter substances, especially glutamate, and decreasing the sensitivity of the NMDA receptor. If Ca^{2+} is increased at baseline, perhaps by stimulating the IP_3 receptor, NMDAR activity will be inhibited. Regulating modulatory levels of postreceptor events by Ca^{2+}/calmodulin, lowering activity of kinase cascades, raising concentrations of certain phosphatases, interfering with IEG activation, and diminishing the number and activity of postsynaptic structures, such as dendrites, scaffolding proteins, and intercellular adhesion molecules, could all be targets for therapeutic intervention (Figure 64). Altering levels of some postreceptor molecules, e.g., cyclic AMP with forskolin, apparently has too broad an effect to be useful in receptor profiling but is often quite useful in augmenting an agent that inhibits AC and increases cAMP. Forskolin is occasionally effective as monotherapy in the hypervigilant patient.

Another kinase group that is activated by phosphorylation is mitogen-activated protein kinase, or MAPK, which is part of a kinase cascade I shall attempt to discuss here. Part of the importance of MAPK is that it is activated by neurotrophins, which are probably elevated in FMS (Russell IJ, personal communication, 2001). Substances of relevance in neurosomatic disorders, such as tyrosine hydroxylase and phospholipase A_2 (PLA$_2$), are substrates for MAPK. Synapsin I is also phosphorylated by the MAPK cascades. This molecule anchors synaptic vesicles to the nerve terminal cytoskeleton in a type of "cage." When it is phosphorylated (by MAPK, PKA, or CaMKII) it releases the vesicles, or "decages" them, so that they can migrate to the neuronal membrane and be available for exocytosis. Various neurotransmitters bind to the presynaptic membrane and cause phosphorylation or dephosphorylation of synapsin I, thereby increasing or decreasing neurotransmitter release.

AA and another eicosanoid, 12-hydroperoxycicosatetraenoic (12-HPETE), activate p38 MAPK kinase activity. MAPK p42/p44 is the best known and is active in LTP. p30 MAPK is a parallel signaling pathway that induces mGluR LTD without involving phosphatase activation.

MITOGEN-ACTIVATED
PROTEIN KINASES (MAPKs)

Major Major Major Major

Joseph Heller (1961)
Catch-22

Even though molecular neurobiology never stops becoming more complicated, this book does, and it's doing so with the MAPKinase cascade. It so happens that this family of closely related proline-targeted serine/threonine kinases, also known as extracellular signal-related kinases (ERKs) or mitogen-activated protein kinases (MAPKs), also known as microtubule-associated protein kinases is *very important.* "MAPKs regulate almost all cellular processes from gene expression to cell death" (Chang L, Karin M, 2001).

When I first read about MAPK, I immediately thought of the character who leads off this section—poor Major Major. He spent almost his entire life unaware of the cruel trick his parents had played upon him; he thought his first name was Caleb. MAPK used to be another name for ERK. Now ERK is just one of the MAPK family.

MAPK is often linked to G-protein-coupled receptors (GPCRs) that have increasingly been shown to integrate an intricate network of multiple cellular signaling pathways (Marinissen JM, Gutkind JS, 2001). I will start with the membrane-associated small G protein "Ras" (there are several others) (Mochizuki N et al., 2001). There are three Ras proteins, Harvey Ras, Kirsten Ras, and neural Ras, isolated from rat sarcoma viral oncogenes in the days before in vitro fertilization. Inactive Ras binds GDP and is regulated by other proteins. Ras begets Raf. In the meantime, inactive MAPK is activated by phosphorylation by another protein kinase, termed MAPK kinase, which is in turn activated by still another protein kinase, termed MAPK kinase kinase, which is where Ras and Raf come in. After GTP is activated and bound to Ras, MAPK kinase kinase is drawn to the plasma membrane where it may be activated by MAPK kinase kinase kinase.

This process is important because MAPK kinase kinase kinase is translocated to the nucleus, where it is perhaps the major activator of immediate early genes. ERKs are activated by neurotrophin and related growth factors. The MAPK kinases responsible for phosphorylation and activation of the ERKs are referred to as ERK kinases II, or, as some prefer to call them, MEKs. Raf incestuously activated MEK, because Raf is a group of protein serine/threonine kinases that are also MAPK kinase kinases (see Figure 65).

Many MAPKs activate specific receptor kinases—MAPK-activated protein kinases, abbreviated as MAPKAPKs—and are inactivated by MAPK phosphatases.

Ras is activated by most of the neurotrophins and insulin, which bind to cytoplasmic receptors that process intrinsic tyrosine kinase in their domains. Nonreceptor tyrosine kinases include Src, which can be activated by GPCRs to form Src-2 homology domains, launching sites of the primary pathways for Trk signal transduction. These include PLC; PI-3K, or phosphatidylinositol-3 kinase, which I almost discussed in the IP_3 section; and Shc, an adapter protein, short for Src homology and collagen. Shc, Ras, Trk, and GTP all affect one another, with the end result being the activation of Ras.

This mind-numbing plethora of information about MAP kinases may actually have clinical application in neurosomatic disorders some day. First, we shall have to discover the substrates for the four general types of MAP kinases. As of now, we know only one substrate, which is not relevant to neurobiology. But the p42/44 MAPK pathway regulates LTP in the mammalian hippocampus, as well as controlling the biosynthesis of the presynaptic protein syntaxin. There is mGluR-dependent LTD in the hippocampus, involving inhibition of N-type Ca^{2+} channels by bradykinin acting at excitatory synapses between CA3 and CA1 pyramidal neurons. Methods currently exist in the laboratory to facilitate or inhibit the activity of all known players in these pathways (Bolshakov VY et al., 2000). A transient application of p38 MAPK leads to *sustained* LTD. It is suggested that the prolongation of action occurs because of p38 MAPK-activated PLA_2, which generates arachidonic acid as a retrograde messenger. AA also activates MAPK pathways, and so the two cascades may act in a positive feedback manner to amplify and prolong the initial signals. Pharmacologic induction of LTD could be beneficial in neurosomatic disorders.

GABAPENTIN

In a chronic-constriction rat model of trigeminal neuralgia, gabapentin was found to be superior to lamotrine (Lamictal) (Christensen D et al., 2001). This finding is of interest because LTG inhibits glutamate release by stabilizing the inactivated conformation of a subtype of Na^+ channels. Both baclofen, a $GABA_B$ agonist, and GBP, which has numerous described modes of action, were superior to LTG in antinociception but only after *repeated* use (not my experience). The necessity for repetitive administration is not understood. A small percentage of my patients respond to subchronic dosing of GBP, LTG, and numerous other substances that usually have an immediate onset of action, and I have assumed a genomic mode of action rather than a receptor/postreceptor cascade mechanism was the neuropharmacologic difference.

We have known that GBP inhibits SP and CGRP, and perhaps the release of glutamate, for some time. We also realize that GBP *opens* the K_{ATP} channel, thereby slowing neural conduction and release of neurotransmitters such as NE, a function also accomplished by its attachment to the alpha$_2$-delta subunit of the L-type Ca^{2+} channel. We have not known how GBP affects the release of glutamate induced by SP, which facilitates the in vitro release of glutamate in slice preparations containing an excess of K^+.

Maneuf and colleagues (2001) have explained this process. Not only is the antihyperalgesic effect of GBP blocked by D-serine (and, therefore, cycloserine), but persistent activation of the NK_1 receptor by SP removes the Mg^{2+} block of the NMDA-receptor channel (Urban L et al., 1994). This process contributes to postsynaptic central sensitization, as does a presynaptic hyperglutamatergic state.

SP acts presynaptically through the NK_1 receptor, and this action is blocked by GBP (Maneuf YP et al., 2001). The cited article also gives some guidelines (and some reason) for measuring serum GBP levels, which are 80 percent of cortical levels. To block substance P, levels of 30 to 100 micromoles (mM) are required. This range is the same as is therapeutic for the treatment of epilepsy. Pregabalin, the S-(+)-isomer of 3-isobutyl-GABA, has the same effect as GBP in this model. The experiment from which I derived this information was performed on slices of the spinal trigeminal nucleus, impelling me to investigate whether preparation of GBP eyedrops and nose drops is feasible (probably not). GBP has no effect on baseline secretion of glutamate and no effect on acute pain (Taylor CP et al., 1998). The researchers conclude that the GBP "binding site" is the alpha$_2$-delta subunit. How this molecule relates to the K_{ATP} channel must relate to K^+ efflux blocking Ca^{2+} influx. There is certainly clinical overlap with the other agents that act at the K_{ATP} channel, especially minoxidil, which I initially try as 1 percent in PLO and find to be very effective. I shall be trying diazoxide in PLO next.

GBP acts on dorsal horn neurons by stimulating the glycine coagonist site of their NMDA receptors, probably by an allosteric mechanism. It only affects cells in which PKC is elevated. It is analgesic, however, by virtue of its acting only on NMDA receptors synapsing with GABAergic interneurons already excited by injury or inflammation. "A chemical whose effect depends on the state of a receptor molecule will not only give more specific spatial actions, but will be temporally selective for certain cell conditions," conclude Gu and Huang (2001). If these findings are correct, it makes stalking the wily GBP mode of action even more challenging.

ZOLPIDEM

In previous works, I have compared CFS to Parkinson's disease. Zolpidem, as a $GABA_A$ agonist, may selectively suppress overactive neurons in the globus pallidus that might overly inhibit the thalamus and cortex (Farver DK, Khan MH, 2001).

Zolpidem might induce selective inhibition of GABAergic inhibitory neurons in the internal globus pallidus and the substantia nigra pars reticulata. This mechanism should activate both the thalamus, with the supplementary motor area, and the pedunculopontine nucleus with the reticulospinal and vestibulospinal pathways. If so, zolpidem could provide a pharmacological equivalent of posteroventral pallidotomy (Daniele A et al., 1997).

Zolpidem has also treated levodopa-induced dyskinesias. Receptors for this compound are found in the ventral pallidum, SNr, and the thalamus. Zolpidem decreases stress-induced DA release and produces a decrease in DA use in the prefrontal cortex of rats. Because basal ganglia circuitry is largely GABAergic, zolpidem may produce different behavioral results by acting at different areas in the network (Ruzicka E et al., 2000). Zolpidem also relieves catatonia (for about four hours) in a manner similar to the benzodiazepines (Thomas P et al., 1997), and a zopiclone metabolite is undergoing clinical trials in treating anxiety disorders.

LAMOTRIGINE

Lamotrigine (Lamictal) attenuates glutamate release by inhibition of use-dependent Na^+ channels, P-type and N-type Ca^{2+} channels, and effects on K^+ channels. It also increases GABA and is a carbonic anhydrase inhibitor. Lamotrigine may be useful in excitotoxic neuronal degenerative disorders. Lamotrigine, by inhibiting presynaptic glutamate release, can also antagonize the effects of ketamine (Anand A, Charney DS, et al., 2000). I use lamotrigine to reverse glutamate and ketamine in my office. It works much better for this purpose than the glutamate-release inhibitor riluzole (Rilutek). I have tried Parafon Forte (chlorzoxazone), and it works surprisingly well. Other ways to reverse ketamine are with nicotine patches, glutamate nasal spray, pindolol, nicotine, and cholinesterase inhibitors. Honey bee venom can be given in a desperate situation, as can pentazocine (Talwin), dopamine agonists, flumazenil, aminophylline, furosemide, atypical neuroleptics, cycloserine, dynorphin, SP, CGRP, and NGF. I am sure there would be more if I thought harder. In the office, I use lamotrigine first, then tacrine, and then cycloserine. Ketamine makes some people jittery. This effect can be prevented by clonidine and reversed by BZDs. Ketamine can be prepared in a transdermal gel that has an onset in two to three minutes. It works in 1 second by eyedrops, 10 seconds by nose drops, and 15 seconds by oral swirl. Ketamine may be given p.o. t.i.d. in doses of 10 to 100 mg (as high as I go). It has more adverse reactions and is not as effective this way, probably because sufficiently high brain levels are not achieved. I guess someone somewhere has been addicted to ketamine, but I have not seen addiction after giving this drug at least 1,000 times, usually in a dose of 50 mg in 500 ml normal saline over three hours. Controlling the rate usually controls the ADRs. I do not usually give IV ketamine more than weekly, but the dose and administration must be adjusted to the clinical needs of the patient. I allow the use of 1:10 to 1:1 ketamine nasal spray, up to every four hours. Such a regimen has kept hopeless patients functional. Ketamine may be combined in the same IV bag with lidocaine, ascorbate, $MgSO_4$, and Ca gluconate. It is my treatment of choice in the office management of acute suicidal depression. Lidocaine is almost tied with ketamine for effectiveness in neurosomatic disorders and can be used daily if necessary, by the IV route. I wrote a section on IV lidocaine in *Betrayal*. Patients who respond to lidocaine will often respond to Talwin, TRH, lamotrigine, Topamax, nicotine, Mexitil (not often enough), hydergine, dopaminergic agents, pindolol, stimulants, Wellbutrin, reboxetine, Zantac, amantadine, AEDs, cholinesterase inhibitors, oxytocin, TRH, and lidocaine 20 percent subcutaneously.

The dose of IV lidocaine is 5 mg/kg over two to three hours as tolerated (only minimal side effects). The dose of subcutaneous lidocaine is 5 mg/kg. I have seen too many patients, who had a good response to lidocaine infused in my office over two to three hours, receive the full IV dose in 30 minutes elsewhere. The rapid infusion is usually quite unpleasant, and, typically, the patient will never respond to lidocaine again.

PENTAZOCINE (TALWIN)

Talwin was originally thought to be an opioid but is now recognized to be a sigma$_1$ agonist. There are also sigma$_2$ ligands that appear to be anxiolytic without inducing sedation and withdrawal anxiogenesis (Sanchez C et al., 1997). Sigma ligands are not antagonized by NTX. Sigma ligands do not bind to the PCP site in the pore of the NMDA receptor and are distinct from such compounds as ketamine. Haloperidol is an antagonist at the sigma$_1$ site, which may have several subtypes. Pentazocine antagonizes ketamine, as do pindolol and lamotrigine.

Sigma$_1$ receptors have neuromodulatory effects on the cholinergic and glutamatergic systems. In some situations they may potentiate NMDA-evoked activity at CA3 hippocampal neurons or stimulate NE release. My experience is that they function more as NMDA partial antagonists, and as such have been found to have neuroprotective effects against NMDA-induced excitotoxicity. DHEA and pregnenolone are anxiolytic in some situations. This anxiolysis is thought to be mediated by the sigma$_1$ receptor (Noda et al., 2000). DHEA and pregnenolone may be metabolized in the brain into anxiolytic compounds.

OXYTOCIN

I've never had the wrong kind [of orgasm]. My worst one was right on the money.

Woody Allen (1979)
Manhattan

Oxytocin is a nonapeptide (nine amino acids) used in general medical practice to enhance uterine contractions during labor. It also causes milk ejection from the nipple in a nursing mother. I use oxytocin routinely in my practice, which does not include obstetrics. Because one of my goals in writing this piece is to illustrate the theory and practice of neurosomatic medicine, I would like to use the patient who has a beneficial response to systemically administered oxytocin as an example.

I first review the mechanisms to stimulate, or simulate, the effect of OXT. These include the following:

1. Alpha$_2$ agonists (Diaz-Cabale Z et al., 2000)
2. Alpha$_1$ agonists, only after a noxious stimulus (Onaka T, 2000)
3. NO agonists or antagonists (Kadekaro M, Summy-Long JY, 2000); however, no antagonists are available for use clinically yet, except possibly dantrolene
4. Estrogen, with or without progesterone—or testosterone
5. GABA$_A$-receptor antagonists (Onaka T, 2000)
6. NMDA-receptor agonists (glutamate stimulates OXT secretion)
7. Naltrexone (morphine inhibits OXT secretion) (Li J et al., 2001)

8. Increasing allopregnenolone, either with natural progestone or flu-oxetine, which I hardly ever use
9. Cycloserine, an NMDA/glycine agonist and somewhat of an indirect opioid antagonist
10. Buspirone (Serres F et al., 2000)
11. Lamotrigine, riluzole, and chlorzoxazone because OXT presynap-tically inhibits glutamate secretion (Pittman QJ et al., 2000)

I would try lamotrigine first, because it is much less expensive than riluzole and does not require periodic liver-function tests. Patients are much less concerned about developing a rash than a liver problem. If the patient has previously responded to lidocaine, then lamotrigine (Lamictal) would also be a good choice. Its effect can be immediate or may take six weeks until the average daily dose for bipolar responders (278 mg) is reached. Lidocaine also inhibits glutamate release. Chlorzoxazone, although inexpensive, is less effective than lamotrigine.

If the patient is hypertensive, anxious, has ADHD, or experiences night-mares, guanfacine would be a good choice. If perimenopausal or low in tes-tosterone, hormonal therapy would be helpful. Such patients usually have a good response to nitroglycerin, the active form of which is nitric oxide. Or-gasm centrally requires estrogen or testosterone, NO, OXT, and norepi-nephrine, plus a little dopamine acting at D_1 receptors. Arousal requires DA, OXT, testosterone, and NO. Testosterone induces NO synthesis, which then stimulates DA release in the medial preoptic nucleus, which facilitates arousal and penile erection. Oxytocin is required for penile erection. The thoracolumbar spinal cord provides innervation to the sympathetic chain. Lumbar nerves innervate the corpus cavernosum of the penis. OXT is trans-ported from the paraventricular hypothalamic nucleus to the pro-erectile thoracolumbar spinal cord (Veronneau-Longueville F et al., 1999), in which binding sites (in the rat) are numerous and diffuse. Both sympathetic and parasympathetic preganglionic neurons are labeled, but primarily sympa-thetic ones. It should be obvious why neurosomatic male patients, who have NE-dependent ejaculation-related processes, commonly relapse for up to a week after having sex. Because DA is depleted after ejaculation, there is a marked increase in central prolactin concentration, thought to account for the refractory period after orgasm in men (Exton MS et al., 2001). Large volumes of NE are secreted in several areas, including the hypothalamus, thoracolumbar cord, and during intromission and ejaculation (Meston CM, Frohlich PF, 2000). Peripheral mechanisms of erection, ejaculation, and their pharmacotherapy are fairly well understood (Bivalacqua TJ et al., 2001).

Serotonin receptors are found on OXT neurons, and serotonin-reuptake inhibitors can inhibit the ability to ejaculate by decreasing the sensitivity of these receptors. As males reach the threshold for ejaculation, OXT is released from the posterior pituitary in a pulsatile manner. The ability of the DA to stimulate ejaculation can be blocked by an OXT antagonist (Cantor JM et al., 1999). OXT is the best way to reverse SRI-induced ejaculatory dysfunction and increase NE levels. Sexual arousal in males as seen on PET is associated with activation of the bilateral temporal regions, the right insular and inferior frontal cortex, and the left anterior cingulate (Stolero S et al., 1999).

Oxytocin sometimes makes neurosomatic women multiorgasmic, often for the first time. Gonadotropin-releasing hormone is also involved in the sexual response, but its secretion is pulsatile and would not be mimicked by nafarelin (Synarel), although I have not tested nafarelin in sexually active males. GnRH in the form of Synarel does not alter sexual behavior after acute and subchronic administration in healthy young males (Perras B et al., 2001). There is no effect acutely, and after 21 days only an increase in the ability for focused attention or motor task perseveration is noted.

The easiest way to antagonize the $GABA_A$ receptor is with furosemide (Lasix). Its duration of action as a diuretic (about 3 hours) has no relation to its $GABA_A$ antagonism (24 to 48 hours). It should be used with caution in people with anxiety disorders. Twenty mg is usually sufficient (the lowest-dose tablet). Flumazenil is very costly but may be effective in about 10 seconds in the form of a 1:10 to 1:1 nasal spray.

A simple method to stimulate the NMDA receptor is with cholinesterase inhibitors. Several of them are used in the treatment of Alzheimer's disease. Other effective NMDA agonists are cycloserine (a glycine-site coagonist), a nicotine patch, and pindolol. There are other techniques, but it should not be necessary to consider them in the usual clinical situation. If rapid stimulation is required, glutamate nasal spray 1:25 → 1:1 is often effective.

Because OXT secretion is inhibited by mu-opioid agonists, naltrexone is a good way to stimulate it. Unfortunately, naltrexone cannot be targeted solely to oxytocinergic neurons and is infrequently used on a chronic basis in neurosomatic medicine. Many patients are exquisitely sensitive to it, perhaps because their endogenous opioids are decreased, at least in peripheral blood. Opioids often help neurosomatic symptoms, and each opioid has slightly different properties. There are multiple mu_1-opioid receptors and splice variants, which makes it sensible to combine or rotate them (Pasternak GW, 2001).

OPIOIDS

There are several distinct families of opioids and their receptors. The endogenous opioid peptides include the enkephalins, the dynorphins, the endomorphins (mu-opioid agonists), and beta-endorphin. They act through three classes of receptors: mu, delta, and kappa. Most opioids in clinical use act at the mu receptor(s). The kappa receptor, highly specific for dynorphin A, an NMDA agonist, can produce psychotomimesis and dysphoria and is increased after running. Dynorphins may have a role in producing neurosomatic symptoms. Oxycodone (Percocet, Oxycontin) is a partial kappa agonist that can synergize with pure mu-opioid agonists. Delta-receptor agonists are still experimental except for clonidine. Its alpha$_{2/3}$ receptor effects are inhibited by a delta-receptor antagonist (Gyires R et al., 2000). Methadone has the unique property of being a mu-opioid agonist, an NMDA-receptor antagonist, and a serotonin-reuptake inhibitor. A fourth opioid receptor was cloned by several groups in 1994. Its endogenous ligand is orphanin FQ, also known as nociceptin (OFQ/N). This receptor is not clinically important at present. It has been found to enhance DA release in the striatum (Konija H et al., 1998) and, perhaps, to have anxiolytic effects. Kappa agonists have an action opposite of cocaine (Thompson AC et al., 2000) on dopamine uptake by the nucleus accumbens and may actually *induce* pain and other neurosomatic symptoms (Vanderah TW et al., 2001), in part by inducing the release of SP and CGRP.

Potentiating opioid effect is frequently desirable because adverse reactions are often dose related. Interestingly, the hedonic effects of morphine can be dissociated from its analgesic properties by using an SP antagonist. Such a combination should greatly reduce the chance of addiction (Hunt SP, Mantyh PW, 2001).

Opioids have a stimulatory effect on many neurosomatic patients. This stimulatory effect is associated with increased hedonia and, perhaps, increased motivational salience. Patients with fibromyalgia are more likely to experience a stimulatory effect from opioids than are patients without fibromyalgia. This observation may be because fibromyalgia patients have elevated levels of substance P in their cerebrospinal fluid, while patients with CFS without fibromyalgia do not (Murtra P et al., 2000).

Rats who lack the substance P (NK1) receptor have a much-reduced reward from opiates. This reduction is not related to expression of dopamine receptors nor to the density of mu-opioid receptors. Substance P receptor knock-out mice, however, do not have an increase in Fos-B positive neurons in both the core and shell zones of the nucleus accumbens, as do wild-type mice. These results of Fos-B activation may be linked to the expression of opiate-dependent reward and suggest that a *synapse* occurs between collaterals of SP-releasing populations of VTA projection neurons and large cholinergic neurons of the nucleus accumbens and nucleus basalis that express the NK1 receptor. These neurons are implicated in associative learning and respond to stimuli that trigger a learned and rewarded task. They also participate in opioid-mediated sexual arousal. Substance P is often elevated by stress, and, although experiments in treating pain with substance P antagonists have not been particularly positive, it is highly likely that substance P antagonists will be effective antidepressants and may also deal with other stress-related syndromes. All existing antidepressants antagonize SP.

The only currently available fairly "clean" SP-receptor antagonist is lidocaine. This agent is certainly one of the most effective medications I use in the treatment of neurosomatic disorders.

One caveat in prescribing opioids: Methadone inhibits the ability of other mu-opioids to decrease forskolin-induced adenyl cyclase activation. This effect of methadone apparently occurs via activation of PKC. Also, methadone, but not morphine, causes a desensitization of the delta-opioid receptor (Liu JG et al., 1999). Methadone should probably not be prescribed with other opioids, although in my practice it is the opioid of choice. It has mu- and delta-agonist actions, is an NMDA antagonist, and is an SRI. Unfortunately, rotation of methadone with morphine does not work. Methadone patients are cross-tolerant to the antinociceptive effects of morphine (Doverty M et al., 2001). Amazingly, they are also hyperalgesic to some stimuli, e.g., the cold pressor test. I cannot recall any patient who had increased pain after methadone. I shall specifically inquire henceforth.

Among the numerous opioid augmentation techniques (e.g., NMDA antagonists of all sorts, cannabinoids, clonidine, tricyclics, gabapentin, minoxidil, venlafaxine, atypical neuroleptics, to name a few that come to mind) is ultra-low-dose NTX, 20 picograms per day. Two of my patients had withdrawal symptoms even at this dose and are now taking femtogram amounts, almost homeopathic at this dilution. Ultra-low-dose NTX is not usually beneficial but is harmless and worth a try, as is low-dose NTX for intractable pruritus refractory to antihistamines (almost always effective) 2 to 5 mg per day (Schmelz M, 2001). This dose of NTX at bedtime may stimulate daytime secretion of endogenous opioids. Low-dose naloxone, 0.5 to 3 mg per day, may be used for opioid-induced constipation. These doses of oral naloxone are often useful in treatment-refractory constipation, such as that seen in severe irritable bowel syndrome. For intractable diarrhea, if all else fails, one can try Sandostatin (octreotide). It is important to keep the dose of opioid antagonist below the threshold of significant inhibition of endogenous opioids, which have numerous other physiologic effects beyond analgesia, including stimulating behavior, anxiolysis, acting as antidepressants, regulating maternal and sexual behavior, and acting at (usually) inhibitory opioid receptors on other neurons. Endogenous opioid levels are reduced in many neurosomatic patients with enhanced sensation of pain (Lembo T et al., 2000). NTX can produce panic attacks (Maremanni I et al., 1998). Naltrexone has been advocated for the treatment of dissociative symptoms in patients with borderline personality disorder (BPD) (Bohus MJ et al., 1999). I have used this agent many times in such patients, never with a positive result and usually provoking anxiety, depression, pain, and feelings of unreality. Bohus and colleagues report that at least "three days of treatment are required before any effects were reported," with a dose of 25 to 100 mg q.i.d. Nine patients were treated. All nine reported a decrease ("marked reduction") in dissociative symptoms. My totally opposite clinical experience may be related to the absence of stress-induced analgesia in my patients, which occurs during fear, not anxiety. Opioid activity is low in individuals with BPD (Pickar D et al., 1982). The authors suggested BPD patients might have increased sensitivity of kappa-opioid receptors with stress-induced activation of the endogenous opioid system favoring increased levels of dynorphin. This way of explaining the pathophysiology of BPD sounds very reasonable to me. Initially, some of the experimental patients "experience more difficulty coping with intense sensations" at the onset of NTX treatment. "Unless patients are assisted in coping with their altered perception, an increased incidence of suicide in this patient population may occur" (Bohus MJ et al., 1999).

Hypothetically, fluoxetine (Prozac) should stimulate OXT because it increases the production of allopregnanolone, a GABAergic neurosteroid. It is even marketed as a PMS-preventing product to be taken for two weeks after ovulation (Sarafem); however, it has not helped any of my PMS patients. Similarly, melatonin stimulates oxytocin secretion, although few of the several types of melatonin receptors (which ultimately act by stimulating protein kinase C) are found on the magnocellular neurons of the supraoptic and paraventricular nuclei of the posterior hypothalamus. There is potential for considerable synaptic plasticity in oxytocin neurons, and more neuronal inputs are received at times of heightened activity, for example, parturition and nursing. These neurons manufacture oxytocin, which is bound to proteins called "neurophysins" and transmitted down two tracts to the posterior pituitary, where it enters capillaries.

As might be expected, the highest density of melatonin receptors is found in the suprachiasmatic nucleus (SCN), which regulates circadian rhythms.

Opioid antagonists can also decrease the effects of diazepam (Swift R et al., 1998) and nicotine (Brever LH et al., 1999) and may find occasional use in treatment-refractory depression (Amiaz R et al., 1999). They have an approved use for alcohol addiction and are often prescribed for self-injurious behavior, particularly in the developmentally disabled. NTX plus fluoxetine enhances retention rates in a naltrexone-only treatment for narcotic addicts (Landoboso MA et al., 1998).

OXYTOCIN, HYPOTHALAMIC FUNCTION, AND CIRCADIAN RHYTHMS

The paraventricular nucleus has been considered by some to be the primary stress response-integrating nucleus in the hypothalamus (Figure 66). The medial preoptic nucleus may supersede the stress-regulatory functions of the PVN in neurosomatic patients with (possibly) decreased CRH levels (Altemus M et al., 2001). The PVN regulates much of the sympathetic outflow to the thoracolumbar cord, with OXT participating, as well as CRH, vasopressin (VPR), SS, enkephalin (ENK), POMC, and atrial natriuretic factor (ANF). They all seem to use the same pathway. Ascending fibers are both peptidergic (CRH, VPR, OXT SS, ENK, VIP) and catecholaminergic (Palkovits M, 1999). The PVN sends noradrenergic afferents to $beta_3$ receptors in white fat, may increase caloric expenditure, and perhaps transform some white fat to brown fat, which radiates excess calories as heat. The use of OXT as an antiobesity agent is not established, however. It currently appears that the best way to lose weight is increasing the activity of one of the NE-regulated uncoupling proteins that uncouples mitochondrial activity from caloric intake (Figure 67). One could then eat much more and still stay thin, especially if one were a nonhuman primate (Diano S et al., 2000). Nonhuman primates with increased activity of such a protein can eat much more than controls and not become obese (Diano S et al., 2000). CRH analogs and melanin-concentrating hormone are promising antiobesity candidates, as are GnRH and OXT (Havel PJ, 2000). Other such substances include glucagon-like peptide-2 (Tang-Christensen M et al., 2000) and inhibitors of acetyl-CoA carboxylase 2 (Abu-Elheiga L et al., 2001).

The only other areas aside from the SCN in which melatonin receptors are located are the anterior pituitary pars tuberalis and the midline thalamic nuclei. The melatonin receptors are very specific and have a high affinity for melatonin. Melatonin, "the hormone of darkness," is manufactured in the pineal gland from serotonin in a simple two-step process. The tonic secretion of melatonin is inhibited by light acting on retinal cones.

There are direct glutamatergic projections to the SCN and *intergeniculate leaflet* (IGL), a small, ventral projection of the lateral geniculate nucleus of the thalamus. The IGL sends axons secreting GABA and neuropeptide Y to the core of the SCN (Figure 68). The SCN has a shell as well, like the nucleus accumbens (Figure 69), but knowing the functional neuroanatomy of the SCN has not thus far enhanced the efficacy of my therapeutic interventions. The NAc shell is part of the "extended amygdala," which also includes the bed nucleus of the stria terminalis and the central nucleus of the amygdala (Figure 15). I believe the IGL is more likely to be dysfunctional than the retinohypothalamic tract, since it is also nonphotically regulated, e.g., by feeding times or activity (Figure 70). The phase delay (sleepy in the daytime, more awake at night) of neurosomatic disorders is not altered by phototherapy. Melatonin is usually ineffective, even though it stimulates OXT secretion. Serotonin neurons of the midbrain dorsal raphe densely innervate the SCN core and have an effect opposite to melatonin afferents. 5-HT neurons to the SCN may be the dominant regulatory input in neurosomatic patients. The SCN innervates the sympathetic superior cervical ganglion, which then innervates the pineal, stimulating melatonin production by two-step enzymatic conversion from serotonin. Because most neurosomatic patients have a degree of dysautonomia, pineal innervation is probably dysregulated. Circadian oscillators in the cortex may also play a role. I discuss these ahead.

VPR and OXT are differentially secreted in stressful situations depending on the social context. In a social defeat situation, VPR is secreted widely throughout the brain, while OXT is increased primarily in the septum and the hypothalamus as well as in the general circulation. Thus, the secretion of the two hormones in behavioral situations is regulated independently (Insel TR, Young LJ, 2001). Further fine-tuning occurs when OXT is released after (1) CCK elevation and (2) a noxious stimulus, resulting in adenosine's acting at the facilitory A_2 receptor and releasing NE. Adenosine, acting at the A_1 receptor, also releases NE. Facilitation of the VPR response after noxious stimuli is DA mediated. Conditioned fear or novelty releases OXT and not VPR. A predictable stimulus does not produce DA release. The conditioned fear response attenuates as NE is depleted or if NE antagonists are administered (Onaka T, 2000). Even though rats are not people, their brains are quite similar to ours, and the results of this experiment fit well into the model developed in this book.

The primary neurotransmitter producing oxytocin release is glutamate, acting on both NMDA and non-NMDA receptors. Glutamate secretion is inhibited presynaptically by mu- and delta-opioid receptors (Ostermeier AM et al., 2000). Estrogen acts at the oxytocinergic NMDA receptor to release OXT. OXT may act as a retrograde transmitter to decrease secretion from glutamatergic neurons. $GABA_A$ receptors on OXT neurons reduce OXT secretion, while OXT receptors on GABA neurons reduce GABA secretion. OXT receptors on the VMH promote sexual activity, while DA-regulated tonic OXT expression in the central nucleus of the amygdala is anxiolytic but supposedly has no effect on sexual behavior.

Rat oxytocin neurons produce five of the many rat synaptic GABA$_A$-receptor subunits. Subunit composition can determine channel kinetics, i.e., how rapidly and for how long does the hyperpolarizing inhibitory chloride channel stay open to allow chloride ions to enter the cell? Pregnant rats demonstrate *subunit switching* to achieve the necessary *synaptic plasticity* for the inhibition of their OXT neurons. Synaptic plasticity describes the ability of individual synapses to alter the strength of their transmission. These are reversible changes that can occur in the adult brain and have been studied most intensely at the NMDA receptor. OXT neurons in the pregnant rat change the ratio of alpha$_1$/alpha$_2$ GABA$_A$ subunits during pregnancy to favor alpha$_1$, which allows more chloride ion through the pore. Neurosteroids facilitate this process. At the onset of labor, OXT neurons become less inhibited, and increased OXT secretion promotes uterine contractions. We shall increasingly recognize subunit switching as an important aspect of synaptic plasticity in other neurons as well (Brussard AB, Herbison AE, 2000).

Vasopressin and OXT are lately viewed as acting similar to classical neurotransmitters. Both can affect neuronal excitability by opening nonspecific cationic channels or by closing K$^+$ channels (Raggenbass M, 2001).

Another possible cause for a delayed sleep-wake cycle concerns VPR and GABA. VPR is stimulatory to most neurons and when secreted by the SCN increases GnRH release from the MPOA (Figure 71) but decreases corticosterone production via the PVN through the ANS, going directly to the adrenal cortex and bypassing CRH and ACTH. VPR seems to be secreted in excess. Many VPR neurons from the SCN also contain GABA. Thus, GABA inhibits autonomic afferents to the pineal and also inhibits daytime melatonin secretion. In a hyperglutamatergic state, neurosomatic patients may resemble nocturnal animals more than diurnal ones and contain increased glutamate instead of GABA in SCN terminals, shortening the phase of surrounding nuclei that maintain a sympathetic/parasympathetic balance (Buijs RM, Kalsbeck A, 2001; Figure 72).

The diffusible messenger that functions as an output molecule of the SCN circadian clock may have been identified. *Prokineticin 2* is an 81-amino acid protein which had previously been identified as a regulator of gastrointestinal movements. It is regularly secreted in the SCN of mice, and its expression is activated by the illumination of the retina (Hastings MH, 2002; Cheng MY et al., 2002). The prokineticin 2 receptor (PK2R) is found in all of the neuroanatomically defined SCN targets. PK2 functions to signal daytime, and mRNA for this small protein is also found in the NAc shell, MPOA, and islands of Calleja. The only area of oscillation in the concentration of PK2 is the SCN, however. Daytime levels are at least fifty times greater than nighttime levels, when PK2 is virtually undetectable. Tuning the levels of PK2 should have profound implication for neurosomatic disorders.

OTHER EFFECTS OF OXYTOCIN

The effect of OXT that has received the most attention in the past decade has involved social bonding. Oxytocin and related peptides are termed "amnesic" in one context because they activate inhibitory interneurons in the hippocampus, the structure most involved in making new memories. This behavior is particularly noted on investigation of stranger mice. Two hours later, the mouse acts as if the stranger mouse is unknown to him or her. This behavior may be related to the anxiolytic activity of OXT in some species. If the stranger mouse is not viewed as threatening, there is much less motivation to remember it. If memory is eroded, it occurs through $alpha_2$ receptors in the olfactory bulb. I have not noticed OXT to impair memory in my patients. Intranuclear OXT is secreted via $alpha_1$ adrenergic or H_1 and H_2 receptors. Alpha blockade decreases histamine-induced OXT release.

OXT, acting at the periventricular hypothalamic nucleus, induces mating ("lordosis") behavior in estrogen-primed female rodents. One of them, the prairie vole, mates for life with its male partner. This behavior is unusual among animals, since male and female promiscuity is the norm. Such affiliation is thought to be due to the reward influences of both DA and NE (acting at the beta receptor) which helps to induce a very powerful memory of an event that is novel, rewarding, or threatening, called a "flashbulb" memory (Hartfield T, McGaugh JL, 1999). A familiar example of a flashbulb memory to almost all members of my generation would be what they were doing when they heard President Kennedy was shot. For my parents, it may have been FDR's death or the bombing of Pearl Harbor. John Lennon's death is often cited by those younger. For most adults alive in 2001, the World Trade Center bombings in New York City may always be remembered. I hate to cite morbid flashbulb memories, but enjoyable ones are too variable to be attributed to an entire generation. For newborn chicks, it is their mother (imprinting).

Oxytocin is also involved in mother-child bonding. It induces breast ductal tissue to contract, ejecting milk while nursing. OXT secreted into the brain activates the ventral tegmental area, which secretes dopamine into the nucleus accumbens, the primary area in the brain involved in anticipation of reward, as well as by thoughts and feelings about the reward after it occurs. The nucleus accumbens also fires if the expected reward does not occur, but to a lesser degree. Oxytocin is viewed by some, perhaps simplistically, as the "hormone of affiliation" (Insel TR, Young LJ, 2001).

OXT is also analgesic, particularly during parturition (labor and delivery) (Petersson M et al., 1996). It is another of several analgesic substances that act by a nonopioid mechanism; i.e., it is not naloxone reversible.

OXT binds to other sites in stimulating maternal behavior at parturition. These include the paraventricular nucleus of the hypothalamus, the bed nucleus of the stria terminalis, and a neural network regulating maternal behavior in the ventromedial hypothalamus (VMH). Oxytocin facilitates social learning only. Motherhood involves the (1) medial preoptic area, perhaps the key hypothalamic structure in neurosomatic disorders; (2) the overlying bed nucleus of the stria terminalis, an amygdala projection; and (3) the ventral tegmental area, which secretes dopamine for the NAc, mesolimbic, and mesocortical tracts. Prolactin stimulates maternal care and nest building while OXT facilitates the onset of maternal care, involving inhibition of the normal aversion to neonatal odors by the olfactory bulb. Prairie voles are monogamous for life and release OXT when they mate. Injection of OXT has the same effect on two prairie voles who do not have the opportunity to mate. D_2 receptors in the NAc are involved in this partner preference, which appears to use the same hedonic pathways as stimulant drugs. NAc dopamine receptors use dopamine pathways associated with reinforcement.

Oxytocin receptors (OTRs) have region-specific functions and regulation. In the VMH, estrogen-dependent expression of OTRs requires PKC and modulates sexual behavior in female rats but has no effect on anxiety. In contrast, in the central nucleus of the amygdala, induction of OTRs is controlled by tonic secretion of DA through activation of PKA. OXT in this area has anxiolytic properties but does not affect female sexual behavior. Different signal transduction pathways can determine effects of ligand-receptor interaction (Bale TL et al., 2001).

Oxytocin decreases feeding behavior and increases satiety (Diaz-Cabale Z, Narvaez JA, et al., 2000). OXT is antagonized by alpha$_2$ agonists and facilitated by 5-HT$_{1A}$ agonists. Buspirone, a 5-HT$_{1A}$ agonist, is also effective at the SCN, and the primary metabolite of buspirone, 1-PP, is an alpha$_2$ antagonist, similar to yohimbine.

It is thought that most of the actions of buspirone occur through 1-PP. Both 5-HT$_{1A}$ and alpha$_2$ agonists could reduce feeding. The recently introduced atypical neuroleptic ziprasidone (Geodon) has the highest 5-HT$_{1A}$ affinity of any known substance. Geodon has produced mania in three patients and anxiety in two or three others. Because I am not aware that Geodon produces the alpha$_2$ antagonist 1-PP, I assume its anxiogenic and mania-inducing properties are due to its very strong 5-HT$_{1A}$ agonism plus 5-HT$_2$ antagonism. I find Geodon to be the most useful atypical neuroleptic. It has few adverse reactions and does not cause weight gain. It is rapidly effective, sometimes on the first dose, and may ameliorate neurosomatic symptoms.

Oxytocin can be delivered in several ways: by a compounded nasal spray, a compounded 10 unit wax-matrix tablet, or a 10 unit vial for daily injection mixed with 0.5 ml of lidocaine so it won't sting very much.

Oxytocin and vasopressin, available most conveniently as DDAVP 0.2 mg tablets, are closely related polypeptides manufactured in the same hypothalamic nuclei. Their actions are usually antagonistic, however. If a patient has an adverse reaction to oxytocin that exacerbates chronic symptoms, DDAVP 0.1 mg daily will occasionally be an effective treatment.

Candidates for a good response to OXT include those who are benefitted by DA eyedrops or nasal spray, hydergine, nitroglycerin, lidocaine, noradrenergic agents, and glutamatergic agonists. TRH responders often respond to OXT because they both release intracellular Ca^{2+}. I can often predict fairly accurately who will respond to what medication just by noting which drugs they had taken prior to their initial visit with me and whether they had a beneficial or an adverse response to them.

Oxytocin is a stress hormone. In stressed male rats OXT is released only in the CNS, not peripherally. OXT acts through integrative networks, converging on the paraventricular nucleus, from which corticotropin-releasing hormone is also secreted. OXT inhibits CRH (Engelmann M et al., 1999). It also has nonopioid analgesic effects (Kang YS, Park JH, 2000). Because CRH may not be particularly elevated in neurosomatic disorders, the MPOA may influence the PVN more than it usually does.

Oxytocin is the drug of choice for pervasive developmental disorder spectrum illnesses. These include autism, Asperger syndrome, and social and emotional (nonverbal) learning disorder. These illnesses involve "theory of mind," an inability to conceive of what another person might be thinking or (especially) feeling. It is similar to having a lack of empathy or social affiliation. It therefore follows that OXT and functionally related substances (especially NE-reuptake inhibitors) would improve PDD spectrum disorders—and they do. The effect is fairly immediate. Vagal nerve stimulation holds promise.

MODAFINIL (PROVIGIL)

Modafinil is a recently marketed drug recommended as a treatment of narcolepsy, for which it is well suited. The research literature in the first three years after its introduction was ambiguous about its mode of action. I suspected it was an NMDA agonist. Modafinil is taken once a day in the morning, although some patients complain of its wearing off too soon and take it twice daily. Its half-life is eight to twelve hours.

Rats will not self-administer modafinil, so it is not classed as an abusable substance. I find its efficacy to be one notch below Adderall, one and a half notches below Dexedrine, two notches below Ritalin (methylphenidate), and probably superior to pemoline (Cylert). Beta-blockers may be added if necessary and can augment the result. Modafinil may be combined with other stimulants, NE-reuptake inhibitors, Tasmar, desipramine, midodrine, tranylcypromine (safely), and any other antidepressant or mood stabilizer.

Modafinil binds to the dopamine transporter in a manner similar to methylphenidate and, to a slightly lesser extent, amphetamine. This effect, as with a dopamine-reuptake inhibitor, prolongs the action of secreted DA (Wisor JP et al., 2001). Modafinil also binds to the tuberomammillary nucleus, which secretes the excitatory transmitter histamine, and to orexin (hypocretin-Hcrt) neurons in the perifornical area of the hypothalamus. Hcrt neurons project excitatory inputs to sympathetic ganglia, especially the LC, and thereby increase the secretion of NE. Hcrt neurons are absent in some narcoleptic and hypersomnic families and may have decreased activity in many narcoleptics (Scammell TE et al., 2001).

An interesting aspect of modafinil's pharmacology is that it might have neuroprotective effects as well as antiparkinson effects in MPTP (1-methyl-4-phenyl-1,2,3,6-tetrahydropyridine)-treated animals. Modafinil is a neuroprotectant in striatal ischemia. At the highest dose in rats it completely reverses MPTP-induced neural toxicity in the nigrostriatal dopaminergic system. When given prophylactically, it prevents MPTP-induced neurodegeneration.

Modafinil (Provigil) somewhat surprisingly raises 5-HT levels in the rat frontal cortex (Ferraro L et al., 2000). The effects of modafinil are more pronounced when an SRI is used. Fenfluramine causes more 5-HT release, but it is neurotoxic and no longer available. In the presence of a 5-HT$_{1A}$ agonist, modafinil has no effect on 5-HT release, demonstrating that its mode of action is electroneurosecretory coupling via mechanisms that do not involve the reuptake process in its 5-HT-enhancing effect.

Modafinil also has a noradrenergic effect that can be antagonized by clonidine, an alpha$_{2ABC}$ agonist. It antagonizes most typical and atypical neuroleptics except raclopride. In my practice I find that atypical neuroleptics reliably antagonize modafinil; modafinil, as a dopamine agonist, synergizes with apomorphine, which is also a DA agonist (Sebban C et al., 1999).

Neurons containing the neuropeptide Hcrt are located exclusively in the lateral hypothalamus and send axons to major nuclei in the brain, including those involved in sleep production. Modafinil activates Hcrt-containing neurons. Hcrt helps to regulate sleep and wakefulness, and Hcrt knock-out mice (they don't make Hcrt) are a model of human narcolepsy, a disorder primarily of REM sleep dysregulation. The narcoleptic tetrad consists of (1) sleep attacks with immediate dreaming; (2) cataplexy, loss of muscle tone when feeling strong emotions; (3) hypnagogic (falling asleep) and hypnopompic (waking up) hallucinations, usually visual, a continuation of the visual aspects of dreams into the waking state; and (4) sleep paralysis—while falling asleep or waking up, an individual can't move a muscle. This terrifying experience may last 5 to 10 minutes. In addition, (5) there may be a feeling of a "presence" in the room as a patient is falling asleep—a tetrad plus one.

Modafinil also increases cortical activation as seen on EEG. Thus, modafinil acts like a somewhat different form of stimulant. It releases 5-HT, but so does cocaine. It should probably not be used in patients with NE and DA intolerance, e.g., panic disorder, until the panic disorder is well controlled. It can synergize with antidepressants, particularly those with noradrenergic activity, and does not seem to cause panic attacks in patients who have never had them previously, as yohimbine can. It is *not* an effective treatment for ADHD but has a niche in neurosomatic medicine, primarily as an add-on to those who have had ADRs to sympatholytics and typical neuroleptics. It mixes fairly well with ketamine, lidocaine, TRH, pentazocine, OXT, hydergine, amantadine, midodrine, tolcapone, yohimbine, high-dose Effexor (to get the NE effect), DA eyedrops and nasal spray, BuSpar via 1-PP, and intravenous amantadine. It is usually not necessary to exceed 400 mg q.d. Adverse reactions are few and are often dose related. They include disorder of initiative and maintaining sleep (DIMS), dysphoria, nausea, tachycardia, elevated blood pressure, and paradoxical sleepiness, especially in a neurosomatic population, who is more apt to fall asleep from a stimulant than to become more alert and energetic by about five to two.

VENTROLATERAL PREOPTIC NUCLEUS (VLPO)

In considering narcolepsy and the rapid changes in behavioral states between wakefulness and sleep, I shall discuss a recent article by Clifford B. Saper and associates (2001). Saper, a neurologist at Harvard, is unusual in that he has strong academic credentials and has written scholarly articles of interest to the practicing clinician conversant with neurobiology.

Saper believes in some forms of the ascending reticular activating system. I have discussed its basic mode of action when considering arousal receptors in sleep. He notes the division of the ARAS into a projection that innervates the thalamus and one that goes to the hypothalamus. Recall that arousal-promoting neurons are noradrenergic (from the LC), serotonergic (from the dorsal raphe), and histaminergic, from the tuberomammillary nucleus (TMN) (see Figure 73). All three groups (in normals) nearly stop firing in REM sleep. Axons from the ventrolateral preoptic nucleus are surrounded by a more diffuse extension from the nucleus, termed the "extended" VLPO. These axons densely innervate the TMN, as well as the dorsal and median raphe nucleus (5-HT) and the LC. VLPO neurons make lesser contact with cholinergic arousal systems that project more to the thalamus, i.e., the pedunculopontine and laterodorsal tegmental nuclei (PPT-LDT).

Nearly 80 percent of the retrogradely labeled VLPO neurons contain both the GABA-synthesizing enzyme glutamic acid decarboxylase and the neuropeptide galanin, both of which are inhibitory. The VLPO nucleus regulates non-REM sleep, while the extended VLPO regulates REM (see Figures 72 and 73).

The relationship between VLPO and monoaminergic cell groups has been termed "flip-flop" (Figure 74). Because it would not promote survival of a mammal to be half awake and half asleep, when one side is firing briskly, the other side is inhibited. Increasing sleep pressure might gradually shift the relative balance of mutual inhibition. When the pressure becomes great enough, a flip-flop occurs, producing a rapid change in firing patterns. This sort of network, or loop, is described as "bistable." If the VLPO is dysfunctional, sleep and wake drive are weaker and produce more wake and sleep bouts, causing narcolepsy.

Orexin/hypocretin neurons in the lateral hypothalamus innervate all components of the ascending arousal system, including the cerebral cortex (Figure 75). Orexin neurons stimulate the neurons more toward wakefulness. In the absence of orexin, and with a dysfunctional VLPO, there would be earlier and more frequent transitions into REM sleep, which is what occurs in narcolepsy (Saper CB et al., 2001). I have devoted extra space to this chapter, because I see it as an almost ideal interface of neurobiology and clinical medicine.

LIDOCAINE

What is the mechanism of action of systematically administered lidocaine in neurosomatic pain or, indeed, any chronic pain? The scientific literature is mute on this subject except for the frequent appearance of the word "unknown." The best explanation is given for neuropathic pain and then for peripheral pain. Injured nerves generate spontaneous ectopic discharges (aberrant action potentials) that are conducted via sodium channels. Sodium channels, of which there are about ten different types, increase in an injured nerve or cluster around the site of a local nerve injury. Lidocaine is a sodium-channel blocker that, when administered systemically, can stop the generation of ectopic discharges without blocking nerve conduction (Mao J,

Chen LC, 2000). Intravenous lidocaine also blocks TNF-alpha (Junger H et al., 2000).

Neuropathic pain behaviors responding to systemic lidocaine include hyperalgesia and allodynia, with a range from no effect to complete response. Many patients become tolerant to the effects of intravenous lidocaine, which may help fatigue, mood, alertness, and visceral hyperalgesia. It may even produce a complete remission of every neurosomatic symptom in an individual patient. Responses may occur only while the lidocaine is infusing or for as long as six months. Although lidocaine is cleared rapidly from systemic circulation, it can persist in the cerebrospinal fluid for days. Mexiletine is much less effective (Attal N et al., 2000). It is obviously necessary for lidocaine to exert its effects by central mechanisms, but those might still involve blocking Na^+ channels, as I shall discuss shortly.

IV lidocaine has been used to treat central pain for 20 years, but I encountered tremendous resistance in the medical community when I first began to use it in 1994 or so. The resistance is still powerful but no longer tremendous. I have given IV lidocaine to thousands of patients. The two worst reactions have been urticaria, after which IV lidocaine was no longer effective in the affected individuals. I have seen no seizures, no arrhythmias, and no need for cardiac monitoring, and it is not expensive (although some facilities charge $1,500 per treatment). Lidocaine 20 percent may be given subcutaneously in a dose of 5 mg/kg. The results are much inferior to IV lidocaine. The injections are painful, produce scar tissue, and last for only eight to 12 hours. Almost no patients wish to continue them or do so only when the beneficial effects of their previous lidocaine IV have worn off and they cannot immediately receive another one. Lidocaine 15 percent in PLO is fairly effective but messy and lasts only two to three hours. There is no need to use a lidocaine bolus. Physicians should infuse it at a rate that does not cause any ADRs. Too rapid infusion may cause a mild delirium and relapse, after which the lidocaine will never work again.

In addition to blocking Na^+ channels, lidocaine inhibits the binding of SP to NK-1 receptors, altering central sensitization (Terada H et al., 1999). It also inhibits glutamate secretion (similar to lamotrigine), and the possibility of its modulating the algogenic action of NGF and BDNF has been suggested (Holthusen H et al., 2000; Cummins TR et al., 2000). Local anesthetics such as procaine, lidocaine, and cocaine cause acute limbic system activation in animals and humans (Post RM, 1992). An endogenous pentapeptide acts as a Na^+-channel blocker (Brinkmeier H et al., 2000).

To understand the mode of action of lidocaine in neurosomatic disorders, we must go back to basics. Recall the model of the hyperactive NMDA receptor maintained by increased retrograde transmission. I have not yet discussed that "[a]ctive propagation of axonally initiated action potentials back into the dendritic tree may provide this retrograde message" (Stuart GJ, Hausser M, 2001). LTP occurs when an EPSP (from the dendrites) precedes action potentials, and LTD results when EPSPs are evoked after action potentials. The timing is critical for plasticity of synaptic strength. At distal dendrites, where this effect is usually small, EPSPs amplify backpropagating action potentials threefold, if the timing is precisely correct, and require the simultaneous activation of only a small number of synaptic inputs.

Backpropagating action potentials are generated by Na^+ channels, and most Na^+ channels are blocked by tetrodotoxin. TTX therefore blocks most backpropagating action potentials. Blocking K^+ channels has the reverse effect. This model was found applicable to NMDA synapses, and lots of them: "we estimate that up to 42% of all excitatory synapses in neocortical layer 5 pyramidal neurons would experience amplification of backpropagating action potentials by appropriately timed EPSPs" (Stuart GJ, Hausser M, 2001; Figure 76).

Activating dendritic sodium channels can work similar to NO and is probably more consistent. Desensitization is not a problem, either. The backpropagation must be decremental, and the dendrites must express Na^+ channels. This finding is the rule, not the exception, and may be the most common mechanism for retrograde messages. Amplification requires a number of synaptic inputs. It is quite difficult to amplify a single dendrite— a very large EPSP is required. To recapitulate: the EPSP must occur a few milliseconds before or be coincident with the action potential of increased synaptic strength at excitatory synapses. I have discussed this type of neural synchrony and oscillation previously when explaining LTP, and it appears to be necessary for LTP to occur. Oscillations in the dendritic membrane potential stimulate the modulation of backpropagating action potentials,

> as amplification of action potentials occurs primarily in the distal apical dendrites that receive associational inputs from other cortical areas. This raises the possibility that the amplification mechanism we describe provides a selection mechanism for potentiation of only those synapses that have contributed to the generation of synchronous network activity. (Stuart GJ, Hausser M, 2001)

Most of my treatment interventions aim at decreasing overlearned LTP. NMDA antagonists, such as ketamine, block the activation of the NMDA receptor so that a (usually) chemical retrograde messenger would not be generated in massive quantities. Lidocaine blocks glutamate release and the Na^+ channel involved in LTP by backpropagation. IV ketamine and IV lidocaine are the two most effective treatments for neurosomatic disorders that I have found so far. The next two are IV amantadine and (possibly) IV guaifenesin (see 855.2 in Chapter 9 regarding their effect on IBS).

GONADOTROPIN-RELEASING HORMONE (GnRH) AND DYSREGULATION OF CIRCADIAN RHYTHMS

(See 827.2, 827.5, and 827.7 in Chapter 9 for more information on this peptide.)

GnRH neurons are regarded by some neuroendocrinologists as the final nervous pathway of melatonin action. GnRH-secreting neurons do not express melatonin receptors, but GnRH mRNA is transiently increased by melatonin treatment. This effect occurs through a "relay" transmitter between the target of melatonin and the GnRH neurons. Melatonin decreases levels of NE and DA and up-regulates NMDA receptors on GnRH neurons. Although there are many other ways to explain circadian rhythm dysfunction in neurosomatic disorders (usually phase delay), the simplest way is usually the best. Sleep-phase disturbances in neurosomatic patients are difficult to treat. They do not respond to photic reentrainment, melatonin therapy, or "sleep hygiene." Because the major transmitters in the retinohypothalamic tract are NAAG and glutamate, the latter of which is continuously hypersecreted to varying degrees, light therapy should not be effective, and melatonin might make neurosomatic disorders worse. Removal of the SCN causes phase advance; overactivation might cause phase delay.

Postreceptor mechanisms of GnRH are similar to those of TRH, i.e., PLC stimulation, inositol phosphate generation, production of IP_3 which increases $[Ca^{2+}]_i$, and DAG formation which activates PKC. TRH is also secreted into the brain from the MPOA and is involved in such diverse processes as regulating body temperature, appetite, weight, mood, fatigue, nociception, respiration, and water intake. Patients who respond to OXT are more likely to respond to TRH, as they are to lidocaine, hydergine, lamotrigine, and catecholaminergic agonists. The SCN has a high density of TRH, Ach, NMDA, and NPY receptors. It contains mRNA for vasopressin, somatostatin, vasoactive intestinal peptide, gastrin-releasing peptide (GRP), SP, GABA, and peptide histidine isoleucine (PHI) (Figure 77). Secretion of VIP and GRP is rhythmically driven by light/dark cycles via the retinohypothalamic tract. Release of VIP and GRP have autocrine/paracrine effects modulating photic entrainment of the circadian pacemaker. None of the identified RNAs in the SCN are diffusible substances that regulate circadian rhythmicity. Injecting VIP or GRP into the SCN or stimulating secretion of glutamate from the retinohypothalamic tract in the latter part of the subjective night causes a phase advance. These three substances mimic the effect of light on photic entrainment, an ineffective mode of habituation in my patients. Because neurosomatic patients are usually phase delayed, a phase advance would be desirable. VIP, GRP, and glutamate produce a phase advance in the early part of the subjective night, which is usually around noon. Blocking the NMDA receptor at any daylight or early evening hour with intravenous ketamine does not cause a phase shift. This finding inclines me more to the GABAergic geniculohypothalamic tract (GHT) projection to the SCN or other circadian oscillators as being dysfunctional in neurosomatic patients.

When I began to write this book, one of my self-imposed rules to make it easier for the reader and less lengthy for the publisher, was "You're not going to discuss molecular genetics!" This refrain was frequently in mind until I got to the SCN and NADH. It should come as no surprise that there is much more to the subject than has been described so far.

In 2001, familial advanced sleep-phase syndrome (FASPS) was linked to an altered gene for the protein PER2. The mutation blocks a phosphorylation site that is thought to be a substrate of CK1ε. This work is the first to discover the genetic basis of a sleep disorder in humans (Toh KL et al., 2001). It showed that familial genetic circuitry controls rhythmic behavior in humans.

Genes controlling circadian rhythms have been found in humans, Drosophila, Neurospora, and Chlamydomonas. The genes most relevant to humans are found in Drosophila. It appears that circadian genes arose independently several times during evolution. The other circadian-gene regulators are quite different (Young MW, Kay SA, 2001).

Recall that PER and its partner protein TIM accumulate rhythmically in the fruit fly and regulate their own expression (Figure 78). Clock (CLK) and Cycle (CYC) are transcription factors that coordinately activate *per* and *tim* genes, an activity suppressed by nuclear PER. Separating intervals of activation and suppression creates self-sustaining oscillations for which stepwise delays are necessary. CK1ε is essential to create these delays in the fly.

Phase delay in the fly is caused, at least in part, by exposure to light of CRY, which then complexes with cytoplasmic TIM to cause rapid TIM degradation by a proteosome-mediated pathway. If the TIM is degraded in the nucleus, the fly is phase advanced. Phase advance may be entrained nonphotically in the hamster using a $5-HT_{1A/7}$ agonist (8-OH-DPAT) administered in the hamster's mid-subjective day only. The phase advance was accompanied by reduced levels of *Per1* and *Per2* mRNA levels in the SCN (Horikawa K et al., 2000). I have been unable to phase reset my patients with the $5-HT_{1A}$ agonists that are available to me.

Neurosomatic patients are often phase delayed and would be diagnosed with a circadian rhythm sleep disorder, delayed sleep phase type, by DSM-

IV-TR criteria. They are most awake in the nighttime and sleepy in the daytime. I doubt that cytoplasmic TIM degradation is the cause, however. A second kinase, "Shaggy," regulates nuclear translocation of the PER/TIM complex. The activity of Shaggy can also determine circadian rhythms.

Shaggy can be inactivated by another phosphoprotein, "Disheveled," a target for CK1ε. When Disheveled is phosphorylated, it exerts a much-reduced effect on Shaggy. Other players are involved, of course: the Wnt signal transduction pathway, Armadillo, ß-catenin, GSK3, and the bZIP transcription factor VRI.

In the FASPS human, the PER2 phosphorylation site for CK1ε is defective. A serine-glycine substitution in the human PER2 protein suppresses phosphorylation of CK1ε targets in PER2 in vitro.

CLK levels rise as PER/TIM levels fall. It has been suggested that CLK suppresses its own transcription, a process blocked by PER/TIM. At any rate, the basic mechanisms of circadian regulation involve rising and falling levels of gene production and gene activation acting in multiple auto-regulatory loops as seen for CLOCK:BMAL1.

I would have not digressed further into circadian molecular genetics unless I thought there might be some treatment clues. In this case, a method to stimulate the activity of CK1ε would cause a FASPS-like syndrome by increasing the phosphorylation of PER2 (Figure 79).

Because PER has a positive autoregulatory role of rhythmically produced CLOCK:BMAL1 complexes in both mice and flies, and presumably humans, circadian physiology requires an agent to turn off the *Per* genes. This job is performed by the cryptochromes, which bind flavins and pterins and promote redox reactions upon absorbing light. CRY1 and CRY2 repress *Per* transcription. CRY, rather than TIM, also physically associates with PER to increase its susceptibility to phosphorylation by CK1ε. Researchers were beginning to write off TIM in mammals until they found mouse TIM to be associated with CRYs in the SCN.

The bottom line, again, is that photic entrainment of circadian rhythms is not too important in neurosomatic patients. Rather, redox sensitivities may establish mechanisms for metabolic entrainment. Signs suggest that circadian molecular genetics has broader physiological and behavioral implications. Circadian genes are necessary for cocaine sensitization in Drosophila (Andretic R et al., 1999). They also regulate learning and memory (Belvin MP et al., 1999). Knock-out mice for *Per1* and *Per2* are denoted *mPer1, mPer2,* where *m* denotes *murine,* the scientific adjective for mouse. There is also an *mPer3,* which does not seem to be a fundamental feature of the circadian mechanism in mice. *mPer1* and *mPer2* knock-outs indicated that they regulated many downstream genes, even those as basic as *mAlas1* and *mAlas2.* These genes express the rate-limiting enzymes for heme biosynthesis, which is required for an enormous number of biological functions, thereby connecting the circadian clock rather directly to cellular biochemistry and physiology (Zheng B et al., 2001).

(846.22) Application of AMPA and SP to the SCN in vitro can produce phase shifts. Blocking Na^+ channels does not cause phase shifts, so lidocaine would not be an effective treatment for this disorder. Both SP and AMPA cause phase delays. SP antagonists or topiramate, which blocks AMPA receptors, could cause phase advance. I have not observed this treatment effect in my patients. With the information available to me at the time of this writing, I am able to neither confidently explain nor treat neurosomatic circadian rhythm disorders, except in the context of general symptomatic improvement which is neurochemically individual (Cravchik A, Goldman D, 2000). The pathway that best lends itself to therapeutic intervention is that from the SCN → dorsal hypothalamus (DH) → locus coeruleus. This loop is discussed next. It is often difficult to treat symptoms, and circadian dysregulation is no exception. In this case, however, an elegant hypothesis is that the retinohypothalamic tract is always hyperactive, causing the commonly encountered phase delay.

(846.6) The dorsomedial hypothalamic nucleus links the SCN and the LC. The LC has circadian rhythms to its NE secretion. The SCN → DMH → LC pathway is probably dysfunctional in neurosomatic disorders. In rats, tract-tracing studies have shown that the DMH is also connected to the rostral ventrolateral medulla, the NTS, the pontine parabrachial nucleus, the hypothalamic PVN, VMH, and lateral hypothalamic area. The lateral hypothalamic area secretes orexins, and its fibers also project to the LC. The VMH is massively innervated by amygdala CRH neurons. The PVN and VMH, as well as the DMH, are part of a CNS noradrenergic circuit regulating food intake. The PVN receives NE projections from the NTS and RVLM, as well as from the LC. I have discussed these noradrenergic circuits in the content of neurosomatic dysautonomic symptoms in previous works. It is difficult to integrate this information as yet into the pathophysiology of phase-shift disorders.

Light therapy is ineffective, and I have seen neither adverse nor beneficial reactions to melatonin. Lesions of the SCN either prevent the suppressive effect of melatonin on GnRH or do not alter it, depending on the type and species of animal tested. SCN lesions do not accentuate melatonin treatment effects. In addition to the SCN, which has the highest content of melatonin receptors, other sites of high density include the POA, cerebral cortex, and thalamus, where they are involved in sleep induction.

Photic entrainment through the retinohypothalamic tract is the primary "zeitgeber" (time giver, entrainment stimulus) and cannot be superseded by melatonin. In the absence of activity through the retinohypothalamic tract, melatonin becomes a zeitgeber, along with food, temperature, and other activities. To be effective, melatonin must be injected into the SCN around dawn or dusk.

The SCN projects to the paraventricular nucleus of the hypothalamus, and this nucleus projects to the superior cervical ganglion (SCG) via the rostral ventrolateral medulla and spinal cord. I have discussed in previous works that the SCG may have other functions than are generally attributed to it. If there is a preexisting NE deficiency, projection to the pineal gland from the SCG may be inadequate and could delay melatonin secretion, causing a "phase delay" if melatonin were more important to setting sleep-wake phases than it seems to be in my patients.

Another consideration for entrainment of circadian rhythms by non-photic input relates to activation of the $5-HT_7$ receptor, either on the SCN itself or on the terminals of the tuberomammillary nucleus, which leads to release of HA, which activates H_2 receptors on the neurons of the SCN. Both routes result in activation of the cAMP-PKA pathway and induction of phase advances (Figure 80).

H_1 and H_2 densities vary over the phases of the light-dark cycle. In this case, the densities would be the inverse of each other. Any receptor agonist or antagonist must be evaluated at or near the level of the SCN. Histamine-induced phase delays in hamsters are more like what I suspect occurs in humans. There is a direct activation of the NMDA receptors, possibly at the polyamine binding site in these animals, which is independent of the H_1 and H_2 receptors.

A rudimentary neural circuit (SCN-DMH-LC) regulates the circadian rhythmicity of sleep-wake cycles (Aston-Jones G et al., 2001). The dorsomedial nucleus of the hypothalamus, where much of the orexin is manufactured, is a relay station that transfers signals from the SCN to the LC. Lesioning the DMH eliminates circadian variations in LC spike activity. The LC is more active during waking states, less active in REM, and inactive in non-REM sleep. Pseudorabies virus was used for retrograde tracing, and the PVN and MPOA were also labeled. Prefrontal regulation of hypothalamic nuclei such as the MPOA, as well as the LC, might gate the strength of the regulatory influences of the SCN on behavioral arousal. NE deficiency could thus be responsible for the phase delay commonly encountered in the assessment of neurosomatic patients.

A great deal has been discovered about SCN genes and gene products in the last few years. Almost every article I read makes the previous one obsolete. Less progress has been made on "signaling outside the clockwork," which is more relevant to clinical practice. The ANS and secretion of corticosteroids may cause circadian dysregulation (Hastings MH, 2000), and NADH is involved.

The SCN receives GABAergic inhibitory projections from the geniculo-hypothalamic tract, the area of the thalamus that receives visual input. It is more likely that the GHT is malfunctioning in neurosomatic disorders, since it is a connection in the regularly dysfunctional corticostriatal-thalamo-cortical circuit. The PVN has numerous inputs that could be abnormal, but the GHT probably furnishes inappropriate photic input to the SCN, which would supersede the effects of melatonin. Current opinion suggests that the SCN primarily establishes circadian rhythms by secretion of a small protein, "prokineticin," which can sustain circadian rhythms even in the face of pinealectomy (see 846.6).

PYRROLIDINES

The "-acetams," of which only piracetam is available to me, are classed as pyrrolidone derivatives. There are a large number of pyrrolidone drugs, eight of which are discussed in a recent review in *Lancet* (Shorvon S, 2001). Each of the drugs, although structurally similar, has somewhat different functions. They all share a lack of effect on DA, 5-HT, NE, A_1, or mu-opioid receptors. Despite their structural similarity to GABA, they have little GABAergic effect. Some of the pyrrolidines, including piracetam and aniracetam, are AMPA agonists. Many of them are AEDs, particularly levetiracetam (Keppra), which differs from all other AEDs in that it has no effect on GABA, glutamate, or Ca^{2+}-channel conductance. Levetiracetam and piracetam are excellent treatments for myoclonus and are effective after the first dose.

Pyrrolidines are being investigated as treatments for mild cognitive impairment, stroke, anxiety, and recently for myoclonus (piracetam and levetiracetam). The mode of action is still not well understood thirty years after the discovery of piracetam. I can also prescribe levetiracetam, but it is devoid of most effects I seek, except antimyoclonic.

Pyrrolidones are excreted unmetabolized (like Neurontin). They have no more adverse reactions than placebo. Piracetam is often combined with clonazepam. The dose I usually prescribe is 800 mg t.i.d., but some studies have given ten times that. Levetiracetam is given in a dose of 500 to 1,500 mg b.i.d. It is also well tolerated and very safe.

Case Report

I usually find the "magic bullet" sooner or later. In this case, it was later. I first saw this Caucasian female patient when she was a high-school student. She had been very high performing in a private school and had been admitted to one of the best universities in the country. She had a typical history: "When I was twelve years old, I got the flu and couldn't get back into the swing of things." She endorsed most of the symptoms on the CFS questionnaire and was often unable to attend school. She was depressed and disgusted with herself. There was a family history of mood disorders.

She initially felt much better on nitroglycerin (I don't use it on people with migraines), Neurontin, baclofen, and naphazoline eyedrops. She improved with oxytocin, and intravenous lidocaine helped her to be well enough to return to school. She relapsed in hot weather. Adding bupropion and midodrine increased her energy. She began college as a disabled student and took two or three classes each semester. She felt better, actually too much better, with IV ketamine, which caused hypomania the one time it was infused.

Over the next several semesters, she gradually improved, both spontaneously and by fine-tuning of her medications. Her cognition improved, and her sleep became more restorative. Her overall symptomatology still waxed and waned. Modafinil, as it does sometimes, increased her energy but caused marked dysphoria. Other stimulants were better tolerated but caused occasional panic attacks. Five years after I first saw her, her symptoms were still exacerbated by stress and overexertion. When she was fatigued, she became anxious about her life circumstances and her future social and professional prospects. If completely sedentary, she had almost no symptoms, but such a lifestyle was neither desirable nor feasible.

She was concerned about applying to graduate school. Her workload would necessarily increase, and she would be teaching undergraduates. She was still limited by a mild neurocognitive disorder. Fortunately, by this time, I had developed the rationale and experience to use antagonists at the glycine coagonist site of the NMDA receptor. These proved to be her most effective medications. With a combination of guaifenesin, probenecid, diltiazem, and trihexyphenidyl (similar to atropine), she felt greatly improved. She was no longer "fuzzy headed" and had more energy and stamina. She looked forward to performing well in graduate school.

FATIGUE

Most neurosomatic illnesses are characterized by fatigue to some degree. I doubt that fatigue is a unitary process, but at a basic level it is part and parcel of neurosomatic dysfunction. First, let us consider what we already may know.

1. Lack of NE and DA. Norepinephrine and dopamine are not made in sufficient amounts, are not released appropriately, or are used up too rap-

idly, exceeding the rate of maximum production by the rate-limiting enzyme tyrosine hydroxylase, which is difficult, but not impossible, to do. These possibilities account for various kinds of synaptic fatigue, and there are examples of catecholamines, e.g., NE in the rat forebrain, decreasing after exercise. There may also be an imbalance between D_1 and D_2 receptors, possibly including D_3 and/or alpha$_1$/alpha$_2$ noradrenergic receptors and subtypes. An alternative way of looking at dopamine depletion might be shifting predominance of the D_1 and D_2 receptors, D_1 activating adenyl cyclase and D_2 inhibiting it, in the manner discussed for the individualistic reaction to delta-9-THC (Marinol). Hypersensitivity of DA/NE autoreceptors is a distinct possibility. Ca^{2+} influx causes exocytosis of neurotransmitter-filled docked vesicles. Only a few of the docked vesicles are released by exocytosis. Recall that exocytosis is regulated by rab3, a low-molecular weight G protein in synaptic vesicles. In the absence of rab3, many more synaptic vesicles are released. Two other synaptic proteins (there are more than 40 of them) interact with rab3 when it is bound to GTP. Together they help to regulate synaptic vesicle fusion with the neuronal membrane. BDNF is often required for exocytosis (Figure 81a-c).

2. Dysfunction of the VLPO/MPOA/VBST. These areas regulate sleepiness, are susceptible to NE deficiency, and help to regulate levels of DA.

3. NMDA hyperactivity. When the NMDA receptor is activated, Ca^{2+} pours in through the receptor channel and through voltage-sensitive Ca^{2+} channels. Calcium influx activates a cascade of phosphorylation reactions. Increasing numbers of molecules are recruited at each step presynaptically. When synaptic transmission occurs, with a flow of ionic current across the cell membrane, the most energy is consumed. Ion pumps are responsible for over half of the brain's energy consumption (Ames A, 1997). In an insect retina, 7.5×10^9 ATP molecules are consumed, translating 1,000 bits of information across a photoreceptor membrane (Laughlin TM et al., 1998), or 7.5×10^6 ATP molecules per bit. The subsequent phosphorylation cascade consumes somewhat less ATP than this. The process is rendered much more energy expensive if there is a lot of "noise" transmitted as well. It costs a chloride pump one to three ATP molecules to transfer one chloride ion.

Reuptake of the neurotransmitter and refilling of the vesicles costs 10 percent of the ATP expended in synaptic transmission. Even with the amount of noise in a normal brain (stochastic resonance), the energy cost rises extremely rapidly with noise, compelling the brain to be energy efficient by dividing information in parallel pathways, each of low capacity, and using energy-efficient neural codes (Levy WB, Baxter RA, 1996).

The energy consumption of the human brain is 20 percent of that of the entire body, even though the brain weighs only three pounds. This degree of energy consumption probably shaped the evolution of the brain (Aeillo LC,

Wheeler P, 1995). Energy costs of all signaling systems are so expensive because a protein molecule codes information by changing conformation, similar to a switch. How fast can it switch, and how much energy is needed? Much energy is consumed by the molecular motors kinesin and dynein so that they can propel substances along microtubules. Kinesins do so rapidly (fast axonal transport). There are numerous types of kinesin- and dynein-related proteins subserving different functions. Of course, they all have inhibitors. Some dyneins are involved in whipping flagella. Others are cytoplasmic. One dynein-related protein is named "dynamitin" (Figure 82).

The motor protein kinesin can cycle its information about 100 times per second, using one ATP molecule per cycle. If the kinesin molecule were not part of the cell, it could be ten times more efficient. When molecules are organized into cellular systems, costs skyrocket. Noise is introduced, and energy is required to distribute signals over relatively large distances. Signaling accounts for 80 percent of the total energy consumption in the cortex. Signaling cost goes predominantly to Na^+/K^+ pumps, which are concentrated in the axons and at synapses. Reversal of ion fluxes are often the last stage of an amplification process, e.g., sensory transduction $\rightarrow$ axonal transmission $\rightarrow$ synaptic transmission.

Energy usage is tightly coupled to neural performance. Signal quality depends on signal-to-noise ratio and "bandwidth," a measure of speed of response. Raising SNR and bandwidth requires extra energy. I discussed the low SNR in neurosomatic disorders extensively in *Betrayal*. The brain is organized to transmit information efficiently at the lowest possible energy cost. Spike coding increases SNR but is more costly than analogue coding. A mixture of the two produces energy-efficient neural codes.

Energy availability penalizes excessive synaptic connections, excessive lengths of neurons, and the use of excessive numbers of ion channels. The neural "pruning" that begins at puberty makes the adult brain more energy efficient and able to think in new ways. "Action potentials can improve efficiency by reducing noise in complicated networks" (Laughlin SB, 2001).

Endothelin

When $[Ca^{2+}]_i$ exceeds the storage capacity of the IP_3 and ryanodine-gated compartments, the next stop is the mitochondria, which may use their own ATP to keep Ca^{2+} out (Figure 81c). With a massive inflow of Ca^{2+} short of excitotoxity, as may occur in neurosomatic disorders, dealing with $[Ca]_i$ may consume considerable energy. Other hypotheses about the nature of fatigue (not just CFS fatigue) abound. I put one forth in *Betrayal*, that fatigue could be caused by excess secretion of endothelin, which releases substance

P, LH, follicle-stimulating hormone (FSH), VP, and GH. Endothelin, being one of the most vasoconstrictive substances known, could account for the increased global cerebral hypoperfusion seen after fatiguing stimuli, notably exercise but also after mental tasks. ET levels are increased in the CSF of FMS patients (Goldstein JA, 1996). ET releases dopamine in ischemic states, acting at the ET_A receptor. ET acting at the ET_B receptor may both stimulate and have neurotoxic actions on striatal DA receptors, which are activated by the release of glutamate acting at striatal NMDA receptors. There is a reciprocal stimulation/repression of DA between the NMDA receptors of the PFC and striatum. Endothelin levels in the CSF in depression are half normal (Hoffman A et al., 1989) but show a trend to elevation in CFS. ET-1 can stimulate release of OXT and VP but not CRH. It has been proposed that ET-3, acting presynaptically, promotes the secretion of tachykinins such as substance P through the prejunctional action of ET_B receptors. Endothelin remains a good candidate for a fatiguing substance, and more of the story remains to be told.

A considerable amount of experimental evidence indicates that endothelin plays a role in neurosomatic disorders. It stimulates NGF secretion (high in FMS CSF) and activates phospholipase A_2, PKC, and the MAP kinase pathway (Desagher S et al., 1997). It can cause edema, reversible by Ca^{2+}-channel blockers, which also normalize ET-mediated vasoconstriction in peripheral tissues (Filep JG et al., 1996). It can modulate sympathetic neurotransmission at both vascular and nonvascular junctions and may act in the CNS as a neurotransmitter, provoking the release of "neurohormones" and neurotransmitters (mainly NE). ET can also alter behavior and nociception (D'Amico M et al., 1996). Glutamate produces analgesia when injected into the PAG area, which is rich in NMDA receptors. These receptors are involved in ET-1-induced behavioral effects. When ET-1 is injected into the PAG of a rat, the animal manifests a complex of aversive reactions but develops antinociception nonetheless, similar to an intra-PAG injection of NMDA. NMDA antagonism of afferents to certain structures, such as the amygdala and hippocampus, is beneficial in most neurosomatic patients. NMDA antagonism within them might not be.

ET-1 acts via NMDA, and its effects can be blocked by NMDA antagonists, as well as by prazosin, an alpha$_1$-receptor antagonist. Non-NMDA glutamate antagonists have no effect on ET-1-induced antinociception. Alpha$_1$-receptor antagonists have little use in neurosomatic disorders aside from relaxing the urethral sphincter.

Endothelin may be neurotoxic via an increase in Ca^{2+} in association with glutamate agonists. This effect can be prevented by Ca^{2+}-channel blockers. ETs (there are three of them, 1-3, and two receptors, A and B) can regulate secretion of prolactin and vasopressin (Kiozumi S et al., 1994). ETs also increase NO/cGMP formation in the adrenal medulla via the ET_B subtype (Mathison Y, Israel A, 1998), as well as stimulating secretion of ANF, aldosterone, and epinephrine from adrenal chromaffin cells. There is a significant amount of ET mRNA in pheochromocytoma cells. Phorbol esters stimulate PKC and are found in tung oil. Phorbol esters stimulate the production of ET-1 six- to tenfold.

When ET is injected outside certain regions of the CNS, it is nociceptive, as NMDA would usually be. Given intraperitoneally (i.p.) it causes abdominal spasms and aversive reactions, which can be antagonized by morphine administered centrally. The pain is not affected by NSAIDs or acetaminophen and seems to be related to the potent ability of ET to constrict smooth muscle (Raffa RB et al., 1996). ET-induced nociception is quite novel, in that it is relieved by benzodiazepines, which are not known for analgesic effects except in neurosomatic disorders. At low doses, ET, acting through the ET_A receptor, potentiates capsaicin-induced nociception. At higher doses, apparently acting through the ET_B receptor, it blocks 5-HT-induced hyperalgesia (Piovezan AP et al., 1998). Nociception caused by ET-1 occurs at the ET_A receptor and can be prevented by preadministration of the mixed ET_A/ET_B antagonist bosentan, or a specific ET_A antagonist, injected into a joint primed with carageenan, an inflammatory substance. Subsequently, however, this joint becomes hypersensitive to ET. Seventy-two hours later, when all pain behavior has long since ceased, normally ineffective doses of ET-1 or other algogenic substances cause a significant pain response. This time, both ET_A and ET_B receptors are involved.

If peripheral endothelin played an important role in neurosomatic disorders, most patients would be hypertensive. Hypotension is actually more common. If endothelin has an effect, it is in the brain. Postganglionic sympathetic neurons release large amounts of ET-3 into the circulation during exercise (Maeda S et al., 1997), although ET-1 is also released. Endothelin leaves its receptors very slowly. The monotonously reproducible findings of global cerebral hypoperfusion on brain SPECT after exercise ergometry seem now, more than ever, to be due to endothelin release. Because postexertional relapse is probably related to depletion of catecholamines, and because ET is secreted from postsynaptic sympathetic neurons, which may not have had enough "dockable" NE to begin with, it is reasonable to implicate ET in this process, particularly since it stimulates the secretion of NMDA, the most culpable neurotransmitter for production and exacerbation of neurosomatic symptoms. It might be more than a coincidence that most agents which worsen neurosomatic symptoms induce endothelin secretion, and vice versa. ET levels are increased by TGF-beta, TNF-alpha, IL-1, insulin, NE, angiotensin II (ATII), and BK. Expression of ET-1 mRNA is inhibited by NO, prostacyclin, ANF (via inhibition of phosphatidylinositol metabolism), heparin, and warfarin. ET activates PLA_2 and MAP kinase and is activated by phorbol esters. The $ET_{A/B}$ receptor antagonist bosentan has been most thoroughly studied, primarily in the treatment of congestive heart failure (Mayauchi T, Guto K, 1999). Its potential toxicity is too great for routine use in neurosomatic medicine. Perhaps most germane to neurosomatic pathophysiology, endothelin closes the K_{ATP} channel, the opposite action of gabapentin and other therapeutically valuable K_{ATP} openers.

Although fatigue is not sleepiness, particularly in a state of hypervigilance, fatigued patients are often sleepy. One reason (besides the accumulation of adenosine during wakefulness) is that endogenous hypocretin (Hcrt) promotes wakefulness and is secreted from the lateral hypothalamus to areas of the brainstem and basal forebrain that produce alerting substances. Hcrt, of course, increases REM sleep latency and decreases REM density. This Hcrt function is constitutive in the pontine reticular formation. The densest projection of $Hcrt_1$ is to the LC, which is usually quiescent during REM and increases the firing rate in the LC via the $Hcrt_1$ receptor. Hcrt is certainly involved in homeostatic sleep mechanisms and may help to regulate circadian rhythms as well. There are two kinds of Hcrt, 1 and 2, and it appears that $Hcrt_1$ is consumed during prolonged wakefulness. $Hcrt_2$ receptors are not found in the LC but are dense in the tuberomammillary nucleus, where the activating substance histamine is produced. Hcrt is desensitized by beta-arrestin in a similar manner to that of beta receptors, which I discussed in *Betrayal*. $Hcrt_1$ receptors are also found in the dorsal raphe and tegmental neurons, where they increase the activity of tyrosine hydroxylase. Galanin may also be secreted in excess from the VLPO.

SLEEP

Sleep disorders are almost ubiquitous in patients with neurosomatic illnesses. I have discussed their pathophysiology in previous works and will update the topic here. Fortunately, just before I wrote this section, the third edition of *Principles and Practice of Sleep Medicine* (2000) became available. I enjoyed reading the first two editions and commend the third to the reader. Because the references in the text are current to 1999, about the time of the marketing of modafinil in the United States, I shall review and discuss selected passages which should be of interest to the physician practicing neurosomatic medicine. At the end of this section, I will highlight articles of interest written in the next two years.

Because my practice involves the application of basic science to clinical medicine, my favorite chapter in the previous editions has been "Basic

Mechanisms of Sleep-Wake States," by Barbara E. Jones. In *Sleep Medicine,* as in this book, the concept of the ascending reticular activating system, or some version of it, is used.

Glutamate is the predominant neurotransmitter in the ARAS and in thalamocortical circuits. Ach projections are also important, as is NE from the LC, which projects widely and is activating. There is a shift from sympathetic to parasympathetic regulation with sleep onset, and activating systems must be damped. The nucleus of the solitary tract, an extension of the vagus into the brainstem, as well as anterior hypothalamic and medial preoptic areas, are important in sleep onset and maintenance. On transverse section, the MPOA is located between the anterior commissure and the optic chiasm.

Inhibition of activating systems is affected by GABAergic neurons as well as muscarinic and nicotinic ascending input, resulting eventually in hyperpolarization of thalamocortical systems, which is reflected in spindle and slow-wave activity on the EEG. Somatostatin is often colocalized with GABAergic neurons. I have administered SS to numerous neurosomatic patients without benefit. Jones distinguishes the roles of DA and NE neurons. The former play a role in behavioral arousal; the latter play an integral role in cortical activation. Catecholamines do not produce arousal by themselves but are integrated into a more complex system of wakefulness. LC neurons decrease their rate of firing in slow-wave sleep (SWS) and cease firing in REM sleep. This dictum is probably not obeyed in neurosomatic sleep.

I shall not discuss the cholinergic activating system here, since, at least in its muscarinic manifestation, it does not appear to be involved in the symptoms of most neurosomatic patients. The presynaptic nicotinic cholinergic receptors excite LC/NE inputs to the dorsal raphe and increase 5-HT. During REM, when the LC is turned off, this same presynaptic input may facilitate 5-HT self-inhibition by the raphe neurons themselves (Hobson JA et al., 1998).

I shall not invoke histamine, an activating neurotransmitter, since no histamine agonist is available for clinical use and histamine does not have much of a role in sleep-wake transition. Perhaps the first activating histaminergic agent will be thioperamide or an analogue, an H_3 autoreceptor antagonist.

Glutamate is hypersecreted in neurosomatic disorders, from both the thalamocortical and corticothalamic circuits and, perhaps to a lesser degree, when the ARAS is stimulated. Of course, the situation is not that simple. NMDA-receptor activation has been implicated in burst discharges of cortical pyramidal cells during SWS. I am not aware of any increase in burst discharges in neurosomatic patients. The primary electrophysiologic evidence of overactivation in such individuals is the alpha-wave intrusion into SWS (also called delta sleep because of the large, slow "delta" waves on EEG for non-REM). Whether alpha-delta sleep causes nonrestorative sleep or other symptoms is currently a matter of some dispute. The overall situation is complicated because the function of sleep, except pertaining to memory consolidation, is speculative. Because brain metabolism decreases by 25 percent in SWS, cells could have an opportunity for "housekeeping" functions.

Spontaneous reactivation of memory traces, occurring while the brain is not processing external input, as in SWS, may be necessary to assign synaptic weights to recent experiences so they can be incorporated into long-term memory. This process is termed memory consolidation and occurs in the hippocampus with cholinergic mediation. The memories are recorded, temporally compressed, and processed via Ach, and then when Ach input ceases, they are "played back" into heteromodal association areas. This activity can be blocked by an AMPA antagonist (Sutherland GR, McNaughton B, 2000). When memory is retrieved, there is a coherence in pattern reactivation between recorded hippocampal and heteromodal (e.g., posterior parietal) neurons. The length of time of compression of electrical activity from a recent memory is about that of one hippocampal theta wave, the time required for NMDA-dependent LTP. It is thought that during REM sleep, there is a weakening of hippocampal synapses for already consolidated memories and a strengthening for those associated with new memories. Retrieval of old memories is not usually impaired in neurosomatic disorders, but recent memory commonly is.

Peptides purportedly involved in wakefulness are SP, CRH, and TRH. SP, elevated in the CSF of FMS patients, is localized in Ach neurons. Administering cholinesterase inhibitors for FMS patients usually (but not always) either has no effect or makes them worse. Giving muscarinic Ach-receptor antagonists has almost never been of benefit, except to reverse an adverse reaction to a cholinesterase inhibitor, to ameliorate irritable bladder, to reduce motion sickness, or as an NMDA/glycine antagonist.

5-HT has a minor role in sleep induction. The ionotropic excitatory $5\text{-}HT_3$ receptor is found on GABAergic neurons in the cortex and forebrain. The "major inhibitory post-synaptic receptor $(5\text{-}HT_{1A})$ is found on many projection neurons and notably on the cholinergic basal forebrain neurons, which are hyperpolarized and inhibited by this receptor" (Jones EG, 2000). Whether the $5\text{-}HT_{1A}$ receptor is the major inhibitory postsynaptic receptor is debatable. Ziprasidone, the most potent $5\text{-}HT_{1A}$ agonist available, does not usually make people sleepy.

Adenosine is definitely important to sleep. I have discussed its role in *Betrayal* and elsewhere in this book, as I have the GABA receptor.

An interesting condition termed "idiopathic recurring stupor" is apparently caused by elevated levels of an endogenous benzodiazepine-like substance in the CSF of affected individuals (Rothstein JD et al., 1992). Although I have previously reported that administering the BZD antagonist flumazenil to CFS patients without panic disorder has had no effect, I have had some luck using furosemide, a $GABA_A$-receptor antagonist, in patients with "stuporous" episodes. Such individuals are uncommon, even in my practice, in which one or two patients are often asleep in the waiting room. Because flumazenil is so expensive, those who fit into the "stupor spectrum" use it in a nasal spray, a form that is fairly effective and rapidly acting.

Growth hormone-releasing hormone (GHRH) is secreted in the hypothalamus and promotes SWS. My experience with GH secretagogues has been that they are not particularly useful. GHRH is not available to the clinician, and the increased marketing of $5\text{-}HT_2$-receptor antagonists, e.g., atypical neuroleptics, nefazodone (Serzone), and mirtazapine (Remeron), may enhance non-REM sleep but not restorative sleep.

There is a laundry list of other endogenous sleep-inducing substances, especially galanin, most of which I have previously discussed. The role of prolactin is considered elsewhere in this book. The sleep disorders of neurosomatic medicine are explicable in the context of NMDA hyperactivity. A disorder of initiating and maintaining sleep occurs because of hypervigilance. Once the patient falls asleep, the GABAergic-Ach thalamocortical shutdown is poorly maintained. Glutamatergic activation, both top-down and bottom-up, interrupts it. A modicum of NE and DA secretion must continue to occur in an attempt to modulate the NMDA hyperactivity, also accounting for hypervigilance during sleep and perhaps for nocturnal panic attacks. Nonrestorative sleep, although it may be viewed as inadequate metabolism of adenosine, alpha-delta intrusion, or some problem with mitochondrial oxidation, is best described as inadequate restoration of NE and DA stores or inadequate biosynthesis of CREB. This deficiency produces continued synaptic fatigue and continued widening of receptive fields, an overflow of working memory, poor selective attention, and inappropriate determination of salience with consequent improper synaptic weighting of too many percepts which supersaturate neural networks to which they are inappropriately admitted. Thus, neurally regulated systems are *dys*regulated and the process is self-perpetuating. An opposing view is that impaired catabolism of monoamines should result in an increased need for sleep, called "homeostatic" in sleep research. Aspartate aminotransferase (AST), in this case an enzyme which catabolizes monoamines rather than being a hepatocellular enzyme, rises after several hours in the sleep-deprived rat (Cirelli C, Tononi G, 1998). Such could also be the case in the neurosomatic patient when monoamines are secreted to the point of synaptic fatigue.

The section about sleep physiology in *Sleep Medicine* is not particularly helpful to the neurosomatic practitioner. A tantalizing tidbit in the chapter "Respiratory Physiology: Neural Control," by John Orem and Leszek Kubin, informs me that NE is inhibitory at the level of medullary respiratory neurons. The LC acts phasically when it perceives novel situations. "Thus, by extrapolation from the behavior of these neurons, noradrenergic effects on breathing may be phasic and particularly relevant during states of emotional or sensory stimulation during wakefulness" (Orem J, Kubin L, 2000). Could phasic NE secretion by an overly taxed LC be responsible for the tidal volume randomness observed in submaximal exercise of FMS patients? The regulation of tidal volume is so complex that at this point one cannot say that this hypothesis is even probable.

Respiratory irregularities are the norm in REM sleep and occur during stages 1 and 2 of non-REM (NREM) sleep. There is a pervasive belief that NREM is "restorative," because metabolic activity decreases and switches to the "parasympathetic" mode. Just how it might be restorative is as yet unknown. NREM can be substantially increased by $5\text{-}HT_2$ antagonists without the patient's feeling any more refreshed than usual on arising. Delta sleep refers to stages 3 and 4 of NREM when there are large, slow delta waves. Persons with chemoreceptors sensitive to hypocapnia are more apt to develop irregular breathing at the onset of NREM sleep. Those who exercise develop hypocapnia, and in 1990 the "hyperventilation provocation test" propounded by the British expert C. M. Bass was used to diagnose CFS, which was assumed to be caused by somatization hypocapnia. I critiqued this work in *Limbic Hypothesis* in 1993. This simple-minded hypothesis has been discredited, since many normal subjects had abnormal responses to hyperventilation, but central pCO_2 misinterpretation may contribute to tidal-volume irregularities. However, many patients exercised so minimally that pCO_2 was scarcely lowered. The NE-novelty hypothesis fits the situation better. The insula regulates tidal volume as well, and dysfunction in this region would fit well into the neurosomatic paradigm.

Prolactin levels undergo a major elevation at sleep onset and culminate around mid-sleep. Decreased dopaminergic inhibition of tonic prolactin secretion with onset of sleep is thought to be responsible for PRL elevation. Because PRL rises after ejaculation, and because arousal and/or ejaculation may cause neurosomatic relapse, PRL levels during sleep would be interesting to obtain. It probably would be decreased, however, in those patients with microarousals, even if they are the microarousals of alpha-delta sleep, since there is a close temporal relationship between PRL secretion and delta sleep.

Serum growth hormone and prolactin were measured hourly during sleep in 25 healthy women and 21 controls. Sleep architecture was similar between the groups. Women with FMS had significantly lower mean concentrations of PRL and GH. There was no difference in IGF-1 levels (Landis CA et al., 2001). The significance of this study is obscure. It would suggest a DA excess during FMS sleep, although numerous other factors regulate PRL. Decreased PRL levels might impair restorative sleep. Recall that PRL rises after orgasm, indicating DA depletion and producing transitory somnolence. This sleep study suggests DA depletion in FMS is not the cause of synaptic fatigue. Rather, docking of DA synaptic vesicles may be impaired. Using inappropriate vesicular translocation as a hypothesis, which actually makes more sense anyway, we can de-emphasize precursor loading and focus attention more on (dys)regulation of synaptic neurophysiology.

A common occurrence among neurosomatic patients is night sweats or shivering. Night sweats have been phantasmagorically associated to a dysregulated cystic fibrosis transmembrane conductance regulator (CFTR). The normal function of CFTR is regulation of Na^+ channels in epithelial cells (Englebienne P et al., 2001). In this paper, ankyrin, a cytoskeletal constituent, is shown to be dysfunctional by altering the function of ion channels and inhibition of the Rnase-L ankyrin-like domain. All CFS symptoms are thereby elucidated and explained.

Temperature regulation, awake or asleep, occurs adjacent to the MPOA in the preoptic anterior hypothalamic (POAH) nuclei. Night sweats in postmenopausal women occur in stage 4 sleep. Although thermoregulatory responses are markedly inhibited in REM sleep, an exception may occur during active dreaming. The back-and-forth movement of the eyes during REM sleep is like scanning and must involve the frontal eye fields and thus the entire attentional network. There is also increased sympathetic activity during the transition from NREM to REM.

Those who deal with neurosomatic patients on a regular basis know that their dreams are very vivid, even if their sleep architecture is not much different than normal. It appears to me that they are hypervigilant while dreaming and are thus more likely to have arousal symptoms, which could be noradrenergically mediated concomitantly with cholinergically mediated dream states. The DLPFC is shut down, while the limbic system, still active, is demodulated. There is activation during dreaming of the anterior cingulate and both amygdala. Infusion of Ach into the POAH reduces temperature. One would expect NE to increase temperature. The combination could produce chills and sweats. Vivid dreams or nightmares are usually eliminated or reduced in intensity by a dose of clonidine or an alpha-blocker at bedtime. This preoptic area is the same that is involved in copulatory behavior. It is fitting that it should play an important role in nocturnal penile tumescence (lateral POA). Penile erection while awake occurs via the MPOA.

Several chapters are devoted to chronobiology, sleep homeostasis, and the circadian aspect of sleep regulation. The suprachiasmatic nucleus consists of several thousand cells that regulate almost all circadian events. It is obvious that SCN function is dysregulated in neurosomatic disorders, but how it is dysregulated and how to reregulate it is not clear at all. Most patients have a delayed sleep phase, i.e., they are more alert when they should be asleep (at night) and sleepy when they should be alert (the rest of the time). This phase delay is very difficult to treat. It does not respond to sleep hygiene, bright light, average room light (180 lux), or increasing serotonin, either in general or at the 5-HT_{1A} receptor located in the SCN. The inputs and outputs and their interactions between photic and nonphotic entrainment stimuli are so complex that I shall not review them here, because there are no effective ways of altering circadian rhythms in neurosomatic patients other than by decreasing NMDA activity, or perhaps increasing NE transmission in the SCN → DH → LC loop.

The retinohypothalamic tract to the SCN is entrained by light. Its neurotransmitter is glutamate. I assume that hypersecretion of glutamate occurs in the retinohypothalamic tract without a decrease in NMDA-receptor sensitivity. Because photic entrainment is more powerful than any other kind, it may be nearly maximal all the time. Chronically heightened glutamatergic input to the SCN would cause phase delay because levels of prokineticin and TNF-alpha are probably elevated. Activity of the NMDA receptor affects CREB, thus activating IEGs such as c-fos and others. This genetic activity must lead to changes in clock phase by oscillations of genes and proteins in SCN neurons.

I shall discuss the molecular genetic basis for mammalian circadian rhythms very basically. They are fairly well understood and should be accessible in any physiology textbook, as well as in the *Sleep Medicine* chapter "Genetic Control of Circadian Rhythms," by Lawrence H. Pinto, Martha Hotz Vitaterna, and Fred W. Turek, which is concise and relatively current. Two proteins (gene products) activate Clock and BMAL1. There are two other genes, *tim* and *per.* Their gene products, TIM and PER, inhibit the ability of Clock: BMAL1 (a "heterodimer") to activate the transcription of *tim* and *per,* thus completing the loop of oscillatory signaling, which takes 24 to 26 hours.

I have avoided explaining detailed neurobiologic mechanisms when they cannot be modified by treatment. Such was the case for the SCN pacemaker until the summer of 2001 when two papers from the McKnight group at University of Texas Southwestern Medical Center in Dallas appeared in *Science* (Reick M et al., 2001; Rutter J et al., 2001). These papers were discussed by Ueli Schibler, Juergen A. Ripperger, and Steven A. Brown from the University of Geneva, who supplied an illustration of the process (Figure 78).

They discuss two master CLOCK proteins, the transcription factors NPAS2 and Clock. The binding of these proteins to their DNA recognition sequences depends on the ratio of NAD^+ to NADH. Because these molecules are essential components of the respiratory chain, as discussed in the section about nicotinamide and amphetamines, the ratio fluctuates according to cellular metabolism. The *clock* gene expresses the transcription factor Clock which forms a heterodimer with BMAL1 (Clock:BMAL1), another transcription factor, and binds to CACTG DNA motifs to stimulate the expression of other pacemaker components such as PER1 and PER2, and the "cryptochromes" CRY1 and CRY2 which are associated with a FAD cofactor. These cryptochromes repress the transcription of *clock* and *BAML1* genes. Thus, there is a negative feedback loop involving *Per* and *Cry* gene expression which switches off Clock:BMAL1 transcriptional activity. NPAS2 can substitute for clock but is not expressed in the rat SCN. It is found in mammalian forebrain structures such as the somatosensory cortex, caudate-putamen, piriform cortex, visual cortex, auditory cortex, striatum, NAc, and dentate gyrus. NPAS2:BMAL1 is expressed at night in rats, their period of greatest activity, and stimulates *Per1, Per2,* and *Cry1* gene expression, while repressing *BMAL1*. This process ensures reliable clock oscillation.

The *LdhA* gene is also turned on by NPAS2:BMAL1 to make the A isoform of lactate dehydrogenase (LDHA). LDHA catalyzes the transformation of pyruvate to lactate, during which NADH is oxidized to NAD^+ under anaerobic conditions. In an aerobic environment, the usual situation, pyruvate is taken up by mitochondria and enters the glycolytic pathway. NAD cofactors affect the levels of NPAS2. NAD^+ lowers them, and NADH increases them. BMAL1 is not affected by NAD cofactors and can form a homodimer, BMAL1:BMAL1, which does not activate transcription. Thus, the amount of NPAS2 made (which has a heme cofactor), depends on how much NADH (or NADPH) is available. Cryptochromes can thereby inhibit Clock and NPAS2 by redox electron transfer through NAD^+ and NADH. The electron jumps from NPAS1-NADH to CRY-FAD and then to the heme cofactor of NPAS1, so that FAD can remain oxidized. In this manner, cell metabolism regulates circadian rhythms.

Human casein kinase 1 epsilon (hCK1ε) can phosphorylate hPER1. This phosphorylation causes a decrease in the protein stability of hPER1, producing a half-life of 12 hours. Unphosphorylated hPER1 remains stable in the cell for longer than 24 hours. Per1 undergoes a daily oscillation in abundance and phosphorylation state in its role in determining circadian rhythms (Keesler GA et al., 2000).

It has been of great importance for organisms to survive periods of starvation. We eat during the day and starve at night, but most animals, including humans in many countries today, often starve for longer periods. Lactate is used as energy during these times in anaerobic glycolysis, requiring that NADH be converted to NAD$^+$. When the NADH/NAD$^+$ ratio is high, we are aroused and consume food, an activity which is a zeitgeber. When the ratio is low, we sleep and are in a starvation mode. When aroused, our neurons secrete glutamate, which is taken up by astrocytes to produce lactate and then transferred to neurons, which use it as their principal energy source.

Neuronal activity decreases during NREM sleep, which may entrain the neurons. Despite glucose homeostasis in the brain, there may be decreased astrocytic lactate transported during NREM sleep. LDHA would decrease as well, but in a circadian manner. NADH would be higher than NAD$^+$ during periods of arousal and vice versa, producing "balanced oscillation of intracellular redox potential, thereby executing biochemical entrainment of the molecular clock" (Rutter J et al., 2001).

Many regions of the brain involved in neurosomatic disorders express NPAS1. Some of them might misinterpret signals or respond to aberrant neurotransmission which would result in a delayed sleep-wake cycle. A starvation mode may account for the pronounced rapid weight gain seen in many patients after the onset of their illness, as may decreased body temperature, also regulated by the MPOA. Exogenous nicotinamide or NADH has not helped my patients who have taken these agents, but perhaps I should try them more often in those with phase-delay symptoms. NADH may be purchased as a nutritional supplement. The rationale for using it for symptoms other than sleep-phase disorder is that NADH is necessary for the synthesis and regeneration of tetrahydrobiopterin (BH$_4$), which is an essential cofactor for tyrosine hydrolase, the rate-limiting enzyme in the biosynthesis of DA. When applied to rat striatal slices in vitro, evoked DA release was doubled. This effect was not observed in vivo, however (Pearl SM et al., 2000). Other factors that regulate NADH/NAD$^+$ in addition to light/dark availability of lactate and glucose, such as neurotransmitters, should be examined more closely. Amphetamines, unlike the usual case in normal subjects, do not phase shift or often cause weight loss in obese phase-delayed neurosomatic patients. Uncoupling agents and other substances that act at the mitochondrial level have not even had human safety trials, but they may regulate premitochondrial processes more directly. This problem may be closer to a solution when my next book is written.

The LC sends a projection to the dorsomedial nucleus of the hypothalamus, which relays it to the SCN. The LC-DMH-SCN circuit is eliminated by lesioning the DMH. Because the LC also has a circadian rhythm to its impulses, it probably participates in the regulation of arousal and sleep.

Other noradrenergically mediated functions, such as cognition, also show circadian variability.

As in most neural connections, there is probably retrograde innervation of LC dendrites by DMH neurons. The SCN is like other hypothalamic nuclei, having numerous intercommunications, particularly with the PVN, MPOA, and LPOA. The DMH is one of the brain regions that expresses Hcrt, which strongly innervates the LC, activating it. LC stimulation affects the entire neuraxis, causing EEG activation and increased wakefulness. For the most part, LC circadian rhythms are regulated by the SCN. If the LC is highly driven to regulate hyperglutamatergic activity in certain areas of the brain, other regions involved in sleep onset and maintaince may receive excess input. LC overactivity and fluctuations may cause the disorder of initiating and maintaining sleep that troubles many neurosomatic patients, is related to other aspects of their dysautonomia (Aston-Jones G et al., 2001), and may contribute to synaptic fatigue.

Perhaps the simplest way to view neurosomatic phase delay is this: Extirpation of the SCN causes phase advance; thus, hyperfunction of the SCN induced by increased glutamatergic input from one or more sources causes secretion of numerous substances through the SCN output pathway, including prokineticin and TNF-alpha. The SCN has many targets, including the medial preoptic area, or as called by some, the medial preoptic nucleus (MPN). Its "slave oscillators" also include peripheral organs such as the kidneys and liver (Reppert SM, Weaver DR, 2002).

It is important to realize that there is a propensity to sleep a certain amount, termed "sleep homeostasis." There are times to sleep and to be awake, termed "circadian," and there is an apportionment of the NREM and REM stages during the sleep cycle, termed "ultradian." NREM EEG "slow waves" are caused by hyperpolarization of thalamocortical neurons. Sleep deprivation results in an enhancement of slow-wave activity when sleep is again allowed, even to the exclusion of REM in the first night of recovery. REM rebound is noted more prominently when subjects have been specifically deprived of REM. The REM pressure will decrease the time in NREM until full recovery occurs. The interactions between REM and NREM have been described in several complex models. It is interesting to me that the prevalence of slow waves is maximal at frontal EEG derivations in the initial phase of sleep. If NREM sleep is to be considered the "recovery" phase of sleep, then the PFC, the most active part of the brain during wakefulness, needs the most recovery.

As has been suggested in the chapter "Sleep Homeostasis and Models of Sleep Regulation," by Alexander A. Borbely and Peter Achermann, diminishing the firing of activating neuronal structures after sleep onset decreases the activity of the phosphorylation cascade. Thus, phosphorylation of transcription factors and induction of IEGs becomes less effective, requiring less cellular energy. Perhaps as a result, the level of mitochondrial RNAs that are transcribed and translated into subunits of respiratory enzymes is considerably higher during waking than during sleep. "Restorative" sleep may thus restore energy.

Hypnotics and stimulants each were allotted two chapters in *Sleep Medicine*. Interesting points I have not made elsewhere are that injections of triazolam (Halcion) into the MPOA consistently enhance sleep, an anatomically specific effect obtainable nowhere else in the brain. Similar results are obtained with phenobarbital, ethanol, and adenosine. Researchers are beginning to think that the tendency to sleep resides in the MPOA, which is cholinergic, and coordinates reproductive and homeostatic functions in the basal hypothalamus. As might be expected, there are many inputs, outputs, and transmitters, but the MPOA may coordinate sleep with other systems, and may be the locus of action of GABAergic hypnotics. The MPOA projects primarily to other hypothalamic nuclei. It is situated just anterior to the ventral bed nucleus of the stria terminalis, and the MPOA/VBST project to the VTA, PAG, and the lateral septum. Further support that neurons responsible for the onset of sleep are in the preoptic area comes from identification of homogenous sleep-promoting neurons in vitro in the ventrolateral preoptic neurons. These neurons must be inhibited by systems of arousal during the waking state (Gallopin T et al., 2000). VLPO neurons probably contain GABA. They are inhibited by Ach and NE. They are somewhat inhibited by 5-HT but not at all by histamine. It is proposed that there are reciprocal inhibitory interactions of these VLPO neurons with the NE, Ach, and 5-HT waking systems to which they project.

Modafinil, which must have just become available in the United States as *Sleep Medicine* went to press, was noted to increase c-fos immunoreactivity in the SCN but not in numerous other areas activated by amphetamine. Modafinil also increases glutamate release in areas of the rat thalamus and hippocampus and decreases GABA release in the MPOA. These changes are hypothesized to reflect an action of a 5-HT_3 antagonist, such as ondansetron (Zofran). Ondansetron should have numerous benefits in addition to that of an antiemetic in neurosomatic disorders. It is a glycine-site antagonist, like kynurenate, but is not an effective hypnotic. The 5-HT system interacts directly with the DA system in the SN and VTA (Barnes JM et al., 1992), providing a rationale for the use of 5-HT_3 antagonists in the treatment of tardive dyskinesia and schizophrenia (Sirota P et al., 2000). Ondansetron has reduced pain in several of my patients when given as an analgesic, similar to the reported benefit of a related agent, tropisetron (Stratz T et al., 2000) which is not available in the United States. Tropisetron is a member of the "tropeine" family, which ondansetron is not

(Maksay G et al., 1999). Ondansetron potentiates cocaine-induced behaviors in the NAc of the rat (Herges S, Taylor DA, 2000) but has been shown to block the motor hyperactivity induced by central administration of amphetamine and DA (Costall B et al., 1987). The ability of DA to inhibit glutamatergic efferents from the mPFC is potentiated by 5-HT$_3$ agonists and inhibited by 5-HT$_3$ antagonists (Costall B et al., 1990), although ondansetron antagonizes the effect of ketamine. The 5-HT$_3$ receptor may have subtypes with different properties. Odansetron may also be a treatment for bulimia, perhaps because 5-HT$_3$ antagonists decrease afferent vagal activity (Faris PL et al., 2000).

Treating "idiopathic central nervous system hypersomnia" (a disorder somewhat similar to primary disorder of vigilance) is an activity more likely than most to attract unwanted scrutiny. Because this disorder is common in my practice, I particularly appreciated the chapter on this topic by Christian Guilleminault and Rafael Pelayo of Stanford University. This illness consists of excessive daytime sleepiness with no "auxiliary" manifestations of narcolepsy, i.e., cataplexy, sleep paralysis, hypnagogic hallucinations, a feeling of a "presence" in the room, and nocturnal sleep disruptions, often with terrifying nightmares. Narcolepsy is due to a hypercholinergic/hypomonaminergic imbalance and an absolute or relative deficiency of the hypocretins. It is tempting to consider modafinil having an agonist effect at Hcrt receptors. Modafinil can be antagonized by clonidine and olanzapine. Modafinil is one way to treat idiopathic CNS hypersomnia. At times, patients with this disorder nap or engage in automatic behavior. In the latter case, dissociative disorder may be in the differential diagnosis. Polysomnography demonstrates a normal or long sleep record, with a very short time to fall asleep on multiple sleep latency testing, but no sleep onset REM phenomena (SOREMP). With these findings, physicians should prescribe stimulants without fear.

Guilleminault and Pelayo describe three subtypes of idiopathic CNS hypersomnia. Subtype I is familial and dysautonomic. It is associated with the HLACW2 antigen. Subtype II is postviral, just like many cases of neurosomatic disorders. Subgroup III has no family or viral antecedents.

The dysautonomic subtype I often presents with migraine headaches. The headaches, as well as many of the other symptoms, respond to stimulants (my experience also). I found the D$_1$/D$_2$ agonist, mazindol, to be most effective for this disorder when it was still being marketed.

Sometimes hypersomnic patients will have SOREMPs but no "auxiliary symptoms." For this situation, Guilleminault and Pelayo advise treatment and long-term observation. These patients are diagnosed as having excessive daytime sleepiness (EDS) with sleep-onset REM periods.

The most common differential diagnosis is between OSA or upper-airway resistance syndrome (UARS). The latter disorder is seen in individuals who have a small posterior airway space (from the back of the tongue to the cervical spine). Such patients have repetitive transient alpha-EEG arousals lasting 3 to 14 seconds, which regularly interrupt their abnormally high inspiratory efforts. There usually will be increases in snoring before the episode, but some women with this disorder do not snore. During an "arousal" there is an increase in inspiratory time and a decrease in expiratory time. If the sleep specialist is not looking for this abnormality, he or she may not consider it. Definitive diagnosis is made by measuring esophageal pressure, an indication of respiratory effort. I have seen only one patient who had this test performed prior to our initial visit. Continuous positive airway pressure (CPAP) must be titrated by measuring snoring and esophageal pressure. The treatment for UARS is with CPAP or surgery. With idiopathic CNS hypersomnia, it is with medication. If referring a patient of normal weight who has a receding chin and a high arched palate for PSG, the physician should also write R/O (rule out) UARS. Hopefully the sleep specialist will know what that means and call if not.

Guilleminault has little use for CFS in his universe. He writes "there is a very poor correlation between the severity of the complaint and the severity of the neuropsychological test results . . . the patients have more tiredness than true sleepiness" (p. 691). If he knew which neuropsychological tests to perform (Sandman C et al., 1993), he would appreciate how severe the disorder was.

There are chapters about restless leg syndrome (RLS), which occurs before falling asleep, periodic limb movement disorders, and bruxism. All three are very common in my practice, with bruxism often antedating the full neurosomatic illness by many years. Patients with RLS have dysesthesias in their legs relieved by vigorous movement. The differential includes akathisia from neuroleptic medications or formication ("ants under my skin") often caused by dopaminergic hyperactivity or excessive stimulant use.

Patients with RLS may also have PMLS, "rhythmical extensions of the big toe and dorsiflexions of the ankle with occasional flexions of the knee and hip, each movement lasting approximately 0.5 to 5.0 seconds with a frequency of about one every 20 to 40 seconds" (Montplaisir J et al., 2000, p. 742).

RLS may be associated with neuropathy, uremia, iron-deficiency anemia, rheumatoid arthritis, magnesium deficiency, and possibly ADHD. Iron is a cofactor in the action of tyrosine hydroxylase, which catalyzes the production of dopa from tyrosine.

Similar but unrelated conditions are the "painful legs and moving toes" syndrome (not relieved by activity) and nocturnal leg cramps, which are usually responsive to gabapentin, baclofen, or clonidine.

The best treatment for RLS and periodic leg movements in sleep (PLMS) is a dopamine agonist such as pramipexole (Mirapex) or ropinirole (Requip) at bedtime. Dopamine agonists are more effective in these conditions than in others because RLS and PLMS are brainstem mediated with a limbic component. DA agonists do not access the mesocortical tract very well and thus are only occasionally useful in most neurosomatic disorders. They do not always work in RLS and PLMS, either. Clonazepam, opioids (stimulate DA), tramadol (Ultram), and gabapentin are also quite effective.

PLMS is similar to the Babinski reflex. Interestingly, the Babinski reflex could be elicited in 50 percent of normal subjects during NREM sleep. RLS and PLMS are caused by dopamine deficiency, not unexpected in neurosomatic patients. Such an individual may have a Meyerson sign, i.e., when an examiner taps the patient's forehead with his or her finger, it will take some time before the patient habituates to the stimulus and stops blinking. Meyerson sign is also seen in Parkinson disease and is thought to be due to a decrease in intracortical inhibition. It is also known as the "glabellar reflex," probably a product of the eponym revulsion of the 1970s.

Both dopamine agonists and propranolol have been reported to be effective in reducing bruxism, which has been found to be unrelated to stress. BZDs reduce bruxism, tricyclic antidepressants are not helpful, and SRIs make it worse. Numerous mechanical devices and behavioral therapies are available to alleviate bruxism. I would suppose that injections of botulinum toxin would be a last resort.

The major idea I took away from reading *Sleep Medicine* is that some cases of idiopathic CNS hypersomnia might stem from insufficient NE input to the MPOA. It is but a short hop from there to implicate the MPOA in many fatiguing disorders in the neurosomatic spectrum.

In order for the MPOA to have an important role in neurosomatic disorders, it must be involved in the modulation of pain. Evidence for this role has been elusive until recently (Jiang M, Behbehani MM, 2001). It has been known for several years that MPOA stimulation produces analgesia, even though there are no direct projections to the spinal cord.

There are intensely stained retrograde and anterograde pathways to the nucleus raphe magnus and the periaqueductal gray. Furthermore, MPOA projections to the PAG terminate in PAG regions that project to the NRM, which acts as a relay between the forebrain and the spinal cord. PAG stimulation, often viewed as an aspect of descending noxious inhibitory control, is mediated through the NRM. Both PAG and NRM are rich in glutamatergic neuronal components. We have seen how activation of glutamatergic afferents to the PAG produce analgesia. The activation of many NRM neurons is blocked by interrupting transmission from the PAG.

In addition to glutamate, the PAG contains neurotensin and SP, which have a facilitatory action in DNIC of up to two hours after intra-PAG injection. Fibers of passage through the MPOA contribute to the PAG-NRM-spinal cord DNIC. Intra-PAG neural networks significantly modulate this process.

CONCLUSION

I know that for many readers the information and conjecture in this book has been confusing, and my reasoning may seem confused. The systems I am discussing are more complex than I can comprehend, and the amount of information available about them is more than I can assimilate, much less compress into these pages. The functional neuroanatomy may be confusing (Figure 83a-b). Some questions I have not been able to answer. I can only speculate that dysfunction of the intergeniculate leaflet, LC, or increased retinohypothalamic tract activity causes the almost ubiquitous phase delay. The origin of elevated substance P and nerve growth factor in the spinal fluid may be the thalamus, the caudate nucleus, or more of a diffuse CNS abnormality. I have deliberately concentrated on molecular neuropharmacology at the expense of functional neuroanatomy because of the tremendous advances in the former discipline since I wrote *Betrayal*.

It still seems quite obvious that the pathophysiology of neurosomatic disorders is primarily cortical. The neural network involved is the corticostriatalthalamocortical plus the extended amygdala with feedforward and feedback projections. The striatum receives input from the entire cortex, and functionally related cortical areas project in overlapping fashion to several striatal areas. It would be foolhardy to posit one particular circuit, but the D_1 receptor-expressing pathway from the caudate nucleus to the globus pallidus interna and substantia nigra pars reticulata must be involved. It contains SP, dynorphin, and GABA and is probably functionally segregated from the D_2-expressing pathway containing GABA and enkephalin, which terminates in the globus pallidus externa. All five dopamine receptors are G-protein coupled. Injection of the D_2 agonist quinpirole into the dorsolateral striatum of rats reduces pain in the formalin test, one model for fibromyalgia pain (Magnusson JE, Fisher K, 2000). The D_1 receptor stimulates adenyl cyclase and may potentiate excitatory cortical glutamatergic input to striatal neurons (Figure 83b). The D_2 receptors may have the opposite effect (Figure 84). Basal ganglia experts are still somewhat divided about whether the circuits are convergent or parallel and segregated, since different areas of the cortex project to specific regions of the striatum (caudate/putamen), pallidum and substantia nigra, thalamic nuclei, and then back to the same cortical region (Figure 85). The globus pallidus externa may inhibit or focus the effect of the striatal projection to the globus pallidus interna. In a finding unlike any I have seen thus far in neurosomatic patients clinically or in the literature, burning mouth syndrome (BMS), a condition I have treated in association with other symptoms quite successfully, is associated with decreased uptake of 6-[^{18}F] Fluorodopa (FDOPA) bilaterally in the putamen only in a study from Finland (Jaasklainen SK et al., 2001). Radioreceptor ligands have been available for over a decade, but not one has been approved for use by the FDA. Their unavailability has markedly hampered my understanding of neurosomatic pathophysiology.

This finding reflects the dopaminergic function of the presynaptic terminals of projection neurons from the substantia nigra pars compacta (SNpc) to the striatum. The substantia nigra pars reticulata is primarily a GABAergic output structure which receives inhibitory GABAergic projections from the caudate and putamen. Its output is decreased by gabapentin and other gabamimetic AEDs (Bloms-Funke P, Loscher W, 1996). The putamen is usually associated with basal ganglia motoric function, but experimental evidence shows the existence of purely nociceptive nigrostriatal neurons. Striatal projections to the SNpc are usually regarded as GABAergic and, therefore, inhibitory, and this influence is probably mediated by the cerebral cortex. Because there are overlapping multiple cortical excitatory projections to the putamen, just as there are in the caudate, the somatosensory cortex and other functionally related cortical areas project to a single striatal zone. I discussed nonmotoric functions of the basal ganglia in relation to perception, cognition, and behavior in *Betrayal,* pages 95-111. My opinions have not substantially changed since I wrote that chapter in 1995. They have become more complex but not different. The FDOPA experiment indicates that the nigrostriatal pathway, as part of a corticostriatalthalamocortical loop, is "involved in the processing and sensory gating of nociceptive information" (Jaasklainen SK et al., 2001, p. 259). Most patients with neurosomatic disorders have a dopamine deficiency, but since it does not involve neuronal loss, is not as severe as Parkinson's disease, and involves the VTA as well as the SN, dopamine-agonist therapy is not usually effective. As I have mentioned and as noted in the Finnish study, abnormal habituation of the blink reflex (glabellar reflex) is seen in neurosomatic pain patients, particularly those with atypical facial pain, RLS, and PMLS.

NMDA receptors are colocalized with DA and GABA receptors on striatal medium spiny neurons (Figure 83b). These neurons can be divided into two groups, suggesting that the population containing dynorphin and

SP and expressing D_1 receptors may be implicated in neurosomatic disorders. Some researchers believe that the actions of systemically administered NMDA-receptor antagonists occur primarily at the level of the medium spiny neurons. When DA secretion is decreased, tyrosine phosphorylation by tyrosine kinase of the NR2B subunit of the NMDA receptor occurs, potentiating and sensitizing it (Oh JD et al., 1998). This finding is an aspect of my hypothetical pathophysiology of neurosomatic disorders and is the reason why genistein, a tyrosine kinase inhibitor, is on my list of treatments. I have discussed the phosphorylation cascade in some detail in this book because of its relevance to NMDAR sensitivity. The striatal medium spiny neuron is a major anatomic locus for modulation of cortical information flow through the basal ganglia and may also be a major influence on neurosomatic symptomatology. Dopaminergic output from the VTA to the NAc might play an even more important role, since the NAc innervates the mesolimbic and mesocortical dopaminergic tracts. Chronically stressed rats have a decreased output of DA from the NAc compared to controls after being administered cocaine (Gambarana C et al., 1999), a deficit that is reversed by daily imipramine administration during the stressful period. Dopamine also tonically acts in the cortex to produce antinociception (Burkey AR et al., 1999), especially via descending tracts from the rostral agranular insular cortex.

Although functional brain imaging does not usually implicate the anterior cingulate cortex in neurosomatic disorders as it does, for example, in depression, the ACC has dense projections to the ventral pallidum, ventral striatum, and the mediodorsal thalamus and then back to the anterior cingulate. Symptoms could be increased or decreased by altering the activity of several subcortical or cortical areas. In the future, pharmacologic treatment may be combined with some form of rTMS (Helmuth L, 2001), resonance modification, EMDR, and CBT. Some researchers believe that the perception of pain occurs in such a widely distributed neural network that localized lesions, inhibition, or activation have no effect, and that all such studies which purport resultant analgesia are technically flawed. They conceive of pain as being a complex balance existing between various sensory systems and cite the variability of response to pain treatment ("neurochemical individuality") as being a clinical example of this process (Jabbur J, Saade NE, 1999). This viewpoint is not too different from my own and is illustrated by the transient efficacy at best of neurosurgical lesions to treat the pain of neurosomatic disorders.

Long-term rTMS in rats increases expression of BDNF and CCK mRNA (Muller MG et al., 2000). Most neurotrophins are made in excess in neurosomatic brains, and CCK is a panicogen. These factors may contribute to the ineffectiveness of rTMS in almost all my patients who have wangled their way into an experiment.

The fact that neurosomatic disorders must be managed on an individual, case-by-case basis is beginning to be recognized in the general medical community (Cravchik A, Goldman D, 2000). Practice has been heretofore oriented toward making the diagnosis and selecting the proper treatment. This approach has worked well for infectious diseases ("bug and drug") but is inadequate to treat the patients I see every day. For that reason, I developed receptor profiling, an attempt to identify an individual patient's neurochemical dysfunction. This approach has been so successful that most previously treatment-refractory patients are markedly improved or asymptomatic after four days of medication trials in the office. Perhaps diagnosis will matter when SP antagonists are identified and employed in the treatment of fibromyalgia and irritable bowel syndrome. NGF blockers might have too many adverse reactions for clinical use. Dynorphin antagonists already exist in the form of acetaminophen and mu-opioid agonists (Sandrini M et al., 2001), but they are hardly panaceas. High doses of acetaminophen raise brain 5-HT levels and inhibit the $5HT_{2A}$ receptor (Srikiatkhachorn A et al., 1999). Acetaminophen is also a COX-3 antagonist.

I have some difficulty with my hypothesis that neurosomatic disorders are related to NMDA-receptor hyperactivity which is insufficiently modulated by submaximal secretion of DA, NE, and GABA with resultant synaptic fatigue of the LC, VTA, and possibly the superior cervical ganglion, which I discussed in *Betrayal*. Bilateral ganglionectomy induces mast-cell hyperplasia in the brain, a possible cause of increased SP and NGF levels in FMS (Bergerot A et al., 2000).

Although NE levels may be too low in neurons modulating the NMDA synapse, they are probably too high elsewhere, contributing to dysautonomic symptoms. Although using agents which decrease synaptic transmission in one way or another is generally beneficial in neurosomatic disorders, such gross interventions can be counterproductive, depending on the location of pharmacologic action. For example, ketamine usually potentiates the effect of morphine. Activation of off cells in the rostroventrolateral medulla by NMDA receptors is required for morphine to be an effective analgesic (Heinricher MM et al., 2001). I have discussed the function of the rostroventrolateral medulla extensively in previous writings (Goldstein JA, 1993). Still, ketamine is the one treatment that is effective in the most patients. One of the primary effects of gabapentin (Neurontin), the most effective oral medication, is to decrease neocortical norepinephrine release (Dooley DJ et al., 2000), perhaps by opening the K_{ATP} channel and hyperpolarizing the neuron, thereby inhibiting synaptic transmission, a great benefit in a hyperglutamatergic state with overflow compensatory noradrenergic activity in certain regions of the CNS. This effect is due to P/Q-type Ca^{2+}-channel blockade, AMPA-receptor antagonism, and K^+ efflux (Dooley DJ et al., 2000), perhaps mimicked by the endogenous neuropeptide galanin.

Variations in receptor subunit construction, which may be dynamic ("subunit switching"), are increasingly being discovered. Gabapentin alters the conformation of Ca^{2+} channels by binding to the alpha$_2$-delta subunit, of which there are now three subtypes. Gabapentin binds to subtypes 1 and 2. Mefenamic acid (Ponstel), the most underused medication on my list besides dipyridamole, potentiates or inhibits $GABA_A$ receptors according to their subunit profiles (Halliwell RF et al., 1999). Chronic cycloserine use alters subunit composition of the NMDA receptors (Bovetto S et al., 1997) so that reduced affinity for glycine and glutamate develops.

Although gabapentin is effective in migraine headache prophylaxis, particularly if the V_1 neurons are expressing PKC (Christensen D et al., 2001), opinion is still divided about whether it increases GABA levels. Tiagabine (Gabitril) definitely does. It is a GABA-reuptake inhibitor and has the highest GABAergic potency of any antiepileptic drug. I am starting to prescribe it for acute migraine therapy, like I do the triptans or certain NSAIDs (Leniger T et al., 2000).

Ketamine may be the most effective medication for neurosomatic disorders, but when the NMDA receptor is blocked, more glutamate is available to act as a ligand at non-NMDA glutamate receptors. As researchers from Yale note: "Dissociative cognitive and perceptual alterations commonly occur at the time of traumatization and as an enduring feature of post-traumatic stress disorder (PTSD)" (Chambers RA et al., 1999). They relate subsequent dissociative experiences to synaptic remodeling caused by increased corticothalamic glutamate. So far, so good. They go on to speculate that since drugs like ketamine can cause dissociation as an adverse reaction, dissociation must occur by glutamate stimulation of AMPA, kainate, or metabotropic glutamate receptors. They suggest the use of medications that inhibit presynaptic glutamate release, such as lamotrigine (Lamictal), which counteracts many of ketamine's effects, so that hyperactive corticolimbic glutamatergic neurotransmission may be more appropriate. This hypothesis approximates my own but implicates other glutamate receptors besides NMDA in the pathophysiology of dissociative disorder.

One of the DSM-IV-TR diagnoses I use frequently is dissociative disorder in its numerous manifestations with its close relative, panic disorder. I suppose that pseudoseizures and blackout spells are the most common varieties. The experience of extreme depersonalization that occurs with ketamine administration excess ("I'm on the ceiling looking down at myself") rarely occurs in my fairly large population of dissociating patients, but mild depersonalization is common. I have not done functional brain imaging on a patient receiving a ketamine infusion (Figure 86, PET of ketamine infusion), but I seriously doubt that it would resemble that of dissociation. Why? Because ketamine, when effective, ameliorates dissociative symptoms as it does all the rest, even in patients with PTSD. Functional brain imaging has been helpful in understanding PTSD. Two groups of women were compared: one had been victims of child abuse but did not develop PTSD, and the other child abuse group did develop PTSD. The abused women with PTSD had PET scans during guided imagery, as did the non-PTSD group. The PTSD group had greater increases in orbitofrontal and anterior temporal activation and decreases in left inferior frontal activation. One group of Vietnam veterans with PTSD was exposed to combat sounds during brain SPECT. They had greater increases in medial prefrontal cortical activity than two control groups, perhaps representing a failure of extinction. It seems paradoxical if one reads only the adjectives, but ketamine, a dissociative anesthetic (only in high doses) is an effective treatment for dissociative disorder.

PTSD patients hypersecrete CRH but have hypocortisolemia extremely sensitive to dexamethasone suppression. These findings distinguish them from any other diagnostic category. There is elevated morning plasma cortisol in children with PTSD. Elevated cortisol from HPA axis hyperfunction could eventually down-regulate the entire system, as is seen in neurosomatic disorders. Relative hyperthyroidism is also seen in adults with PTSD. NE levels also increase with physical exercise or trauma-related stimulus exposure. Yohimbine, an alpha$_2$ antagonist which increases NE, reliably produces panic attacks in patients with PTSD but not nearly as often in neurosomatic patients. An NMDAR antagonist administered after predator exposure does not alter PTSD in animals but is often effective in humans.

There is more evidence of a 5-HT dysfunction in PTSD, since the disorder responds fairly well to SRIs, unlike the neurosomatic illnesses. GABA agonists are not as effective as one would expect them to be in relieving hyperarousal symptoms. This lack of response suggests down-regulation of GABA$_A$ receptors (Sacerdote F et al., 1999). Hypersecretion of CRH in the face of hypocortisolemia suggests a deficit at the ACTH (corticotrophin) level in the pituitary. There may be down-regulation of CRH receptors or alteration of postreceptor events. There may also be a deficit in production of ACTH from propiomelanocortin. One might expect to see reduced levels of CSF beta-endorphin in such a population, but measurements of this substance have yielded inconsistent results. The various other ways that POMC and ACTH production in the PVN could be inhibited are complex and not very relevant to neurosomatic disorders, except for alpha-MSH, which binds to the melanocortin-4 receptor and may reduce obesity.

Even though I am trying to de-emphasize the HPA axis, some further explanation of its role in neurosomatic disorders is necessary. The PVN is the crucial locus for HPA regulation, and I have suggested that in many hypocortisolemic disorders, perhaps due to low secretion of CRH and/or ACTH, that the MPOA might play a more important role. Prolonged stress in such disorders apparently does not lead to the large increase in expression of CRH mRNA in the PVN, although AVP mRNA is still increased.

Brainstem catecholaminergic drive from areas such as the RVLM promotes HPA secretory activity following hemorrhage, hypotension, and respiratory distress, acting via alpha adrenoceptors. These responses are not mediated by higher centers.

Other stressors are regulated by projections from the amygdala, hippocampus, and PFC. The amygdala can secrete massive amounts of CRH and glutamate and is, as noted, involved in fear conditioning. The medial or central amygdalar nuclei appear to be most involved in this response but not in the HPA response to either, suggesting "stressor specificity" in amygdalar stress pathways (Herman JP, Cullinan WE, 1997).

Excitation of the PVN may also be conveyed by the BST, which also links the MPOA and the hippocampus. The BST, being a part of the "extended amygdala," should activate the HPA axis when stimulated.

Inhibiting the stress response is more relevant to our interests. Inhibition, of course, occurs by negative feedback to the HPA but can occur in absence of this signal, implying the existence of neuronal inhibitory pathways for maintenance of basal HPA tone. Activation of the hippocampus decreases HPA tone, a fact known for many years. The role of the hippocampus in this process has been a focus of the work of David de Wied and colleagues for the past two decades. Such a finding fits in well with the concept of overlearning and absence of hippocampal atrophy in neurosomatic disorders. The PFC and the lateral septum have individual, yet integrated, roles in the stress response which are "stressor specific," as are all "limbic" stress-inhibiting circuits.

Stimulation of the MPOA and medial BST inhibit the stress response. Both regions have high numbers of GABA-containing neurons. GABA inhibits the release of CRH, ACTH, and corticosteroids in vivo. The medial parvocellular region of the PVN has a significant number of GABA terminals and $GABA_A$ receptors.

"The literature suggests that the stress-regulatory circuit activated by a particular stressor is crucially dependent on stimulus attributes. In general, limbic stress pathways are most sensitive to stressors involving higher order sensory processing" (Herman JP, Cullinan WE, 1997). These stressors are not potentially life threatening, but their salience has been conditioned by comparison with previous experience. They are multisynaptic and multimodal. Specific stressors elicit characteristic patterns of limbic activation, unless the stress response has become overlearned and overly generalized. Even so, the impact of the overlearned stress response should have an individual impact on the PVN according to the distinct set of limbic relays it employs.

The structures (PFC, hippocampus, amygdala, other limbic sites) involved in the multimodal stress response do not, in most instances, project directly to the PVN. There is at least one intermediary structure, which, especially in the case of the hippocampus, is GABAergic. The MPOA is a prime example of how hippocampal activation can cause inhibition of the PVN and reduction in CRH and HPA activity.

Conversely, the activated amygdala secretes GABA and inhibitory neuropeptides. These projections have the capacity to inhibit the GABAergic projection neurons from the MPOA and the BST, resulting in disinhibition of the PVN, increased CRH, and increased HPA activity.

On the basis of this functional neuroanatomy, it appears that whatever role the amygdala had in fear and/or anxiety learning in the neurosomatic patient, this information has been transferred to other cortical areas, resulting in the predominance of the PFC-hippocampal circuit I described in *Betrayal,* with resultant hypocortisolism because of excitatory projections to the GABAergic MPOA and BST. The pieces are coming together.

Ketamine administered to normal subjects causes them to be forgetful and decreases attention (Figure 86). Neurosomatic patients report the opposite effects, suggesting that they attend better to relevant stimuli and do not overload working memory after receiving ketamine. Riluzole (Rilutek) decreases the secretion of presynaptic glutamate as its major effect yet is not nearly as effective as lamotrigine, which also increases GABA and blocks carbonic anhydrase and Na^+ and Ca^{2+} channels. Riluzole is less useful than chlorzoxazone which is occasionally analgesic. Physicians planning to administer ketamine to a patient with dissociative disorder should consider an informed consent signature so that other physicians may be less apt to question their judgment.

Because kynurenate has become better known in the neuroscience community (I use probenecid to prevent its central excretion), it is increasingly being used as a generic NMDA antagonist rather than a glycine coagonist-site antagonist. Many do not seem to realize how many sites the NMDA receptor possesses that could modify its action (Figure 87). Glycine-site antagonists vary in their effects on neurosomatic symptoms. Guaifenesin is the best; diltiazem is next. Ondansetron has been disappointing. Patients who respond to probenecid have no assured propensity to derive benefit from diltiazem or ondansetron. Nootropics often antagonize probenecid among their other actions, despite their putative classification as NMDA/

glycine antagonists. The most reliable probenecid and guaifenesin antagonist is D-cycloserine, a glycine-site partial agonist which sometimes acts as a mu-opioid antagonist. Other glycine-site antagonists include verapamil, felbamate, nimodipine, and atropine.

Phentermine, which I thought was a fairly safe stimulant, turns out to be a neurotoxic MAO-A inhibitor (Ulus IH et al., 2000). MAO-A inhibition is increased when pseudoephedrine or estradiol are added, and one might expect serotonin syndrome to have been reported from use of these agents. Perhaps the best way to treat serotonin syndrome is not with cyproheptadine (Periactin) but with a specific 5-HT$_{2A}$-receptor antagonist related to ritanserin, such as the atypical neuroleptics. A 5-HT$_3$ antagonist could be added to the atypical neuroleptic. Clozapine, the first atypical neuroleptic used in humans, has inherent 5-HT$_3$ antagonisms. Serotonin syndrome is produced, at least in part, by marked elevation of anterior hypothalamic NE (Nisijima K et al., 2001).

The CNS actions of levetiracetam (Keppra) and guaifenesin are poorly understood. They may work in opposite ways. Guaifenesin, used as an intravenous anesthetic in large animals, synchronizes the patterns of electroencephalogram in pigs, as may occur in NREM sleep (Haga HA et al., 2000). It appears to be in the same league as IV ketamine, lidocaine, and amantadine when a 250 mg dose is infused over two to three hours. The need for institutional review board approval was trumped when a 49-year-old woman said she was going back to Louisiana the next day. She had adequate responses to several treatments over the preceding five years but no "magic bullet." She informed me she was going to "end it all" if she did not feel well when she got home. IV guaifenesin eliminated all symptoms. So far, it has about a 50 percent success rate in treatment-refractory patients. Adverse drug reactions have not been a problem. Using the route of oral swirl or nasal spray, guaifenesin is often transiently effective when a patient needs a "pick-me-up" to complete a task requiring alertness.

Like levetiracetam (Keppra), zonisamide (Zonegran) also has a poorly understood mode of action. Zonisamide is known to block Na$^+$ channels, to allosterically modulate the GABA$_A$ receptor, and to attenuate voltage-sensitive Ca^{2+} channels. Zonisamide also inhibits the depolarization induced by neuronal excitation, i.e., it opens K$^+$ channels, allowing K$^+$ efflux. None of the properties of levetiracetam or zonisamide particularly lend themselves to receptor profiling, and neither new AED is very effective in treatment-refractory neurosomatic disorders. Levetiracetam has the advantage of not producing serious adverse drug reactions.

PTSD is thought to have considerable relevance to neurosomatic medicine because of the increased reporting of child abuse of various sorts among patients, which perhaps causes them to be hypervigilant or hyper-aroused. They do not usually report reexperiencing the traumatic event(s), amnesia for it, or a reluctance to discuss it. Their dissociative episodes and exaggerated startle response represent PTSD-like disturbances in neuro-cognitive processing (Newport DJ, Nemeroff CB, 2000).

A recent study that used self-reported childhood victimization as a risk factor for depression in adult life compared 295 depressed women to 612 controls (Wise LA et al., 2001). These results corroborated what had been found many times before in similar surveys. "Compared with women who re-ported no abuse, relative risk estimates were substantially increased for women who reported experience or fear of: any abuse as a child or adoles-cent, physical abuse only, sexual abuse only, and physical and sexual abuse. Risk of depression was highest in women who reported both physical and sexual abuse" (Weiss EL et al., 1999). Although I do not wish any child to be abused, it is nevertheless reassuring to read that I had not been subtly shifted into a parallel time track just prior to reading a paper by Raphael and col-leagues (2001).

The authors of the Wise and colleagues paper did admit, "We can only speculate about presence and magnitude of recall bias." They also hypothe-sized that the twofold greater incidence of depression among women may be related to a higher rate of childhood victimization (about 22 percent).

As this book goes to press, the issue of nature versus nurture remains un-resolved. I have decided that I want to read no more retrospective studies of the effects of self-reported childhood victimization unless some highly reli-able discriminator is included. I cannot say at present what such an item would be.

Do Children Learn to Be Hypervigilant?

Learning theory is a brand of psychology that had its first clinical appli-cation in behavior modification, beginning in the 1960s. Learning theory has two conceptual paradigms: classical conditioning, developed by Pavlov in the 1920s, and operant conditioning, enunciated most cogently by B. F. Skinner in the 1950s. Both of these paradigms viewed brain function as a "black box." Pavlov and Skinner realized that cognition influenced behavior but were ill equipped to measure its properties in relation to the behavior they were shaping. Cognitive therapy, a type of conditioning, was first sys-tematized in the 1950s and 1960s by Aaron Beck, a former psychoanalyst. Since then, numerous others have made significant contributions, and now these three models, as well as several others, have been combined in modern learning theory.

Classical conditioning, the oldest, is still in many ways the best. Its principles are simple. An unconditioned stimulus is a normal physiological response. In Pavlov's experiments, he used the example of a dog salivating when a piece of meat was placed before it. A conditioned stimulus involves pairing the physiologic response with a new stimulus. Pavlov used a bell and rang it when the meat appeared. After several trials, the dog would salivate when it heard the bell ring. The pairing of an US with a CS can have complex permutations.

Operant conditioning is conceptually straightforward. The experimenter, or therapist, waits until a behavior occurs spontaneously and then rewards it. Different rewards are appropriate for various organisms, and for people as well. The spontaneously occurring behavior is said to be "emitted," and the reward can be any event that occurs after the response is emitted. The reward is termed a "reinforcement" and is not always apparent. People can emit seemingly meaningless responses for no evident reinforcement, but if the investigator observes what occurs immediately after the response is emitted, that event is, by definition, a reinforcer.

Cognitive therapy seeks to alter attitudes, inferences, and/or expectations that are illogical. Beck gives the example of an anxious person going into a party where he doesn't know anyone and thinking, "I'm worried that no one will like me." The depressed person in the same situation will think, "I know no one will like me."

The cognitive model is used to define cognitive therapy: disorders are characterized by dysfunctional thinking derived from dysfunctional beliefs; improvement results from cognitive change. This model is almost all encompassing, and I shall not explain it further here. A recent book reads like a melding of philosophy and psychology (*Scientific Foundations of Cognitive Theory and Therapy of Depression,* Clark DA, Beck AT, Alford BA, 1999). It is notable for a complete absence of neurobiological content to demonstrate physiology, pathophysiology, and treatment, but it is a remarkable work nonetheless.

Beck postulates different types of "schemas" that correspond to different functions or aspects of an individual: (1) cognitive-conceptual, (2) affective, (3) physiological, and (4) behavioral. Although all four schemas apply to neurosomatic disorders, the *physiological schemas* seem most relevant. That "they are involved in processing enteroceptive stimuli and their operation . . . is particularly apparent in certain psychopathological conditions such as panic disorder and hypochondriasis" (Clark DA et al., 1999, p. 85). He would place most neurosomatic disorders in the category of depression.

> Depression is viewed in terms of the activation of a cluster of interlocking schemas dealing with primal concerns of loss or deprivation.

This primal loss mode is characterized by (a) cognitive conceptual schemas leading to the actual or threatened loss of one's vital resources; (b) affective schemas representing the subjective state of dysphoria or sadness; (c) physiological schemas involving a perceived state of fatigue or physiological deactivation; (d) motivational schemas associated with a state of helplessness, lack of goal-directedness, or loss of pleasurable engagement; and (e) behavioral schemas representing a response action plan characterized by withdrawal or inactivity. (Clark DA et al., 1999, pp. 110-111)

Although these schemas are not fully applicable to most of my patients, after reading Beck's book it is more amazing to me than ever that I can take a patient completely out of a "primal loss mode" in seconds or minutes with the appropriate medication.

With this skimpy introduction, consider how a child learns to be hypervigilant. I had always assumed that it was because the child felt unsafe. If he had an alcoholic father, he never knew when Daddy would come home and be inexplicably angry, perhaps physically abusive. Such children, I and many others thought, would develop neural networks that placed a premium on sensory novelty or threat, to the extent that the confluence of their genetic programming, intrauterine environment, and immediate postnatal relationship with a mothering figure allowed.

Patients with neurosomatic disorders report a high incidence of various kinds of child abuse which were intermittently or chronically stressful for them and resulted in feeling unsafe during the years when the brain was developing major axonal and dendritic connections, or "hardwiring." Numerous published studies validated the association of neurosomatic symptoms, particularly those involving pain and the autonomic components of anxiety (Goldenberg DL, 1989).

Those with fibromyalgia had lower musculoskeletal pain thresholds than normal (Lorenz J et al., 1996). Patients with IBS had heightened visceral sensitivity. IBS with diarrhea was compared to panic disorder (Mayer EA et al., 2001). A number of studies have reported an association between child abuse and adult functional pain, particularly fibromyalgia, chronic pelvic pain syndrome, chronic low back pain, and chronic headache. These associations were found by patient self-report and by population sampling (reviewed in Raphael KG et al., 2001). So many of my patients had reported child abuse that I included an item about it in my CFS questionnaire to assess the effect of this variable on symptoms and treatment response. Although almost half of my patients endorse this section and describe the type of their abuse, the difference (if any) between the two groups has not leapt out at me. I have not been able to afford to hire someone to perform the types of factor analysis I would like. We have begun to study by chart review which other medications patients who benefit from gabapentin respond to. I viewed an abstract by Jon Russell reporting no increased incidence of child abuse in fibromyalgia as a chance aberration and thought a similar article (Taylor ML et al., 1995) to be so contrary to my clinical experience and scientific reasoning that I disregarded it, as well.

Conjecture, no matter how brilliant or profound, cannot substitute for application of the experimental method. Some recent articles have changed my point of view. Keogh and colleagues (2001) note that "pain and anxiety are intrinsically linked, since both are associated with increased attentional vigilance for negative stimuli," citing previous references to that effect. They find that those who pay more attention to their pain are more disabled by it and more likely to exhibit disrupted attentional performance than healthy controls, citing the work of Eccleston and colleagues (1997). This group from the United Kingdom and Belgium finds "attentional disruption lies in the tendency of those who report high negative affect to be more hypervigilant to bodily sensations and to report more health complaints." They find that high-intensity pain plus high somatic awareness produce the greatest attentional disruption. Why, they ask, is pain given attentional priority? Perhaps fear of pain and pain severity interact (Crombez G et al., 1998), hypothesize Eccleston's group.

In animals, however, fear inhibits pain while anxiety enhances it (Rhudy JL, Meagher MW, 2000). Fear results in stress-induced analgesia, which has been linked to the release of endogenous opioids. "Fear is an immediate alarm reaction to present threat, characterized by impulses to escape, and typically results in a surge of sympathetic arousal" (Barlow DH et al., 1996). Anxiety, on the other hand, is a future-oriented emotion characterized by negative affect and apprehensive anticipation of potential threats, and results in hypervigilance and somatic tension. The hypervigilance appears to be restricted to pain-related fear and pain vigilance (Peters ML et al., 2000). Hypervigilance is defined as "a readiness to select out and respond to a certain kind of weak or infrequent stimulus from the external or internal environment" (Chapman R, 1986). Many authors lump fear and anxiety together, unlike Rhudy and Meagher. Prior to their cited article, the most prevalent model was that pain-related fear and pain catastrophizing are predictive of somatosensory vigilance (Peters ML et al., 2000). Most authors agree, however, that attention to pain in FMS patients is stimulus specific and involves central pain-modulating mechanisms and/or cognitive processing. It is not necessarily comorbid with generalized anxiety disorder or a variant thereof, or to anxiety sensitivity (Asmundson GJG et al., 1997; Keogh E et al., 2001), but involves being hypervigilant for pain-related material. Such a state requires a certain *context* for assigning *salience* to potentially pain-related stimuli or cognitions so that *attention* is allocated to them. Patients with low pain-related anxiety may shift attention away from pain-related environmental stimuli, a coping strategy termed "cognitive avoidance" in which one distracts from, or ignores, pain (Jensen PM et al., 1991). The degree to which a person attends to pain-related stimuli is increasingly being regarded as a "trait," a disposition one is born with or perhaps acquires as a result of dysfunctional maternal-neonate interaction. Traits can be amplified by "states," or reactions to environmental circumstances such as stress.

Cognitive-behavioral therapy associates measures of pain beliefs and measures of functioning among patients with chronic pain (Jensen MP et al., 1999). Pain beliefs, in a large number of studies, are associated with measures of psychological functioning, physical functioning, coping efforts, pain behavior, and pain-treatment outcomes. I have found none of these to predict response to treatment in my office, but CBT is perhaps the most widely promoted treatment for neurosomatic disorders. Catastrophizing cognitions, hopelessness, and a markedly decreased self-efficacy are common. Chronic-pain patients are said to believe damage is occurring, that they are necessarily disabled by pain, and that family members should be solicitous when they are hurting. These beliefs reflect patient function and are thought to be amenable to CBT.

I do not necessarily disagree with cognitive theory and refer selected patients for CBT with EMDR. I *know* that the neurosomatic model ("cognitive therapy in a pill," as I once termed gabapentin) works much faster and with a much greater degree of improvement. Many therapists who do CBT with EMDR are inflexible in their approach, i.e., "one size fits all"; I avoid referring patients to these individuals.

A slightly different take on the situation is that of M. W. Stroud and associates (2000). They also find that pain beliefs and cognitions are related to chronic pain adjustment. In addition, their results indicate that negative cognitions are more predictive of outcome than pain beliefs. "Negative self-statements were consistently related to less adaptive adjustment to chronic pain. . . . such as 'I am useless, I am going to become an invalid,' and 'I can no longer do anything.'" Negative self-statements are related to catastrophizing. New patients make these kinds of statements to me almost daily. Negative cognitions such as these, as well as negative expectations about the potential efficacy of my treatment, have no bearing on the (usually very good) outcome that ensues in one to four days. Recall that in the late 1980s two well-trained psychologists worked with me doing CBT. One was my wife. The other did her doctoral dissertation on an aspect of CFS. They did well at first but eventually had to leave because most patients found treatment with medications to be faster, better, and more cost effective.

It is more scientific, in my view, to apply cognitive neuroscience to cognitive theory. Learning occurs when a stimulus or behavior is paired with a reward or a punishment (safety behaviors are rewarding), termed a "reinforcer." Learning requires that the delivery of the reinforcer be predictable to some extent and requires a "prediction error" to support it. When the reinforcer is omitted, unlearning, or "extinction," is said to take place. If the reinforcer is presented only very occasionally ("intermittent reinforcement"), extinction may take very long, even a lifetime. Expected reinforcers do not support learning because they do not generate prediction errors. Neurons responding to prediction errors will modify their synapses to produce associative learning.

DA neurons are activated by novel rewards, but not by fully predicted rewards, and decrease their firing if the predicted rewards are omitted. They almost cease firing if there is an inescapable aversive stimulus but increase firing if escape ("coping") is possible. I have discussed DA at length because its activity is a critical aspect of neurosomatic illness.

In a classical conditioning model, if the original US is *always* paired with the CS, there will be no rise in DA (actually, a fall). If the US then is omitted and the CS is presented by itself, no learning occurs because there is no prediction error. VTA DA neurons acquire stronger responses as a result of intermittent reinforcement (Waelti P et al., 2001). DA neurons show more activation with rewards with a high prediction error, because they were more novel, than with those with a small prediction error. A stimulus that is somewhat similar to the US may also produce DA activation due to stimulus generalization. "DA neurons themselves code the reward prediction error during the differential process of behavioral and neuronal learning" (Waelti P et al., 2001). The generation and action of the hypothetical DA teaching signal probably involves the mesolimbocortical tracts. Chains of predictive stimuli can exist in "higher order conditioning," and predictive value could be assigned to a stimulus quite different from the initial US. Chronically stressed rats have a deficit in spatial working memory, which is ameliorated by injection of a D_1-receptor agonist into the PFC (Mizoguchi K et al., 2000). Pretreatment with a D_1-receptor antagonist prevents the improvement. One cannot always generalize from rats to humans, but the only agent that may soon be available for clinical use in this manner is the D_1/D_2 agonist apomorphine. Mazindol, a D_1/D_2 agonist which is no longer available, although helpful for certain patients, was no panacea. If a selective D_1 agonist were approved for clinical use, I wonder whether its effects in the striatum might conflict with its action in the PFC. At any rate, chronically stressed children or adults develop deficits in working memory due, at least in part, to a DA deficiency. Patients with neurosomatic disorders appear to have a DA deficiency whether they are currently stressed or not, and all have deficits in working memory. Did some early childhood influence cause a hypodopaminergic state in their PFCs, or is a hypodopaminergic PFC determined by genetic, intrauterine, or early postnatal condition? Perhaps it is a mixture of both, as I have long believed, frequently writing that feeling unsafe as a child contributes to the brain's being hardwired to be hypervigilant. Are neurosomatic patients even hypervigilant?

A Different Reality

The debate over the relative influence of heredity and environment has been taking place for centuries, ever since Aristotle ("psyche" = soul). It has ranged from the literal "tabula rasa" of John Locke to the deterministic ideas of Baron d'Holbach, the latter expressed in a different context by Sigmund Freud.

Locke wrote, "Let us then so suppose the mind [at birth] be, as we say, white paper, void of all characters, without any ideas, how comes it to be furnished?" (Durant W, Durant A, 1956, p. 746). Locke thought ideas came from experience, and was the progenitor of British empiricism as well as the Declaration of Independence ("all men are created equal"). He was reacting to the Scholastic philosophers as well as the later Cambridge Platonists who believed in innate ideas present at birth, which may be available to us by introspection.

Helvétius followed Locke but advanced a new corollary. He believed that there were no inborn differences in neonatal minds: "All are endowed with a strength and power of attention sufficient to raise them to the rank of illustrious men. . . . The inequality of their capacity is always the effect of the difference in situations in which chance has placed them" (Durant W, Durant A, 1956, p. 683). Helvétius was widely read in his time. His ideas helped to motivate both the American and French Revolutions and suggested the perfectability of man in a socialist welfare state.

Freud's theory of the unconscious could have paraphrased d'Holbach:

> [Man's] organization in no wise depends on himself; his ideas come to him involuntarily; his habits are in the power of those who cause him to contract them. He is unceasingly modified by causes visible or concealed, over which he has no control, which necessarily regulate his mode of existence, give a color to his thinking and determine his manner of acting. He is good or bad, happy or miserable, wise or foolish, reasonable or irrational, without his will counting for anything in these various states. (Durant W, Durant A, 1956, p. 702)

Denis Diderot, a leading encyclopedist, put forth a view more in tune with our times:

> Man is not born blank. True, he is born without ideas and without directed passions; but from the first moment of his life he is endowed with a predisposition to *conceive, compare,* and *retain* some ideas [my italics] with more relish than others; and with dominant tendencies resulting in actual passions. (Durant W, Durant A, 1956, p. 690)

This work was not published until 100 years later *(Refutation of Helvétius)* and argued that sensations are transformed differently in different individuals by inherited differences in the structure of the brain (Durant W, Durant A, 1965).

René Descartes (1596-1650), in his *Treatise on the Passions,* expressed a view even more consonant with my own:

> Now that we have studied them [the passions], WE SEE THAT WE HAVE MUCH LESS REASON TO FEAR THEM THAN BEFORE. For we see that they are all good by nature and all we need do is avoid their excesses or bad uses. And these can be cured by separating in oneself the motions of the blood and spirits from the ideas they are usually linked with. (Durant W, Durant A, 1956, p. 346)

It looks like *Tuning the Brain* was a novel idea in the seventeenth century, although a theory of humors had been described as early as Paracelsus. I have most enjoyed the work of David Hume, but I find myself being a Cartesian, at least in regard to neuropsychopharmacology.

In recent years, with few exceptions, such as Dienstbier (1989), I. J. Russell, and the duo of Hudson and Pope (1995), almost all researchers and clinicians have accepted the apparently overwhelming mass of evidence that childhood maltreatment results in many problems sooner or later, a position compatible with the views of both Locke and d'Holbach. Much of this work on child abuse, particularly in regard to whether it is remembered or forgotten, has been discussed in a recent book by Daniel L. Schacter (2001). Evidence indicates that people can voluntarily suppress nontraumatic memories but may have no particular ability to suppress memories for traumatic events or cues. This inability is quite evident in women who report repressed or recovered memories of childhood sexual abuse to Schacter's group (McNally RJ et al., 2001). It may even be that women with post-traumatic stress disorder are more prone to false memory (Bremner JD et al., 2000). False-memory fabrication appears to be a fairly common phenomenon (Porter S et al., 1999). Women with recovered memory of childhood sexual abuse (those prompted to recall it by some process, psychothera-peutic or otherwise) score higher than those who continuously remember it or believe they had repressed it on measures of fantasy proneness and disso-ciation. Repressed-memory patients are the most distressed (McNally RJ, Clancy SA, Schacter DL, Pitman RK, 2000). The nature of childhood mem-ories recalled depends somewhat on the context in which the memory is re-activated (Winkielman P, Schwarz N, 2001). Traumatized individuals with and without PTSD are equally prone to false recall on a word association test. The impact of their false recall is related to their degree of anxiety and is thought to be due to a deficit in monitoring the accuracy of their retrieval memory.

Many of my patients have dissociative disorders of various types, and many of these report childhood abuse. A causal relationship has been doubted in the work of H. Merckelbach and P. Muris (2001). They found that individuals who scored high on the Dissociative Experiences Scale were subject to fantasy proneness, heightened suggestibility, and suscepti-bility to "pseudomemories." They state: "Correlates of dissociation may promote a positive response bias to retrospective self-report instruments of traumatic experiences." This conclusion relates to the term "effort after meaning" used by Hudson and Pope (1995). "Effort after meaning refers to the tendency of suffering individuals to seek some sort of explanation for their plight," as they define it (a restatement of the phrase, "man's search for meaning") (p. 161). Such persons may more assiduously search their mem-ories for traumatic or negative experiences in an attempt to establish a causal relationship, and this tendency may have a genetic basis. By "ge-netic" Hudson and Pope seem to mean that fibromyalgia patients (whom they were discussing) are more likely to have family members with neuro-somatic disorders. When a memory is retrieved, however, it is much more susceptible to alteration than when it is in its consolidated state (Nader K et al., 2001). Individuals may have a genetic predisposition to alterations in retrieval memory, which could be activated or amplified by state-dependent processes. Memory for autobiographical ("semantic") facts was tested in adolescents with an alleged history of trauma and in controls. The adoles-cents who reported trauma were found to have more difficulty with seman-tic personal memory than control adolescents (Meesters C et al., 2000).

False memories are characterized by a failure to recollect detailed infor-mation about the event, or its "perceptual vividness" (Dodson CS et al., 2000; Gonsalves B, Paller KA, 2000, 2002). They can sometimes be distin-guished by lesser activation during functional brain imaging or evoked re-sponses. Vision has the highest priority for encoding among all sensory in-put. Even though imagined visual images activate the same regions of the occipital cortex as percepts, which are actually seen, the latter do so more intensely. Perhaps activation by imaginary scenes is highest in the fantasy-prone individual.

It is possible to review the false-memory literature, but it would be impossible to scan and summarize the mountain of work purportedly demonstrating that child abuse of some sort results in dysfunctional adults all, much, or most of the time. I still believe it must be so. Studies in identical and fraternal twins reared together and reared apart usually demonstrate an environmental role in determining behavior, health, and illness. When the variable being studied is *pain,* the results until recently have been more ambiguous. It has not been easy to establish the relationship of child abuse to adult pain syndromes, and almost all studies have relied on patient self-report. There is an increasing trend among health professionals to not accept patient-reported child abuse unless there is corroborating testimony from multiple sources. The only reason to obtain such information is if the patient's disorder could be improved by a therapeutic process directed at the recalled child abuse. This issue is not relevant in neurosomatic medicine, in which the goal is to make the patient feel normal in the shortest possible time. Child abuse would not be an issue in CBT with EMDR, which deals with matters in the present time, although patients are often directed to reexperience such events by misguided, overzealous therapists. Recalling a dysfunctional environment, neglect, or abuse is one thing, demonstrating that it has a causal role to play in adult disorders is another matter. One of the bases of psychoanalysis was enabling the return of repressed memories. The work of Franz Alexander and George Engel used psychodynamic theory to explain which organs would be "chosen" to express conflict. A large number of intelligent individuals subscribed to such paradigms.

A paper authored by Karen G. Raphael, Cathy Spatz Widom, and Gudrun Lange, from the Department of Psychiatry at New Jersey Medical School in Newark has shaken the foundations of my beliefs about the etiology of many disorders, not only those that are neurosomatic. Titled "Childhood Victimization and Panic in Adulthood: A Prospective Investigation" (2001), it really "knocked my socks off." I can't recall any one article in recent years that had such a profound effect on me.

These researchers used a prospective cohort design with documented cases of sexual abuse, physical abuse, and neglect presented in a court of law in a midwestern city between 1967 and 1971. The children selected were less than 11 years of age at the time of the abuse or neglect incident. They compared these cases to a control group matched for age, sex, race, and social class. There was an attempt to interview all cases and controls 20 years later using structured and semi-structured rating scales, including the Diagnostic Interview Schedule (DIS) from the National Institute of Mental Health, which used DSM-III-R diagnostic criteria. Interviewers and subjects were blind to the purpose of the study. Seventy-six percent were located and able to participate out of an original sample of 1,575. Subjects completed a form which assessed self-reported childhood victimization, subdivided into sexual abuse, physical abuse, and neglect. Of the sample, 62 percent reported some history of childhood victimization. The frequency and type of pain complaints were evaluated using items from the somatization module of the DIS and from other measures. Participants did not have a physical examination, nor were they checked for tender points. There was no difference in any pain measure between those who experienced any type of childhood victimization and those with no trauma.

Because it has long been suggested that unexplained pain is a mechanism through which major depressive disorder expresses childhood trauma, these variables were correlated. There was no concordance between MDD and pain symptoms among those who experienced child abuse, but the non-abused group demonstrated a significant comorbidity of MDD and unexplained pain symptoms. However, "Based on *retrospective self-reports of childhood victimization,* we found a significant relationship between childhood victimization and adult pain complaints" (Raphael KG et al., 2001, emphasis added).

Thus, there is no correlation between documenting child abuse and unexplained pain complaints in adulthood, but self-reported retrospective histories of child abuse are more frequently given by those with unexplained pain. In this book, of course, "unexplained pain" is explained neurobiologically. Similarly, child abuse does not predispose a person to MDD and unexplained pain. Of those with documented abuse, 73 percent had a continuous memory of the abuse and reported it. Of those without documented victimization, 49 percent also self-reported victimization. There may have been undocumented victimization in the control group, and 27 percent of those with documented victimization did not recall it when questioned. I can find no error or flaws in the methods section or in the way the data was analyzed, other than those noted by the authors.

What are the implications of these findings? Raphael and colleagues discuss some of them: (1) a childhood experience of abuse leads to hypoalgesia or a decreased tendency to somatize distress; (2) the abused child may become desensitized to distress, i.e., he or she may develop better coping skills and become hardier; (3) the adult patient who self-reports child victimization may be more health-care seeking and may perceive his or her symptoms to be mysterious and uncontrollable. This type of chronic stress is potentially damaging, and this attitude (supposedly) mitigates against successful therapeutic intervention.

I shall play the devil's advocate and try to explain the findings of Raphael and colleagues from a neurosomatic perspective. Although this study was a massive undertaking, it requires replication because it is potentially paradigm shifting. When confronted with novel biological information that I cannot explain, I try to view it from an evolutionary perspective. How does this function or behavior increase the organism's chances of survival? Does the abused child become a hardy adult?

For almost the entire existence of homo sapiens, survival has not been guaranteed, or even likely. The average age span of primitive humans was about 25. Causes of mortality were frequent, numerous, apparently random, and almost omnipresent. For most children in primitive societies life was quite unsafe, and they could be abandoned or left exposed in crisis situations. Children had to deal with the rigors of such a lifestyle in order to survive to adulthood. Modern civilization has made the environment much more comfortable in industrialized countries, but the human genotype has not changed. Most people alive today would have died at a young age if they had been born 20,000 years ago. Those who somehow lived would have had to thrive despite extreme adversity, which might be compared to the child victimization of today. One method of doing so would have been to modulate the stress response or the response to it. Secretion of neurotransmitters, hormones, and other substances, which might have been lifesaving during a "fight-or-flight" situation, should be rapidly decreased when the stress terminates. Such a "deactivation" would be dependent on which stimuli were perceived as potentially dangerous. A context must be developed to determine salience and allocate attention. If stimuli were dealt with in an improper context, one result might be anxiety, which "leads to increased environmental and somatic scanning that facilitates sensory receptivity" (Rhudy JL, Meagher MW, 2000). I have emphasized this point in my book. What is involved in turning off the acute alarm reaction that characterizes fear?

There is a broad consensus that fear activates the amygdala. The context in which fear is experienced involves a widely distributed neural network in which the hippocampus and DLPFC play a prominent role. If there is a conflict in expectation or prediction, the anterior cingulate becomes activated. Other cortical regions, particularly the parietal, determine salience and attentional allocation. Thalamic nuclei participate, especially the lateral geniculate (for vision), as do various hypothalamic nuclei, the superior colliculus, the LC, the VTA, and the brainstem nucleus paragigantocellularis, which helps to regulate LC output (Buchel C, Dolan RJ, 2000). Phobics deactivate their amygdalae more slowly than controls, while the posterior regions of the ACC and insula are activated by pain anticipation. More anterior areas are involved in pain sensation. Joseph LeDoux, an expert in the amygdala, believes, like Robert Post, that the amygdala is a rapid subcortical processing unit for aversive information that should be under supervision of more sophisticated cortical regions lest there be too high a "false alarm rate." A decline in amygdala activation occurs when the cortex has appropriately modified synaptic connections to learn the aversive associations. Most studies find that neurosomatic patients are hypersensitive to musculoskeletal pain-related stimuli and their anticipation, a finding that is correlated with increased negative expectations (anxiety) about the painful stimulus. One experiment found that fibromyalgia patients did not differ from controls in being hypervigilant to innocuous stimuli as determined by ERP, but this study was flawed because many in the patient group had been prescribed and were taking psychotropic medications (Lorenz J et al., 1996). The patients, as numerous other experiments have shown, were hypersensitive to painful stimuli, perhaps due to a dysfunction in the DLPFC-hippocampal-amygdala network, which would process information to confirm their inappropriate contexts.

"Fear extinction" is the term used in the literature to describe elimination of anxiety about certain kinds of stimuli. The individual need not feel anxious but should have many of the autonomic (usually sympathetic) concomitants of an anxiety disorder. Extinction requires new learning, both in the amygdala and the hippocampus, which is NMDA mediated (Corcoran KA, Maren S, 2000; Collins DR, Pare D, 2000; Falls WA et al., 1992). Contiguous areas of the rat dorsomedial PFC modulate fear reactivity in response to fear conditioning; the more anterior modulates extinction (Morgan MA, LeDoux JE, 1995).

Much of the problem can be explained by a DA deficiency in the mesolimbocortical tracts, which emanate from the VTA. There is a circuit from the entorhinal cortex of the hippocampus (perhaps more important in memory than the hippocampus itself) through the ventral subiculum to the NAc. This circuit modulates the efficacy, and perhaps nature, of contextual information on conditioned responses (Burhans L et al., 2000). Stimulation of DA receptors by systemic injection of apomorphine, however, reduces both fear learning and fear extinction, perhaps because of a nonspecific site of action, or because it is a D_2 agonist as well as a D_1 agonist. D_1 agonists potentiate GABAergic inhibition in the lateral amygdala (Johnson LR, LeDoux JE, 2000). DA in general is an NMDA antagonist, and if it acted in the hippocampus and amygdala, it would impair new learning.

Increased DA in the PFC should decrease glutamatergic projections to both the hippocampus and amygdala and also alter the context in which stimulus salience is determined. VTA DA projections inhibit glutamate secretion in the PFC by synapsing on cortical glutamate neurons and indirectly by synapsing on GABAergic interneurons in the mPFC. These interneurons contact glutamate neurons in the mPFC (Beyer CE, Steketee JD, 1999). PFC DA is low and glutamate is high in patients with neurosomatic disorders.

Of course, mGluRs are involved. Administering an antagonist of the mGluR5 receptor prevents the acquisition of the conditioned fear response in rats (Fendt M et al., 2000). A group II mGluR agonist blocks fear-potentiated startle in rats (Stanek L et al., 2000). Vagal nerve stimulation also blocks fear-potentiated startle in rats and should be available to treatment-refractory neurosomatic patients. It is thought to have this effect by increasing parasympathetic activity (Markus TM et al., 2000).

It is always important to note that humans are not rats. Chronic unavoidable stress, which simulates the life situation or physiologic responses of neurosomatic patients, decreases DA in the NAc shell of rats and makes them hyporeactive to aversive stimuli, quite the opposite of my patient population (Masi F et al., 2000).

Stress increases the incidence of false memory, as does chronic anxiety (Payne JD et al., 2002). False memory is thought to occur (other than effort for meaning) by deficits in retrieval (hippocampal), content (PFC), and strategic memory (ACC). Stress-related hippocampal dysfunction may bring a false sense of familiarity to inexperienced situations (déjà vu). False memories may thereby be accepted as real and elaborated upon long before a neurosomatic illness develops. Then, working memory fills up and new memories are hard to form. False memory may be analogous to bruxism, which often precedes FMS by many years.

What do I believe? After reading the Raphael and colleagues article, I am less likely to causally attribute chronic diffuse pain, and perhaps the entire panoply of neurosomatic symptoms (I rarely see a patient with just one or two), to child abuse. Frequent family clustering, "postviral" onset, and absence of psychopathology in many individuals now inclines me more to a genetic, intrauterine, and/or immediate postnatal etiology. Anxiety, hypervigilance in the absence of anxiety, and chronic autonomic dysfunction, all due to a cortical hyperglutamatergic state, are still compatible with the false-memory literature. The finding that child abuse victims become fairly intact adults, possibly better able to cope with stress is anathema to me, yet it is understandable. The relationship between development of coping skills to childhood experiences needs to be investigated further. Patients with a primary disorder of vigilance may represent a different population or may be a human example of the chronically stressed, hyporesponsive rats. Whatever the case, the presumed etiology of the disorder seems to have little bearing on response to treatment, which is usually quite successful.

Patients with CFS and FMS do not have mismatch negativity of the P50 time point on auditory evoked responses, but PTSD patients do. The amplitude of the P100 wave is increased in PTSD. It is decreased, if anything, in neurosomatic disorders. Both findings illustrate impaired sensory gating in PTSD, and schizophrenia as well, in which abnormal prepulse inhibition of the P50 wave is consistently found. There are no consistent decreases in hippocampal or amygdala size found in neurosomatic disorders, but these are characteristic of PTSD. Reduced activation of the prefrontal cortex, which inhibits the amygdala and thereby modulates the stress response, is found in both disorders but also occurs in depression and schizophrenia (Duncan J, Owen AM, 2000). These same prefrontal areas are activated by widely differing cognitive tasks (Figure 88). "This common network of active regions includes mid-dorsolateral, mid-ventrolateral and dorsal anterior cingulate regions. Whatever the function of these regions, they seem to be recruited by modest increases in demands as diverse as response selection, working memory maintenance and stimulus recognition" (Duncan J, Owen AM, 2000). These areas show further reduction in blood flow on brain SPECT in neurosomatic disorders when patients are performing cognitive tasks. The frequent activation in ventrolateral and anterior cingulate cortex, described in depression, is usually absent in baseline brain SPECT.

In fact, if a patient has a neurosomatic disorder, his or her pattern of cerebral blood flow will not reflect the existence of any comorbid Axis I diagnosis, such as panic disorder, which manifests an increase in left hippocampal and parahippocampal glucose metabolism on PET, and decreased metabolism in the right inferior parietal and right superior temporal cortices (Bisaga A et al., 1998).

It may appear that neurosomatic patients have conditioned fears and anxieties that they are unable to extinguish. These may manifest, for example, as catastrophizing. Mesoprefrontal DA neurons are involved in coordinating the normal extinction of a fear response (Morrow BA et al., 1999). If DA is deficient, fear responses, even for specific sensations, may not be extinguished (Keogh E et al., 2001) and could cause an attentional bias for pain-related stimuli. The patients may be more sensitive to potentially painful stimuli such as windup, increased pain sensation with each repetitive stimulus to a certain area (Staud R et al., 2001). Windup may be a manifestation of central sensitization of one or more wide dynamic range neurons as a result of long-term potentiation via NMDA receptors (Gjerstad J et al., 2001).

Neurosomatic patients often relapse after cognitive tasks. I have previously suggested that this type of symptom exacerbation is due to prolonged focusing of attention by increasing secretion of DA and NE in order to raise signal-to-noise ratio. Evidence now indicates sustained activation of the human mesolimbic dopamine system during performance of cognitive tasks (Fried I et al., 2001) even though brain energy consumption is not increased. These results imply that the brain is not a muscle; thinking does not necessarily deplete ATP, and decreased ATP does not arouse the sensation of brain fatigue. Dopamine also potentiates the firing of delay-active neurons in the PFC, which are important for working memory. The increase in dopamine release can be up to 100 percent and may involve the amygdala and hippocampus as well. Dopamine secretion is important for directing attention to salient stimuli. Inadequate dopamine secretion could lead to misperception of salience. During learning, the increase in extracellular dopamine is sustained and could possibly lead to synaptic fatigue in an individual whose dopamine resources were already overcommitted. Goal-directed motor tasks produce extended dopamine elevation in the striatum, as shown by PET done while playing a video game. Dopamine is also necessary for concentration. It stabilizes active neural representations and protects them from interfering stimuli. It acts as a sustained facilitator of information processing in the brain.

Another pharmacologic method to increase dopamine is with amphetamine. Amphetamine has an excitatory effect on DA neurons as do glutamatergic afferents by inducing bursts of DA secretion. The excitation mediated by (mostly) NMDA receptors is followed by an inhibitory pause mediated by mGluR1 in the normal course of events. Amphetamine produces a selective inhibition of mGluR1 receptors primarily by activation of postsynaptic alpha$_1$ adrenergic receptors (Paladini CA et al., 2001). Amphetamine may block the DA transporter, increasing extracellular DA, which then acts on alpha$_1$ adrenoceptors to inhibit the hyperpolarization caused by mGluRs. Endogenous NE may also act separately from DA to affect the firing of DA neurons. Because inhibitory mGluRs are blocked, excitation caused by AMPA and NMDA receptors is enhanced. Stimulating the LC electrically can increase firing of DA neurons.

DA neurons are not generally activated by salient stimuli, which require attentional allocation, but they may code attentional components associated with rewards (Schultz W, 2001). DA neurons fail to discriminate between rewards and fire only when a reward is surprisingly present or absent, to alert the organism to a new contingency. DA is secreted in short puffs from synchronous neurons in the frontal cortex and striatum as a signal to the neighboring neurons, including the NAc, for optimal processing of stimuli and actions leading to reward. DA acts at these neurons by diffusion, in a paracrine manner, after enough short puffs, and alters their responsiveness. Omission of reward suppresses DA secretion and subsequent tonic stimulation of neighboring DA receptors. A prediction error signal is thus generated once a mismatch is detected, which can lead to synaptic changes, new learning, and changes in predictions and behavioral outcomes.

DA release during a reward prediction error is fast, occurring within 100 to 300 msec. With other behaviors such as eating, stress, social behavior, and sex, the dopamine responses last from seconds to minutes. The slowest DA responses are tonic and paracrine and continuously "enable function of a large variety of motor, cognitive, and motivational processes which are deficient in Parkinsonian patients" (Schultz W, 2001) and perhaps those with neurosomatic disorders.

A sophisticated supplement with excellent illustrations was published by *Trends in Neurosciences* in 2000, edited by C. Warren Olanow, Jose A. Obeso, and John G. Nutt. Titled "Basal Ganglia, Parkinson's Disease, and Levodopa Therapy," it illustrates the complexities of dopaminergic regulation in the Parkinsonian patient. Although the mesocorticolimbic tracts work somewhat differently than the basal ganglia, many of the same principles apply to both. Interested readers are referred to this issue. I shall discuss a few highlights.

DA exerts a bimodal influence on glutamate-mediated synaptic transmission. Low DA preferentially activates D_1 receptors, which increase NMDA receptor-mediated currents by opening L-type Ca^{2+} channels. Higher concentrations activate D_2 receptors, which suppress AMPA-mediated currents. D_1 postreceptor events involve cAMP, PKA, and DARPP-32 signal transduction cascades. D_1 and D_2 receptors facilitate each other in a complex process in this setting. Phasic DA secretion in anticipation of reward would stimulate both receptors. Additive D_1 and D_2 stimulation is inhibitory. In a situation in which DA neurons would be chronically stimulated, an attenuated DA-mediated inhibitory action on D_2 receptors would occur, since they are located within the synapse. As a result, when a phasic burst is required, less DA would be secreted. "Therefore, the system appears to be designed to attenuate phasic DA-mediated responses under conditions in which the dopaminergic system is being tonically overdriven" (Onn S-P et al., 2000). The tonic low-level secretion of DA can provide stimulation to DA autoreceptors and also to D_2/D_4 heteroreceptors on corticostriatal glutamatergic afferents. Decreased DA activity increases (Figures 89a-b) corticostriatal glutamatergic activity, a point I have emphasized throughout this book. No medication will selectively stimulate D_4 receptors and decrease this glutamatergic transmission. Blocking the D_4 receptor, as perhaps may be accomplished with olanzapine, does not have a profound effect on neurosomatic disorders. The role of noradrenergic receptors in regulation of this system remains to be established.

The tonic enabling function requires low, sustained concentrations of extracellular DA in the appropriate areas. If DA is too high or too low, regional brain function will not be optimal. Other neurotransmitters, such as glutamate, aspartate, GABA, and adenosine, have a similar paracrine effect in many regions of the brain. If ambient DA is too low, enabling functions might be impaired. If it is too high, anxiety or paranoia might ensue.

It is difficult to isolate DA in the pathophysiology and treatment of neurosomatic symptoms. NE, especially acting at alpha$_1$ noradrenergic receptors, often synergizes with DA, and DA neurons express excitatory alpha$_1$ receptors. Both transmitters affect contextual shifts in the PFC and lower the STN ratio. NE, in particular, may be deficient in the hyperglutamatergic PFC of the neurosomatic patient but secreted in excess elsewhere, accounting in part for the ameliorative effects of many agents that reduce axonal transmission and transmitter release, or those that modulate excitatory receptors.

Stimulant drugs often make fatigued neurosomatic patients feel worse. Further catecholamine depletion could exacerbate a preexisting hyperglutamatergic state that was being inadequately modulated by DA and NE. Transient enhancement of DA secretion in the presence of hypersensitive D$_2$/D$_3$ autoreceptors could lead to prolonged suppression of DA release from the same neuron(s). Important work has been published about the D$_3$ receptor, which has enhanced my understanding about the mesocorticolimbic dopaminergic tracts. The basic finding is quite novel: The expression of the D$_3$ receptor is regulated by the neurotrophin brain-derived neurotrophic factor. D$_3$ receptors are normally expressed in the NAc shell. If the dopamine neurons on one side of the brain are chemically destroyed, the amount of D$_3$ RNA goes down. I would expect it to increase or to be up-regulated in a dopamine-deficit state. However, if BDNF is infused into the shell, the expression of D$_3$ receptors is restored. It appears that D$_3$ expression is not dependent on regional DA, but on levels of cosecreted BDNF. This idea is new to me in classical transmitter neurochemistry (Guillin O et al., 2001).

BDNF knock-out mice were bred to investigate the situation further with the remarkable finding that levels of D$_1$ and D$_2$ receptors are fine, as are levels of D$_3$ receptors in the islands of Calleja, just below the NAc (White FJ, 2001).

Neurons in the VTA produce both DA and BDNF and project them to the NAc, a cozy relationship. If DA-producing neurons in the VTA are damaged, BDNF does not reach the NAc and D$_3$ declines. Those in the islands of Calleja are unaffected. If the rats with the damaged VTA are injected with the anti-Parkinsonian compound L-dopa repeatedly, D$_3$ neurons are again expressed in the NAc along with TrkB, the receptor for BDNF. The BDNF in this situation came from the frontal cortex, where it is expressed by D$_1$ and D$_5$ receptors activated by L-dopa, the precursor of DA. The BDNF is transported to the NAc where there are TrkB receptors to which it can attach. The BDNF/TrkB induce the expression of the D$_3$ receptor. The number of NAc D$_3$ receptors is not determined only by endocytosis or manufactured via the neuronal terminal but can rapidly respond to stimulus contingencies by moment-to-moment variations of BDNF production in the PFC. For me, this process is a concrete example of a mechanism by which NAc function can vary. Depending only on DA, glutamate, and GABA levels in the mPFC and VTA really wasn't doing the job. Although I'm sure there is more to be told in this story, I feel much better about it now. I had been thinking for a while now that BDNF might be one of the "good" neurotrophins in neurosomatic medicine. It facilitates synaptic vesicle exocytosis, too. BDNF levels in CSF have not been measured yet, but I hope they will be soon.

I am ineluctably drawn to the conclusion that DA receptors are dysfunctional in neurosomatic disorders. The primary dysfunction appears to be in the NAc DA autoreceptor, which may be D_2/D_3 in type (Shafer RA, Levant B, 1998). It is preferentially located in the limbic system and affects locomotion and perhaps reinforcement and reward. D_5 receptors may also be involved, since D_3 blocking agents do not have much effect on neurosomatic symptoms, and neither do D_2/D_3 agonists such as pramipexole, which alleviates RLS, PMLS, and bruxism. Drugs such as pramipexole should have DA transmission responses analogous to pindolol and ziprasidone in the 5-HT system, but they do not seem to.

PFC pyramidal-cell glutamatergic hyperactivity could increase the activity of GABA interneurons within the VTA and thereby increase GABA-mediated inhibition of DA activity. Furthermore, a glutamatergic cortico-accumbens pathway induces subsequent feedback regulation of the VTA (Harden DG et al., 1998). In this instance, both stimulation of monosynaptic mPFC → NAc neurons and stimulation of the NAc itself inhibits VTA DA cell firing. Thus, a hyperglutamatergic PFC could excite local inhibitory neurons within the VTA and/or an inhibitory projection from the NAc to the VTA. The number of cells firing may be regulated primarily by the stimulation of cell-body autoreceptors. A basic deficit in VTA DA secretion may be due to an inability of hypersensitive autoreceptors to compensate. Thus, physical, mental, or emotional stress could not produce an augmented response, and in the case in which increased DA secretion is imposed upon the system, as with amphetamines or ejaculation, the DA secretion could be diminished even further and the patient would relapse.

This explanation does not consider the effects of postsynaptic signal transduction abnormalities. Patients with neurosomatic disorders may also have diminished postsynaptic dopamine responsivity, the opposite of what is seen in euthymic patients with bipolar disorder (Anand A, Verhoeff P, et al., 2000). Pathophysiology, at least in a subgroup, might not be caused by decreased DA secretion. Such patients might be more difficult to treat and could respond to agents that decreased DA secretion, perhaps via alpha noradrenergic receptors, to those that up-regulated postsynaptic DA receptors, or to stimulants, which could flog the hyporesponsive receptors into greater activity. After all, some neurosomatic patients *do* respond to stimulants. The deficit might be anywhere in the panoply of the G-protein-coupled postsynaptic mechanisms discussed in this book. All five DA receptors are coupled to inhibitory or stimulatory G proteins.

The redox-modulating site of the NMDAR directly regulates its function. If it is reduced, NMDAR function is potentiated; reduction can be blocked by an oxidizing agent. Reduction enhances long-lasting allodynia produced by dynorphin. Oxidation greatly reduces allodynic time. Reducing agents potentiate the NMDAR-induced increase in $[Ca^{2+}]_i$ and neurotransmitter release. These effects can be blocked by oxidizing agents. Ascorbic acid, lipoic acid, and, under certain circumstances, NO can decrease NMDA responses. Fully oxidized NMDA receptors remain functional (Laughlin SB et al., 1998). I have discussed my clinical use of ascorbate in *Betrayal* and previously in this book. I find it to be more effective for alertness and cognition than I do for pain in the typical patient, if there is such an entity in neurosomatic medicine.

"Now Wai-ai-ait a Minute . . ."
(Isley Brothers, "Shout," 1959)

Perhaps some aspect of perceiving "unexplained" pain leads to self-reported childhood victimization, thus segregating this symptom from other neurosomatic disorders. I have suggested a relationship to false-memory syndrome. Perhaps each recollection of childhood leads to successive alteration of childhood memory in the more labile retrieval mode to ascribe meaning, or cause, to current pain. Because pain seems to be more associated with inappropriate secretion of neurotrophins than other types of neurosomatic disorders, the stimulus to remake synaptic connections in chronic "unexplained" pain may be greater. Thus, false memories at least could have a neurobiological rationale in the individual with fibromyalgia syndrome, chronic pelvic pain, painful irritable bowel or irritable bladder syndrome, chronic headache, and numerous other painful conditions.

Prospective studies have looked at the effect of parental behavior on various childhood outcomes, but aside from numerous twin studies (identical vs. fraternal, reared together vs. reared apart), I have not read a long-term longitudinal study conducted to investigate the role of maladaptive parental behavior in the association between parent and offspring psychiatric, or any other, disorder until quite recently (Johnson JG et al., 2001).

Rapid expansion in our understanding of neurotrophin neurobiology has led to the "neurotrophin hypothesis," which "proposes that repetitive neuronal activity enhances the expression, secretion, and/or actions of NTs at the synapse to modify synaptic transmission and connectivity" (Schinder

AF, Poo M-M, 2000, p. 639), and thus provides a connection between neuronal activity and synaptic plasticity.

NTs are usually secreted from dendrites and act as retrograde messengers (not classed among the "atypicals" yet) at presynaptic terminals to induce long-lasting modifications. Transcription of NT genes is regulated by neuronal activity: increased by excitation, decreased by inhibition. The secretion of NGF is constitutive, while that of BDNF is activity dependent. The secretions of NT-3 and NT-4 are not related to neuronal depolarization. BDNF is said to "instruct" the presynaptic terminal to increase transmitter secretion. We have already seen this action in relationship to cytoskeletal proteins and synaptic vesicles.

NTs also are secreted presynaptically in an anterograde manner. This process potentiates glutamatergic synaptic activity and has been ascribed to NT-3 and NT-4 and BDNF. These neurotrophins decrease GABAergic transmission in cortical neurons. NT secretion can, by itself, promote synaptic modifications. Acute modulation occurs at the level of presynaptic vesicular release. Chronic activity-dependent secretion of BDNF in cortical cultures decreases the postsynaptic response of glutamatergic neurons to excitatory inputs while increasing their responsiveness to GABAergic interneurons. The effect of chronic BDNF secretion is entirely postsynaptic.

NTs increase the length and complexity of dendritic trees in cortical neurons. This effect is prevented by blockade of neuronal spiking, synaptic transmission, or L-type Ca^{2+} channels. NTs are important regulators of nociceptive function (Bennett DLH, 2001). The sensitivity of the peripheral nociceptive system appears to be under tonic regulation by NGF. Increasing NGF produces hyperalgesia, both directly and indirectly, by provoking mediator release from mast cells, activation of sympathetic efferents, and (not relevant to neurosomatic disorders) activation of the 5-lipoxygenase pathway. NGF can, over a longer term, regulate receptors for VR1, bradykinin, and the proteins for Na^+ channels (Fjell J et al., 1999). Expression of neuropeptides within sensory neurons such as SP and CGRP are strongly regulated by NGF (Figure 90). A subset of NGF-sensitive nociceptors has been shown to constitutively express BDNF. The central integrative processing of peripheral nociceptive input occurs first in the dorsal horn, where the action of NTs on pain has been most studied. BDNF is thought to regulate the "gain" of the system by phosphorylation of intracellular targets by TrkB. This process occurs in NMDA-mediated responses, which are significantly enhanced by BDNF. More rostral loci may function in a similar manner.

Thus, there is a neurobiological substratum for the coupling of pain and memory, even though we don't seem to recall specific pain sensations very well. The patient with fibromyalgia syndrome has particular neurochemical propensities to falsely self-report childhood victimization. This disease-specific tendency does not obviate the longitudinal study of 592 biological parents and their offspring from 1975 to 1993. The conclusions of this study were these: Maladaptive parental behavior is associated with increased risk for the development of psychiatric disorders among the offspring of parents with and without psychiatric disorders. Maladaptive parental behavior appears to be an important mediator of the association between parental and offspring psychiatric behaviors. The offspring of parents with psychiatric disorders were not at risk for psychiatric disorders unless there was a history of maladaptive parental behavior (Johnson JG et al., 2001). The sample size was too small to include many subjects with schizophrenia or bipolar disorder, for whom the etiology is presumed to be more strongly genetic. This study was carefully done but did not focus on child abuse or neglect per se. Surprisingly, it found no correlation between parental and child psychiatric disorder of any sort once the variable of maladaptive behavior was controlled for. These results are as astonishing as those of the Raphael and colleagues study and suggest no relationship between genetic predisposition and psychiatric disorder, at least until early adulthood. This finding remains to be replicated, allows no facile rejoinder, and, although it does not address pain, is otherwise the opposite of the Raphael and colleagues study.

Conclusion

Closing the Circuit:
The Role of the Nucleus Accumbens
in Neurosomatic Disorders

I have made a valiant attempt to avoid discussing the functional neuro-anatomy of the NAc, but despite such intentions, my plans must be modified. The NAc is one of the key dysfunctional areas in neurosomatic pathophysiology. I begin with some interesting "pearls." Numerical citations are from the abstracts of the Society for Neuroscience Conference in 2000.

The VTA supplies dopaminergic neurons to the NAc, PFC, and nigrostriatal areas. I shall omit discussion of the latter system, since, although dysfunctional in neurosomatic disorders (Meyerson's sign), it is primarily involved with habits and other learned motor behaviors. All DA neurons from the VTA have release-modifying autoreceptors, and the DA transporter appears to be of the D_2 variety. The mPFC DA neurons have an enhanced rate of DA synthesis and turnover and lack autoreceptors modulating synthesis (Cass WA, Gerhardt GA, 1995). The mPFC DA neurons are more sensitive to stress and have fewer transporters than those in the NAc.

Morphine causes decreased Ach in the NAc, and morphine withdrawal causes Ach to increase. Aversive stimuli also cause an increase in NAc Ach (Rada PV et al., 1996). When rats self-administer cocaine, there is a diffuse increase in phasic (burst) firing in all accumbens subterritories according to one group (Uzwiak AJ et al., 1997), but according to another, there is hyperactivity in the shell and hypoactivity in the core (Parkinson JP et al., 1999). Sexual activity increases DA transmission in the female rat NAc, but NAc activity does not enhance female rat copulatory receptivity (Pfaus JG et al., 1995). Indeed, there is no evidence that female rats even enjoy the experience.

The NAc shell is prominently involved in the aversive behavioral effects of kappa-opioid receptor (KOR) agonists, including dynorphin, the KOR endogenous ligand. These receptors are usually directly apposed to glutamatergic varicosities and are thus thought to decrease postsynaptic responses to glutamate in the NAc shell (Svingos AL et al., 1999). They also down-regulate activity at presynaptic and postsynaptic D_2 receptors in the manner of quinpirole (Acri JB et al., 2001). When CI-988, a CCK_B antagonist, is perfused into the NAc, it increases DA overflow, but so do CCK_A and CCK_C antagonists (Corwin RL et al., 1995). Both ethanol and cocaine increase extracellular DA in the NAc, ethanol more so. This finding (293.9) may account for the alcohol intolerance so frequently encountered in neurosomatic patients (DA depletion).

The accumbens output neurons express NMDA receptors. Perfusion of the NAc with an NMDA-receptor antagonist causes a decrease in GABA in the NAc and VTA but not in the PFC. Presumably as a consequence, DA increases in the NAc, VTA, and PFC, as determined by dual-probe neurodialysis (528.12). According to this experiment, glutamatergic efferents from the PFC inhibit NAc and VTA DA secretion by stimulating GABAergic interneurons.

mGluRs operate predominantly by modulating voltage-gated Ca^{2+} channels or events regulating Ca^{2+}-mediated neurotransmission downstream from the Ca^{2+} channels. In this manner, they operate somewhat like autoreceptors and are intimately related with autoreceptor function, a poorly understood phenomenon. It is generally accepted, however, that autoreceptors modulate release by regulating Ca^{2+} channels. The action of synthesis-modifying autoreceptors is even less well understood, although the machinery for classical neurotransmitter synthesis usually is present in the nerve terminal so that transmitters do not require manufacture in the cell body and then axonal transport. It may be that D_2-autoreceptor activation results in reduction of both basal- and forskolin-stimulated activity of tyrosine hydroxylase via reduction of the activity of adenyl cyclase (Lindgren N et al., 2001). When dealing with a patient made sleepy by stimulants or who develops rapid tolerance to them, there is always the question of whether to desensitize the D_2 autoreceptors with a D_2/D_3 agonist (some autoreceptors are of the D_3 variety) or to block hypersensitive autoreceptors with haloperidol, which, unfortunately, is not D_2-selective enough for this purpose, blocking D_3 receptors also. I am uncertain to what degree it blocks D_4 autoreceptors, which may also be involved in this process. Its use is limited, because it blocks postsynaptic D_2/D_3 receptors as well, perhaps vitiating its autoreceptor effect.

DA autoreceptors may be subtype specific (53.12). The D_2 subtype is thought to function as an autoreceptor inhibiting both synthesis and release from DA terminals as well as modulating the DA transporter. Assessment of modulators of DA release is complicated by interactions of multiple DA receptors. D_1-receptor activation decreases NAc DA; blocking it increases NAc DA neurotransmission (532.7). In perhaps a related manner, D_1-receptor activation enhances depolarization-evoked $GABA_A$ release and Ca^{2+} entry, as well as stimulating neural transmission in general by inhibiting inwardly rectifying potassium conductance (IRK). D_1-receptor activation enhances NMDA-receptor function, at least in some cases by direct protein-protein binding between the NR2A subunit and the D_1R (532.3).

The D_3 receptor, highly concentrated in limbic regions, especially in the NAc, increases DA reuptake when activated. D_1-receptor activation inhibits the ability of the D_3 receptor to activate GIRK channels. This inhibition may occur by phosphorylation of the D_3 receptor. GIRK currents induced by quinpirole are inhibited by cAMP. D_1 agonists increase cAMP; D_1 and D_3 receptors are coexpressed in vivo (533.2). D_3 antagonists block the effects of NMDA antagonists (533.10).

D_4 receptors are found in the striatum, where they modulate the direct and indirect pathways. These receptors are not found on striatal interneurons (533.7). DA is thought to modulate glutamate release by activating D_4 receptors. These receptors are located on corticostriatal projections to the striatum and NAc (Gerfen CR, 2000). D_2-like receptors may function similarly.

Blocking the 5-HT_3 receptor antagonizes many of the effects of cocaine and amphetamines. Activation of the 5-HT_{1B} receptor augments the effect of cocaine in increasing NAc DA (676.3), suggesting the use of triptans and stimulants. Although D_1 receptors increase NMDA-channel activity, D_2 receptors decrease it, at least in part by transactivation of PDGF receptors. These receptors are coupled to phosphorylase C and then to a PKC/Ca^{2-} calmodulin signaling system. Some monoamine transporters are regulated by Na^+ channels. Cocaine-like agents such as procaine have a rapid pharmacologic effect on these channels, producing a pressor effect, but lidocaine does not (845.23).

The distribution of the DAT was studied in thalamic and hypothalamic areas as part of an investigation of hypodopaminergic disorders of arousal. DAT concentrations were highest (to my surprise) in the RTN, with the nonspecific thalamic nuclei coming in second. The perifornical area, from which springs orexin, also had high DAT levels. Dopaminergic influences can produce behavioral activation which can suppress generations of stage II sleep spindles.

The foregoing having been said, there is little in the literature about what transpires when the activity of the DA autoreceptor is pharmacologically modified. The clearest contemporary presentation of its function is in a work by S.-P. Onn and colleagues (2000). Their hypothesis is presented in Figure 47b. Autoreceptors are usually formed in an environment in which there is tonic secretion of a neurotransmitter that diffuses in a paracrine manner. I have provided examples of how DA meets this criterion.

Onn and colleagues note that low concentrations of DA preferentially activate D_1 receptors because they are closer to the synapse. Activated D_1 receptors cause an increase in NMDA-mediated currents, whereas high concentrations of DA that activate D_2 receptors suppress AMPA-mediated currents. D_1 receptor facilitation of NMDA currents involves cAMP, PKA, and DARPP-32 signal transduction cascades. Simultaneous stimulation of D_1 and D_2 receptors would produce additive inhibitory effects. With less firing, there would be an attenuated stimulation of D_2 autoreceptors, located primarily within the synapse. "Therefore, the system appears to be designed to attenuate phasic DA-mediated responses under conditions in which the dopaminergic system is being tonically over-driven" (Onn S-P et al., 2000).

I have tried every way I can think of to change DA autoreceptor hypersensitivity and can still not quite get it right. I still believe I can, using the proper medications. One such would be sulpiride, a D_2 antagonist which has antidepressant effects. Sulpiride will block D_2 autoreceptors and postsynaptic receptors in the NAc and VTA, but importantly, also in the PFC, a property which haloperidol apparently does not possess (Kaneno S et al., 2001).

I may not have used D_2/D_3 agonists for a long enough period of time, although several of my patients chronically use pramipexole (Mirapex) for RLS. Behavioral sensitization to the locomotor stimulant effect of amphetamine or quinpirole has been induced by intermittent drug administration (Muscat R et al., 1993). Multiple-pulse stimulation of isolated NAc enhances DA release in quinpirole-sensitized rats but decreases DA release in amphetamine-sensitized rats. The difference probably relates to different modes of drug action. Amphetamine works by blocking the inward uptake through the DAT and releasing DA into the synaptic cleft through the same DAT in a nonvesicular manner by reverse transport. Amphetamine also decreases stimulation-dependent vesicular DA release by redistributing DA from the vesicles to the cytosol (Schmitz Y et al., 2001). There are conflicting results about whether amphetamine-induced DA release activates the D_2 autoreceptor. I and others think it does, but one group (Ruskin DN et al., 2001) finds that it does not.

An experimental D_2/D_3 antagonist named *DS121* preferentially binds to autoreceptors. It increases locomotor activity as monotherapy in rats and greatly enhances that produced by cocaine. It works best when there are supersensitive DA autoreceptors (Ellinwood EH et al., 2000). DS121 is the medication I have been searching for, or at least something like it, because the D_2/D_3 autoreceptors in the NAc mediate psychomotor activation (Canalese JJ, Iverson SD, 2000). Human trials of this substance have not been performed as of this writing (Ellinwood EM, personal communication, 2001). Arvid Carlsson's group has begun human trials with a similar medication.

Dopaminergic autoreceptors were discovered in the early 1970s by Arvid Carlsson and his group at Gotheburg, Sweden. Carlsson won the Nobel Prize in 2000 for his work on chemical neurotransmission. He has developed a partial dopamine-receptor agonist called aripiprazole which has been shown to possess antipsychotic properties in phase III clinical trials on schizophrenics. His group has also developed preferential dopamine autoreceptor antagonists, one of which, OSU6162, has been used in human trials (Carlsson A, 2001). He is currently working with a $5\text{-}HT_{2A}$-receptor antagonist, M100,907. This compound has been shown to lower glutamatergic function. Carlsson's group finds it to have antipsychotic properties in schizophrenic patients. If neurosomatic disorders are hyperglutamatergic, OSU6162 may ameliorate them. Carlsson's figure of CSTC loops in schizophrenia bears some relation to the hypothesis described in this book.

Presynaptic DA may not be entirely removed by reuptake or enzymes but may accumulate at low levels in a "tonic dopamine pool" which is constantly present in extrasynaptic space where it may act by diffusion. This pool is tightly regulated by multiple feedback systems (Onn S-P et al., 2000) and is of such low concentration that it can stimulate only autoreceptors, not postsynaptic receptors. It thus acts to limit glutamate-stimulated DA release. In a hyperglutamatergic state, as I have postulated for neurosomatic disorders, the D_2 and other autoreceptors would be hypersensitive, limiting DA secretion in the phasic phase which is more relevant to human behavior. Indeed, it has been demonstrated experimentally that stimulation of the prefrontal cortex at physiologically relevant frequencies inhibits DA release in the nucleus accumbens (Jackson ME et al., 2001). Lesions of the fornix-fimbria, which interfere with input from the hippocampal formation, do not lead to firing of accumbens output neurons as is normally the case. This finding has led the Grace group at the University of Pittsburgh (most recently, Floresco SB et al., 2001) to show that hippocampal afferents "gate" the prefrontal throughput in the accumbens, perhaps by regulating activity of VTA DA neurons. Hippocampal gating nicely complemented my speculations about dysfunction of the PFC-hippocampal circuit in *Betrayal,* just before I had become acutely aware of the role the accumbens shell played in stress and drug-seeking behavior (Kalivas PW, Duffy P, 1995).

Since that time, hundreds of articles have been published about the nucleus accumbens, 147 articles between December 2000 and December 2001. I cannot review this literature here but shall mention some interesting points:

1. $5\text{-}HT_{1B/1D}$ agonists may increase NAc DA release.
2. Nicotinic cholinergic blockade reduces cocaine sensitivity.

3. PFC DA depletion produces adrenergic hyperactivity in the NAc.
4. Stimulation of mGluRs is required for NAc DA release.
5. Amygdala regulation of the NAc is regulated by the PFC.
6. Inescapable aversive hypothalamic stimulation releases Ach in the NAc shell; escape from the stimulation reverses it.
7. The NAc is topographically organized in regard to the origin of afferent stimuli. For example, areas with particular cytoarchitectural or immunohistochemical characteristics may receive input from the hippocampus or the amygdala, but not both.
8. Different neural networks within the nucleus accumbens are activated depending on the circumstances (Heimer L et al., 1997).
9. Subregions of the NAc vary in their autoregulation of DA synthesis (Heidbreder CA, Baumann MH, 2001).

There is much more. We'll have the nucleus accumbens and its relationships to kick around more in the future, but a proper appreciation of accumbal dysfunction due to hyperglutamatergic input allows me to close this book with a sense of completion.

Appendix

Criteria for Hypomanic Episode

A.   A distinct period of persistently elevated, expansive, or irritable mood, lasting throughout at least 4 days, that is clearly different from the usual nondepressed mood.

B.   During the period of mood disturbance, three (or more) of the following symptoms have persisted (four if the mood is only irritable) and have been present to a significant degree:

   (1)   inflated self-esteem or grandiosity
   (2)   decreased need for sleep (e.g., feels rested after only 3 hours of sleep)
   (3)   more talkative than usual or pressure to keep talking
   (4)   flight of ideas or subjective experience that thoughts are racing
   (5)   distractibility (i.e., attention too easily drawn to unimportant or irrelevant external stimuli)
   (6)   increase in goal-directed activity (either socially, at work or school, or sexually) or psychomotor agitation
   (7)   excessive involvement in pleasurable activities that have a high potential for painful consequences (e.g., the person engages in unrestrained buying sprees, sexual indiscretions, or foolish business investments)

C.   The episode is associated with an unequivocal change in functioning that is uncharacteristic of the person when not symptomatic.

D.   The disturbance in mood and the change in functioning are observable by others.

E.   The episode is not severe enough to cause marked impairment in social or occupational functioning, or to necessitate hospitalization, and there are no psychotic features.

F.   The symptoms are not due to the direct physiological effects of a substance (e.g., a drug of abuse, a medication, or other treatment) or a general medical condition (e.g., hyperthyroidism).

   Note: Hypomanic-like episodes that are clearly caused by somatic antidepressant treatment (e.g., medication, electroconvulsive therapy, light therapy) should not count toward a diagnosis of Bipolar II Disorder.

Diagnostic criteria for 301.13 Cyclothymic Disorder

A. For at least 2 years, the presence of numerous periods with hypomanic symptoms (see p. 368) and numerous periods with depressive symptoms that do not meet criteria for a Major Depressive Episode. **Note:** In children and adolescents, the duration must be at least 1 year.

B. During the above 2-year period (1 year in children and adolescents), the person has not been without the symptoms in Criterion A for more than 2 months at a time.

C. No Major Depressive Episode (p. 356), Manic Episode (p. 362), or Mixed Episode (see p. 365) has been present during the first 2 years of the disturbance.

   Note: After the initial 2 years (1 year in children and adolescents) of Cyclothymic Disorder, there may be superimposed Manic or Mixed Episodes (in which case both Bipolar I Disorder and Cyclothymic Disorder may be diagnosed) or Major Depressive Episodes (in which case both Bipolar II Disorder and Cyclothymic Disorder may be diagnosed).

D. The symptoms in Criterion A are not better accounted for by Schizoaffective Disorder and are not superimposed on Schizophrenia, Schizophreniform Disorder, Delusional Disorder, or Psychotic Disorder Not Otherwise Specified.

E. The symptoms are not due to the direct physiological effects of a substance (e.g., a drug of abuse, a medication) or a general medical condition (e.g., hyperthyroidism).

F. The symptoms cause clinically significant distress or impairment in social, occupational, or other important areas of functioning.

Criteria for Panic Attack

Note: A Panic Attack is not a codable disorder. Code the specific diagnosis in which the Panic Attack occurs (e.g., 300.21 Panic Disorder With Agoraphobia [p. 441]).

A discrete period of intense fear or discomfort, in which four (or more) of the following symptoms developed abruptly and reached a peak within 10 minutes:

   (1) palpitations, pounding heart, or accelerated heart rate
   (2) sweating
   (3) trembling or shaking
   (4) sensations of shortness of breath or smothering
   (5) feeling of choking
   (6) chest pain or discomfort
   (7) nausea or abdominal distress
   (8) feeling dizzy, unsteady, lightheaded, or faint
   (9) derealization (feelings of unreality) or depersonalization (being detached from oneself)

(10) fear of losing control or going crazy
(11) fear of dying
(12) paresthesias (numbness or tingling sensations)
(13) chills or hot flushes

Diagnostic criteria for 300.02 Generalized Anxiety Disorder

A. Excessive anxiety and worry (apprehensive expectation), occurring more days than not for at least 6 months, about a number of events or activities (such as work or school performance).

B. The person finds it difficult to control the worry.

C. The anxiety and worry are associated with three (or more) of the following six symptoms (with at least some symptoms present for more days than not for the past 6 months). **Note:** Only one item is required in children.

(1) restlessness or feeling keyed up or on edge
(2) being easily fatigued
(3) difficulty concentrating or mind going blank
(4) irritability
(5) muscle tension
(6) sleep disturbance (difficulty falling or staying asleep, or restless unsatisfying sleep)

D. The focus of the anxiety and worry is not confined to features of an Axis I disorder, e.g., the anxiety or worry is not about having a Panic Attack (as in Panic Disorder), being embarrassed in public (as in Social Phobia), being contaminated (as in Obsessive-Compulsive Disorder), being away from home or close relatives (as in Separation Anxiety Disorder), gaining weight (as in Anorexia Nervosa), having multiple physical complaints (as in Somatization Disorder), or having a serious illness (as in Hypochondriasis), and the anxiety and worry do not occur exclusively during Posttraumatic Stress Disorder.

E. The anxiety, worry, or physical symptoms cause clinically significant distress or impairment in social, occupational, or other important areas of functioning.

F. The disturbance is not due to the direct physiological effects of a substance (e.g., a drug of abuse, a medication) or a general medical condition (e.g., hyperthyroidism) and does not occur exclusively during a Mood Disorder, a Psychotic Disorder, or a Pervasive Developmental Disorder.

Diagnostic criteria for 300.81 Somatization Disorder

A. A history of many physical complaints beginning before age 30 years that occur over a period of several years and result in treatment being sought or significant impairment in social, occupational, or other important areas of functioning.

B. Each of the following criteria must have been met, with individual symptoms occurring at any time during the course of the disturbance:

(1) *four pain symptoms:* a history of pain related to at least four different sites or functions (e.g., head, abdomen, back, joints, extremities, chest, rectum, during menstruation, during sexual intercourse, or during urination)

(2) *two gastrointestinal symptoms:* a history of at least two gastrointestinal symptoms other than pain (e.g., nausea, bloating, vomiting other than during pregnancy, diarrhea, or intolerance of several different foods)

(3) *one sexual symptom:* a history of at least one sexual or reproductive symptom other than pain (e.g., sexual indifference, erectile or ejaculatory dysfunction, irregular menses, excessive menstrual bleeding, vomiting throughout pregnancy)

(4) *one pseudoneurological symptom:* a history of at least one symptom or deficit suggesting a neurological condition not limited to pain (conversion symptoms such as impaired coordination or balance, paralysis or localized weakness, difficulty swallowing or lump in throat, aphonia, urinary retention, hallucinations, loss of touch or pain sensation, double vision, blindness, deafness, seizures; dissociative symptoms such as amnesia; or loss of consciousness other than fainting)

C. Either (1) or (2):

(1) after appropriate investigation, each of the symptoms in Criterion B cannot be fully explained by a known general medical condition or the direct effects of a substance (e.g., a drug of abuse, a medication)

(2) when there is a related general medical condition, the physical complaints or resulting social or occupational impairment are in excess of what would be expected from the history, physical examination, or laboratory findings

D. The symptoms are not intentionally produced or feigned (as in Factitious Disorder or Malingering).

Diagnostic criteria for
300.82 Undifferentiated Somatoform Disorder

A. One or more physical complaints (e.g., fatigue, loss of appetite, gastrointestinal or urinary complaints).

B. Either (1) or (2):

(1) after appropriate investigation, the symptoms cannot be fully explained by a known general medical condition or the direct effects of a substance (e.g., a drug of abuse, a medication)

(2) when there is a related general medical condition, the physical complaints or resulting social or occupational impairment is in excess of what would be expected from the history, physical examination, or laboratory findings

C. The symptoms cause clinically significant distress or impairment in social, occupational, or other important areas of functioning.

D. The duration of the disturbance is at least 6 months.

E. The disturbance is not better accounted for by another mental disorder (e.g., another Somatoform Disorder, Sexual Dysfunction, Mood Disorder, Anxiety Disorder, Sleep Disorder, or Psychotic Disorder).

F. The symptom is not intentionally produced or feigned (as in Factitious Disorder or Malingering).

Diagnostic criteria for 300.11 Conversion Disorder

A. One or more symptoms or deficits affecting voluntary motor or sensory function that suggest a neurological or other general medical condition.

B. Psychological factors are judged to be associated with the symptom or deficit because the initiation or exacerbation of the symptom or deficit is preceded by conflicts or other stressors.

C. The symptom or deficit is not intentionally produced or feigned (as in Factitious Disorder or Malingering).

D. The symptom or deficit cannot, after appropriate investigation, be fully explained by a general medical condition, or by the direct effects of a substance, or as a culturally sanctioned behavior or experience.

E. The symptom or deficit causes clinically significant distress or impairment in social, occupational, or other important areas of functioning or warrants medical evaluation.

F. The symptom or deficit is not limited to pain or sexual dysfunction, does not occur exclusively during the course of Somatization Disorder, and is not better accounted for by another mental disorder.

Specify type of symptom or deficit:

With Motor Symptom or Deficit
With Sensory Symptom or Deficit
With Seizures or Convulsions
With Mixed Presentation

Diagnostic criteria for Pain Disorder

A. Pain in one or more anatomical sites is the predominant focus of the clinical presentation and is of sufficient severity to warrant clinical attention.

B. The pain causes clinically significant distress or impairment in social, occupational, or other important areas of functioning.

C. Psychological factors are judged to have an important role in the onset, severity, exacerbation, or maintenance of the pain.

D. The symptom or deficit is not intentionally produced or feigned (as in Factitious Disorder or Malingering).

E.   The pain is not better accounted for by a Mood, Anxiety, or Psychotic Disorder and does not meet criteria for Dyspareunia.

Code as follows:

307.80   Pain Disorder Associated With Psychological Factors: psychological factors are judged to have the major role in the onset, severity, exacerbation, or maintenance of the pain. If a general medical condition is present, it does not have a major role in the onset, severity, exacerbation, or maintenance of the pain. This type of Pain Disorder is not diagnosed if criteria are also met for Somatization Disorder.

Specify if:

Acute: duration of less than 6 months

Chronic: duration of 6 months or longer

307.89 Pain Disorder Associated With Both Psychological Factors and a General Medical Condition: both psychological factors and a general medical condition are judged to have important roles in the onset, severity, exacerbation, or maintenance of the pain. The associated general medical condition or anatomical site of the pain (see below) is coded on Axis III.

Specify if:

Acute: duration of less than 6 months

Chronic: duration of 6 months or longer

Note: The following is not considered to be a mental disorder and is included here to facilitate differential diagnosis.

Pain Disorder Associated With a General Medical Condition: a general medical condition has a major role in the onset, severity, exacerbation, or maintenance of the pain. (If psychological factors are present, they are not judged to have a major role in the onset, severity, exacerbation, or maintenance of the pain.) The diagnostic code for the pain is selected based on the associated general medical condition if one has been established (see Appendix G) or on the anatomical location of the pain if the underlying general medical condition is not yet clearly established—for example, low back (724.2), sciatic (724.3), pelvic (625.9), headache (784.0), facial (784.0), chest (786.50), joint (719.4), bone (733.90), abdominal (789.0), breast (611.71), renal (788.0), ear (388.70), eye (379.91), throat (784.1), tooth (525.9), and urinary (788.0).

Diagnostic criteria for 300.7 Hypochondriasis

A.   Preoccupation with fears of having, or the idea that one has, a serious disease based on the person's misinterpretation of bodily symptoms.

B.   The preoccupation persists despite appropriate medical evaluation and reassurance.

C.   The belief in Criterion A is not of delusional intensity (as in Delusional Disorder, Somatic Type) and is not restricted to a circumscribed concern about appearance (as in Body Dysmorphic Disorder).

D. The preoccupation causes clinically significant distress or impairment in so-cial, occupational, or other important areas of functioning.

E. The duration of the disturbance is at least 6 months.

F. The preoccupation is not better accounted for by Generalized Anxiety Dis-order, Obsessive-Compulsive Disorder, Panic Disorder, a Major Depressive Episode, Separation Anxiety, or another Somatoform Disorder.

Specify if:

> **With Poor Insight:** if, for most of the time during the current episode, the person does not recognize that the concern about having a serious illness is excessive or unreasonable

---

Diagnostic criteria for 307.42 Primary Insomnia

A. The predominant complaint is difficulty initiating or maintaining sleep, or nonrestorative sleep, for at least 1 month.

B. The sleep disturbance (or associated daytime fatigue) causes clinically sig-nificant distress or impairment in social, occupational, or other important ar-eas of functioning.

C. The sleep disturbance does not occur exclusively during the course of Narcolepsy, Breathing-Related Sleep Disorder, Circadian Rhythm Sleep Disorder, or a Parasomnia.

D. The disturbance does not occur exclusively during the course of another mental disorder (e.g., Major Depressive Disorder, Generalized Anxiety Dis-order, a delirium).

E. The disturbance is not due to the direct physiological effects of a substance (e.g., a drug of abuse, a medication) or a general medical condition.

**Diagnostic criteria for
301.83 Borderline Personality Disorder**

A pervasive pattern of instability of interpersonal relationships, self-image, and affects, and marked impulsivity beginning by early adulthood and present in a variety of contexts, as indicated by five (or more) of the following:

(1) frantic efforts to avoid real or imagined abandonment. **Note:** Do not include suicidal or self-mutilating behavior covered in Criterion 5.

(2) a pattern of unstable and intense interpersonal relationships characterized by alternating between extremes of idealization and devaluation

(3) identity disturbance: markedly and persistently unstable self-image or sense of self

(4) impulsivity in at least two areas that are potentially self-damaging (e.g., spending, sex, substance abuse, reckless driving, binge eating). **Note:** Do not include suicidal or self-mutilating behavior covered in Criterion 5.

(5) recurrent suicidal behavior, gestures, or threats, or self-mutilating behavior

(6)   affective instability due to a marked reactivity of mood (e.g., intense episodic dysphoria, irritability, or anxiety usually lasting a few hours and only rarely more than a few days)

(7)   chronic feelings of emptiness

(8)   inappropriate, intense anger or difficulty controlling anger (e.g., frequent displays of temper, constant anger, recurrent physical fights)

(9)   transient, stress-related paranoid ideation or severe dissociative symptoms

Research criteria for mild neurocognitive disorder

A.   The presence of two (or more) of the following impairments in cognitive functioning, lasting most of the time for a period of at least 2 weeks (as reported by the individual or a reliable informant):

(1)   memory impairment as identified by a reduced ability to learn or recall information

(2)   disturbance in executive functioning (i.e., planning, organizing, sequencing, abstracting)

(3)   disturbance in attention or speed of information processing

(4)   impairment in perceptual-motor abilities

(5)   impairment in language (e.g., comprehension, word finding)

B.   There is objective evidence from physical examination or laboratory findings (including neuroimaging techniques) of a neurological or general medical condition that is judged to be etiologically related to the cognitive disturbance.

C.   There is evidence from neuropsychological testing or quantified cognitive assessment of an abnormality or decline in performance.

D.   The cognitive deficits cause marked distress or impairment in social, occupational, or other important areas of functioning and represent a decline from a previous level of functioning.

E.   The cognitive disturbance does not meet criteria for a delirium, a dementia, or an amnestic disorder and is not better accounted for by another mental disorder (e.g., a Substance-Related Disorder, Major Depressive Disorder).

Research criteria for premenstrual dysphoric disorder

A.   In most menstrual cycles during the past year, five (or more) of the following symptoms were present for most of the time during the last week of the luteal phase, began to remit within a few days after the onset of the follicular phase, and were absent in the week postmenses, with at least one of the symptoms being either (1), (2), (3), or (4):

(1)   markedly depressed mood, feelings of hopelessness, or self-deprecating thoughts

(2)   marked anxiety, tension, feelings of being "keyed up," or "on edge"

(3) marked affective lability (e.g., feeling suddenly sad or tearful or increased sensitivity to rejection)

(4) persistent and marked anger or irritability or increased interpersonal conflicts

(5) decreased interest in usual activities (e.g., work, school, friends, hobbies)

(6) subjective sense of difficulty in concentrating

(7) lethargy, easy fatigability, or marked lack of energy

(8) marked change in appetite, overeating, or specific food cravings

(9) hypersomnia or insomnia

(10) a subjective sense of being overwhelmed or out of control

(11) other physical symptoms, such as breast tenderness or swelling, headaches, joint or muscle pain, a sensation of "bloating," weight gain

Note: In menstruating females, the luteal phase corresponds to the period between ovulation and the onset of menses, and the follicular phase begins with menses. In nonmenstruating females (e.g., those who have had a hysterectomy), the timing of luteal and follicular phases may require measurement of circulating reproductive hormones.

B. The disturbance markedly interferes with work or school or with usual social activities and relationships with others (e.g., avoidance of social activities, decreased productivity and efficiency at work or school).

C. The disturbance is not merely an exacerbation of the symptoms of another disorder, such as Major Depressive Disorder, Panic Disorder, Dysthymic Disorder, or a Personality Disorder (although it may be superimposed on any of these disorders).

D. Criteria A, B, and C must be confirmed by prospective daily ratings during at least two consecutive symptomatic cycles. (The diagnosis may be made provisionally prior to this confirmation.)

TREATMENT ALGORITHM

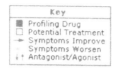

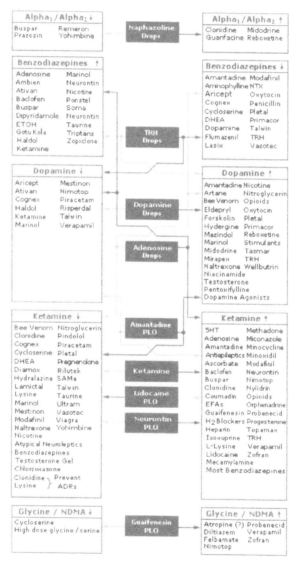

MEDICATION LIST: PRESENT AND NEAR-FUTURE TREATMENT OPTIONS FOR NEUROSOMATIC DISORDERS

[ ] Abecarnil
[ ] Acamprosate (polyamine NMDA site antagonist)
[ ] Acular ophth. solution (ketorolac)
[ ] Adderall (amphetamine salts)
[ ] Adenocard nasal spray 1:10, 1:1
[ ] Agmatine (NMDA, NOS, alpha$_2$, and possibly Neurontin antagonist)
[ ] Allopregnanolone (gabergic neurosteroid)
[ ] Amantadine p.o. (NMDA antagonist)
    [ ] 400 mg/gm in PLO gel
    [ ] 200 mg IV over 3 hours
[ ] Ambien (zolpidem)
[ ] Amerge (naratriptan, Marinol antagonist)
[ ] Amiloride (Na$^+$ channel blocker, nAchR blocker)
[ ] Aminophylline (synergizes with forskolin)
[ ] 4-aminopyridine (K$^+$ channel blocker)
[ ] Amoxapine (glycine/NMDA antagonist)
[ ] Amperozide (5HT$_2$ antagonist, D$_{1-4}$ agonist)
[ ] AndroGel (increases DA and NO, testosterone topical gel)
[ ] Antalarmin (CRHR1 antagonist)
[ ] Aricept (donepezil, NMDA agonist)
[ ] Artane (trihexyphenidyl)
[ ] Arvanil (CB$_1$ partial agonist)
[ ] Ascorbate I.V.
[ ] Atenolol
[ ] Ativan p.o. (lorazepam)
    [ ] IM 2 mg/ml
    [ ] nasal spray 1:10 (to abort panic attacks)
[ ] Atropine (may block glycine coagonist site of NMDA receptor)
[ ] Baclofen p.o. (antagonizes forskolin)
    [ ] 10% in PLO gel
[ ] Biaxin (clarithromycin, GABA antagonist, motilin agonist)
[ ] Biphosphonates (potential analgesics)
[ ] Bosentan (endothelin antagonist)
[ ] Bright light/sunlight 2 hours/day for 2 weeks (to stop daytime secretion of melatonin)
[ ] BuSpar (buspirone, pindolol antagonist, clonidine antagonist)
[ ] Butalbital
[ ] C1 and C2 nerve stimulation (affects trigeminal subnucleus caudalis)
[ ] CCK$_B$ receptor antagonist (e.g., L365260)
[ ] Celexa (citalopram, antagonizes baclofen)
[ ] Citrate (for alkalinization)

[ ] Clonidine p.o. (Antagonizes yohimbine and oxytocin, mu opioid agonist)
    [ ] 0.2% in PLO
[ ] Cognex (tacrine, NMDA agonist)
[ ] Coumadin (to inhibit secretion of NGF and activation of cPLA$_2$)
[ ] Cycloserine (ketamine/glycine-site agonist)
[ ] D$_2$/D$_3$ autoreceptor antagonist OSU6162 (in human trials)
[ ] Danocrine (has antimanic properties, for PMS and rapid-cycling bipolar disorder)
[ ] Dantrolene (blocks calcium release, NO antagonist)
[ ] Darvocet
[ ] DDAVP (may antagonize oxytocin and act as a stimulant)
[ ] Delta-opioid agonists (clonidine only one available)
[ ] Depakote (sodium valproate)
[ ] Dexedrine (dextroamphetamine)
[ ] Dextromethorphan (weak NMDA antagonist)
[ ] DHEA
[ ] Diamox (acetazolamide)
[ ] Diazoxide gel (opens K$_{ATP}$ channels)
[ ] Diltiazem (5HT$_3$ antagonist, decreases dysmenorrhea, glycine/NMDA antagonist)
[ ] Dipyridamole (Persantine, adenosine-reuptake inhibitor, weak PDE5 inhibitor)
[ ] Dopamine 40 mg/ml
    [ ] nasal spray 1:10
    [ ] ophthalmic solution 1:10
[ ] Doxazosin (Cardura, ∝-1 antagonist)
[ ] ECT
[ ] Effexor XR (venlafaxine, antagonized by naltrexone)
[ ] Felbatol (agonist at glycine/NMDA site)
[ ] Finasteride (indirect Talwin antagonist)
[ ] Flumazenil
    [ ] IV
    [ ] nasal spray 1:10 (to reverse BZDs)
[ ] Forskolin (cyclic AMP agonist via AC inhibition)
[ ] FRFamide agonists or antagonists (modulates N-type Na$^+$ channels)
[ ] Furosemide (as a GABA$_A$ antagonist, duration 24 hours)

[ ] Gabitril (tiagabine, may be used acutely for migraine)
[ ] Galanin congeners (e.g, galnon)
[ ] Galantamine (Reminyl, muscarinic and nicotine cholinergic agonist)
[ ] Gamma globulin IV (probably dopaminergic)
  [ ] IM
[ ] Genistein (? tyrosine kinase inhibitor, direct glycine site blocker)
[ ] Glipizide (to block K^+ channels)
[ ] Glutamate NS 1:25 ➜ 1:1 (reverses NMDA antagonists)
[ ] Gotu kola (CCK antagonist)
[ ] Growth hormone
[ ] Guaifenesin po (glycine/NMDA antagonist)
  [ ] 10% in PLO
  [ ] IV (dose must be individualized)
[ ] Guanfacine (alpha$_{2A}$R agonist)
[ ] Haloperidol nasal spray 1:10
[ ] HCG IM (as sodium-channel blocker)
[ ] Heparin (to block release of intracellular calcium, antagonizes oxytocin, NMDA antagonist)
[ ] Histogranin (peptide nonopioid analgesic via NMDA antagonism)
[ ] Honey bee venom (modulates PLA_2)
[ ] Hydergine (ergoloid mesylates, DA agonist)
[ ] Hydralazine (cGMP agonist)
[ ] Hydroxyzine (as GABA agonist)
[ ] Ifenprodil (NR$_2$B antagonist)
[ ] IGF-1 nasal spray
[ ] Imitrex SQ (sumatriptan)
  [ ] p.o.
  [ ] nasal spray
  [ ] ophth. solution
[ ] Indocin p.o. (indomethacin)
  [ ] vaginal
  [ ] 10% in PLO
[ ] Inositol or Isoprinosine (antagonizes Depakote and lithium, anxiolytic and antidepressant at 10 gm qd x 30 days)
[ ] Isoxuprine gel 4% (polyamine NMDA site antagonist)
  [ ] oral 20 mg (reversed by SAMe; beta$_2$ agonist)
[ ] Ketamine p.o. 10-100 mg (Talwin antagonist)
  [ ] gel 80 and 240 mg/gm in PLO
  [ ] I.V.
  [ ] nasal spray 50 mg/ml 1:10
  [ ] ophth. solution 1:10
[ ] KKCA gel
[ ] Klonopin (clonazepam)

[ ] Kutapressin (polypeptide porcine liver extract, BK antagonist)
[ ] Kynurenate (endogenous glycine-site NMDA blocker; at present, only increased by probenecid)
[ ] L-leucine (gabapentin antagonist)
[ ] Lamictal (ketamine antagonist, lidocaine agonist)
[ ] Levetiracetam (an AED with an unknown mode of action)
[ ] Lidocaine IV (Na^+ channel and SP antagonist; inhibits glutamate release)
  [ ] sublingual tablet
  [ ] gel 5% and 15%
  [ ] SQ
  [ ] trigger-point injection
[ ] Lithium (antagonized by inositol)
[ ] Loreclezole (allosteric modulation at the GABA$_A$ beta subunit)
[ ] Lupron (leuprolide, modulates NE, GnRH modulates sympathetic function)
[ ] Luvox (fluvoxamine)
[ ] Lysine (to reduce EAA secretion and open K$_{ATP}$ channel)
[ ] Marinol (delta-9-THC, antagonizes forskolin, may augment Lamictal and Rilutek, reversed by Amerge and verapamil)
[ ] Mecamylamine (nicotine and NMDA antagonist)
[ ] Memantine (NMDA antagonist)
[ ] Meprobamate (adenosine agonist)
[ ] Meridia (sibutramine-SNRI)
[ ] Mestinon (pyridostigmine)
[ ] Methadone ($\propto$ 3/β4 nAchR blocker) (mu-opioid, NMDA antag., SRI)
[ ] Methergine (5HT$_1$ agonist, 5HT$_2$ antagonist, active metabolite of Sansert)
[ ] Methylphenidate—immediate release
  [ ] once-daily dose
[ ] Mexiletine (a second-rate oral lidocaine)
[ ] mGluR agonists or antagonists
[ ] Midodrine (ProAmatine, $\propto$-1 agonist)
[ ] Milnacipran (SNRI)
[ ] Minocycline (as NMDA antagonist)
[ ] Minoxidil gel (to open K^+ channels—sometimes is superior to Neurontin)
[ ] Mirapex (pramipexole, NMDA antagonist, DA agonist of choice for bruxism, RLS, PLMS)
[ ] MMAI (? nontoxic serotonin releaser)
[ ] Modafinil (Provigil, Zyprexa and clonidine antagonist)
[ ] MS Contin (oxytocin antagonist)

[ ] Mysoline (primidone, for tremors and mood stabilization)

[ ] NADH (increases DA, many other actions, disappointing thus far)

[ ] Naloxone 1mg (1-3 mg qd for opioid-induced constipation)

[ ] Naltrexone 50-100 mg (may synergize with anxiolytics)

    [ ] 20 picograms (to prevent opioid tolerance)

[ ] Naphazoline ophth. solution

[ ] Nardil (phenelzine)

[ ] NEP-APN blockers (to increase met-enkephalin, e.g., RB101)

[ ] Neuromedin B (anxiolytic bombesin antagonist)

[ ] Neurontin p.o. (gabapentin, antagonized by glipizide)

    [ ] gel 400 mg/gm in PLO

[ ] Neuropeptide Y agonists or antagonists

[ ] Niacinamide (to augment stimulants)

[ ] Nicotine patch (increases DA, GABA, NMDA, 5-HT, NE; decreases CGRP)

[ ] Nimodipine (inhibits $5-HT_3$, NMDA, and nicotine Ach receptors; acts chronically as a $5-HT_2$ antagonist)

[ ] Nitroglycerin

[ ] Nociceptin (another endogenous opioid)

[ ] Norflex 10% in PLO (orphenadrine citrate, NMDA antagonist)

[ ] Nylidrin gel 1.2% (polyamine NMDA site antagonist, NR1/2B blocker)

    [ ] oral 6 and 12 mg

[ ] Omega-3 and -6 fatty acids (inhibit protein kinase C)

[ ] Opipramol (anxiolytic sigma agonist)

[ ] Orexin (A and B agonist and antagonist)

[ ] Oseltamivir (Tamiflu)

[ ] Oxcarbazepine (Trileptal)

[ ] OxyContin po (oxycodone)

    [ ] gel (partial kappa-opioid agonist)

[ ] Oxytocin IM 10 units (alpha$_2$ blocker, antagonized by haloperidol and clonidine, increases intracellular Ca^2 via activation of IP_3)

    [ ] p.o. 10 units

    [ ] nasal spray

[ ] Papaverine (inhibits AC and adenosine reuptake)

[ ] Parafon Forte (chlorzoxazone—decreases glutamate secretion)

[ ] Parnate (tranylcypromine)

[ ] Passionflower/valerian

[ ] Paxil (paroxetine)

[ ] Penicillin (as a GABA antagonist)

[ ] Pentoxifylline (Trental, TNF-alpha antagonist, inhibits adenosine reuptake)

[ ] Periactin (cyproheptadine, as a serotonin antagonist)

[ ] Phentermine (neurotoxic, MAOI)

[ ] Pindolol (BuSpar and ketamine antagonist)

[ ] Piracetam (or related nootropics)

[ ] Pletal (cilostazol)

[ ] Ponstel (mefenamic acid, GABA agonist NSAID)

[ ] Prazosin (∝-1 antagonist)

[ ] Prednisone

[ ] Pregabalin (son of Neurontin)

[ ] Pregnenolone

[ ] Primacor nasal spray (milrinone) 1:10 or 1:1

[ ] Probenecid (inhibits kynurenate excretion)

[ ] Progesterone 10% MIC/cream gm

    [ ] natural

[ ] Proglumide (CCK inhibitor)

[ ] Propranolol

[ ] Protein kinase C activators (e.g., phosphatidylserine) and inhibitors (e.g., bisindolylmaleimides)

[ ] Prozac (fluoxetine)

[ ] Reboxetine (may antagonize baclofen)

[ ] Relaxin (made during pregnancy, a "nutraceutical" now)

[ ] Remeron (mirtazapine)

[ ] Requip (ropinirole)

[ ] Rilutek (riluzole)

[ ] Risperdal (risperidone)

[ ] Rivastigmine (Exelon—inhibits two cholinesterases)

[ ] Rolipram (once-daily dose, PDE4 inhibitor)

[ ] Salagen (pilocarpine tablets for xerostomia and xerophthalmia)

[ ] SAMe (reverses nylidrin and isoxsuprine)

[ ] Sansert (methysergide—related to LSD)

[ ] Selegiline p.o.

    [ ] 2% in PLO

[ ] Senktide (SP antagonist)

[ ] Seroquel (quetiapine, anxiolytic, possible analgesic)

[ ] Serzone (nefazodone, $5-HT_2$ antagonist)

[ ] Soma (caprisodol, adenosine agonist)

[ ] Sonata (zaleplon, almost worthless)

[ ] Suramin-like agents (to block ATP)

[ ] Synarel (nafarelin, for PMS)

[ ] Talwin (pentazocine, sigma$_1$ agonist)

[ ] Tamoxifen (for PMS and rapid cycling)

[ ] Tamsulosin (Flomax, peripheral ∝-antagonist)

[ ] Tasmar (tolcapone, LFTs required)

[ ] Taurine (may block polyamine site, putative GABA$_A$ agonist)
[ ] TCAs
[ ] Tegaserod (5HT$_4$ antagonist)
[ ] Tetrahydrobiopterin (NO synthase cofactor, requires SAMe for biosynthesis)
[ ] Thioperamide (H$_3$ [autoreceptor] antagonist, increases histamine)
[ ] Thyroid
[ ] Topamax (topiramate, AMPA antagonist, piracetam antagonist)
[ ] Transcranial magnetic stimulation
[ ] Trazodone (a sleeping pill)
[ ] TRH IV (benzodiazepine antagonist)
　　[ ] SQ
　　[ ] nasal spray 500 u 1:10 dilution
　　[ ] ophth.solution 500 u 1:10 dilution
[ ] Triestrogen 5 mg/gm VAN crm gm
[ ] Ultram (tramadol, analgesic, antidepressant, Rx for RLS)
[ ] Vagal nerve stimulation (excitatory or inhibitory)
[ ] Valtrex (valacyclovir, as GABA antagonist)
[ ] Vasotec (enalapril, ACE inhibitor, BK agonist, may synergize with forskolin)
[ ] Verapamil (Marinol and DA antagonist)
[ ] Viagra (sildenafil, PDE5 inhibitor)
[ ] Vicodin (hydrocodone/acetaminophen)
[ ] Vinpocetine (inhibits PDE1, Na$^+$ channel blocker)
[ ] Wellbutrin (bupropion)
[ ] Xanax (alprazolam)
　　[ ] Xanax-SR (no cognitive impairment)
[ ] Yohimbine (antagonizes clonidine)
[ ] Zanaflex (tizanidine, almost worthless, but not quite)
[ ] Zantac (ranitidine, NMDA antagonist, cholinesterase inhibitor)
[ ] Ziprasidone (Geodon, most potent 5-HT$_{1A}$ agonist)
[ ] Zofran (ondansetron, blocks glycine coagonist site of NMDA receptor, 5-HT$_3$ antagonist, NMDA-receptor agonist, antagonizes stimulants and ketamine)
[ ] Zoloft (sertraline)
[ ] Zonisamide (looking for a use, rarely analgesic)
[ ] Zopiclone (longer half-life than Ambien + possible anxiolytic)
[ ] Zyprexa (olanzapine, antagonizes ketamine)
[ ] _____

[ ] _____
[ ] _____
[ ] _____
[ ] _____
[ ] _____
[ ] _____
[ ] _____
[ ] _____
[ ] _____
[ ] _____
[ ] _____
[ ] _____
[ ] _____
[ ] _____
[ ] _____
[ ] _____
[ ] _____
[ ] _____
[ ] _____
[ ] _____
[ ] _____
[ ] _____
[ ] _____
[ ] _____
[ ] _____
[ ] _____
[ ] _____
[ ] _____
[ ] _____
[ ] _____
[ ] _____
[ ] _____
[ ] _____
[ ] _____
[ ] _____
[ ] _____
[ ] _____
[ ] _____
[ ] _____
[ ] _____
[ ] _____
[ ] _____
[ ] _____
[ ] _____
[ ] _____
[ ] _____
[ ] _____
[ ] _____
[ ] _____
[ ] _____
[ ] _____
[ ] _____
[ ] _____
[ ] _____
[ ] _____
[ ] _____
[ ] _____
[ ] _____

CFS SYMPTOM CHECKLIST

This symptom checklist is not sufficient to diagnose chronic fatigue syndrome unless other disorders have been ruled out by appropriate assessment.

A. Did your illness begin: ☐ abruptly? ☐ gradually?
    at what age? _____ age now? _____

B. Did your illness begin with a flu-like episode? ☐ yes ☐ no

    If yes: were lab tests done? _____
             what tests? _____
                         _____
             were abnormalities found? _____

C. Were you treated for psychological problems prior to the onset of this illness? ☐ yes ☐ no

    If yes: psychotherapy? ☐ yes ☐ no
             medication: _____

D. Did your illness follow exposure to new carpet/paint, tung oil, industrial solvents, pesticides, or other environmental toxins? ☐ yes ☐ no

    If yes, please describe: _____
                            _____

E. Do any medications make you feel better or worse? ☐ yes ☐ no

    If yes, please describe: _____
                            _____

F. Were you subject to prolonged stressors during childhood (e.g., abusive or dysfunctional home)? ☐ yes ☐ no

    If yes, please describe: _____
                            _____

G. Were you subject to unusual or extreme stressors in your life immediately prior to the onset of illness? ☐ yes ☐ no

    If yes, please describe: _____
                            _____

H. What is your occupation? _____

I.   Are you disabled (unable to work?) ☐ yes ☐ no

    If yes, what is the date you last worked? _____

J.   Are your symptoms worse: ☐ in the summer? ☐ in the winter?
    ☐ no difference?

Rate the severity of your symptoms from 0 to 10.

1.   ____Fatigue—usually made worse by physical exercise

    Is your level of activity less than 50 percent of normal?
    ☐ yes ☐ no

2.   ____Cognitive function problems

    ____ (a) attention-deficit disorder, including concentration
            problems

    ____ (b) calculation difficulties
            describe: _____
            _____

    ____ (c) memory disturbance
            describe: _____
            _____

    ____ (d) spatial disorientation, getting lost in familiar locations,
            problems judging distances

    ____ (e) frequently saying the wrong word

3.   ____ Psychological problems

    ____ (a) depression

    ____ (b) anxiety—which may include panic attacks and phobias
            (irrational fears)

    ____ (c) personality changes—usually a worsening of a previ-
            ous mild tendency

    ____ (d) emotional lability (mood swings)

    ____ (e) psychosis

4.   ____ Other nervous system problems

    ____ (a) sleep disturbance

    ____ (b) headaches

    ____ (c) changes in visual acuity

    ____ (d) seizures

_____ (e) numb or tingling feelings

_____ (f) lightheadedness—feeling "spaced out"

_____ (g) disequilibrium

_____ (h) frequent unusual nightmares

_____ (i) difficulty moving your tongue to speak

_____ (j) ringing in ears

_____ (k) paralysis

_____ (l) severe muscular weakness

_____ (m) blackouts

_____ (n) intolerance of bright lights

_____ (o) intolerance of alcohol

_____ (p) alteration of taste, smell, and hearing

_____ (q) nonrestorative sleep

_____ (r) decreased libido

_____ (s) twitching muscles ("benign fasciculations")

5. _____ Recurrent flu-like illnesses—often with chronic sore throat

6. _____ Painful lymph nodes—especially on sides of neck and under the arms

7. _____ Severe nasal and other allergies—often worsening of previous mild problem

8. _____ Weight change—usually gain

9. _____ Muscle and joint aches with tender "trigger points" or fibromyalgia

10. _____ Abdominal pain, diarrhea, nausea, intestinal gas—"irritable bowel syndrome"

11. _____ Low-grade fevers or feeling hot often

12. _____ Night sweats

13. _____ Heart palpitations

14. _____ Severe premenstrual syndrome (PMS)

15. _____ Rash of herpes simplex or shingles

16. _____ Uncomfortable or recurrent urination—pain in prostate

17. _____ Other symptoms

_____ (a) rashes

_____ (b) hair loss

_____ (c) impotence

_____ (d) chest pain

_____ (e) dry eyes and mouth

_____ (f) cough

_____ (g) TMJ syndrome

_____ (h) endometriosis

_____ (i) frequent canker sores

_____ (j) cold hands and feet

_____ (k) serious rhythm disturbances of the heart

_____ (l) carpal tunnel syndrome

_____ (m) pyriform muscle syndrome causing sciatica

_____ (n) thyroid inflammation

_____ (o) various cancers

_____ (p) periodontal (gum) disease

_____ (q) mitral valve prolapse

_____ (r) easily getting out of breath ("dyspnea on exertion")

_____ (s) symptoms worsened by extremes of temperature

_____ (t) multiple sensitivities to medicine, food, and other substances

Additional comments: _____

_____

_____

_____

_____

_____

_____

_____

_____

_____

_____   _____

Patient's signature   Date

References

Aarflot T, Bruusgaard D (1996). Association between chronic widespread musculo-skeletal complaints in thyroid autoimmunity, results from a community survey. *Scandanavian Journal of Primary Health Care* 14(2):111-115.

Abel T, Lattal KM (2001). Molecular mechanism of memory acquisition, consolidation, and retrieval. *Current Opinion in Neurobiology* 11(2):180-187.

Abu-Elheiga L, Matzuk MM, Abo-Hashema K, Wakil SJ (2001). Continuous fatty acid oxidation and reduced fat storage in mice lacking acetyl-CoA carboxylase 2. *Science* 291:2613-2616.

Acri JB, Thompson AC, Shippenberg TS (2001). Modulation of pre- and post-synaptic dopamine D_2 receptor function by the selective kappa-opioid receptor agonist U69593. *Synapse* 39:343-350.

Aicher SA, Sharma S, Pickel VM (1999). N-methyl-D-aspartate receptors are present in vagal afferents and their dendritic tracts in the nucleus tractus solitarius. *Neuroscience* 91(1):119-132.

Aiello LC, Wheeler P (1995). The expensive tissue hypothesis: The brain and the digestive system in human and primate evolution. *Current Anthropology* 36: 199-221.

Alagarsamy S, Sorensen S, Conn PJ (2001). Coordinate regulation of metabotropic glutamate receptors. *Current Opinion in Neurobiology* 11(3):357-362.

Alberts KR, Bradley LA, Alarcon GS, Mountz JM, Sotolongo A, Liu H-G (2000). Anticipation of acute pain and high arousal feedback in women with fibromyalgia (FM): High pain anxiety and high negative affectivity (NA) evokes increased pain and anterior cingulate cortex (ACC) activity without nociception. *AFSA Update* 7(2):5.

Alleva E, Aloe L, Cirulli F, De Acetis L, Padoa Schioppa C (1997). Postnatal NGF administration causes adult hyperalgesia and overreactivity to social stimuli but does not reverse capsaicin induced hypoalgesia. *Psychoneuroendocrinology* 22(8):591-602.

Alleva E, Petruzzi S, Cirulli F, Aloe L (1996). NGF regulatory function in stress and coping of rodents and humans. *Pharmacology, Biochemistry and Behavior* 54(1):65-72.

Allgaier C, Schiebler P, Muller D, Fuerstem TJ, Illes P (1999). NMDA receptor characterization and subunit expression in rat cultured mesencephalic neurons. *British Journal of Pharmacology* 120:121-130.

Almeida LE, Pereira EF, Alkondon M, Fawcett WP, Randall WR, Albuquerque EX (2000). The opioid antagonist naltrexone inhibits activity and alters expression of alpha7 and alpha4beta2 nicotinic receptors in hippocampal neurons: Implications for smoking cessation programs. *Neuropharmacology* 39:2740-2755.

Altemus M, Dale JK, Michelson D, Demitrack MA, Gold PW, Straus SE (2001). Abnormalities in response to vasopressin infusion in chronic fatigue syndrome. *Psychoneuroendocrinology* 26:175-188.

Altier N, Stewart J (1997). Tachykinin NK-1 and NK-3 selective agonists induce analgesia in the formalin test for tonic pain following intra-VTA or intra-accumbens neuroinfusions. *Behavioral Brain Research* 89:151-165.

Amandusson A, Hallbeck M, Hallbeck AL, Hermanson O, Blomqvist A (1999). Estrogen-induced alterations of spinal cord enkephalin gene expression. *Pain* 83:243-248.

Ameri A (1999). The effects of cannabinoids on the brain. *Progress in Neurobiology* 58:315-348.

Ames A (1997). Energy requirements of brain function: When is energy limiting? In Beal MF, Howell N, Bodis-Wollner I (Eds.), *Mitochondria and free radicals in neurodegenerative disease* (pp. 17-27). New York: Wiley-Liss.

Amiaz R, Stein O, Dannon PN, Grunhaus L, Schreiber S (1999). Resolution of treatment-refractory depression with naltrexone augmentation of paroxetine—A case report. *Psychopharmacology* 143:433-434.

Anand A, Charney DS, Oren DA, Berman RM, Hu XS, Cappiello A, Krystal JH (2000). Attenuation of the neuropsychiatric effects of ketamine with lamotrigine. *Archives of General Psychiatry* 57:270-276.

Anand A, Verhoeff P, Seneca N, Zoghbi S, Seibyl JP, Charney DS, Innis RB (2000). Brain SPECT imaging of amphetamine-induced dopamine release in euthymic bipolar disorder patients. *American Journal of Psychiatry* 157:1108-1114.

Andersson H, Lindquist E, Olson L (1997). Plant-derived amino acids increase hippocampal BDNF, NGF, c-fos, and hsp mRNAs. *NeuroReport* 8:1813-1817.

Andretic R, Chaney S, Hirsch J (1999). Requirement for circadian genes for cocaine sensitization in *Drosophila*. *Science* 285:1066-1068.

Arbogast LA, Hyde JF (2000). Estradiol attenuates the forskolin-induced increases in hypothalamic tyrosine hydroxylase activity. *Neuroendocrinology* 71:219-227.

Arinami T, Li L, Mitsushio H, Itokawa M, Hamaguchi H, Toru M (1996). An insertion/deletion polymorphism in the angiotensin converting enzyme gene is associated with both brain substance P contents and affective disorders. *Biological Psychiatry* 40:1122-1127.

Arnsten, AFT (1998). Catecholamine modulation of prefrontal cortical cognitive function. *Trends in Cognitive Sciences* 2:436-447.

Asmundson GJG, Kuperos JL, Norton GR (1997). Do patients with chronic pain selectively attend to pain-related information? Preliminary evidence for the mediating role of fear. *Pain* 72:27-32.

Aston-Jones G, Chen S, Zhu Y, Oshinsky ML (2001). A neural circuit for circadian regulation of arousal. *Nature Neuroscience* 4:732-738.

Aston-Jones G, Rajkowski J, Cohen J (1999). Role of locus coeruleus in attention and behavioral flexibility. *Biological Psychiatry* 46:1309-1320.

Ataka T, Kumamoto E, Shimoji K, Yoshimura M (2000). Baclofen inhibits more effectively C-afferent than Adelta-afferent glutamatergic transmission in substantia gelatinosa neurons of adult rat spinal cord slices. *Pain* 86(3):273-282.

Attal N, Brasseur L, Guirimand F, Dupuy M, Parker F, Gaude V, Bouhassira D (2000). Effects of intravenous lidocaine on spontaneous and evoked pains in patients with CNS injury. In Devor M, Rowbotham MC, Wiesenfeld-Hallin Z (Eds.), *Proceedings of the Ninth World Congress on Pain,* Volume 16 (pp. 863-874). Seattle, WA: IASP Press.

Avery RA, Franowicz JS, Studholme C, van Dyck CH, Arnsten AF (2000). The alpha-2A-androceptor agonist, guanfacine, increases regional cerebral blood flow in dorsolateral prefrontal cortex of monkeys performing a spatial working memory task. *Neuropsychopharmacology* 23(3):240-249.

Baev C (1997). Highest level automatisms in the nervous system, a theory of functional principles underlying the highest form of brain function. *Progress in Neurobiology* 51:129-166.

Bailey CH, Giustetto M, Huang Y-Y, Hawkins RD, Kandel ER (2000). Is heterosynaptic modulation essential for stabilizing of Hebbian plasticity and memory? *Nature Reviews Neuroscience* 1(1):11-20.

Bajjalieh S (2001). SNAREs take the stage: A prime time to trigger neurotransmitter secretion. *Trends in Neurosciences* 24(12):678-680.

Bale TL, Davis AM, Auger AP, Dorsa DM, McCarthy MM (2001). CNS region-specific oxytocin receptor expression: Importance in regulation of anxiety and sex behavior. *Journal of Neuroscience* 21:2546-2552.

Barañano DE, Ferris CD, Snyder SH (2001). Atypical neural messengers. *Trends in Neurosciences* 24(2):99-106.

Barkley RA (1997). Behavioral inhibition, sustained attention, and executive functions: Constructing a unified theory of ADHD. *Psychological Bulletin* 121:65-94.

Barlow DH, Chorpita BF, Turovsky JC (1996). Fear, panic, anxiety, and disorders of emotion. In Hope DA (Ed.), *Nebraska symposium on motivation: Perspectives on anxiety, panic, and fear,* Volume 43 (pp. 251-328). Lincoln, NE: University of Nebraska Press.

Barnes JM, Barnes NM, Cooper SJ (1992). Behavioral pharmacology of 5-HT$_3$ receptor ligands. *Neuroscience and Biobehavioral Reviews* 16:107-113.

Barrows D (1995). Functional capacity of people with chronic fatigue immune dysfunction syndrome. *American Journal of Occupational Therapy* 49(4):327-337.

Bauer M (1997). High-dose thyroxin in prophylaxis resistant affective disorder. *Biol Psychiatry* 42:78S-79S.

Baughman KL (2002). B-type natriuretic peptide—A window to the heart. *New England Journal of Medicine* 347:158-159.

Baxter MG, Murray EA (2002). The amygdala and reward. *Nature Reviews Neuroscience* 3:563-573.

Beggs JM, Brown TH, Byrne JH, Crow T, LeDoux JE, LeBar K, Thompson RF (1999). Learning and memory: Basic mechanisms. In Zigmond MJ, Bloom FE, Landis SC, Roberts JL, Squire LS (Eds.), *Fundamental Neuroscience* (pp. 1411-1454). San Diego, CA: Academic Press.

Beique JC, Blier P, de Montigny C, Debonnel G (2000). Potentiation by (-) pindolol of the activation of postsynaptic 5-HT$_{1A}$ receptors induced by venlafaxine. *Neuropsychopharmacology* 23:294-306.

Belvin MP, Zhou H, Yin JC (1999). The *Drosophila dCREB2* gene affects the circadian clock. *Neuron* 22:777-787.

Belzung C, Le Guisquet AM, Agmo A (2000). Anxiolytic-like effects of meprobamate: Interactions with an opioid and an opiate antagonist in Swiss and BALB/C mice. *Pharmacology, Biochemistry, and Behavior* 65(3):465-474.

Bennett DLH (2001). Neurotrophic factors: Important regulators of nociceptive function. *The Neuroscientist* 7(1):13-17.

Bereiter DA, Bereiter DF (2000). Morphine and NMDA receptor antagonism reduce c-*fos* expression in the spinal trigeminal nucleus produced by an acute injury to the TMJ region. *Pain* 85:65-77.

Bergado JA, Fernández CI, Gómez-Soria A, González O (1997). Chronic intraventricular infusion with NGF improves LTP in old cognitively-impaired rats. *Brain Research* 770:1-9.

Bergeron R, de Montigny C, Debonnel G (1999). Pregnancy reduces brain sigma receptor function. *British Journal of Pharmacology* 127:1769-1776.

Bergerot A, Reynier-Rebuffel A-M, Callebert J, Aubineau P (2000). Long-term superior cervical sympathectomy induces mast cell hyperplasia and increases histamine and serotonin content in the rat dura mater. *Neuroscience* 96(1):205-213.

Bergles DE, Roberts DB, Somogyi P, Jah CE (2001). Glutamatergic synapses on oligodendrocyte precursor cells. *Nature* 405:187-191.

Berman RM, Capiello A, Anand A, Oren DA, Heninger GR, Charney DS, Krystal JH (2000). Antidepressant effects of ketamine in depressed patients. *Biological Psychiatry* 47:351-354.

Bernasconi R, Mathivet P, Bischoff S, Marescaux C (1999). Gamma-hydroxybutyric acid: An endogenous neuromodulator with abuse potential? *Trends in Pharmacological Sciences* 20:135-141.

Bevilaqua LR, Cammarota M, Paratcha G, de Stein ML, Izquierdo I, Medina JH (1999). Experience-dependent increase in cAMP-responsive element binding protein in synaptic and non-synaptic mitochondria of the rat hippocampus. *European Journal of Neuroscience* 11:3753-3756.

Beyer CE, Steketee JD (1999). Dopamine depletion in the medial prefrontal cortex induces sensitized-like behavioral and neurochemical responses to cocaine. *Brain Research* 833:133-141.

Bezzi P, Volterra A (2001). A neuron-glia signaling network in the active brain. *Current Opinion in Neurobiology* 11:387-394.

Bicalacqua TJ, Hellstrom WJ, Kadowitz PJ, Champion HC (2001). Increased expression of arginase II in human diabetic corpus cavernosum: In diabetic-associated erectile dysfunction. *Biochemical and Biophysical Research Communications* 283(4):923-927.

Birnbaum S, Gobeske KT, Auerbach J, Taylor JR, Arnsten AF (1999). A role for norepinephrine in stress-induced cognitive deficits: α-1 adrenoceptor mediation in the prefrontal cortex. *Biological Psychiatry* 46:1266-1274.

Bisaga A, Katz JL, Antonini A, et al. (1998). Cerebral glucose metabolism in women with panic disorder. *American Journal of Psychiatry* 155:1178-1183.

Bito H, Deisseroth K, Tsien RW (1996). CREB phosphorylation and dephosphorylation: A Ca^{2+} and stimulus-duration dependent switch for hippocampal gene expression. *Cell* 87:1203-1214.

Bitran D, Dowd JA (1996). Ovarian steroids modify the behavioral and neurochemical responses of the central benzodiazepine receptor. *Psychopharmacology* 125:65-73.

Blakely RD (2001). Dopamine's reversal of fortune. *Science* 293:2407-2409.

Blaustein MP, Golovina VA (2001). Structural complexity and functional diversity of endoplasmic reticular Ca^{2+} stores. *Trends in Neurosciences* 24:602-608.

Blessing WW (1997). Inadequate frameworks for understanding bodily homeostasis. *Neuroscience* 20:235-239.

Blier P, Bergeron R, de Montigny C (1997). Selective activation of postsynaptic $5-HT_{1A}$ receptors induces rapid antidepressant response. *Neuropsychopharmacology* 16:333-338.

Blobe GC, Schiemann WP, Lodish HG (2000). Role of transforming growth factor beta in human disease. *New England Journal of Medicine* 342(18):1350-1358.

Bloch M, Schmidt PJ, Danaceau M, Murphy J, Nieman L, Rubinow DR (2000). Effects of gonadal steroids in women. *American Journal of Psychiatry* 157:924-930.

Bloms-Funke P, Loscher W (1996). The anticonvulsant gabapentin decreases firing rates of substantia nigra pars reticulata neurons. *European Journal of Pharmacology* 316:211-218.

Bohus MJ, Lanwehrmeyer GB, Stiglmayr CE, et al. (1999). Naltrexone in the treatment of dissociative symptoms in patients with borderline personality disorder: An open-label trial. *Journal of Clinical Psychiatry* 60:598-603.

Bolshakov VY, Carboni L, Cobb MH, et al. (2000). Dual MAP kinase pathways mediate opposing long-term plasticity at CA3-CA1 synapses. *Nature Neuroscience* 3:1107-1112.

Bolyard LA, Van Looy JW, Vasko MR (2000). Sensitization of rat sensory neurons by chronic exposure to forskolin or "inflammatory cocktail" does not downregulate and requires continuous exposure. *Pain* 88:277-285.

Bonetta L (2001). Scientists battle obesity overload. *Nature Medicine* 7:387.

Bordi F, Quartaroli M (2000). Modulation of nociceptive transmission of NMDA/ glycine site receptor in the ventropostero-lateral nucleus of the thalamus. *Pain* 84:213-224.

Borowitz JL, Gunasekar PG, Isom GE (1997). Hydrogen cyanide generation by mu-opiate receptor activation: Possible neuromodulatory role of endogenous cyanide. *Brain Research* 768:294-300.

Bovetto S, Boyer P-A, Skolnick P, Fossom LH (1997). Chronic administration of a glycine partial agonist alters the expression of *N*-methyl-D-aspartate receptor subunit mRNAs. *Journal of Pharmacology and Experimental Therapeutics* 283:1503-1509.

Boyce S, Hill RG (2000). Discrepant results from preclinical and clinical studies on the potential of substance P-receptor antagonist compounds as analgesics. In Devor M, Rowbotham MC, Wiesenfeld-Hallin Z (Eds.), *Proceedings of the Ninth World Congress on Pain* (pp. 313-324). Seattle, WA: IASP Press.

Brake WG, Sullivan RM, Flores G, Srivastava LK, Gratton A (1999). Neonatal ventral hippocampal lesions attenuate the nucleus accumbens dopamine response to stress: An electrochemical study in the adult rat. *Brain Research* 831:25-32.

Brändli P, Löffler B-M, Breu V, Osterwalder R, Maire J-P, Clozel M (1996). Role of endothelin in mediating neurogenic plasma extravasation in rat dura mater. *Pain* 64:315-322.

Brefczynski JA, DeVoe EA (1999). A physiological correlate of the "spotlight" of visual attention. *Nature Neuroscience* 2:370-374.

Bremner JD, Innis RB, Southwick SM, Staib L, Zoghbi S, Charney DS (2000). Decreased benzodiazepine receptor binding in prefrontal cortex in combat-related posttraumatic stress disorder. *American Journal of Psychiatry* 157:1120-1126.

Brever LH, Behm FM, Westman EC, et al. (1999). Naltrexone blockade of nicotine effects in cigarette smokers. *Psychopharmacology* 143:339-346.

Brezina V, Weiss KR (1997). Analyzing the function consequences of transmitter complexity. *Trends in Neurosciences* 20(11):538-543.

Brinkmeier H, Aulkmeyer P, Wollinsky KH, Rudel R (2000). An endogenous pentapeptide acting as a sodium channel blocker in inflammatory autoimmune disorders of the central nervous system. *Nature Medicine* 6:2000-2006.

Broberger C (1999). Hypothalamic cocaine- and amphetamine-regulated transcript (CART) neurons: Histochemical relationship to thyrotropin-releasing hormone, melanin-concentrating hormone, orexin/hypocretin and neuropeptide Y. *Brain Research* 848:101-113.

Brosamlee C (1998). The making, changing, and breaking of contacts. *Trends in Neurosciences* 21:3:91-94.

Bruning JC, Gautam D, Burks DJ, Gillette J, Schubart M, Orban PC, Kelin R, Krone W, Muller-Wieland D, Kahn CR (2000). Role of brain insulin receptor in control of body weight and reproduction. *Science* 289:2122-2125.

Brussard AB, Herbison AE (2000). Long-term plasticity of postsynaptic $GABA_A$-receptor function in the adult brain: Insights from the oxytocin neurons. *Trends in Neurosciences* 23:190-195.

Buchel C, Dolan RJ (2000). Classical fear conditioning in functional neuroimaging. *Current Opinion in Neurobiology* 10:219-223.

Buijs RM, Kalsbeck A (2001). Hypothalamic integration of central and peripheral clocks. *Nature Reviews Neuroscience* 2:521-525.

Burhans L, Taylor C, Gabriel M (2000). Ventral subicular lesions, neuronal activity, and extinction of avoidance responses with novel contextual and cue stimuli. *Society for Neuroscience Abstract Bulletin:* 74.3.

Burkey AR, Carstens E, Jasmin L (1999). Dopamine reuptake inhibition in rostral agranular insular cortex produces antinociception. *Journal of Neuroscience* 19: 4169-4179.

Burnstock G (2001). Purine-mediated signalling in pain and visceral perception. *Trends in Pharmacological Sciences* 22:182-188.

Burstein R, Malick A (2000). Trigeminohypothalamic and reticulohypothalamic tract neurons in the upper cervical spinal cord and caudal medulla of the rat: II. Axonal mapping in the midbrain, diencephalons, and basal ganglia. *Abstracts of the Society for Neuroscience:* 433.

Byrne JH (1999). Postsynaptic potentials and synaptic integration. In Zigmund MJ, Bloom FE, Landis SC, Roberts JL, Squire LS (Eds.), *Fundamental Neuroscience* (pp. 345-362). San Diego, CA: Academic Press.

Cabib S, Puglisi-Allegra S (1996). Different effects of repeated stressful experiences or mesocortical and mesolimbic dopamine metabolism. *Neuroscience* 73(2):375-380.

Calabresi P, Pisani A, Merevri NB, Bernardi G (1996). The corticostriatal projection: From synaptic plasticity to dysfunction of the basal ganglia. *Trends in Neuroscience* 19:19-24.

Calder AJ, Lawrence AD, Young AW (2001). Neuropsychology of fear and loathing. *Nature Reviews Neuroscience* 2(5):352-363.

Calon F, Tahar AH, Blanchet PJ, Morissette M, Grondin R, Goulet M, Doucet JP, Robertson GS, Nestler E, Di Paolo T, Bedard PJ (2000). Dopamine-receptor stimulation: Biobehavioral and biochemical consequences. *Trends in Neuroscience* 23(10, Suppl.):S92-S100.

Canales JJ, Iversen SD (2000). Psychomotor-activating effects mediated by dopamine D_2 and D_3 receptors in the nucleus accumbens. *Pharmacology, Biochemistry and Behavior* 67:161-168.

Cantor JM, Binik YM, Pfaus JG (1999). Chronic fluoxetine inhibits sexual behavior in the male rat: Reversal with oxytocin. *Psychopharmacology* 144:355-362.

Carlsson A (2001). A paradigm shift in brain research. *Science* 294:1021-1024.

Carpenter PA, Just MA, Raichle ED (2000). Working memory and executive function: Evidence from neuroimaging. *Current Opinion in Neurobiology* 10:195-199.

Carro E, Nunez A, Busigoma S, Torres-Aleman I (2000). Circulating insulin-like growth factor 1 mediates effects of exercise on the brain. *Journal of Neuroscience* 20:2926-2933.

Cass WA, Gerhardt GA (1995). In vivo assessment of dopamine uptake in rat's medial prefrontal cortex; Comparison with dorsal striation and nucleus accumbens. *Journal of Neurochemistry* 65:201-207.

Castellanos, XF (1999). Stimulants and tic disorders. *Archives of General Psychiatry* 56:337-338.

Cecchi M, Passani MB, Bacciotini L, et al. (2001). Cortical acetylcholine release elicited by stimulation of histamine H_1 receptors in the nucleus basals magnocellularis: A dual-probe microdialysis study in the freely moving rat. *European Journal of Neuroscience* 13:68-78.

Chakravoty SG, Halbriech U (1997). The influence of estrogen on monoamine oxidase activity. *Psychopharmacology Bulletin* 33(2):229-233.

Chambers RA, Bremner JD, Moghaddam B, et al. (1999). Glutamate and post-traumatic stress disorder: Toward a psychobiology of dissociation. *Seminars in Clinical Neuropsychiatry* 4:274-281.

Chang L, Karin M (2001). Mammalian MAP kinase signaling cascades. *Nature* 410:37-40.

Chapman R (1986). Pain, perception, and illness. In Sternbach RA (Ed.), *The Psychology of Pain.* New York: Raven Press.

Chasin MR, Galvin RW, National Roundtable on Health Care Quality (1998). The urgent need to improve health care quality. *JAMA* 280(11):1000-1005.

Chemilli RM, Willie JT, Sinton CM, Elmquist JK, Scammell T, Lee C, Richardson JA, Williams SC, Xiong Y, Kisanuki Y, et al. (1999). Narcolepsy in orexin knockout mice: Molecular genetics of sleep regulation. *Cell* 98:437-451.

Chen BT, Avshalumav MV, Rice ME (2001). H_2O_2 is a novel, endogenous modulator of synaptic dopamine release. *Journal of Neurophysiology* 85:2468-2476.

Chen JF, Beilstein M, Xu YH, Turner TJ, Moratalla R, Standaert DG, Alloyo VJ, Fink JS, Schwarzschild MA (2000). Selective attenuation of psychostimulant-induced behavioral responses in mice lacking A_{2A} adenosine receptors. *Neuroscience* 97:195-204.

Cheng MY, Bullock CM, Li C, et al. (2002). Prokineticin2 transmits the behavioral circadian rhythm of the suprachiasmatic nucleus. *Nature* 417:405-410.

Cherubini E, Conti F (2001). Generating diversity of GABAergic synapses. *Trends in Neurosciences* 24:155-162.

Chizh BA, Headly PM, Tzsehentke TM (2001). NMDA receptor antagonists as analgesics: Focus on the NR2B subtype. *Trends in Pharmacological Sciences* 22:636-641.

Choi YB, Tenneti L, Le DA, Ortiz J, Bai G, Chen HS, Lipton SA (2000). Molecular basis of NMDA receptor-coupled ion channel modulation by S-nitrosylation. *Nature Neuroscience* 3(1):15-21.

Christensen D, Gautron M, Guilbaud G, Kayser V (2001). Effect of gabapentin and lamotrigine on mechanical allodynia-like behavior in a rat model of trigeminal neuropathic pain. *Pain* 93:147-153.

Chun MM, Phelps EA (1999). Memory deficits for implicit conceptual information in amnesic subjects with hippocampal damage. *Nature Neuroscience* 2:844-847.

Cirelli C, Tononi G (1998). Changes in gene expression after long-term sleep deprivation in rats. *Society of Neuroscience Abstracts* 24:1430.

Clark DA, Beck AT, Alford BA (1999). *Scientific Foundations of Cognitive Theory and Therapy of Depression*. New York: John Wiley.

Clark KB, Naritoku DK, Smith DC, Browning RA, Jenson RA (1999). Enhanced recognition memory following vagus nerve stimulation in human subjects. *Nature Neuroscience* 2(l):79-87.

Codor M, Bjijou Y, Carlhol B, Stinus L (1999). D-amphetamine-induced behavioral sensitization: Implication of a glutamatergic medial prefrontal cortex-ventral tegmental innervation. *Neuroscience* 94:705-721.

Cohen JD, Botvanick M, Carter CS (2000). Anterior cingulate and prefrontal cortex: Who is in control? *Nature Neuroscience* 3(5):421-423.

Cole JC, Littleton JM, Little HJ (2000). Acamprosate but not naltrexone, inhibits conditioned abstinence behavior associated with repeated ethanol administration and exposure to a plus-maze. *Psychopharmacology* 147:403-411.

Collins DR, Pare D (2000). Differential fear conditioning induces reciprocal changes in the sensory responses of lateral amygdala neurons to the CS(+) and CS (-). *Learning and Memory* 7:97-103.

Colwell CS, Levine MS (1997). Histamine modulates NMDA-dependent swelling in the neostriatum. *Brain Research* 766:205-212.

Congar P, Leinekugal X, Ben-Ari Y, Crépel V (1997). A long-lasting calcium-activated non-selective cationic current is generated by synaptic stimulation of exogenous activation of group I metabotropic glutamate receptors in CA1 pyramidal neurons. *Journal of Neuroscience* 17:5366-5379.

Constantinidis C, Franowicz MN, Goldman-Rakic PS (2001). The sensory nature of mnemonic representation in the primate prefrontal cortex. *Nature Neuroscience* 4:311-316.

Contreras-Vidal JL (1999). The gating functions of the basal ganglia movement control. *Progress in Brain Research* 121:21-276.

Corchero J, Garcia-Gil L, Manzanares J, Fernandez-Ruiz JJ, Fuentes JA, Ramos JA, (1998). Perinatal delta9-tetrahydrocannibinol exposure reduces proenkephalin gene expression in the caudate-putamen of adult female rats. *Life Science* 63(10): 843-850.

Corcoran KA, Maren S (2000). Hippocampal inactivation disrupts contextual retrieval of fear memory after extinction. *Journal of Neuroscience* 21:1720-1726.

Cordero-Erausquin M, Marubio LM, Klink R, Changeux J-P (2000). Nicotinic receptor function: New perspectives from knockout mice. *Trends in Pharmacological Sciences* 21:211-217.

Corr DB, Sesack SR (2000). Projections from the rat prefrontal cortex to the ventral tegmental area: Target specificity in synaptic associations with mesoaccumbens and mesocortical neurons. *Journal of Neuroscience* 20:3864-3873.

Corwin RL, Jorn A, Hardy M, Crawley JN (1995). The CCK-B antagonist CI-988 increases dopamine levels in microdialysate from the rat nucleus accumbens via a tetrodotoxin- and calcium-independent mechanism. *Journal of Neurochemistry* 65(1):208-217.

Cossart R, Dinocourt C, Hirsch JC, Merchan-Perez A, DeFelipe J, Ben-Ari Y, Esclopez M, Bernard C (2001). Dendritic but not somatic GABAergic inhibition is decreased in experimental epilepsy. *Nature Neuroscience* 4:52-62.

Costall B, Domeney AM, Naylor RJ, Tyers MB (1987). Effects of the 5-HT$_3$ receptor antagonists, GR38032F, on raised dopaminergic activity in the mesolimbic system of the marmoset and the rat. *British Journal of Pharmacology* 92:881-894.

Costall B, Naylor RJ, Tyers MB (1990). The psychopharmacology of 5-HT$_3$ receptors. *Pharmacologic Therapeutics* 47:181-202.

Cotrina ML, Nedergaard M (2000). ATP as a messenger in astrocyte-neuronal communication. *Neuroscientist* 6:120-126.

Courmel K (1996). *Companion Volume to Dr. Jay A. Goldstein's Betrayal by the Brain: A Guide for Patients and Their Physicians.* Binghamton, NY: The Haworth Press.

Cox CL, Sherman SM (1999). Glutamate inhibits thalamic reticular neurons. *Journal of Neuroscience* 19(15):6694-6699.

Crabtree JW, Collingridge GL, Isaac JTR (1998). A new intrathalamic pathway linking modality-related nuclei in the dorsal thalamus. *Nature Neuroscience* 1(5):389-394.

Craig AD (1998). A new version of the thalamic disinhibition hypothesis of central pain. *Pain Forum* 7:1-14.

Craig AD, Chen K, Bandy D, Reiman EM (2000). Thermosensory activation of insular cortex. *Nature Neuroscience* 3:184-190.

Cravchik A, Goldman D (2000). Neurochemical individuality: Genetic diversity among human dopamine and serotonin receptors and transporters. *Archives of General Psychiatry* 57:1105-1114.

Crestani F, Lopez M, Baer K, Essrich C, Benke D, Laurent JP, Belzyny C, Fritschy J-J, Luscher B, Mohler H (1999). Decreased $GABA_A$ receptor clustering results in enhanced anxiety and a bias for threat cues. *Nature Neuroscience* 2:833-839.

Crombez G, Eccleston C, Baeyens F, et al. (1998). When somatic information threatens, catastrophic thinking enhances attentional interference. *Pain* 75:187-198.

Crowley KL, Flores JA, Hughes CN, Iacono RP (1998). Clinical application of ketamine ointment in the treatment of significant allodynia and hyperalgesia associated with chronic neuropathic pain. *International Journal of Pharmaceutical Compounding* 2(2):122-127.

Cummings JL (2000). Cholinesterase inhibitors: A new class of psychotropic compounds. *American Journal of Psychiatry* 157:4-15.

Cummins TR, DB-Hajj SD, Balck IA, Waxman SG (2000). Sodium channels as molecular targets in pain. In Devor M, Rowbotham MC, Wiesenfeld-Hallin Z (Eds.), *Proceedings of the Ninth World Congress on Pain* (pp. 77-91). Seattle, WA: IASP Press.

D'Amico M, Berrino L, Maione S, et al. (1996). Endothelin-1 in periaqueductal gray area of mice induces analgesia via glutamatergic receptors. *Pain* 65:205-209.

Daniele A, Albanese A, Gainotti G, et al. (1997). Zolpidem in Parkinson's disease. *Lancet* 349:1222-1223.

Danysz W, Parsons CG, Kornhuber J, Schmidt WJ, Quack G (1997). Aminoadamantanes as NMDA receptor antagonists and antiparkinson agents: Preclinical studies. *Neuroscience and Biobehavioral Reviews* 21(4):455-468.

Dawson TM (2002). Preconditioning-mediated neuroprotection through erythropoietin? *Lancet* 395:96-97.

De Keyser J, Solter G, Luiten PG (1999). Clinical trials with neuroprotective drugs in acute ischemic stroke: Are we doing the right thing? *Trends in Neurosciences* 22(June):535-540.

de Lima J, Beggs S, Howard R (2000). Neural toxicity of ketamine and other NMDA antagonists. *Pain* 88(3):311-312.

De Sarro G, Gratteri S, Nacceri F, et al. (2000). Influence of D-cycloserine on the anticonvulsant activity of some anti-epileptic drugs against audiogenic seizures in DBA/2 mice. *Epilepsy Research* 40:109-121.

De Souza F, Silva MA, Mattern C, Hacker R, Nogueira PJC, Huston JP, Schwarting RKW (1997). Intranasal administration of the dopaminergic agonists L-dopa, amphetamine, and cocaine increases dopamine activity in the neostriatum: A microdialysis study in the rat. *Journal of Neurochemistry* 68:233-239.

DeBellis MD, Keshavan MS, Spencer S, Hall J (2000). N-acetylaspartate concentrations in the anterior cingulate of maltreated children and adolescents with PTSD. *American Journal of Psychiatry* 157:1275-1277.

deFockert JW, Rees G, Frith CD, Lavie N (2001). The role of working memory in visual selective attention. *Science* 291:1803-1806.

del Olmo S, Bustamante J, del Rio RM, Solis J (2000). Taurine activated $GABA_A$ but not $GABA_B$ receptors in the rat hippocampal CA1 area. *Brain Research* 864: 298-307.

Delfs JM, Zhu Y, Druban JP, Aston-Jones GS (1998). Origin of noradrenergic afferents to the shell subregion of the nucleus accumbens: Anterograde and retrograde tract-tracing studies in the rat. *Brain Research* 806:127-140.

De-Melo JD, Tonussi CR, D'Orleans-Juste P, Rae GA (1998). Articular nociception induced by endothelin-1, carrageenan, and LPS in naive and previously inflamed knee joints in the rat: Inhibition by endothelin receptor antagonists. *Pain* 77:261-269.

Demitrack MA, Dale JK, Straus SE, et al. (1991). Evidence for impaired activation of the hypothalamic-pituitary-adrenal access in patients with chronic fatigue syndrome. *Journal of Clinical Endocrinology and Metabolism* 73:1224-1234.

DePonti F, Tonini M (2000). Irritable bowel syndrome: New agents targeting serotonin receptor subtypes. *Drugs* 61:317-332.

Desagher S, Corcier J, Glowinski J, Tence M (1997). Endothelin stimulates phospholipase D in striatal astrocytes. *Journal of Neurochemistry* 68:78-87.

Dev KK, Nakanishi S, Henley JM (2001). Regulation of mglu(7) receptors by proteins that interact with the intracellular C-terminus. *Trends in Pharmacological Science* 22(7):355-361.

Devinsky O, Morrell JM, Vogt BA (1995). Contributions of anterior cingulate cortex to behavior. *Brain* 118:279-306.

Di Matteo V, De Blasi A, Di Giulio C, Esposito E (2001). Role of $5HT_{2C}$ receptors in the control of central dopaminergic function. *Trends in Pharmacological Sciences* 22:229-232.

Diano S, Urbanski HF, Horvath B, et al. (2000) Mitochondrial uncoupling protein 2 (UCP2) in the non-human primate brain and pituitary. *Endocrinology* 141:4226-4238.

Diaz-Cabale Z, Narvaez JA, Petersson M, Uvnas-Moberg K, Fuxe K (2000). Oxytocin/alpha$_2$-adrenoceptor interactions in feeding responses. *Neuroendocrinology* 71:209-218.

Diaz-Cabale Z, Petersson M, Narvaez JA, Uvnas-Moberg K, Fuxe K (2000). Systemic oxytocin treatment modulates alpha$_2$ adrenoceptors in telencephalic and diencephalic regions of the rat. *Brain Research* 887:421-425.

Dienstbier RA (1989). Arousal and physiological toughness: Implications for mental and physical health. *Psychological Review* 96:84-100.

Dingemanse J (2000). Issues important for national COMT inhibition. *Neurology* 55(11, Suppl. 4):524-532.

Dirksen R, Van Luijtelaar ELJM, Van Rijn CM (1998). Selective serotonin reuptake inhibitors may enhance responses to noxious stimulation. *Pharmacology Biochemistry and Behavior* 60(3):719-725.

Dodson CS, Koutstaal W, Schacter DL (2000). Escape from illusion: Reducing false memories. *Trends in Cognitive Sciences* 4:391-396.

Dooley DJ, Fink KB, Mieske CA, et al. (1999). Inhibition of K+-evoked glutamate release from slices of rat neocortex by gabapentin. *Society for Neuroscience Abstracts:* 896.8.

Dougherty DD, Bonab AA, Spencer TJ, Rauch SL, Madras BK, Fischman AJ (1999). Dopamine transporter density in patients with attention deficit hyperactivity disorder. *Lancet* 354:2132.

Doverty M, Somogyi AA, White JM, et al. (2001). Methadone maintenance patients are cross-tolerant to the antinociceptive effects of morphine. *Pain* 93:155-163.

Drevets WC (2001). Neuroimaging and neuropathological studies of depression; Implications for the cognitive-emotional features of mood disorders. *Current Opinion in Neurobiology* 11:240-248.

Drew AE, Derbez AE, Dudek JD, Werling LL (1999). Regulation of dopamine transporter (DAT) activity by nicotinic receptors in rat prefrontal cortex. *Society for Neuroscience Abstracts:* 801.9.

Du J, Hull EM (1999). Effects of testosterone on neuronal nitric oxide synthase and tyrosine hydroxylase. *Brain Research* 836:90-98.

Duman RS, Heninger GR, Nestler EJ (1997). A molecular and cellular theory of depression. *Archives of General Psychiatry* 54:597-606.

Duncan J (2001). An adaptive coding model of neural function in prefrontal cortex. *Nature Reviews Neuroscience* 2(11):820-829.

Duncan J, Owen AM (2000). Common regions of the human frontal lobe recruited by diverse cognitive demands. *Trends in Neurosciences* 23:475-483.

Dunn AJ, Swiergiel AH (1999). Behavioral responses to stress are intact in CRF-deficient mice. *Brain Research* 845:14-20.

Durant W, Durant A (1956). *The story of civilization.* New York: Simon and Schuster.

Durstewitz D, Seamans JK, Sejnowskii TJ (1999). Dopaminergic modulation of activity states in the prefrontal cortex. *Society for Neuroscience Abstracts:* 488.15.

Eccleston C, Crombez G, Aldrich S, Stannard C (1997). *Pain* 72(1-2):209-215.

Edagawa Y, Saito H, Abe K (1999). Stimulation of the 5-HT$_{1A}$ receptor selectively suppresses NMDA receptor-mediated synaptic excitation in the rat visual cortex. *Brain Research* 827(1-2):225-228.

Eichenbaum H (2000). A cortical-hippocampal system for declarative memory. *Nature Reviews Neuroscience* 1:41-50.

Eisenberg E, Pud D (1998). Can patients with chronic neuropathic pain be cured by acute administration of the NMDA antagonist amantadine? *Pain* 74:337-339.

Elgersma Y, Silva AJ (1999). Molecular mechanisms of synaptic plasticity and memory. *Current Opinion in Neurobiology* 9:209-213.

Ellinwood EH, King GR, Davidson C, Lee TH (2000). The dopamine D_2/D_3 antagonist DS121 potentiates the effect of cocaine on locomotion and reduces tolerance in cocaine tolerant rats. *Behavioral Brain Research* 116:169-175.

Ellis CM, Monk C, Simmons A, et al. (1999). Functional magnetic resonance imaging neuroactivation studies in normal subjects and subjects with the narcoleptic syndrome: Actions of modafinil. *Journal of Sleep Research* 2:85-93.

Enarson MC, Hays H, Woodroffe MA (1999). Clinical experience with oral ketamine. *Journal of Pain and Symptom Management* 17(5):384-386.

Enderg H, Linner L, Svensson TH (1999). Effects of reboxetine on ventral tegmental area neuronal activity and dopamine output in major projection areas. *Society for Neuroscience Abstracts:* 488.22.

Engel AK, Fries P, Singer W (2001). Dynamic predictions: Oscillations and synchrony in top-down processing. *Nature Reviews Neuroscience* 2:704-716.

Engel AK, Singer W (2001). Temporal binding and the neural correlates of sensory awareness. *Trends in Cognitive Sciences* 5(1):16-25.

Engelmann M, Ebner K, Landgraf R, Hulsboer F, Wotjak CT (1999). Emotional stress triggers intrahypothalamic but not peripheral release of oxytocin in male rats. *Journal of Neuroendocrinology* 11:867-872.

Englebienne P, Herst CV, De Smet K, D'Haese A, De Meirleir K (2001). Interactions between Rnase L ankyrin-like domain and ABC transporters as a possible origin for pain, ion transport, CNS and immune disorders of chronic fatigue immune dysfunction syndrome. *Journal of Chronic Fatigue Syndrome* 8(3/4):83-102.

Enserink M (2001). Gulf War illness: The battle continues. *Science* 291:812-816.

Espejo EF (1997). Selective dopamine depletion within the medial prefrontal cortex and its anxiogenic-like effects in rats placed on the elevated plus maze. *Brain Research* 762:281-284.

Evengard B, Nilsson CG, Lindh G, Lindquist L, Evereth P, Frerickson S, Terenius L, Henriksson KG (1998). Chronic fatigue syndrome differs from fibromyalgia. Evidence for elevated substance P levels in cerebrospinal fluid of patients with chronic fatigue syndrome. *Pain* 78:153-155.

Exton MS, Kruger THC, Kock M, et al. (2001). Coitus-induced orgasm stimulates prolactin secretion in healthy subjects. *Psychoneuroendocrinology* 26:287-294.

Fagni L, Chavis P, Ango F, Bockaert J (2000). Complex interactions between mGluRs, intracellular Ca^{2+} stores and ion channels. *Trends in Neurosciences* 23:80-88.

Fairbanks CA, Posthumus IJ, Kitto KF, Stone LS, Wilcox GO (2000). Monoxodine, a selective imidazoline/alpha$_2$ adrenergic receptor agonist synergizes with morphine and deltorphin II to inhibit substance P induced behavior in mice. *Pain* 84:13-20.

Falls WA, Miserendino MJ, Davis M (1992). Extinction of fear-potentiated startle: Blockade by infusion of an NMDA antagonist into the amygdala. *Journal of Neuroscience* 12:854-863.

Faris PL, Kim SW, Meller WH, et al. (2000). Effect of decreasing afferent vagal activity with ondansetron on symptoms of bulimia nervosa: A randomized, double-blind trial. *Lancet* 355:792-797.

Farver DK, Khan MH (2001). Zolpidem for antipsychotic-induced Parkinsonism. *Annals of Pharmacotherapy* 35:435-437.

Feinstein N, Parnas D, Parnas H, Dudel J, Parnas I (1998). Functional and immunocytochemical identification of glutamate autoreceptors of an NMDA type in crayfish neuromuscular junction. *Journal of Neurophysiology* 80(6):2893-2899.

Fendt M, Schweinbacher I, Kock M (2000). Injections of the metabotropic glutamate receptor antagonist MPEP into the lateral amygdala prevent acquisition of the conditioned fear response. *Society for Neuroscience Abstracts:* 75.3.

Fernandez-Chacon R, Konigstorfer A, Gerber SH, Garcia J, Matos MF, Stevens CF, Brose N, Rizo J, Rosenmund C, Sudhof TC (2001). Synaptotagamin I functions as a calcium regulator of release probability. *Nature* 410:41-49.

Ferraro L, Antonelli T, Tanganelli S, O'Connor WT, Perez de la Mora M, Mendez-Franco J, Rambert FA, Fuxe K (2000). Amplification of cortical serotonin release: A further neurochemical action of the vigilance-promoting drug modafinil. *Neuropharmacology* 39(11):1974-1983.

Ferre S (1997). Adenosine-dopamine interactions in the ventral striatum: Implications for the treatment of schizophrenia. *Psychopharmacology* 133(2):107-120.

Ferry B, Roozendaal B, McGaugh JL (1999). Role of norepinephrine in mediating stress hormone regulation of long-term memory storage: A critical involvement of the amygdala. *Biological Psychiatry* 46:1140-1152.

Fields DR, Stevens B (2000). ATP: An extracellular signaling molecule between neurons and glia. *Trends in Neurosciences* 23:628-633.

File SE, Flucke E, Fernandes C (1999). Beneficial effects of glycine (Bioglycin) on memory and attention in young and middle-aged adults. *Journal of Clinical Psychopharmacology* 19:506-512.

Filep JG, Skrobik Y, Fournier A, Foldes-Filep E (1996). Effects of calcium antagonists on endothelin-1-induced myocardial ischemia and oedema in the rat. *British Journal of Pharmacology* 118:893-900.

Fischer M, Kaech S, Wagner V, Brinkhaus H, Matus A (2000). Glutamate receptors regulate actin-based plasticity in dendritic spines. *Nature Neuroscience* 3(9):887-894.

Fisher A, Biggs CS, Starr MS (1998). Differential effects of NMDA and non-NMDA antagonists on the activity of aromatic-amino acid decarboxylase activity in the nigrostriatal dopamine pathway of the rat. *Brain Research* 792:126-132.

Fisher K, Hagen NA (1999). Analgesic effect of oral ketamine in chronic neuropathic pain of spinal origin: A case report. *Journal of Pain and Symptom Management* 18:61-66.

Fisher SK, Agranoff BW (1999). Phosphoinositides. In *Basic neurochemistry: Molecular, cellular, and medical aspects,* Sixth edition (pp. 415-432). Philadelphia, PA: Lippincott.

Fjell J, Cummins TR, Fried K, et al. (1999). In vivo NGF deprivation reduces SNS expression and TTX-R sodium currents in IB4-negative DRG neurons. *Journal of Neurophysiology* 91:803-810.

Flanders KC, Ren RF, Lippa CF (1997). Transforming growth factor betas in neurodegenerative disease. *Progress in Neurology* 54:71-85.

Fletcher PJ, Azampanah A (1999). Stimulation of 5-HT$_{1B}$ receptors in the nucleus accumbens reduces d-amphetamine self-administration. *Abstracts of the Society for Neuroscience:* 1823.

Flood P (1999). Neuronal nicotinic acetylcholine receptors are differentially modulated by intravenous anesthetics. *Society for Neuroscience Abstracts* 25:1242.

Flores CF (2000). The promises and pitfalls of a nicotine cholinergic approach to pain management. *Pain* 88:1-6.

Floresco SB, Todd CL, Grace AA (2001). Glutamatergic afferents from the hippocampus to the nucleus accumbens regulate activity of ventral tegmental area dopamine neurons. *Journal of Neuroscience* 21:4915-4922.

Fossier P, Tauc L, Baux G (1999). Calcium transients and neurotransmitter release at an identified synapse. *Trends in Neurological Sciences* 22:161-166.

Francis DD, Meaney MJ (1999). Maternal care and the development of stress responses. *Current Opinion in Neurobiology* 9:128-134.

Fried I, Wilson CL, Morrow JW, et al. (2001). Increased dopamine release in the human amygdala during performance of cognitive tasks. *Nature Neuroscience* 4:201-206.

Frerking M, Nicoll RA (2000). Synaptic kainate receptors. *Current Opinion in Neurobiology* 10:342-351.

Frey U, Morris RGM (1998). Synaptic tagging: Implications for late maintenance of hippocampal long-term potentiation. *Trends in Neuroscience* 21(5):181-188.

Fritschy JM, Weinmann O, Wenzel A, Benke D (1998). Synapse-specific localization of NMDA and GABA$_A$ receptor subunits revealed by antigen-retrieval immunohistochemistry. *Journal of Comparative Neurology* 390:194-210.

Frye MA et al. (1999). CSF thyrotropin-releasing hormone gender difference: Implications for neurobiology and treatment of depression. *Journal of Neuropsychiatry and Clinical Neuroscience* 11:349-353.

Fryer JD, Lukas RJ (1999). Antidepressants noncompetitively inhibit nicotinic acetylcholine receptor function. *Journal of Neurochemistry* 72:1117-1124.

Galarreta M, Hestrin S (2001a). Electrical synapses between GABA-releasing interneurons. *Nature Reviews Neuroscience* 2:425-433.

Galarreta M, Hestrin S (2001b). Spike transmission and synchrony detection in networks of GABAergic interneurons. *Science* 292:2295-2299.

Galeotti N, Ghelardini C, Morrachi N, et al. (1999). The anorectic effect induced by amphetamine and cocaine is mediated by the alpha-2 adrenoreceptor subtype. *Society for Neuroscience Abstracts:* 749.15.

Galeotti N, Ghelardini C, Vinci MC, Bartolini A (1999). Role of potassium channels in the antinociception induced by agonists of alpha-2 adrenoceptors. *British Journal of Pharmacology* 126(5):1214-1220.

Gallopin T, Fort P, Eggerman E, et al. (2000). Identification of sleep-promoting neurons in vitro. *Nature* 404:992-995.

Gambarana C, Masi F, Tagliamonte A, Scheggi S, Ghiglieri O, De Montis MG (1999). A chronic stress that impairs reactivity in rats also decreases dopaminergic transmission in the nucleus accumbens: A microdialysis study. *Journal of Neurochemistry* 72:2039-2046.

Garcia-Sevilla JA, Escriba PV, Ozaita A, LaHarpe R, Walzer L, Eytan A, Guimon J (1999). Up-regulation of immunolabeled alpha$_{2A}$-adrenoceptors, Ca$_i$ coupling proteins, and regulatory receptor kinases in the prefrontal cortex of depressed suicides. *Journal of Neurochemistry* 72:282-291.

Garcia-Villar R, Dupuis C, Martinoke JP, Fioremonte J, Bueno L (1996). Functional evidence for NO-synthase activation by substance P through a mechanism not involving classical tachykinin receptors in guinea pig ileum in vitro. *British Journal of Pharmacology* 118:1283-1261.

Gardner DM, Schulman KI, Walker SE, Tailor SAN (1996). The making of a user friendly MAOI diet. *Journal of Clinical Psychiatry* 57:99-104.

Gavioli EC, Canteros NS, De Lima TC (1999). Anxiogenic-like effect induced by substance P injected into the lateral septal nucleus. *NeuroReport* 10(6):3399-3423.

Gehring WJ, Knight RT (2000). Prefrontal-cingulate interaction in action monitoring. *Nature Neuroscience* 3(5):516-520.

Genoux D, Haditsch V, Knobloch M, et al. (2002). Protein phosphatase 1 is a molecular constraint on learning and memory. *Nature* 418:970-975.

Gerfen CR (2000). Molecular effects of dopamine on striatal-projection pathways. *Trends in Neurosciences* 23(10)(Suppl.):S64-S70.

Giamberardino MA, Affaiatia G, Valente R, Iezzies VL (1997). Changes in visceral pain reactivity as a function of estrous cycle in female rats with artificial ureteral calculus. *Brain Research* 744:234-238.

Gibbs RB (1999). Treatment with estrogen and progesterone affects relative levels of brain derived neurotrophic factor mRNA and protein in different regions of the adult rat brain. *Brain Research* 844:20-27.

Gifford AN, Gardner EL, Ashby CR (1997). The effect of intravenous administration of delta-9-tetrahydrocannabinol on the activity of A10 dopamine neurons recorded in vivo in anesthetized rats. *Neuropsychology* 36:96-99.

Gilbert SD, Clark TM, Flores CM (2001). Antihyperalgesic effect of epibatidine in the formalin model of facial pain. *Pain* 89:159-165.

Gingrich MB, Junge CE, Traynelis SF (2000). Potentiation of NMDA receptor function by the serine protease thrombin. *Journal of Neuroscience* 20:4582-4595.

Gingrich MB, Traynelis SF (2000). Serine proteases and brain damage—Is there a link? *Trends in Neurosciences* 23(9):399-407.

Gintzler AR, Bohan MC (1990). Pain thresholds are elevated during pseudopregnancy. *Brain Research* 507:312-316.

Giovengo SL, Russell IJ, Larson AA (1999). Increased concentrations of nerve growth factor in cerebrospinal fluid of patients with fibromyalgia. *Journal of Rheumatology* 26:1564-1569.

Gjerstad J, Tjolsen A, Hole K (2001). Induction of long-term potentiation by single wide dynamic range neurons in the dorsal horn is inhibited by descending pathways. *Pain* 91:263-268.

Glanz J (1997). Mastering the nonlinear brain. *Science* 277:1758-1760.

Glazewski S, Gesc KP, Silva A, Fox K (2000). The role of alpha-CaMKII autophosphorylation in neocortical experience-dependent plasticity. *Nature Neuroscience* 3:911-918.

Goadsby PJ, Lipton RB, Ferrari MD (2002). Migraine—Current understanding and treatment. *The New England Journal of Medicine* 346(4):257-270.

Gobert A, Rivet J-M, Cistarelli L, Melon C, Millan JM (1999). Buspirone modulates basal and fluoxetine-stimulated dialyzate levels of dopamine, noradrenaline, and serotonin in the frontal cortex of freely moving rats. Activation of serotonin receptors and blockage at alpha-2 receptors underlie its actions. *Neuroscience* 93:1251-1262.

Goeders NE (1997). A neuroendocrine role in cocaine reinforcement. *Psychoneuroendocrinology* 22(4):237-259.

Gold JI, Shadlen MN (2001). Neural computations that underlie decisions about sensory stimuli. *Trends in Cognitive Sciences* 5(1):10-16.

Goldenberg DL (1989). An overview of psychologic studies in fibromyalgia. *Journal of Rheumatology* 16:12-14.

Goldstein JA (1983). Cimetidine and mononucleosis. *Annals of Internal Medicine* 99(3):410-411.

Goldstein JA (1986). Danazol and the rapidly cycling affective patient. *Journal of Clinical Psychiatry* 47:153-154.

Goldstein JA (1990). *Chronic fatigue syndrome: The struggle for health.* Beverly Hills, CA: Chronic Fatigue Syndrome Institute.

Goldstein JA (1993). *Chronic fatigue syndrome: The limbic hypothesis.* Binghamton, NY: The Haworth Medical Press.

Goldstein JA (1996). *Betrayal by the Brain: The Neurological Basis of Chronic Fatigue Syndrome, Fybromyalgia Syndrome, and Related Neural Network Disorders.* Binghamton, NY: The Haworth Press.

Goldstein JA (1998). The pilgrim's progress. *The National Forum* 1(4):3-6.

Goldstein JA (1999). Instantaneous neural network reconfiguration by pharmacologic modulation of afferent cranial nerve input. *National Forum* 3(1):27-30.

Goldstein JA, Mena I, Jouanne E, Lesser I (1995). The assessment of vascular abnormalities in late life chronic fatigue syndrome by brain SPECT: Comparison with late life major depressive disorder. *Journal of Chronic Fatigue Syndrome* 1:55-80.

Gonsalves B, Paller KA (2000). Neural events that underlie remembering something that never happened. *Nature Neuroscience* 3:1316-1321.

Gonsalves B, Paller KA (2002). Mistaken memories: Remembering events that never happened. *The Neuroscientist* 8:391-395.

Gottschalk WA, Jiang H, Tartaglia N, Feng L, Figurov A, Lu B (1999). Signaling mechanisms mediating BDNF modulation of synaptic plasticity in the hippocampus. *Learning and Memory* 6(3):243-256.

Grachev ID, Apkarian AV (2000). Anxiety in healthy humans is associated with orbital frontal chemistry. *Molecular Psychiatry* 5:482-488.

Graver E, Alkalai D, Kapun J, et al. (2000). Stress does not enable pyridostigmine to inhibit brain cholinesterase after parenteral administration. *Toxicology and Applied Pharmacology* 164:301-304.

Greene YM, Tariot PRN, Wishart H, Cox C, Holt CJ, Schwid S, Noviasky J (2000). A 12 week open trial of donepezil hydrochloride in patients with multiple sclerosis and associated cognitive impairments. *Journal of Clinical Psychopharmacology* 20:350-356.

Grillner P, Berretta N, Bernardi G, Svensson TH, Mercuri NB (2000). Muscarinic receptors depress GABAergic synaptic transmission in rat mid brain dopamine neurons. *Neuroscience* 96(2):299-307.

Grillner S (1997). Ion channels and locomotion. *Science* 78:1078-1087.

Gronier B, Perry KW, Rasmussen K (2000). Activation of the mesocorticolimbic dopaminergic system by stimulation of muscarinic cholinergic receptors in the ventral tegmental area. *Psychopharmacology* 147:347-355.

Grosche J, Matyash V, Muller T, et al. (1999). Microdomains for neuron-glia interaction: Parallel fiber signaling to Bergmann glial cells. *Nature Neuroscience* 2:139-143.

Grossberg S (2000). The complementary brain: Unifying brain dynamics and modularity. *Trends in Cognitive Sciences* 4:233-246.

Gruzelier J (1996). The state of hypnosis: Evidence and applications. *Quarterly Journal of Medicine* 89(4):313-317.

Gu Y, Huang L-YM (2001). Gabapentin actions on *N*-methyl-D-aspartate receptor channels are protein kinase C-dependent. *Pain* 93:85-92.

Gudelsky GA (1999). Biphasic effect of sigma receptor ligands on the extracellular concentration of dopamine in the striatum of the rat. *Journal of Neural Transmission* 106:849-856.

Guidotti A, Costa E (1998). Can the antidysphoric and anxiolytic profiles of selective serotonin reuptake inhibitors be related to their ability to increase brain 3 alpha, 5 alpha-tetrahydroprogesterone (allopregnalone) availability? *Biological Psychiatry* 44(9):865-873.

Guillery RW, Feig SL, Lozsadi DA (1998). Paying attention to the thalamic reticular nucleus. *Trends in Neurosciences* 21:28-32.

Guillin O, Diaz J, Carroll P, Griffon N, Schwartz JC, Sokoloff P (2001). BDNF controls dopamine D_3 receptor expression and triggers behavioral sensitization. *Nature* 411:86-89.

Gulati A, Kumar A, Morrison S, Shahani BT (1997). Effect of centrally administered endothelin agonists on systemic and regional blood circulation in the rat: Role of sympathetic nervous system. *Neuropeptides* 31(4):301-309.

Gupta T, Dorfman J, Cleeman L, Viorad M (1996). Amiloride, a novel nicotinic acetylcholine receptor (nAChR) by both enantiomers of methadone, a mu opioid receptor agonist. *Society for Neuroscience Abstracts* 25:1240.

Gusnard DA, Raichk NE (2001). Searching for a baseline: Functional imaging and the resting human brain. *Nature Reviews Neurosciences* 2:635-694.

Guzman M, Galve-Roperty I, Sanchez C (2001). Ceramide: A new second messenger of cannabinoid action. *Trends in Pharmacological Sciences* II:19-22.

Gyires R, Mullner K, Ronai E (2000). Functional evidence that gastroprotection can be induced by alpha$_{2B}$-adrenoceptor subtypes in the rat. *European Journal of Pharmacology* 396:131-135.

Haber S, McFarland NR (2001). The place of the thalamus in frontal cortical-basal ganglia circuits. *The Neuroscientist* 7(4):315-324.

Haber SN, Fudge JL, McFarland N (2000). Striatonigro striatal pathways in primates form an ascending spiral from the shell to the dorsal striatum. *Journal of Neuroscience* 20:2369-2382.

Habib KE, Weld RP, Rice KC, Pushkas J, Champoux M, Listwak S, Webster EL, Atkinson AJ, Schulkin J, Contoreggi C et al. (2000). Oral administration of a corticotropin-releasing hormone antagonist significantly attenuates behavioral, neuroendocrine, and autonomic responses to stress in primates. *Proceedings of the National Academy of Sciences* 97:6079-6084.

Haga HA, Moerch H, Soli NE (2000). Effects of intravenous infusion of guiafenesin on electroencephalographic variables in pigs. *American Journal of Veterinary Research* 61:1599-1601.

Hakoas A, Kaukoranta J, Aito M (1999). Effect of estradiol on postpartum depression. *Psychopharmacology* 146(1):108-110.

Halliwell RF, Thomas P, Patten D, James CH, Martinez-Torres A, Miledi R, Smart TG (1999). Subunit-selective modulation of GABA$_A$ receptors by the non-steroidal anti-inflammatory agent, mefenamic acid. *European Journal of Neuroscience* 11:2897-2905.

Harden DG, King D, Finlay JM, Grace AA (1998). Depletion of dopamine in the prefrontal cortex decreases the basal electrophysiological activity of mesolimbic dopamine neurons. *Brain Research* 794:96-102.

Hardingham GE, Arnold FJL, Bading H (2001). Nuclear calcium signaling controls CREB-mediated gene expression triggered by synaptic activity. *Nature Neuroscience* 4(3):261-267.

Harkin A, Nowak G, Paul IA (2000). Noradrenergic lesion inhibits desipramine-induced activation of NMDA receptors. *European Journal of Pharmacology* 389(2-3):187-192.

Hartfield T, McGaugh JL (1999). Norepinephrine infused into the basolateral amygdala posttraining enhances retention in a spatial water maze task. *Neurobiology of Learning and Memory* 71:232-239.

Harvey SC, Li X, Skolnick P, Kirst HA (2000). The antibacterial and NMDA receptor activating properties of aminoglycosides are dissociable. *European Journal of Pharmacology* 381(1):1-7.

Hassel B, Tauboll E, Gjerstad L (2001). Chronic kynurenine treatment increases rat hippocampal GABA shunt activity and elevates cerebral taurine levels. *Epilepsy Research* 43:153-156.

Hastings MH (2000). Circadian clockwork: Two loops are better than one. *Nature Reviews Neuroscience* 1:143-146.

Hastings MH (2002). A gut feeling for time. *Nature* 417:391-392.

Havel PJ (2000). Role of adipose tissue in body-weight regulation: Mechanisms regulating leptin production and energy balance. *Proceedings of the Nutrition Society* 59(3):359-371.

Hayashi A, Nagaoka M, Yamada K, Ichitani Y, Miake Y, Okado N (1998). Maternal stress induces synaptic loss and developmental disabilities of offspring. *International Journal of Developmental Neuroscience* 16(3-4):209-216.

Hebb DO (1949). *The Organization of Behavior.* New York: John Wiley.

Heeger DJ, Ress D (2002). What does fMRI tell us about neuronal activity? *Nature Review Neuroscience* 3(2):142-151.

Heidbreder CA, Baumann MH (2001). Autoregulation of dopamine synthesis in subregions of the rat nucleus accumbens. *European Journal of Pharmacology* 411:107-113.

Heim C, Ehlert U, Hellhammer DH (2000). The potential role of hypocortisolism in the pathophysiology of stress related bodily disorders. *Psychoneuroendocrinology* 25:1-35.

Heimer L, Alheid GF, deOlmos JS, Groenwegen HJ, Haber SN, Harlan RE, Zahn DS (1997). The accumbens: Beyond the core-shell dichotomy. *Journal of Neuropsychiatry and Clinical Neuroscience* 9:354-381.

Heinricher MM, Schouten JC, Jobst EE (2001). Activation of brainstem N-methyl-D-aspartate receptors is required for the analgesic actions of morphine given systematically. *Pain* 92(1-2):129-138.

Heinrichs SC, Menzaghi F, Schulteis G, Koob GF, Stinus L (1995). Suppression of corticotropin-releasing factor in the amygdala attenuates aversive consequences of morphine withdrawal. *Behavioral Pharmacology* 6:74-80.

Helmuth L (2001). Boosting brain activity from the outside in. *Science* 292:1284-1286.

Hendricks JC, Williams JA, Panckeri K, et al. (2001). A non-circadian role for cAMP signaling and CREB activity in drosophila rest homeostasis. *Nature Neuroscience* 4:1108-1115.

Herges S, Taylor DA (2000). Involvement of 5-HT$_3$ receptors in the nucleus accumbens in the potentiation of cocaine-induced behaviours in the rat. *British Journal of Pharmacology* 131(7):1294-302.

Herman JP, Cullinan WE (1997). Neurocircuitry of stress: Central control of the hypothalamo-pituitary-adrenocortical axis. *Trends in Neurosciences* 20(2):78-84.

Hernandez M, Nieto ML, Crespo MS (2000). Cytosolic phospholipase A$_2$ and the distinct transcriptional programs of astrocytoma cells. *Trends in Neurosciences* 23(6):259-264.

Hester JT, Ryder D, Kelly DG, Favorov OV (1999). The cortical pyramidal cell as a set of interacting error backpropagating dendrites: A mechanism for discovering nature's order. *Abstracts of the Society for Neuroscience:* 2258.

Hirtel P, Fagerquist MV, Svensson TH (1999). Enhanced cortical dopamine output and antipsychotic-like effects of raclopride by alpha-2 adrenoceptor blockage. *Science* 286:105-107.

Hobson JA, Stickgold R, Pace-Schott EF (1998). The neuropsychology of REM sleep dreaming. *NeuroReport* 9:R1-R4.

Hoffman A, Keiser HR, Grossman E, et al. (1989). Endothelin concentrations in cerebrospinal fluid in depressives. *Lancet* 2:8678-8679.

Hogervorst E, Boshuisen M, Riedel W, Willeken C, Jolles J (1999). The effect of hormone replacement therapy on cognitive function in elderly women. *Psychoneuroendocrinology* 24(1):43-68.

Holmberg M, Scheinin M, Kurose H, Miettine R (1999). Adrenergic alpha$_{2C}$ adrenoreceptors reside in rat striatal gabaergic projection neuron: Comparison of radioligand binding and immunohistochemistry. *Neuroscience* 93(4):1323-1333.

Holthusen H, Infeld S, Lipfert P (2000). Effect of pre- or post-traumatically applied IV lidocaine on primary and secondary hyperalgesia after experimental heat trauma in humans. *Pain* 88:295-302.

Honey RC, Good M (2000). Associative components of recognition memory. *Current Opinion in Neurobiology* 10:200-204.

Horikawa K, Yokota S, Fuji K, et al. (2000). Nonphotic entrainment by 5-HT$_{1A/7}$ receptor agonists accompanied by reduced *Per1* and *Per2* mRNA levels in suprachiasmatic nuclei. *Journal of Neuroscience* 20:5867-5873.

Horrigan JP, Barnhill LJ (1999). Guanfacine and secondary mania in children. *Journal of Affective Disorders* 54:309-314.

Horvitz JC (2000). Mesolimbocortical and nigrostriatal dopamine responses to salient non-reward events. *Neuroscience* 96:651-656.

Hudson JI, Pope HG (1995). Does childhood sexual abuse cause fibromyalgia? *Arthritis and Rheumatism* 38:161-163.

Human SE, Malenke RC (2001). Addiction and the brain: The neurobiology of compulsion and its resistance. *Nature Reviews Neuroscience* 2:695-703.

Hunt SP, Mantyh PW (2001) The molecular dynamics of pain control. *Nature Reviews Neuroscience* 2:83-91.

Huntsman MM, Munoz A, Jones EG (1999). Temporal modulation of GABA(A) receptor subunit gene expression of in developing monkey cerebral cortex. *Neuroscience* 91(4):1223-1245.

Husi H, Grant SGN (2001). Proteomics of the nervous system. *Trends in Neurosciences* 24:259-266.

Husi H, Word MA, Choudhary JS, Blackstock WP, Grant SGN (2000). Proteonomic analysis of NMDA receptor adhesion protein signaling complexes. *Nature Neuroscience* 3:661-669.

Hutcheon B, Yarom Y (2000). Resonance, oscillation and the intrinsic frequency preferences of neurons. *Trends in Neurosciences* 23:216-222.

Hutchison WD, Davis KD, Lozano AM, Tasker RR, Dostrovsky JO (1999). Pain-related neurons in the human cingulate cortex. *Nature Neuroscience* 2 (5):403-405.

Hyman SE, Malenka RC (2001). Addiction and the brain: The neurobiology of compulsion and its persistence. *Nature Reviews Neuroscience* 2(10):795-703.

Ida T, Nakaharon K, Murakami T, et al. (2000). Possible involvement of orexin in the stress reaction of rats. *Biochemical and Biophysical Research Communications* 220:318-323.

Ikemoto S, Panksepp J (1999). The role of nucleus accumbens dopamine in motivated behavior: A unified interpretation with special reference to reward-seeking. *Brain Research Reviews* 31:6-41.

Insel TR, Young LJ (2001). The neurobiology of attachment. *Nature Reviews Neuroscience* 2:129-136.

Invernizzi RW, Parini S, Saccneti G, et al. (2001). Chronic treatment with reboxetine by osmotic pumps facilitates its effects on extracellular noradrenaline and may desensitize alpha$_2$-adrenoceptors in the prefrontal cortex. *British Journal of Pharmacology* 32:183-188.

Irifune M, Soto T, Kamata Y, Nishikawa T, Doh T, Kawahara M (2000). Evidence for GABA receptor agonistic properties of ketamine: Convulsive and anesthetic behavioral models in mice. *Anesthesia and Analgesia* 91:230-236.

Iversen SD, Muller RU (1997). Cognitive neuroscience: Editorial overview. *Current Opinion in Neurobiology* 7:151-156.

Izzo AA, Mascolo N, Capaso F (2000). Marijuana in the new millennium: Prospectives for cannabinoid research. *Trends in Pharmacological Sciences* 21:281-282.

Jaasklainen SK, Rinne JO, Forsell H, et al. (2001). Role of the dopaminergic system in chronic pain—A fluorodopa-PET study. *Pain* 90:257-261.

Jabbur J, Saade NE (1999). From electrical wiring to plastic neurons: Evolving approaches to the study of pain. *Pain Supplement* 6:587-592.

Jackson A, Uphouse L (1998). Dose dependent effects of estradiol benzoate on 5HT$_{1A}$ receptor agonist action. *Brain Research* 796:299-302.

Jackson ME, Frost AS, Moghaddam B (2001). Stimulation of prefrontal cortex at physiologically relevant frequencies inhibits dopamine release in the nucleus accumbens. *Journal of Neurochemistry* 78:920-923.

Jacobs EH, Yamatodani A, Timmerman H (2000). Is histamine the final neurotransmitter in the entrainment of circadian rhythms in mammals? *Trends in Pharmacological Sciences* 21:293-298.

Jaen JC, Laborde E, Pousch RA, Caprathe BW, Sorensen PJ, Fegus J, Spiegel K, Markl J, Dickerson MR, Davis RE (1995). Kynurenic acid derivatives inhibit the binding of nerve growth factor (NGF) to the low-affinity p75 NGF receptor. *Journal of Medicinal Chemistry* 38(22):4439-4445.

Jenner P, Zeng BY, Smith LA, et al. (2000). Anti-Parkinsonian and neuroprotective effects of modafinil in MPTP-treated common marmoset. *Experimental Brain Research* 133:178-189.

Jennings C, Aamodt S (Eds.) (2000). Computational approaches to brain function. *Nature Neuroscience:* 3(Suppl.).

Jensen MP, Romano JM, Turner JA, Good AB, Wald LH (1999). Patient beliefs predict patient functioning: Further support for a cognitive behavioral model of chronic pain. *Pain* 81:95-104.

Jensen MP, Turner JA, Romano JM, Karoly P (1991). Coping with chronic pain: A review of the literature. *Pain* 47:249-283.

Jentsch JD, Taylor JR, Roth RH (2000). Phencyclidine model of frontal cortical dysfunction in non-human primates. *The Neuroscientist* 6(4):263-270.

Jevtovic-Todorovic V, Wozniak DF, Powell S, Nardi A, Olney JW (1998). Clonidine potentiates the neuropathic pain-relieving action of MK-801 while preventing its neurotoxic and hyperactivity side effects. *Brain Research* 781:202-211.

Jiang M, Behbehani MM. Physiological characteristics of the projection pathway from the medial preoptic to the nucleus raphe magnus of the rat and its modulation by the periaqueductal gray. *Pain* 94(2):139-147.

Jo YH, Schlichter R (1999). Synaptic corelease of ATP and GABA in cultured spinal neurons. *Nature Neuroscience* 2(3):241-245.

Joffe RT (1998). The use of thyroid supplements to augment antidepressant medication. *Journal of Chinical Psychiatry* 59(suppl 51):26-29.

Johnson JG, Cohen P, Kasen S, et al. (2000). Association of maladaptive parental behavior with psychiatric disorder among parents and their offspring. *Archives of General Psychiatry* 58:453-460.

Johnson LR, LeDoux JE (2000). Gabaergic inhibition in the fear conditioning circuit of the lateral amygdala is potentiated by dopamine D_1 agonists. *Society for Neuroscience Abstracts:* 466.1.

Jones EG (2000). Cortical and subcortical contributions to activity-dependent plasticity in primate somatosensory cortex. *Annual Review of Neuroscience* 23:1-37.

Jones EG (2001). The thalamic matrix and thalamocortical synchrony. *Trends in Neurosciences* 24:595-601.

Jones S, Kaver JA (1999). Amphetamine depresses excitatory synaptic transmission via serotonin receptors in the ventral tegmental area. *Journal of Neuroscience* 19:9780-9787.

Jones S, Sudweeks S, Yakel JL (1999). Nicotinic receptors in the brain: Correlating physiology with function. *Trends in Neurosciences* 22:555-561.

Jorge C, Mannainoi G, Gingrich MB, Traynelis SF (1999). Plasmin and thrombin regulation of NMDA receptor function. *Society for Neuroscience Abstracts:* 785.12.

Junger H, Doom CM, Sorkin LS (2000). Mid-axonal TNF causes allodynia and C-nociceptor activity: TNF-induced activity is blocked by low-dose intravenous lidocaine. In Devor M, Rowbotham MC (Eds.), *Proceedings of the Ninth World Congress on Pain* (pp. 241-248). Seattle, WA: IASP Press.

Kaas J, Ebner F (1998). Intrathalamic connections: A new way to modulate cortical plasticity? *Nature Neuroscience* 1(5):341-342.

Kaasinen V, Nagren K, Hietala J, Farde L, Rinne JO (2001). Sex differences in extrastriatal dopamine D_2-like receptors in the human brain. *American Journal of Psychiatry* 158:308-311.

Kadekaro M, Summy-Long JY (2000). Centrally produced nitric oxide and the regulation of body fluid and blood pressure homostases. *Clinical and Experimental Pharmacology and Physiology* 27(5-6):450-459.

Kakh BS, Zhoo X, Sydes J (2000). State-dependent cross-inhibition between transmitter-gated cation channels. *Nature* 406:408-410.

Kalivas PW, Duffy P (1995). Selective activation of dopamine transmission in the shell of the nucleus accumbens by stress. *Brain Research* 675:325-328.

Kalivas PW, Nakamura M (1999). Neural systems for behavioral activation and reward. *Current Opinion in Neurobiology* 9:223-227.

Kaneno S, Fukamauchi F, Komatsu H, Koyama K, Ikawa K (2001). Reversal effect of sulpiride on rotational behavior of rats with unilateral frontal cortex ablation: An alternative explanation for the pharmacological mechanism of its antidepressant effect. *Behavioural Pharmacology* 12:69-73.

Kang J, Tiang L, Goldman SA, Nedergaard M (1998). Astrocyte-mediated potentiation of inhibitory synaptic transmission. *Nature Neuroscience* 1:683-692.

Kang YS, Park JH (2000). Brain uptake and the analgesic effect of oxytocin—Its usefulness as an analgesic agent. *Archives of Pharmacological Research* 23: 391-395.

Kanwisher N, Wojciulik E (2000). Visual attention: Insights from brain imaging. *Nature Reviews Neuroscience* 1:91-98.

Kaplan DR, Cooper E (2001). PI-3 kinase and IP_3: Partners in NT3-induced synaptic transmission. *Nature Neuroscience* 4(1):5-7.

Kaplan DR, Miller FD (2000). Neurotrophin signal transduction in the nervous system. *Current Opinion in Neurobiology* 10:381-391.

Karlsten R, Gordht T (2000). Adenosine, a new analgesic for the treatment of neuropathic pain. *The International Association for the Study of Pain Newsletter* No. 1:3-6.

Kayser V, Berkley KJ, Kita H, Gautron M, Guilbaud G (1996). Estrous and sex variations in vocalization thresholds to hind paw and tail pressure stimulation in rats. *Brain Research* 742:352-354.

Keck ME, Sillaber I, Ebner K, et al. (2000). Acute transcranial magnetic stimulation of frontal brain regions selectively modulates the release of vasopressin, biogenic amines and amino acids in rat brain. *European Journal of Neuroscience* 12:3713-3720.

Keesler GA, Comacho F, Guo Y, et al. (2000). Phosphorylation and destabilization of human period 1 clock protein by human casein kinase 1 epsilon. *NeuroReport* 11:951-955.

Keidel M, Rieschki P, Stude C, et al. (2001). Antinociceptive reflux alteration in acute posttraumatic headache following whiplash injury. *Pain* 92:319-326.

Kemp JA, McKernan RM (2002). NMDA receptor pathways as drug targets. *Nature Neuroscience* 5(Suppl.):1039-1042.

Keogh E, Ellery D, Hunt C, Hannent I (2001). Selective attentional bias for pain-related stimuli amongst pain fearful individuals. *Pain* 91:91-100.

Kim LR, Pomeranz B (1999). The sympathomimetic agent, 6-hydroxydopamine, accelerated cutaneous wound healing. *European Journal of Pharmacology* 376: 257-264.

Kimura H (2000). Hydrogen sulfide induces cyclic sleep and modulates the NE or DA receptor. *Biochemistry and Biophysics Research Communication* 267:129-133.

Kind PC, Neumann PE (2001) Plasticity: Downstream of glutamate. *Trends in Neurosciences* 24:553-554.

Kiozumi S, Katoaka Y, Niwa M, et al. (1994). Endothelin increased $[Ca^{2+}]_i$ in cultured neurones and slices of rat hippocampus. *NeuroReport* 5:1077-1080.

Kiss JP, Vizi ES (2001). Nitric oxide: A novel link between synaptic and non-synaptic transmission. *Trends in Neurosciences* 24:211-215.

Klempner MS, Hu LT, Evans J, Schmid CH, Johnson GM, Trevino RP, Norton D, Levy L, Wall D, McCall J, et al. (2001). Two controlled trials of antibiotic treatment in patients with persistent symtpoms and history of Lyme disease. *New England Journal of Medicine* 345:85-92.

Klintsova AY, Greenough W (1999). Synaptic plasticity in cortical systems. *Current Opinion in Neurobiology* 9:203-208.

Kobasa SC, Maddi SR, Puccetti MC, Zola MA (1985). Effectiveness of hardiness, exercise and social support as resources against illness. *Journal of Psychosomatic Research* 29(5):523-533.

Kofke WA, Bloom MJ, VanCott A, Brenner RF (1997). Electrographic tachyphylaxis to etomidate and ketamine used for refractory status epilepticus controlled with isoflurane. *Journal of Neurosurgical Anesthesiology* 9(3):269-272.

Konija H, Masuda H, Kiyofomi I, et al. (1998). Modification of dopamine release by nociception in conscious rat striatum. *Brain Research* 788:342-344.

Kontas HA, Wei EP (1998). Cerebral arteriolar dilations by K_{ATP} channel activators need L-lysine or L-arginine. *American Journal of Physiology* 274:H974-H981.

Koob GF (1992). Drugs of abuse: Anatomy, pharmacology and function of reward pathways. *Trends in Pharmacological Science* 13(5):177-184.

Koob GF (1999). Drug reward and addiction. In Zigmund MS, Bloom FE, Landis SC, et al., *Fundamental Neuroscience* (pp. 1261-1282). San Diego, CA: Academic Press.

Kretschmer BO (1999). Modulation of the mesolimbic dopamine system by glutamate: Role of NMDA receptors. *Journal of Neurochemistry* 73:839-848.

Krimer LS, Muly EC, Williams GV, Goldman-Rakic PS (1998). Dopaminergic regulation of cerebral cortical microcirculation. *Nature Neuroscience* 1:286-289.

Kryger MH, Roth T, Dement WC (Eds.) (2000). *Principles and practice of sleep medicine.* Philadelphia: W.B. Saunders.

Kubota T, Hirota K, Anzawa N, Yoshida H, Kushikota T, Matsuki A (1999). Physostigmine antagonizes ketamine-induced noradrenaline release from the medial prefrontal cortex in rats. *Brain Research* 840(1-2):175-178.

Kubota T, Hirota K, Yoshida H, Takahashi S, Ohkawa H, Anzawa N, Kushikata T, Matsuki A (1999). Inhibitory effect of clonidine on ketamine-induced norepinephrine release from the medial prefrontal cortex in rats. *British Journal of Anesthesiology* 83:945-947.

Kuhar MJ, Couceyro PR, Lambert PD (1999). Catecholamines. In Siegel GJ, Agranoff BW, Albers RW, Fisher SK, Uhler MD (Eds.), *Basic neurochemistry: Molecular, cellular, and medical aspects,* Sixth edition (pp. 243-262). Philadelphia, PA: Lippincott.

Kuwaki T, Kurihara H, Cao WH, Kurihara Y, Unekawa M, Yazaki Y, Kumada M (1997). Physiological role of brain endothelin in the central autonomic control: From neuron to knock-out mouse. *Progress in Neurobiology* 51:545-579.

Kwak B, Mulhapt F, Myit S, Mach F (2000). HMG-CoA reductase inhibitors as a novel type of immunosuppressor. *Nature Medicine* 6:1399-1402.

Kwan CL, Crawley AP, Mikulis DJ, Davis KD (2000). An fMRI study of the anterior cingulate cortex and surrounding medial wall activations evoked by noxious heat and cold stimuli. *Pain* 83:359-374.

Kyle GJ, DeLander GE (1994). Adenosine kinase and adenosine deaminase inhibition modulates spinal adenosine and opioid agonist induced antinociception in mice. *European Journal of Pharmacology* 271:37-46.

Lagrange AH, Wagner EJ, Ronnekleiv OK, Kelly MJ (1996). Estrogen rapidly attenuates a $GABA_B$ response in hypothalamic neurons. *Neuroendocrinology* 64:114-123.

Landis CA, Lentz MS, Rothermel J, et al. (2001). Decreased nocturnal levels of prolactin and growth hormone in women with fibromyalgia. *Journal of Clinical Endocrinology and Metabolism* 86:1672-1678.

Landoboso MA, Iraurigit, Jimenez-Lerma JM, et al. (1998). A randomized trial of adding fluoxetine to a naltrexone treatment program for heroin addicts. *Addiction* 93:739-744.

Langin D (2001). Diabetes, insulin secretion, and the pancreatic beta-cell mitochondrion. *The New England Journal of Medicine* 345(24):1772-1774.

Lariviere WR, Melzack R (2000). The role of corticotropin-releasing factor in pain and analgesia. *Pain* 84:1-12.

Laughlin SB (2001). Energy as a constraint on the coding and processing of sensory information. *Current Opinion in Neurobiology* 11:475-480.

Laughlin SB, de Ruyter van Stevenick RR, Anderson JC (1998). The metabolic cost of neural information. *Nature Neuroscience* 1:36-41.

Laughlin TM, Kitto KF, Wilcox GL (1998). Redox manipulation of NMDA receptors in vivo: Alteration of acute pain transmission and dynorphin-induced analgesia. *Pain* 80:37-43.

Lawand NB, Lu Y, Westlund KN (1999). Nicotinic cholinergic receptors: Potential targets for inflammatory pain relief. *Pain* 80:291-299.

Lees KR, Aplund K, Carolei A, Davis SM, Diener H-C, Kaste M, Orgogozo J-M, Whitehead J (2000). Glycine antagonist (gavestinel) in neuroptorection (GAIN International) in patients with acute stroke: A randomised controlled trial. *GAIN International Investigators* 3(335):1949-1954.

Lehninger AL, Nelson DL, Cox MM (1993a). Amino acid oxidation and the production of urea. In Lehninger AL, Nelson DL, Cox MM (Eds.), *Principles of biochemistry* (pp. 506-542). New York: Worth.

Lehninger AL, Nelson DL, Cox MM (1993b). Cells. In *Principles of biochemistry* (pp. 21-55). New York: Worth.

Lehninger AL, Nelson DL, Cox MM (1993c). Integration and hormonal regulation of mammalian metabolism. In Lehninger AL, Nelson DL, Cox MM (Eds.), *Principles of Biochemistry* (pp. 736-788). New York: Worth.

Lehninger AL, Nelson DL, Cox MM (1993d). Oxidative phosphorylation and photophosphorylation. In Lehninger AL, Nelson DL, Cox MM (Eds.), *Principles of biochemistry* (pp. 542-597). New York: Worth.

Lembo T, Naliboff BO, Martin K, et al. (2000) Irritable bowel syndrome patients show altered sensitivity to exogenous opioids. *Pain* 87:137-147.

Leniger T, Wiemann M, Bingmann D, et al. (2000). Different effects of gabergic anti-convulsants on 4-aminopyridine-induced spontaneous gabergic hyperpolarizations of hippocampal pyramidal cells—Implication for their potency in migraine therapy. *Cephalalgia* 20:533-537.

Leslie RA (2001). News and comment. *Trends in Neurosciences* 24:566-567.

Levi-Montalcini R, Skaper SD, Dal Toro R, Petrelli L, Leon A (1996). Nerve growth factor: From neurotrophin to neurokine. *Trends in Neurosciences* 19: 514-520.

Levin BE, Donn-Meynell AA, Routh VH (2001). Brain glucosensing and the K_{ATP} channel. *Nature Neuroscience* 4:451-460.

Levitt JB (2001). Function following form. *Science* 292(13):232-233.

Levy WB, Baxter RA (1996). Energy efficient neural codes. *Neural Computation* 8:531-536.

Li J, You Z, Chen E, Song C, Lu C (2001). Chronic morphine treatment inhibits oxytocin release from the supraoptic nucleus slices of rats. *Neuroscience Letters* 300:54-58.

Liberzon I, Young EA (1997). Effects of stress and glucocorticoids on CNS oxytocin receptor binding. *Psychoneuroendocrinology* 22:411-422.

Lidow MS, Williams GV, Goldman-Rakic PS (1988). The cerebral cortex, a case for a common site of action of antipsychotics. *Trends in Pharmacological Sciences* 19:136-140.

Lieberman DN, Mody I (1999). Casein-kinase II regulates NMDA channel function in hippocampal neurons. *Nature Neuroscience* 2:125-132.

Lindgren N, Xu ZQ, Herrera-Marschitz M, Haycock J, Hökfelt T, Fisone G (2001). Dopamine D_2 receptors regulation tyrosine hydroxylase activity and phosphorylation at Ser40 in rat striatum. *European Journal of Neuroscience* 13:773-780.

Linner L, Enderz H, Ohman D, et al. (2001). Reboxetine modulates the firing pattern of dopamine cells in the ventral tegmental area and selectively increases dopamine availability in the prefrontal cortex. *Journal of Pharmacology and Experimental Therapeutics* 297:540-546.

Liu F, Wan Q, Pristupa ZB, Yu XM, Wang YT, Niznik HB (2000). Direct protein-protein coupling enables cross-talk between dopamine D_5 and gamma-aminobutyric acid A receptors. *Nature* 403:274-280.

Liu JG, Liao XP, Gong ZH, Quin BY (1999). The difference between methadone and morphine in regulation of delta-opioid receptors underlies the antagonistic effect of methadone on morphine-mediated cellular mechanisms. *European Journal of Pharmacology* 372:233-239.

Lloyd TE, Bellen HJ (2001). pRIMing synaptic vesicles for fusion. *Nature Neuroscience* 4(10):965-966.

Logothetis NK, Pauls J, Augath MA, Trinath T, Oeltermann A (2001). Neurophysiological investigation of the basis of the fMRI signal. *Nature* 412:150-157.

Lohmann AB, Welch SP (1999). Antisenses to opioid receptors attenuate ATP-gated K^+ channel opener-induced antinociception. *European Journal of Pharmacology* 384:147-152.

Lorenz J, Grasedyck K, Bromm B (1996). Middle and long latency somatosensory evoked potentials after painful laser stimulation in patients with fibromyalgia syndrome. *Electroencephalography and Clinical Neurophysiology* 100:165-168.

Louk J, Vanderschuren MJ, Wardeh J, et al. (1999). Opposing role of dopamine D_1 and D_2 receptors in modulation of rat nucleus accumbens noradrenaline release. *Journal of Neuroscience* 19:4123-4131.

Louk JMJ, Donne-Schmidt E, DeVries TJ, VanMoursel AP, Tilders FJH, Schoffelmeer ANM (1998). A single exposure to amphetamine is sufficient to induce long-term behavioral neuroendocrine and neurochemical sensitization in rats. *Journal of Neuroscience* 19:9579-9586.

Lovick TA (2000). Panic disorder—A malfunction of multiple transmitter control systems within the midbrain periaqueductal grey matter? *Neuroscientist* 6:48-59.

Luo S, Kulak JM, Cartier GE, et al. (1998). Alpha-conotoxin AuIB selectively blocks alpha-3 beta-4 nicotinic acetylcholine receptors and nicotine-evoked norepinephrine release. *Journal of Neuroscience* 18:8571-8579.

Luscher C, Nicoll RA, Malenka RC, Muller D (2000). Synaptic plasticity and dynamic modulation of the postsynaptic membrane. *Nature Neuroscience* 3(6): 545-500.

Lynch G (2002). Memory enhancement: The search for mechanism-based drugs. *Nature Neuroscience* 5(Suppl.):1035-1038.

Ma D, Zhao C, Mayhem TM, Ju G (1997). Response of substance P-immunoreactive nerve fibers in the anterior pituitary to plasma oestrogen levels in the rat. *Journal of Neuroendocrinology* 9:735-740.

MacDonald RL, Olsen RW (1994). $GABA_A$ receptor channels. *Annual Review of Neuroscience* 17:569-602.

Maeda S, Thyauchi T, Goto K, Matsuda M (1997). Differences in the change in the time course of plasma endothelin-1 and endothelin-3 levels after exercise in humans. *Life Sciences* 61:419-425.

Magee JC (2000). Dendritic integration of excitatory synaptic input. *Nature Reviews Neuroscience* 1:181-190.

Maggio R, Riva M, Vaglini F, et al. (1998). Nicotine prevents experimental Parkinsonism in rodents and induces increase of striatal growth factors. *Journal of Neurochemistry* 71:2439-2446.

Magnusson JE, Fisher K (2000). The involvement of dopamine in nociception: The role of D_1 and D_2 receptors in the dorsolateral striatum. *Brain Research* 855: 260-266.

Make B, Jones JM (1998). Impairment of patients with chronic fatigue syndrome. In Klimas N, Patarca-Montero R (Eds.), *Disability and chronic fatigue syndrome: Clinical, legal, and patient perspectives* (pp. 43-55). Binghamton, NY: The Haworth Medical Press.

Maksay G, Laube B, Betz H (1999). Selective blocking effects of tropisetron and atropine on recombinant glycine receptors. *Journal of Neurochemistry* 73(2):802-806.

Malenka RC, Nicoll RA (1999). Long-term potentiation—A decade of progress? *Science* 285:1870-1874.

Malmow R, Mainen Z, Hayashi Y (2000). LTP mechanisms: From S1 level to four-lane traffic. *Current Opinion in Neurobiology* 10:352-357.

Mamiya T, Noda Y, Noda A, et al. (2000). Effect of sigma receptor agonist on the impairment of spontaneous alternation behavior and decrease of cyclic GMP level induced by nitric oxide synthase inhibitors in mice. *Neuropharmacology* 39:2391-2398.

Manabe T (2002). Does BDNF have pre- or postsynaptic targets? *Science* 295: 1651-1652.

Maneuf YP, Hughes J, McKnight AT (2001). Gabapentin inhibits the substance P-facilitated K^+-evoked release of [^{3}H] glutamate from rat caudal trigeminal nucleus slices. *Pain* 93:191-196.

Manzanares J, Corchero J, Romero J, Fernández-Ruiz J, Ramos J, Fuentes J (1999). Pharmacological and biochemical interactions between opioids and cannabinoids. *Trends in Pharmacological Sciences* 20:287-294.

Mao J, Chen LC (2000). Systemic lidocaine for neuropathic pain relief. *Pain* 87:7-17.

Marder E (1997). Computational dynamics in rhythmic neural circuits. *The Neuroscientist* 3:295-302.

Maremmani I, Marini G, Fornai F (1998). Naltrexone-induced panic attacks. *American Journal of Psychiatry* 155:447.

Marinissen MJ, Gutkind JS (2001). G-protein coupled receptors and signaling networks: Emerging paradigms. *Trends in Pharmacological Sciences* 22:368-376.

Markou A, Coston TR, Koob GF (1998). Neurobiological similarities in depression and drug dependence: A self-medication hypothesis. *Neuropsychopharmacology* 18(3):135-174.

Markus TM, Hassert DL, Jensen RA (2000). Reductions of anxiety-related behaviors in rats by electrical stimulation of the vagus nerve. *Society for Neuroscience Abstracts:* 852.10.

Marona-Lewicka D, Selken JR, Nichols DE (1999). Effects of combined treatment with D-amphetamine and the selective 5-HT releasing agent, MMAI on behavior, thermoregulation, and body weight. *Society for Neuroscience Abstracts:* 747.3.

Martinez-Levin M, Hermosillo AG (2000). Autonomic nervous system dysfunction may explain the multisystem features of fibromyalgia. *Seminars in Arthritis and Rheumatism* 29(S):197-199.

Marvin G, Sharma A, Aston W, Field C, Kendall MJ, Jones DA (1997). The effects of busipirone on perceived exertion and time to fatigue in man. *Experimental Physiology* 82(6):1057-1060.

Masi F, Mangiavacchi S, Gamborana C, Tagliamonte A (2000). Persistent behavioral and neurochemical sequelae of chronic stress exposure in rats. *Society for Neuroscience Abstracts:* 852.14.

Mason DJ, Lowe J, Welch SP (1999). Cannabinoid modulation of dynorphin A: Correlation to cannabinoid-induced nociception. *European Journal of Pharmacology* 378:237-248.

Masuda Y (1999). Symptoms of patients suffering from somatoform disorders and ifenprodil. *Psychosomatics* 40:449.

Mathison Y, Israel A (1998). Endothelin ET_B receptor subtype mediates nitric oxide/cGMP formation in rat adrenal medulla. *Brain Reseach Bulletin* 45:15-19.

Mayauchi T, Guto K (1999). Heart failure and endothelin receptor antagonists. *Trends in Pharmacological Sciences* 20:210-217.

Mayer EA, Craske M, Naliboff BD (2001). Depression, anxiety, and the gastrointestinal syndrome. *Journal of Clinical Psychiatry* 62(Suppl 8):28-36.

Mazarati A, Langel V, Bartfai The (2001). Galanin: An endogenous anticonvulsant? *Neuroscientist* 7:506-517.

McBain CJ, Fisahn A (2001). Interneurons unbound. *Nature Reviews Neuroscience* 2:11-23.

McDonald AW, Cohen JD, Stenger VA, Carter CS (2000). Dissociating the role of the dorsolateral prefrontal and anterior cingulate cortex in cognitive control. *Science* 288:1835-1838.

McEwen BS (1998). Protective and damaging effects of stress mediators. *New England Journal of Medicine* 338:171-179.

McEwen BS (1999). The effects of stress on structural and functional plasticity in the hippocampus. In Charney DS, Nestler EJ, Bunney BS (Eds.), *Neurobiology of mental illness* (pp. 475-493). New York: Oxford University Press.

McGaugh JL (2002). Memory consilidation and the amygdala: A systems perspective. *Trends in Neurosciences* 25:456-461.

McGaugh JL, Izquierdo I (2000). The contribution of pharmacology to research on the mechanisms of memory formation. *Trends in Pharmacological Sciences* 21:208-210.

McNally RJ, Clancy SA, Schacter DL (2001). Directed forgetting of trauma cues in adults reporting repressed or recovered memories of childhood sexual abuse. *Journal of Abnormal Psychology* 110:151-156.

McNally RJ, Clancy SA, Schacter DL, Pitman RK (2000). Personality profiles, dissociation, and absorption in women reporting repressed, recovered, or continuous memories of childhood sexual abuse. *Journal of Consulting and Clinical Psychology* 68:1033-1037.

Medani R, Hulo S, Toni N, Medani H, Steimer T, Muller D, Vassalli JD (1999). Enhanced hippocampal long-term potentiation and learning by increased neuronal expression of tissue type plasminogen activator in transgenic mice. *EMBO Journal* 18:3007-3012.

Meesters C, Merckelbach H, Muris P, Wessel I (2000). Autobiographical memory and trauma in adolescents. *Journal of Behavior Therapy and Experimental Psychiatry* 31:29-39.

Mehta MA, Calloway P, Sahakian BJ (2000). Amelioration of specific working memory deficits by methylphenidate in a case of adult attention deficit/hyperactivity disorder. *Journal of Psychopharmacology* 14(3):299-302.

Mel BW (2002). What the synapse tells the neuron. *Science* 295:1845-1846.

Menza MA, Kaufman KR, Castellanos A (2000). Modafinil augmentation of antidepressant treatment in depression. *Journal of Clinical Psychiatry* 61:378-381.

Merckelbach H, Muris P (2001). The causal link between self-reported trauma and dissociation: A critical review. *Behavioral Research and Therapy* 39:245-254.

Mercuri NB, Federici M, Bernardi G (1999). Inhibition of catechol-*o*-methyltransferase (COMT) in the brain does not affect the action of dopamine and levadopa: An in vitro electrophysiological evidence from rat mesencephalic dopamine neurons. *Journal of Neural Transmission* 106:1135-1140.

Meston CM, Frohlich PF (2000). The neurobiology of sexual function. *Archives of General Psychiatry* 57:1012-1030.

Mesulam M-M (2000). *Principles of behavioral and cognitive neurology,* Second edition. New York: Oxford University Press.

Middleton HC, Sharma A, Agouzoul D, Sahakian BJ, Robbins TW (1999). Idazoxan potentiates rather than antagonizes some of the cognitive effects of clonidine. *Psychopharmacology* 145(4):401-411.

Miele M, Mara MA, Enrico P, Esposito G, Serra PA, Nigheli R, Zangani D, Miele E, Desole MS (2000). On the mechanism of d-amphetamine-induced changes in glutamate, ascorbic acid and uric acid release in the stratum of freely moving rats. *British Journal of Pharmacology* 129:582-588.

Mieske CA, Dooley DJ, Pugsley TA (1999). Gabapentin: Novel and selective presynaptic P/Q-type calcium channel modulator of neurotransmitter release? *Society for Neuroscience Abstracts:* 896.5.

Miller EK (2000). The prefrontal cortex and cognitive control. *Nature Reviews Neuroscience* 1:59-65.

Miller GW, Gainetdinov RR, Levy AI, Caron MG (1997). Dopamine transporters and neuronal injury. *Trends in Pharmacological Sciences* 20:424-429.

Mink JW (1999). Basal ganglia. In Zigmund MS, Bloom FE, Landis SC, et al., *Fundamental Neuroscience.* San Diego, CA: Academic Press.

Misgeld U, Zeilhofer HU, Swandulla D (1998). Synaptic modulation of oscillatory activity of hypothalamic neural networks in vitro. *Cellular and Molecular Neurobiology* 18:1:29-38.

Mitchell AC (2001). An unusual case of chronic neuropathic pain responds to an optimum frequency of intravenous ketamine infusions. *Journal of Pain and Symptom Management* 21:443-446.

Miyashita Y, Hayashi T (2000). Neural representation of visual objects: Encoding and top-down activation. *Current Opinion in Neurobiology* 10:187-194.

Mizoguchi K, Yuzurihara M, Ishige A, et al. (2000). Chronic stress induces impairment of spatial working memory because of prefrontal dopaminergic dysfunction. *Journal of Neuroscience* 20:1568-1574.

Mochizuki N, Yamashita S, Kurokawa K, et al. (2001). Spatio-temporal images of growth factor-induced activation of Ras and Rap 1. *Nature* 411:1065-1068.

Molina-Hernandez A, Nunez A, Arias-Montano JA (2000). Histamine H_3 receptor activation inhibits dopamine synthesis in rat striatum. *NeuroReport* 11:163-166.

Molnar E, Baude A, Richmond SA, Patel PB, Somogyi P, McIlhinney RAJ (1993). Biochemical and immunocytochemical characterization of antipeptide antibodies to a cloned GluR1 glutamate receptor subunit: Cellular and subcellular distribution in the rat forebrain. *Neuroscience* 53:307-327.

Montplaisir J, Nicholas A, Goodboot R, Walters A (2000). Restless leg syndrome and periodic limb movement disorder. In Kryger MH, Roth T, Dement WC (Eds.), *Principles and practice of sleep medicine,* Third edition. Philadelphia: W.B. Saunders.

Moore RY (1999). Circadian timing. In Zigmund MS, Bloom FE, Landis SC, et al., *Fundamental neuroscience* (pp. 1189-1206). San Diego, CA: Academic Press.

Morgan MA, LeDoux JE (1995). Differential contributions of the dorsal and ventral medial prefrontal cortex to the acquisition and extinction of conditioned fear in rats. *Behavioral Neuroscience* 109:681-688.

Mori S, Popoli M, Brunello M, Piacagni G, Perez J (2001). Effect of reboxetine treatment on brain cAMP- and calcium/calmodulin-dependent protein kinases. *Neuropharmacology* 40:448-456.

Mormobos S, Fujimaki K, Okuyama N, et al. (1999). Stimulation of adenylyl-cyclase and induction of brain-derived neurotrophic factor and TrKB by NKH477, a novel and potent Forskolin derivative. *Journal of Neurochemistry* 72:2198-2205.

Morris RK, Ahmed M, Wearden AJ, Mullis R, Strickland P, Appleby L, Campbell IT, Pearson D (1999). The role of depression in pain, psychophysiological syndromes and medically unexplained symptoms associated with chronic fatigue syndrome. *Journal of Affective Disorders* 55:143-148.

Morrow BA, Elsworth JD, Rasmusson AM, Roth RH (1999). The role of meso-prefrontal dopamine neurons in the acquisition and expression of conditioned fear in the rat. *Neuroscience* 92:562-564.

Moss SJ, Smart TG (2001). Constructing inhibitory synapses. *Nature Reviews/Neuroscience* 2(April):240-250.

Muller MG, Toschi N, Kresse AE, et al. (2000). Long-term repetitive transcranial magnetic stimulation increases the expression of brain-derived neurotrophic factor and cholecystokinin in mRNA, but not neuropeptide tyrosine mRNA in specific areas of rat brain. *Neuropsychopharmacology* 23:205-215.

Murphy DD, Cole NB, Greenberger V, Segal M (1998). Estradiol increases dendritic spine density by reducing GABA neurotransmission in hippocampal neurons. *Journal of Neuroscience* 18:2550-2559.

Murphy DD, Cole NB, Segal M (1998). Brain derived neurotropic factor mediates estradiol-induced dendritic spine formation in hippocampal neurons. *Proceedings of the National Academy of Science, USA* 95:11412-11417.

Murtra P, Scheasby AM, Hunt SP, De Felipe C (2000). Rewarding effects of opiates in rats and mice blocking the receptor for substance P. *Nature* 405:180-183.

Muscat R, Patel J, Trout SJ, Wieczorek W, Kruk ZL (1993). Dissociation of the effects of amphetamine and quinpirole on dopamine release in the nucleus accumbens following behavioural sensitization: An ex vivo voltammetric study. *Behavioral Pharmacology* 4(4):411-418.

Nader K, Schofe GE, LeDoux JE (2000). Fear memories require protein synthesis in the amygdala for reconsolidation after retrieval. *Nature* 406:722-726.

Nakamura M, Ofuji K, Chikama T, Nishida T (1997). The NKl receptor and its participation in the synergistic enhancement of corneal epithelial migration by substance P and insulin-like growth factor-1. *British Journal of Pharmacology* 120(4):547-552.

Nakamura T, Uramura K, Nambo T, et al. (2000). Orexin-induced hyperlocomotion and stereotypy and mediate by the dopaminergic system. *Brain Research* 873: 181-187.

Navarra P, Dello Russo C, Mancuso C, Preziosi P, Grossman A (2000). Gaseous neuromodulators in the control of neuroendocrine stress axis. *Annals of the New York Academy of Science* 917:638-646.

Ness TJ, Fillingim RB, Randich A, et al. (2000). Low intensity vagal nerve stimulation lowers human thermal pain thresholds. *Pain* 86:81-85.

Ness TJ, San Pedro EC, Richard JS, Kezar L, Liv H-G, Mountz JM (1998). A case of spinal cord injury-related pain with baseline rCBF brain SPECT imaging and beneficial response to gabapentin. *Pain* 78:139-143.

Nestler EJ, Greengard P (1999). Serine and threonine phosphorylation. In Siegel GJ, Agranoff BW, Albers RW, Fisher SK, Uhler MD (Eds.), *Basic neurochemistry: Molecular, cellular, and medical aspects,* Sixth edition (pp. 471-496). Philadelphia, PA: Lippincott.

Nestler ER (2001). Molecular basis of long-term plasticity underlying addiction. *Nature Reviews Neuroscience* 2(1):119-126.

Netzeband JG, Conroy SM, Parsons KL, Gruol DL (1999). Cannabinoids enhance NMDA-elicited Ca^{2+} signals in cerebellar granule neurons in culture. *Journal of Neuroscience* 19:8765-8777.

Newport DJ, Nemeroff CB (2000). Neurobiology of post-traumatic stress disorder. *Current Opinion in Neurobiology* 10:211-218.

Nicole O, Docagne F, Ali C, Margaill I, Carmeliet P, MacKenzie ET, Vivian D, Buisson A (2001). The proteolytic activity of tissue plasminogen activator enhances NMDA receptor-mediated signaling. *Nature Medicine* 7(1):59-64.

Nicolelis M (1997). Dynamic and distributed somatosensory representations as the substrates for cortical and subcortical plasticity. *Seminars in Neuroscience* 9:24-33.

Nijsen MJ, Croiset G, Diamant M, Stami R, Kamphuis RJ, Broijnzeel A, deWied D, Wiegant VM (2000). Endogenous corticotropin-releasing hormone inhibits conditioned-fear-induced vagal activation in the rat. *European Journal of Pharmacology* 389:89-98.

Nisijima K, Yoshino T, Yui K, et al. (2001). Potent serotonin (5-HT$_{2A}$) receptor antagonists completely prevent the development of hyperthermia in an animal model of the 5-HT syndrome. *Brain Research* 890:23-31.

Nobler MS, Oquendo MA, Kegeles LS, Malone KM, Campbell CC, Sackeim HA, Mann JJ (2001). Decreased regional brain metabolism after ECT. *American Journal of Psychiatry* 158(2):305-308.

Noda Y, Kamei H, Kamei Y, et al. (2000). Neurosteroids ameliorate conditioned fear stress: An association with sigma receptors. *Neuropsychopharmacology* 23:276-284.

Northoff G, Eckert J, Fritze J (1997). Glutamatergic dysfunction in catatonia? Successful treatment of three acute akinetic catatonic patients with the NMDA antagonist amantadine. *Journal of Neurology, Neurosurgery, and Psychiatry* 62: 404-406.

Northoff G, Lins H, Boker H, Danos P, Bogerts B (1999). Therapeutic efficacy of *N*-methyl-D-aspartate antagonist, amantadine, in febrile catatonia. *Journal of Clinical Psychopharmacology* 19(5):484-485.

Nunez E, Lopez-Corcuera B, Vazquez J, Gimenez C, Aragon C (2000). Differential effects of the tricyclic antidepressant amoxapine on glycine uptake mediated by the recombinant GLYT1 and GLYT2 glycine transporters. *British Journal of Pharmacology* 129:200-206.

Nusser Z (2000). AMPA and NMDA receptors: Similarities and differences in their synaptic distribution. *Current Opinion in Neurobiology* 10:337-341.

Nyce JW (1999). Insight into adenosine receptor function using antisense and gene-knockout approaches. *Trends in Pharmacological Sciences* 20:79-83.

O'Doherty JO, Kringelbach ML, Rolls ET, Hornak J, Andrew SC (2001). Abstract reward and punishment representations in the human orbitofrontal cortex. *Nature Neuroscience* 4:95-102.

Oh JD, Russell D, Vaughan CL, Chase TN (1998). Enhanced tyrosine phosphorylation of striatal NMDA receptor subunits: Effects of dopaminergic denervation and L-dopa administration. *Brain Research* 813:150-159.

Olanow CW, Obeso JA, Nutt JG (Eds.) (2000). Basal ganglia, Parkinson's disease, and levodopa therapy. *Trends in Neurosciences* 23(10, Suppl.).

Olney JW (1994). Neurotoxicity of NMDA receptor antagonists: An overview. *Psychopharmacology Bulletin* 30:533-540.

Onaka T (2000). Catecholaminergic mechanisms underlying neurohypophysial hormone responses to unconditioned or conditioned aversive stimuli in rats. *Experimental Physiology* Spec No: 1015-1105.

Onn S-P, West AR, Grace AA (2000). Dopamine-mediated regulation of striatal neuronal and network interactions. *Trends in Neurosciences* 23(10 [268]Suppl.): S48-S56.

Orem J, Kubin L (2000). Respiratory physiology: Neural control. In Kryger MH, Roth T, Dement WC (Eds.), *Principles and practice of sleep medicine,* Third edition (pp. 205-220). Philadelphia: W.B. Saunders.

Orser BA, Pennefather PS, McDonald JF (1997). Multiple mechanisms of ketamine blockade of *N*-methyl-D-aspartate receptors. *Anesthesiology* 86:903-917.

Ostermeier AM, Schlosser B, Schwender D, Sutor B (2000). Activation of mu- and delta-opioid receptors cause presynaptic inhibition of glutamatergic excitation in neocortical neurons. *Anesthesiology* 93:1053-1063.

Otake K, Nakamura Y (1999). Site of action of thyrotropin-releasing hormone on central nervous system neurons revealed by the expression of the immediate early gene c-fos in the rat. *Neuroscience* 94:1167-1177.

Pace-Schott EF, Hobson JA (2002). The neurobiology of sleep: Genetics, cellular physiology and subcortical networks. *Nature Reviews Neuroscience* 3:591-605.

Paladini CA, Fiorillo CD, Morikawa H, Williams JT (2001). Amphetamine selectively blocks inhibitory glutamate transmission in dopamine neurons. *Nature Neuroscience* 4:275-288.

Palkovits M (1999). Interconnections between the neuroendocrine hypothalamus and the central autonomic system. *Frontiers of Neuroendocrinology* 20:270-295.

Pan W, Barbes WA, Kastin AJ (1998). Permeability of the blood-brain barrier to neurotrophins. *Brain Research* 788:87-94.

Paoletti P, Ascher P, Neyton J (1997). High affinity zinc inhibition of NMDA, NR1, and NR2 receptors. *Journal of Neuroscience* 17:5711-5725.

Parasuraman R (Ed.) (1998). *The attentive brain.* Cambridge, MA: MIT Press.

Park SK, Chung K, Chung JN (2000). Effects of purinergic and adrenergic antagonists in a rat model of painful peripheral neuropathy. *Pain* 87(2):171-180.

Parkinson J, Fudge J, Hurd Y, Pennortz C, Peoples L (2000). Finding motivation at Seabrook Island: The ventral striatum, learning and plasticity. *Trends in Neurosciences* 23:383-384.

Parkinson JA, Olmstead MC, Burns LH, Robbins TW, Everitt BJ (1999). Dissociation in effects of lesions of the nucleus accumbens core and shell on appetitive pavlovian approach behavior and the potentiation of conditioned reinforcement and locomotor activity by D-amphetamine. *Journal of Neuroscience* 19(6):2401-2411.

Parri HR, Gould TM, Cronelli V (2001). Spontaneous astrocytic Ca^{2+} oscillations *in situ* drive NMDAR-mediated neuronal excitation. *Nature Neuroscience* 4:803-812.

Pasqualini C, Olivier Z, Guibert B, Frain O, Leviel V (1996). Rapid stimulation of striatal dopamine synthesis by estradiol. *Cellular and Molecular Neurobiology* 16(3):411-416.

Pasternak GW (2001). Incomplete cross tolerance and multiple mu opioid receptors. *Trends in Pharmacological Sciences* 22:67-70.

Patapoutian A, Reichardt LF (2001). TRK receptors: Mediators of neurotrophin action. *Current Opinion in Neurobiology* 11(3):272-280.

Pattachini R, Maggi CA, Holzer P (2000). Tachykinin autoreceptors in the gut. *Trends in Pharmacological Sciences* 21:166.

Paul R, Zhang ZG, Elicieri BP, Zing Q, Boccia AD, Zhang RL, Chopp M, Cheresch DA (2001). Src deficiency or blockade of Src activity in mice provides cerebral protection following stroke. *Nature Medicine* 7:222-227.

Paulsen O, Moser EI (1998). A model of hippocampal memory encoding and retrieval: GABAergic control of synaptic plasticity. *Trends in Neurosciences* 21:273-278.

Payne JD, Nadel L, Allen JJ, Thomas KG, Jacobs WJ (2002). The effects of experimentally induced stress of false recognition. *Memory* 10(1):1-6.

Pearl SM, Antion MD, Stanwood GD, et al. (2000). Effects of NADH on dopamine release in rat striatum. *Synapse* 36:95-101.

Pekary AE, Mayerhoff J, Sattin A (1999). Electroconvulsive seizures (ECS) increase levels of prepro-TRH derived peptides in rat hypothalamus, cingulate, and cerebellum. *Society for Neuroscience Abstracts:* 757.11.

Perez-Velasquez JL, Carlea DJ (2000). Neural synchrony through electronic interaction. *Trends in Neurosciences* 23(2):68-74.

Perlmutter SJ, Leitman SF, Garrey MA, Hanborger S, Feldman E, Leonard HL, Swedo SE (1999). Therapeutic plasma exchange and intravenous immunoglobulin for obsessive-compulsive disorder and tic disorders in childhood. *Lancet* 354:1153-1158.

Pernia A, Mico J-A, Calderon E, Torres L-M (2000). Venlafaxine for the treatment of neuropathic pain. *Journal of Clinical Psychiatry* 19:408-409.

Perras B, Smolnik R, Fehm HL, Born J (2001). Signs of sexual behavior are not increased after subchronic treatment with LHRH in young men. *Psychoneuroendocrinology* 26:1-15.

Peters ML, Vlaeyen JW, van Drunen C (2000). Do fibromyalgia patients display hypervigilance for innocuous somatosensory stimuli? Application of a body scanning reaction time paradigm. *Pain* 86(3):283-292.

Petersson M, Alster P, Lundeberg T, Uvnas-Moberg K (1996). Oxytocin increases nociceptive thresholds in a long-term perspective in female and male rats. *Neuroscience Letters* 212:87-90.

Peyron C et al. (2000). A mutation in a case of early onset narcolepsy and a generalized absence of hypocretin peptides in human narcoleptic brains. *Nature Medicine* 6:991-997.

Peyron R, Garcia-Larrea L, Gregoire MC, Convers P, Richard A, Lavenne F, Barral FG, Mauguiere F, Michel D, Laurent B (2000). Parietal and cingulate processes in central pain: A combined positron emission tomography (PET) and functional magnetic resonance imaging (fMRI): Study of an unusual case. *Pain* 84:77-87.

Pfaus JG (1999). Neurobiology of sexual behavior. *Current Opinion in Neurobiology* 9:787-788.

Pfaus JG, Damsma G, Wenkstern D, Fibiger HC (1995). Sexual activity increases dopamine transmission in the nucleus accumbens and striatum of female rats. *Brain Research* 693(1-2):21-30.

Pickar D, Cohen MR, Naber D, et al. (1982). Clinical studies of the endogenous opioid system. *Biological Psychiatry* 17:276-283.

Pierce RC, Kalivas PW (1997). A circuitry model of behavioral sensitization to amphetamine-like psychostimulants. *Brain Research Reviews* 25:192-216.

Pimental M, Chow EJ, Hallegua D, et al. (2001). Small intestinal bacterial overgrowth: A possible association with fibromyalgia. *Journal of Musculoskeletal Pain* 9:114-197.

Pimental M, Chow EJ, Lin HC (2000). Eradication of small intestinal bacterial overgrowth reduces symptoms of irritable bowel syndrome. *American Journal of Gastroenterology* 95:161-164.

Piomelli D, Gioffrida A, Calignano A, deFonseca FX (2000). The endocannibinoid system as a target for therapeutic drugs. *Trends in Pharmacological Sciences* 21:218-224.

Piovenzan AP, D'Orleans-Juste P, Tonussi CR, Rae GA (1998). Effects of endothelin-1 on capsaicin-induced nociception in mice. *European Journal of Pharmacology* 351:15-22.

Pittaluga A, Pattorini R, Andrioli GC, et al. (1999). Activity of putative cognition enhancers in kynurenate test performed with human neocortex slices. *Journal of Pharmacology and Experimental Therapeutics* 290:423-428.

Pittman QJ, Hirosawa M, Mouginot D, Kombian SB (2000). Neurohypophysial peptides as retrograde transmitters in the supraoptic nucleus of the rat. *Experimental Physiology* Spec No: 1395-1435.

Pliszka S, Brown ERG, Wynne SK, et al. (2000). A double-blind, placebo-controlled study of Adderall and methylphenidate in ADHD. *Journal of American Academy of Child and Adolescent Psychiatry* 39(5):619-626.

Pollack MH, Worthington JJ, Manfro GG, Otto MW, Zucher BG (1997). Abecarnil for the treatment of generalized anxiety disorder: A placebo-controlled comparison of two dosage ranges of abecarnil and buspirone. *Journal of Clinical Psychiatry* 58(Suppl. 11):19-23.

Poo M (2001). Neurotrophins as synaptic modulators. *Nature Reviews Neuroscience* 2:24-32.

Popoli P, Reggio R, Pezzola A (1997). Adenosine A_1 and A_2 receptor agonists prevent the electroencephalographic effects induced by MK-801 in rats. *European Journal of Pharmacology* 333:143-146.

Porter S, Yuille JC, Lehman DR (1999). The nature of real, implanted and fabricated memories for emotional childhood events: Implications for the recovered memory debate. *Law and Human Behavior* 23:517-537.

Posner MI, Raichle ME (1995). Precisof images of mind. *Behavioral and Brain Sciences* 18:327-384.

Post RM (1992). The psychobiology of dysphoric mania. *Clinical Neuropharmacology* 15(Suppl. 1, Pt. A):624A-651A.

Post RM (2000). Neural substrates of psychiatric syndromes. In Mesulam M-M (Ed.), *Principles of behavioral and cognitive neurology,* Second edition (pp. 406-438). New York: Oxford University Press.

Pozzo-Miller LD, Gottschalk W, Zhang L, et al. (1999). Impairments in high-frequency transmission, synaptic vesicle docking, and synaptic protein distribution in the hippocampus of BDNF knockout mice. *Journal of Neuroscience* 19:4972-4983.

Pussinen R, Sirvio J (1999). Effects of cycloserine. *Journal of Psychopharmacology* 13:171-179.

Rada PV, Hackel BG (2000). Supra-additive effect of d-fenfluramine plus phentermine on extracellular acetylcholine in the nucleus accumbens: Possible mechanism for inhibition of excessive feeding and drug abuse. *Pharmacology, Biology and Behavior* 65:369-373.

Rada PV, Mark GP, Taylor KM, Hoebel BG (1996). Morphine and naloxone, i.p. or locally, affect extracellular acetylcholine in the accumbens and prefrontal cortex. *Pharmacology Biochemistry and Behavior* 53(4):809-816.

Rademacher DJ, Andres KA, Riley MG, et al. (1999). Determination of the place preference properties of the potent serotonin 5-HT$_2$ receptor antagonist amperozide (FG5606): A comparison with cocaine. *Society for Neuroscience Abstracts:* 746.23.

Raffa RB, Schupsky JJ, Lee DKU, Jacoby HI (1996). Characterization of endothelin-induced nociception in mice: Evidence for a mechanically distinct analgesic model. *Journal of Pharmacology and Experimental Therapeutics* 278:1-7.

Raggenbass M (2001). Vasopressin and oxytocin-induced activity in the central nervous system: electrophysiologic studies using in-vitro systems. *Progress in Neurobiology* 64:307-326.

Rainov NG, Heidecke V, Burkert W (2001). Long-term intrathecal infusion of drug combinations for chronic back and leg pain. *Journal of Pain and Symptom Management* 22:862-871.

Ramachandran VS, Blakeslee S (1998). *Phantoms in the brain: Probing the mysteries of the human mind.* New York: William Morrow.

Rampon C, Tang Y, Goodhouse J, Shimizu E, Kyin E, Tsien JZ (2000). Enrichment induces structural changes and recovery from non-spatial memory deficits in CA1-NMDA R1 knock-out mice. *Nature Neuroscience* 3:238-244.

Raphael KG, Widom CS, Lange G (2001). Childhood victimization and pain in adulthood: A prospective investigation. *Pain* 92:283-293.

Redgold FA, Caldwell CC, Sitkovsky MV (1999). Ecto-protein kinases: Ecto-domain phosphorylation as a novel target for pharmacologic manipulation? *Trends in Pharmacological Sciences* 20:453-458.

Redgrave P, Prescott TJ, Gurney K (1999). The short-latency dopamine response: Too short to signal reward error? *Trends in Neurosciences* 22(4):146-151.

Reick M, Garcia JA, Dudley C, McKnight SL (2001). NPAS2: An analog of clock operative in the mammalian forebrain. *Science* 293:506-509.

Reis DJ, Dejunathan S (2000). Is agmatine a novel neurotransmitter in the brain? *Trends in Pharmacological Sciences* 21:187-193.

Reppert SM, Weaver DR (2002). Coordination of arcadian timing in mammals. *Nature* 418:935-941.

Rhudy JL, Meagher MW (2000). Fear and anxiety: Divergent effects on human pain thresholds. *Pain* 84:65-75.

Rice MA (2000). Ascorbate regulation and its neuroprotective ride in the brain. *Trends in Neurosciences* 23(5):209-216.

Richter DW, Mironov SL, Busselberg D, Lalley PM, Bischoff AM, Wilken B (2000). Respiratory rhythm generation: Plasticity of a neuronal network. *The Neuroscientist* 6(3):188-205.

Richter DW, Spyer KM (2001). Studying rhythmogenesis of breathing: Comparison of in vivo and in vitro models. *Trends in Neurosciences* 24:464-472.

Rinzel J, Rall W (1974). Transient response in a dendritic neuron model for current injected at one branch. *Biophysical Journal* 14:759-790.

Ritz R, Sejnowski TJ (1997). Synchronous oscillatory activity in sensory systems: New vistas on mechanisms. *Current Opinion in Neurobiology* 7:536-546.

Robbins TW (1998). Arousal and attention: Psychopharmacological and neuropsychological studies in experimental animals. In Parasuraman R (Ed.), *The attentive brain* (pp. 189-220). Cambridge, MA: MIT Press.

Robbins TW, Everitt BJ (1996). Neural behavioral mechanisms of reward and motivation. *Current Opinion in Neurobiology* 6:228-236.

Robertson SJ, Ennion SJ, Evans RJ, Edwards FA (2001). Synaptic P2X receptors. *Current Opinion in Neurobiology* 11:378-386.

Roca CA, Schmidt PJ, Rubinow DR (1999). Gonadal steroids and affective illness. *The Neuroscientist* 5(4):227-237.

Rocha AF (1997). The brain as a symbol-processing machine. *Progress in Neurobiology* 53:121-198.

Rogalski SL, Cyr C, Chavkin C (1999). Activation of the endothelin receptor inhibits the G protein-coupled inwardly rectifying potassium channel by a phospholipase A2-mediated mechanism. *Journal of Neurochemistry* 72(4):1409-1416.

Roques BP (2000). Novel approaches to targeting neuropeptide systems. *Trends in Pharmacological Sciences* 21(December):475-483.

Rose CR, Konnerth A (2001a). Exciting glial oscillations. *Nature Neuroscience* 4:773-774.

Rose CR, Konnerth A (2001b). NMDA receptor-mediated Na^+ signals in spines and dendrites. *Journal of Neuroscience* 21:4207-4214.

Rosmond R, Dallman MS, Bjorntorp P (1998). Stress related cortisol secretion in men: Relationships between abdominal obesity and endocrine metabolic and hemodynamic abnormalities. *Journal of Clinical Endocrinology and Metabolism* 83:1853-1859.

Rosniecki JJ, Letourneau R, Sugiultzoglu M, et al. (1999). Differential effect of histamine 3 receptor-active agents on brain, but not peritoneal, mast cell activation. *Journal of Pharmacology and Experimental Therapeutics* 290:1427-1435.

Rothstein JD, Guidotti A, Tinuper P, et al. (1992). Endogenous benzodiazepine receptor density in idiopathic recurring stupor. *Lancet* 340:1002.

Row EJB, Toni I, Josephs O, Frackowiak RSJ, Passingham RE (2000). The prefrontal cortex: Response selection or maintenance within working memory? *Science* 288:1656-1660.

Rudolph U, Crestani F, Mohler H (2001). $GABA_A$ receptor subtypes: Dissecting their pharmacological functions. *Trends in Pharmacological Sciences* 22:188-194.

Rupniak NMJ, Kramer MS (1999). Discovery of the antidepressant and anti-emetic efficacy of substance P receptor (NK_1) antagonists. *Trends in Pharmacological Sciences* 20:485-489.

Rupprecht R, Holsboer F (1999). Neuroactive steroids: Mechanism of action and neuropsychopharmacological perspectives. *Trends in Neurosciences* 22(9): 410-416.

Rupprecht R, Koch M, Montkowski A, Lancel M, Faulhaber J, Harting J, Spanagel R (1999). Assessment of neuroleptic-like properties of progesterone. *Psychopharmacology* 143(1):29-38.

Ruskin DN, Bergstrom DA, Shenker A, et al. (2001). Drugs used in the treatment of attention-deficit hyperactivity disorder affect postsynaptic firing rate and oscillation without preferential dopamine autoreceptor action. *Biological Psychiatry* 49:340-350.

Russ H, Muller T, Woitalla D, et al. (1999). Detection of tolcapone in the cerebrospinal fluid of Parkinsonian patients. *Naunyn Schmiedebergs Archive Pharmacologica* 360:719-720.

Rusworth MFS, Owen AM (1998). The functional organization of the lateral prefrontal cortex. Conjecture or conjunction in the electrophysiology literature. *Trends in Cognitive Science* 2:46-53.

Rutter J, Reick M, Wu LC, McKnight SL (2001). Regulation of clock and NPAS2 DNA binding by the redox state of NAD cofactors. *Science* 293:510-514.

Ruzicka E, Roth J, Jech R, Busek P (2000). Subhypnotic doses of zolpidem oppose dopaminergic-induced dyskinesia in Parkinson's disease. *Movement Disorders* 15:734-735.

Sacchetti E, Guarneri L, Bravi D (2000). H_2 antagonist nizatidine may control olanzapine-associated weight gain in schizophrenic patients. *Biological Psychiatry* 48:167-168.

Sacerdote F, Panerai AE, Frattola L, Ferrarese C (1999). Benzodiazepine-induced chemotaxis is impaired in monocytes from patients with generalized anxiety disorder. *Psychoneuroendocrinology* 24:243-249.

Salami M, Fathollahi Y, Esteky H, Motamedi F, Atapour N (2000). Effects of ketamine on synaptic transmission and long-term potentiation in layer II/III of rat visual cortex in vitro. *European Journal of Pharmacology* 390(3):287-293.

Sanchez C, Arnt J, Costall B, Kelly ME, Meier E, Naylor RJ, Perregaard J (1997). The selective δ_2-ligand Lu 28-179 has potent anxiolytic-like effects in rodents. *Journal of Pharmacology and Experimental Therapeutics* 283:1323-1332.

Sandkuhler J (2000). Learning and memory in pain pathways. *Pain* 88:113-118.

Sandman C, Barron J, Nackhoul K, Goldstein J (1993). Memory deficits associated with chronic fatigue immune dysfunction syndrome. *Biological Psychiatry* 33:618-623.

Sandrini M, Romualdi P, Vitale G, et al. (2001). The effect of a paracetamol and morphine combination on dynorphin A levels in rat brain. *Biochemical Pharmacology* 61:1409-1416.

Sanes JR, Lichtman JW (1999). Can molecules explain long-term potentiation? *Nature Neuroscience* 2:597-604.

Sanne P, Jobe T, Sinha S, Deleon D, Gavira M (1997). Treatment of pseudoseizure patients with histamine (H_2) blocking agents (abstract). *Journal of Neuropsychopharmacology* 904:658.

Saper CB, Chou TC, Scammell TE (2001). The sleep switch: Hypothalamic control of sleep and wakefulness. *Trends in Neurosciences* 24:726-731.

Satoh S, Matsumura H, Hayaishi O (1998). Involvement of adenosine A_{2A} receptor in sleep promotion. *European Journal of Pharmacology* 351:155-162.

Scammell TE, Nishino S, Mignot E, Saper CB (2001). Narcolepsy and low CSF orexin (hypocretin) concentration after a diencephalic stroke. *Neurology* 56(12): 1751-1753.

Scannevin RH, Huganir RL (2000). Post synaptic organization and regulation of excitatory synapses. *Nature Reviews Neuroscience* 1:133-141.

Schacter DL (2001). *The seven sins of memory: How the mind forgets and remembers.* New York: Houghton Mifflin.

Schafe GE, Nader K, Blair HT, LeDoux JE (2001). Memory consolidation of Pavolvian fear conditioning: A cellular and molecular perspective. *Trends in Neurosciences* 24(9):540-546.

Schiah I-S, Yatham LN, Srisurapononet M, Lamb RW, Tam EM, Zis AP (2000). The addition of pindolol accelerates the response to electroconvulsive therapy in patients with major depression: A double-blind, placebo-controlled pilot study. *Journal of Clinical Psychopharmacology* 20:373-378.

Schibler U, Kipperger JA, Brown SA (2001). Chronobiology—Reducing time. *Science* 293:437-438.

Schilman H, Hyman SE (1999). Intracellular signaling. In Zigmund MS, Bloom FE, Landis SC, et al., *Fundamental neuroscience* (pp. 269-316). San Diego, CA: Academic Press.

Schinder AF, Poo M-M (2000). The neurotrophin hypothesis for synaptic plasticity. *Trends in Neurosciences* 23:639-645.

Schmelz M (2001). A neural pathway for itch. *Nature Neuroscience* 4:9-10.

Schmid RL, Sandler AN, Katz J (1999). Use and efficacy of low-dose ketamine in the management of acute postoperative pain: A review of the current techniques and outcomes. *Pain* 82:111-125.

Schmitz Y, Lee CJ, Schmauss C, et al. (2001). Amphetamine distorts stimulation-dependent dopamine overflow: Effects on D_2 autoreceptors, transporters, and synaptic vesicle stores. *Journal of Neuroscience* 21:5916-5924.

Schoffelmeer NAM, Van der Schuren LJMJ, Van Royen DE, Wardeh G, Hogenboom F, Mulder AH (1998). Lack of alpha-2 adrenoceptor autoregulation of noradrenaline release in rat nucleus accumbens slices. *Naunyn Schmiedebergs Arch Pharmacol* 356:89-90.

Schore AN (1994). *Affect regulation and the origin of the self: The neurobiology of emotional development.* Hillsdale, NJ: Lawrence Erlbaum Associates.

Schorf MB, Hauck M, Stover R, McDonald N, Berkowitz D (1998). Effect of gamma-hydroxybutyrate on pain. Fatigue and the alpha sleep anomaly in patients with fibromyalgia. Preliminary report. *Journal of Rheumatology* 251:1986-1990.

Schultz W (2000). Multiple reward signals in the brain. *Nature Reviews Neuroscience* 1:199-207.

Schultz W (2001). Reward signaling by dopamine neurons. *The Neuroscientist* 7:293-302.

Schweitzer PJ (2000). Cannibinoids decrease the K^+ M-current in hippocampal CA1 neurons. *Journal of Neuroscience* 20:51-58.

Scott LV, Medbak S, Dinan TG (1998). Blunted adrenocorticotropin and cortisol responses to corticotrophin-releasing hormone stimulation in chronic fatigue syndrome. *Acta Psychiatrica Scandinavia* 97:450-457.

Seahill L, Chappell PB, Kim YS, et al. (2001). A placebo-controlled study of guanfacine in the treatment of children with tic disorders and attention deficit hyperactivity disorder. *American Journal of Psychiatry* 158:1067-1074.

Sebastiao AM, Ribeiro JA (2000). Fine tuning neuromodulation by adenosine. *Trends in Pharmacological Sciences* 21:341-346.

Sebban C, Zhang XQ, Tesolin-Decros B, Millan MJ, Spedding M (1999). Contrasting EEG profiles elicited by antipsychotic agents in the prefrontal cortex of the conscious rat: Antagonism of the effects of clozapine by modafinil. *British Journal of Pharmacology* 128:1045-1054.

Seifer MJ (1998). *The life and times of Nikola Tesla: Biography of a genius.* New York: Kensington.

Senior K (2002). Anxiety linked to a protein kinase enzyme. *Lancet* 360:1077.

Serres F, Muma NA, Raap DK, Garcia F, Battaglia G, Van de Kar LD (2000). Coadministration of 5-hydroxytryptamine (1A) antagonist WAY-100635 prevents fluoxetine-induced desensitization of postsynaptic 5-hydroxytryptamine (1A) receptors in hypothalamus. *Journal of Pharmacology and Experimental Therapeutics* 294(1):296-301.

Shafer RA, Levant B (1998). The D_3 dopamine receptor in cellular and organized function. *Psychopharmacology* 135:1-16.

Shapiro NA, Verdvin ML, DeGraw JO (2001). Treatment of refractory major depression with tramadol monotherapy. *Journal of Clinical Psychiatry* 62:205-206.

Sharp FR, Tomitaka M, Bernaudin M, Tomitaka S (2001). Psychosis: Pathological activation of limbic thalamocortical circuits by psychomimetics and schizophrenia? *Trends in Neurosciences* 24:330-334.

Shen K, Tervel MN, Connor JH, Shenolikar S, Meyer T (2000). Molecular memory by reversible translocation of calcium/calmodulin dependent protein kinase II. *Nature Neuroscience* 3(9):881-886.

Shepheard SL, Williamson DJ, Williams J, Hiu RG, Hargraves RJ (1995). Comparison of the effects of sumatriptan and the NK1 antagonist CP-99, 994 on plasma extravasation in the dura mater and c-fos mRNA expression in the trigeminal nucleus caudalis of rats. *Neuropharmacology* 34:2555-2561.

Sherman SM (2001). The importance of burst firing in the transmission of information to cortex by thalamic relay cells. *Trends in Neurosciences* 24(2):122-127.

Sherwood NT, Lo DC (1999). Long-term enhancement of central synaptic transmission by chronic BDNF treatment. *Journal of Neuroscience* 19:7025-7036.

Shi WX, Pun CL, Zhang XX, et al. (2000). Dual effects of D-amphetamine on dopamine neurons mediated by dopamine and non-dopamine receptors. *Journal of Neuroscience* 20:3004-3011.

Shimoyama M, Shimoyama N, Gorman AL, Elliot KJ, Inturrisi CE (1999). Oral ketamine in the rat formalin test: Role of the metabolite, norketamine. *Pain* 81:85-93.

Shimoyama M, Shimoyama N, Hori Y (2000). Gabapentin affects glutamatergic excitatory neurotransmission in rat dorsal horn. *Pain* 85:405-414.

Shin M, Kosslyn SM, McNally RJ, Alport NM, Thompson WL, Rauch SI, Macklin ML, Pitman RK (1997). Visual imagery and perception in post-traumatic stress disorder: A positron emission tomographic investigation. *Archives of General Psychiatry* 54:233-241.

Shirayama Y, Mitsushio H, Takashima M, Ichikawa H, Takahashi K (1996). Reduction of substance P after chronic antidepressant treatment in the striatum, substantia nigra and amygdala of the rat. *Brain Research* 739(1-2):70-78.

Shors TJ, Elkabes S, Selcher JC, Black IB (1997). Stress persistently increases NMDA receptor-mediated binding of [^{3}H]PDBV (a marker for protein kinase C) in the amygdala, and re-exposure to the stressful content re-activates the increase. *Brain Research* 750:293-300.

Shorvon S (2001). Pyrrolidone derivatives. *Lancet* 358:1885-1892.

Sibson NR, Dhankar A, Mason GF, et al. (1998). Stoichiometric coupling of brain glucose metabolism and glutamatergic neuronal activity. *Proceedings of the National Academy of Sciences, USA* 95:316-321.

Silver R, Silverman A-J, Vitkovic L, Lederhendler II (1996). Mast cells in the brain: Evidence and functional significance. *Trends in Neuroscience* 19:25-31.

Simon EP, Dahl LF (1999). The sodium pentothal hypnosis interview with follow-up treatment for complex regional pain syndrome. *Pain and Symptom Management* 18:132-136.

Simonian SX, Delaleau B, Caraty A, Herbison AE (1998). Estrogen receptor expression in brain stem noradrenergic neurons of the sheep. *Norendocrinology* 67:392-402.

Simons DG, Travell JG, Simons LS (1999). *Myofascial pain and dysfunction: The trigger point manual.* Baltimore, MD: Williams and Wilkins.

Sirota P, Mosheva T, Shabtay H, Giladi N, Korczyn AD (2000). Use of the selective serotonin 3 receptor antagonist odansetron in the treatment of neuroleptic-induced tardive dyskinesia. *American Journal of Psychiatry* 157:287-289.

Skerry TM, Genever PG (2001). Glutamate signaling in non-neuronal tissues. *Trends in Pharmacological Sciences* 22(4)175.

Skifter DA, Chaika CV, Lewis RE, Monaghan DT (1999). Identification of insulin signaling pathways that modulate NMDA receptor activity. *Society for Neuroscience Abstracts:* 785.11.

Slatkin NE, Rhitier M, Balton TM (2001). Donepizil in the treatment of opioid-induced sedation: Report of six cases. *Journal of Pain and Symptom Management* 21:425-438.

Slemmer JE, Damaj MI, Martin BR (1999). Effect of bupropion on neuronal nicotinic acetylcholine receptors. *Society for Neuroscience Abstracts:* 25:1241.

Smilaowska M, Obuchowicz E, Turchan J, Herman ZS, Przewloki R (1997). Clonidine administration increases neuropeptide-Y immunoreactivity and neuropeptide-Y mRNA in the rat cerebral cortex neurons. *Neuropeptides* 31(3):203-207.

Smith E, Acton L, Sharp T (1997). Enhancement of dopamine-mediated behavior by the NMDA antagonists MK-801 and CPP: Similarities with repeated electroconvulsive shock. *Psychopharmacology* 133:55-94.

Smith SJ (1999). Dissecting dendrite dynamics. *Science* 283:1860-1861.

Smythe JW, Murphy D, Bhatnagar S, Timothy C, Costall B (1996). Muscarinic antagonists are anxiogenic in rats tested in the black-white box. *Pharmacology, Biochemistry and Behavior* 54:57-63.

Soderling TR (2000). CaM-kinases: Modulators of synaptic plasticity. *Current Opinion in Neurobiology* 10:375-380.

Soderling TR, Derkach VA (2000). Post synaptic protein phosphorylation and LTP. *Trends in Neuroscience* 23(2):75-80.

Sorensen J, Bengtsson A, Ahlnar J, Henriksson KG, Ekselius L, Rengtsson M (1997). Fibromyalgia—Are there different mechanisms in the processing of pain? A double-blind crossover comparison of analgesic drugs. *Journal of Rheumatology* 8:1615-1621.

Spanagel R, Weiss F (1999). The dopamine hypothesis of reward: Past and current status. *Trends in Neurosciences* 22(11):521-527.

Spina MJ, Basso AM, Zorrilla EP, Heyser CJ, Rivier J, Vale W, Merlo-Pich E, Koob GF (2000). Behavioral effects of central administration of the novel CRF antagonist astressin in rats. *Neuropsychopharmacology* 22:230-239.

Srikiatkhachorn A, Tarasub N, Govitrapong P (1999). Acetaminophen-induced antinociception via central 5-HT$_{2A}$ receptors. *Neurochemistry International* 34:491-498.

Stahl SM (1998). Basic psychopharmacology of antidepressants, part II: Estrogen as an adjunct to antidepressive treatment. *Journal of Clinical Psychiatry* 59 (Suppl. 4):15-24.

Stahl SM (2000a). The function of nicotine receptors. *Journal of Clinical Psychiatry* 61:628-629.

Stahl SM (2000b). The new cholinesterase inhibitors for Alzheimer's disease. Part 2. Illustrating their mechanisms of action. *Journal of Clinical Psychiatry* 61(11): 813-814.

Stanek L, Walker DL, Davis M (2000). Amygdala infusion of LY354740, a group II metabotropic glutamate receptor agonist, blocks fear-potentiated startle in rats. *Society for Neuroscience Abstracts:* 755.13.

Staud R, Vierck CJ, Cannon RL, et al. (2001). Abnormal sensitization and temporal summation of second pain (wind-up) in patients with fibromyalgia syndrome. *Pain* 91:165-175.

Steere AC (2001). Medical progress: Lyme disease. *New England Journal of Medicine* 345:115-125.

Steriade M (1999). Coherent oscillations and short-term plasticity in cortico-thalamic networks. *Trends in Neuroscience* 22:337-345.

Sternbach H, State R (1997). Antibiotics: Neuropsychiatric effects and psychotropic interactions. *Harvard Review of Psychiatry* 5:214-226.

Stolero S, Gregoire MC, Gerard D, et al. (1999). Neuroanatomical correlates of visually evoked sexual arousal in human males. *Archives of Sexual Behavior* 28:1-21.

Stone TW (2000). Development and therapeutic potential of kynurenic acid and kynurenine derivatives for neuroprotection. *Trends in Pharmacological Sciences* 21:149-154.

Stoop R, Surprenant A, North RA (1997). Different sensitivities to pH of ATP-induced currents at four cloned P2X receptors. *Journal of Neurophysiology* 78: 1837-1840.

Stratakis CA, Karl M, Schulte HM, Chrousos GP (1994). Glucocorticosteroid resistance in humans. Elucidation of the molecular mechanisms and implications for pathophysiology. *Annals of the New York Academy of Science* 746:362-376.

Stratz T, Farber L, Varga B, et al. (2000). Treatment of fibromyalgia with intravenous application of tropisetron. *Journal of Musculoskeletal Pain* 6(4):31-40.

Stroud MW, Thorn BE, Jensen MP, Boothby JL (2000). The relation between pain beliefs, negative thoughts, and psychosocial functioning in chronic pain patients. *Pain* 84:347-352.

Stuart GJ, Hausser M (2001). Dendritic coincidence detection of EPSP and action potentials. *Nature Neuroscience* 4:63-71.

Sudhof TC (1999). Intracellular trafficking. In Siegel GJ, Agranoff BW, Albers RW, Fisher SK, Uhler MD (Eds.), *Basic neurochemistry: Molecular, cellular, and medical aspects,* Sixth edition (pp. 175-190). Philadelphia, PA: Lippincott.

Sullivan RM, Gratton A (1999). Lateralized effects of medial prefrontal cortex lesions on neuroendocrine and autonomic stress responses in rats. *Journal of Neuroscience* 19(7):2834-2840.

Sun MK, Alkon DL (2002). Carbonic anhydrase gating of attention: Memory therapy and enhancement. *Trends in Pharmacological Science* 23(2):83-89.

Sutherland GR, McNaughton B (2000). Memory trace reactivation in hippocampal and neocortical neuronal ensembles. *Current Opinion in Neurobiology* 10:180-186.

Suzuki T, Aoki T, Kato H, Yamakazi M, Misawa M (1999). Effects of the 5-HT$_3$ receptor antagonist ondansetron on the ketamine- and dizocilpine-induced place preferences in mice. *European Journal of Pharmacology* 385:99-102.

Svingos AL, Clarke CL, Pickel VM (1999). Localization of the delta-opioid receptor and dopamine transporter in the nucleus accumbens shell: Implications for opiate and psychostimulant cross-sensitization. *Synapse* 34(1):1-10.

Swift R, Davidson D, Rosen S, et al. (1998). Naltrexone effects on diazepam intoxication and pharmacokinetics in humans. *Psychopharmacology* 135:256-262.

Takahashi S, Sonehara K, Takagi K, Miwa T, Horikomi K, Mita N, Nagase H, Iizuka K, Sakai K (1999). Pharmacological profile of MS-377, a novel antipsychotic agent with selective affinity for sigma receptors. *Psychopharmacology* 145(3)295-302.

Takahashi T, Yamashita H, Zhang Y-X, Nakamura S (1996). Inhibitory effect of MK-801 on amantadine-induced dopamine release in the rat striatum. *Brain Research Bulletin* 41:363-367.

Takenouchi K, Nishijo H, Uwano T, Tamura R, Takigawa M, Ono T (1999). Emotional and behavioral correlates of the anterior cingulate cortex during associative learning in rats. *Neuroscience* 93(4):1271-1287.

Tanda G, Fraur D, Chiara G (1996). Chronic desipramine and fluoxetine differentially affect extracellular dopamine in the rat prefrontal cortex. *Psychopharmacology* 127:83-87.

Tang Y, Shimizu E, Dube G, Rampon C, Kerchner G, Zhuo M, Liu G. Tsien JZ (1999). Genetic enhancement of learning and memory in mice. *Nature* 401:63-69.

Tang-Christensen M, Larsen PJ, Thulesen J, Romber J, Vrang N (2000). The proglucagon-derived peptide, glucagon-like peptide-2, is a neurotransmitter involved in the regulation of food intake. *Nature Medicine* 6:802-807.

Tan-No K, Taira A, Wako K, Niijima F, Nakagawasai O, Tadano T, Sakurada C, Sakurada T, Kisara K (2000). Intrathecally administered spermine produces the scratching, biting, and licking behavior in mice. *Pain* 86:55-61.

Taylor CP, Gee NS, Su TZ, Kocsis JD, Welty DF, Brown JP, Dooley DJ, Boden P, Singh L (1998). A summary of mechanistic hypothesis of gabapentin pharmacology. *Epilepsy Research* 29:231-246.

Taylor CW, Broad LM (1998). Pharmacological analysis of intracellular Ca^{2+} signaling: Problems and pitfalls. *Trends in Pharmacological Sciences* 19:370-375.

Taylor FB, Russo J (2001). Comparing guanfacine and dextroamphatamine for the treatment of adult attention-deficit/hyperactivity disorder. *Journal of Clinical Psychopharmacology* 21:223-228.

Taylor ML, Trotter DR, Csuka ME (1995). The prevalence of sexual abuse in women with fibromyalgia. *Arthritis and Rheumatism* 38:229-234.

Teagarden MA, Rebec GV (1999). Modulation of presumed glutamate/ascorbate heteroexchange by haloperidol in freely moving rats. *Abstracts of the Society for Neuroscience:* 2210.

Terada H, Ohta S, Nishikawa T, et al. (1999). The effect of intravenous or subarachnoid lidocaine on glutamate accumulation during transient forebrain ischemia in rats. *Anesthesia and Analgesia* 89:957-961.

Thoenen H, Sendtner M (2002). Neurotrophins: From enthusiastic expectations through sobering experiences to rational therapeutic approaches. *Nature Neuroscience* 5(Suppl.):1046-1050.

Thomas P, Rascle C, Mastain B, et al. (1997). Test for catatonia with zolpidem. *Lancet* 349:702.

Thompson AC, Zapata A, Justice JB Jr, et al. (2000). Kappa-opioid receptor activation modifies dopamine uptake in the nucleus accumbens and opposes that of cocaine. *Journal of Neuroscience* 20:9333-9340.

Thomson AF (2000). Facilitation, augmentation, and potentiation at central synapses. *Trends in Neurosciences* 23:305-312.

Toh KL, Jones CR, He Y, Eide EJ, Hinz WA, Virshup DM, Ptacek LJ, Fu YH (2001). An hPer2 phosphorylation site mutation in familial advanced sleep phase syndrome. *Science* 291(5506):1040-1043.

Toni T, Lechan RM (1993). Neuroendocrine regulation of thyrotropin-releasing hormone (TRH) in the tuberoinfundibular system. *Journal of Endocrinologic Investigation* 16:715-753.

Travagli RA, Williams JT (1996). Endogenous monoamines inhibit glutamate transmission in the spinal trigeminal nucleus of the guinea-pig. *Journal of Physiology* 491:177-185.

Traynelis SF, Lipton SA (2001). Is tissue plasminogen activator a threat to neurons? *Nature Medicine* 7:17-18.

Treede R-D, Apkoran AV, Bromm B, et al. (2000). Cortical representation of pain: Functional characterization of nociceptive areas near the lateral sulcus. *Pain* 87:113-119.

Tsien JZ (2000). Linking Hebb's coincidence-detection to memory formation. *Current Opinion in Neurobiology* 10:266-273.

Tsutsumi Y, Yamamato K, Matsuura S, Hotas S, Sakai M, Shrakura E (1998). The treatment of neuroleptic malignant syndrome using dantrolene sodium. *Psychiatry and Clinical Neuroscience* 52:433-438.

Turken AU, Swick D (1998). Is response selection in the anterior cingulate cortex specific to output modality? *Society for Neuroscience Abstracts* 23(2):1682.

Turrigiano GG, Nelson SB (2000). Hebb and homeostasis in neural plasticity. *Current Opinion in Neurobiology* 10:358-364.

Tzschentke TM, Schmidt WJ (1998). Does the noncompetitive NMDA receptor antagonist dizocilpine (MK801) really block behavioral sensitization associated with repeated drug administration? *Trends in Pharmacological Sciences* 19: 447-451.

Ugolini A, Corsi M, Bordi F (1997). Potentiation of NMDA and AMPA responses by group I mGluR in spinal cord motoneurons. *Neuropharmacology* 36:1047-1055.

Ulus IH, Maher TJ, Wurtman RJ (2000). Characterization of phentermine and related compounds as monoamine oxidase (MAO) inhibitors. *Biochemical Pharmacology* 59:1611-1621.

Ungless MA, Whistler JL, Malenka RC, Bonci A (2001). Single cocaine exposure in vivo induces long-term potentiation in dopamine neurons. *Nature* 411(6837):583-587.

Urban L, Thompson SWN, Dray A (1994). Modulation of spinal excitability: Cooperation between neurokinin and excitatory amino acid transmitters. *Trends in Neurosciences* 17:432-438.

Uvnas-Moberg K. (1997). The physiological and endocrine effects of social contact. *Annals of the New York Academy of Sciences* 807:146-163.

Uzwiak AJ, Guyette FX, West MO, Peoples LL (1997). Neurons in accumbens subterritories of the rat: Phasic firing time-locked within second of intravenous cocaine self-infusion. *Brain Research* 767(2):363-369.

Vaidya CJ, Austin G, Kirkorian G, et al. (1998). Selective effects of methylphenidate in attention deficit hyperactivity disorder: A functional magnetic resonance study. *Proceedings of the National Academy of Sciences* 95:14494-14499.

Van der Schuren LJMJ, Wardeh G, De Vries TJ, Mulder AH, Schoffelmeer ANM (1999). Opposing role of dopamine D_1 and D_2 receptors in modulation of rat nucleus accumbens noradrenaline release. *Journal of Neuroscience* 19(10):4123-4131.

van Hooft JA, Vijverberg HP (2000). 5-HT_3 receptors and neurotransmitter release in the CNS: A nerve ending story? *Trends in Neurosciences* 23(12):605-610.

Vanderah TW, Ossipov MH, Lai J, et al. (2001). Mechanisms of opioid-induced pain and antinociceptive tolerance: Descending facilitation and spinal dynorphin. *Pain* 92:5-9.

Veesei L, Dibo G, Kiss C (1998). Neurotoxins and neurodegenerative disorders. *Neurotoxicology* 19(45):511-514.

Veronneau-Longueville F, Rampin O, Freund-Mercier M-J, Tang Y, Calas A, Marson L, McKenna KE, Stoeckel M-E, Benoit G, Giuliano F (1999). Oxytocinergic innervation of autonomic nuclei controlling penile erection in the rat. *Neuroscience* 93:1437-1447.

Viggiano D, Sadele AG (2000). Hypertrophic A10 dopamine neurons in a rat model of attention-deficit hyperactivity disorder (ADHD). *NeuroReport* 11:3677-3680.

Volkow NP, Wang GJ, Fowler JS, et al. (1999). Association of methylphenidate-induced craving with changes in right striato-orbitofrontal metabolism in cocaine abusers: Implications in addiction. *American Journal of Psychiatry* 156:19-26.

Volpi R, Chiodera P, Cafferra P, Scaglioni A, Saceani A, Coiro V (1997). Different control mechanisms of growth hormone (GH) secretion between gamma-amino and gamma-hydroxy-butyric acid: Neuroendocrine evidence in Parkinson's disease. *Psychoneuroendocrinology* 22:531-538.

Vorel SR, Lu X, Hayes RJ, et al. (2001). Relapse to cocaine-seeking after hippocampal theta burst stimulation. *Science* 292:1175-1177.

Waelti P, Dickinson A, Schultz W (2001). Dopamine responses comply with basic assumptions of formal learning theory. *Nature* 412:43-48.

Wallenstein GV, Eichenbaum H, Hasselmo ME (1998). The hippocampus as an association of discontiguous events. *Trends in Neurosciences* 21:317-323.

Wan FI, Lin HC, Kang BH, et al. (1999). D-amphetamine induced depletion of energy and dopamine in the rat striatum is attenuated by nicotinamide pre-treatment. *Brain Research Bulletin* 50:167-171.

Wang Z, Rebec GV (1999). Dose-dependent effects of ascorbic acid pretreatment on both the behavioral response to amphetamine and ascorbic acid accumulation in the rat neostriatum. *Society for Neuroscience Abstracts:* 747.4.

Watkins LR, Martin D, Ulrich P, Tracey KJ, Maier SF (1997). Evidence for the involvement of spinal cord glia in subcutaneous formalin induced hyperalgesia in the rat. *Pain* 71:225-235.

Waxham MN (1999). Neurotransmitter receptors. In Zigmund MS, Bloom FE, Landis SC, et al., *Fundamental neuroscience* (pp. 235-268). San Diego, CA: Academic Press.

Waxman J, Zatzkis SM (1999). Fibromyalgia and menopause: Examination of the relationship. *Postgraduate Medicine* 80:165-167.

Wei F, Wang G-D, Kerchner GA, Kim SJ, XU h-M, Chen Z-F, Zhuo M (2001). Genetic enhancement of inflammatory pain by forebrain NR2B overexpression. *Nature Neuroscience* 4(2):164-169.

Wei H, Leeds P, Chen RW, et al. (2000). Neuronal apoptosis induced by pharmacological concentrations of 3-hydroxykynureine: Characterization and protection by dantrolene use and bcl-2 overexpression. *Journal of Neurochemistry* 75:81-90.

Weiss EL, Longhurst JG, Mazure CM (1999). Childhood sexual abuse as a risk factor for depression in women: Psychosocial and neurobiological correlates. *American Journal of Psychiatry* 156:816-828.

West RE, Wu RL, Billah MM, Egen RW, Anthes JC (1999). The profiles of human and primate [3H] N-alpha binding differ from that of rodents. *European Journal of Pharmacology* 377:233-239.

Westerink BHC, Kwint H-F, de Vries JB (1997). Eating induced dopamine release from mesolimbic neurons is mediated by NMDA receptors in the ventral tegmental area: A dual-probe microdialysis study. *Journal of Neurochemistry* 69:662-668.

Westphal RS, Tavalin SJ, Lin JW, Alto NM, Frasier IDC, Langeberg LK, Sheng M, Scott JD (1999). Regulation of NMDA receptors by an associated phosphatase-kinase signaling. *Science* 285:93-96.

White FJ (2001). Dopamine receptors get a boost. *Nature* 411:35-37.

Whittemore ER, Ilyin VI, Konkoy CS, Woodward RM (1997). Subtype-selective antagonism of NMDA receptors by nylidrin. *European Journal of Pharmacology* 337:197-208.

Wickelgren I (1997). Estrogen stakes claim to cognition. *Science* 276:675-678.

Wiedemann K, Jahn H, Yassuridis A, Kellner M (2001). Anxiolytic-like effects of atrial natriuretic peptide on cholecystokinin tetrapeptide-induced panic attacks. *Archives of General Psychiatry* 58:371-377.

Williams RSB, Cheng L, Mudge AW, Harwood AJ (2002). A common mechanism of action for three mood-stabilizing drugs. *Nature* 417:292-295.

Winder DG, Sweatt JD (2001). Roles of serine/threonine phosphatases in hippo-campal synaptic plasticity. *Nature Reviews Neuroscience* 2(7):461-474.

Winkielman P, Schwarz N (2001). How pleasant was your childhood? Beliefs about memory shape inferences from experienced difficulty of recall. *Psychological Science* 12:176-179.

Wirkner K et al. (2000). Inhibition by adenosine A_{2A} receptors of NMDA but not AMPA currents in striatal neurons. *British Journal of Pharmacology* 130:259-269.

Wise LA, Zierlur S, Krieger N, Harlow BL (2001). Adult onset of major depressive disorder in relation to early life violent victimization: A case-control study. *Lancet* 358:881-887.

Wisor JP, Nishino S, Sora I, Uhl GH, Mignot E, Edgar DM (2001). Dopaminergic role in stimulant-induced wakefulness. *Journal of Neuroscience* 21(5):1787-1794.

Wisse BE, Schwartz MW (2001). Role of melanocortins in control of obesity. *Lancet* 358:857-858.

Woolley CS (1999). Effects of estrogen in the CNS. *Current Opinion in Neurobiology* 9(3):349-354.

Wu CC, Wang JH, Chio CW, Yen MH (1999). Comparison between effects of dantrolene and nifedipine on lipopolysaccharide-induced endotoxemia in the Lewis rats. *Chinese Journal of Physiology* 42:211-217.

Wu Y, Wang W, Richerson GB (1999). Nonvesicular GABA release is enhanced by anticonvulsants that increase brain [GABA]. *Society for Neuroscience Abstracts:* 783.5.

Wu YN, Shen KZ, Johnson SW (1999). Presynaptic inhibition preferentially reduces an NMDA receptor mediated component of transmission in rat midbrain dopamine neurons. *British Journal of Pharmacology* 127(6):1422-1430.

Yamazaki H, Arai M, Inoue K, et al. (2000). The roles of TGF-β in the brain on the emergence of central fatigue after exercise. *Abstracts of the Society for Neuroscience:* 478.

Yates SL, Tedford CE, Gregory R, et al. (1999). Effects of selective H_3 histamine receptor antagonists on tele-methylhistamine in rat cerebral cortex. *Biochemical Pharmacology* 57:1059-1066.

Yehuda R (2000). Biology of posttraumatic stress disorder. *Journal of Clinical Psychiatry* 61(Suppl. 7):14-21.

Yonezawa Y, Kuroki T, Kawahara T, Tashiro N, Uchimura H (1998). Involvement of gamma-aminobutyric acid neurotransmission in phencyclidine-induced dopamine release in the medial prefrontal cortex. *European Journal of Pharmacology* 341:45-56.

Young MW, Kay SA (2001). Time zones: A comparative genetics of circadian clocks. *Nature Reviews Genetics* 2:702-715.

Yu L, Liao P-C (1999). Female sexual hormones may distinctively modulate striatal dopamine and serotonin depletions induced by methamphetamine in mice. *Abstracts of the Society for Neuroscience:* 2089.

Yu L, Liao P-C (2000). Estrogen and progesterone distinctively modulate methamphetamine-induced dopamine and serotonin depletions in C57BL/6J mice. *Journal of Neural Transmission* 107(10):1139-1147.

Zametkin AJ, Liutta W (1998). The neurobiology of attention-deficit hyperactivity disorder. *Journal of Clinical Psychiatry* 59(Suppl. 7):17-23.

Zelena D, Kiem DT, Barna I, Makara GB (1999). Alpha$_2$-adrenoceptor subtypes regulate ACTH and beta endorphin secretions during stress in the rat. *Psychoneuroendocrinology* 24:333-343.

Zhang D, Pan ZH, Awobuluyi M, Lipton SA (2001). Structure and function of GABA(C) receptors: A comparison of native versus recombinant receptors. *Trends in Pharmacological Science* 22(3):121-132.

Zheng B, Albrecht U, Kaasik K, et al. (2001). Nonredundant roles of the *mPer1* and *mPer2* genes in the mammalian circadian clock. *Cell* 105:683-694.

Index